Tenth Edition

Volume 1

Competency Based

BD Chaurasia's

Human Anatomy

Regional and Applied **Dissection and Clinical**

As per the latest NMC Guidelines | Competency Based Medical Education (CBME) Curriculum under Graduate Medical Education Regulation

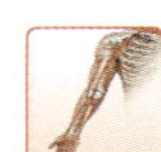 **Upper Limb**

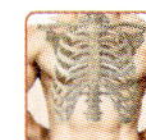 **Thorax**

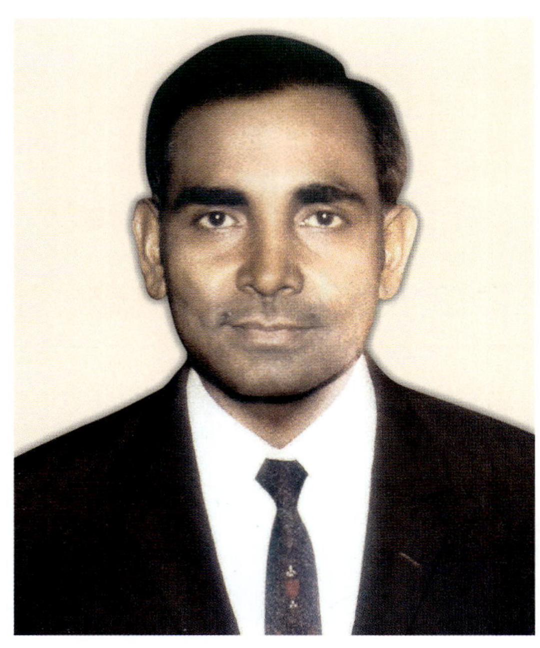

Dr BD Chaurasia (1937–1985)
was Reader in Anatomy at GR Medical College, Gwalior.
He received his MBBS in 1960, MS in 1965 and PhD in 1975.
He was elected fellow of National Academy of Medical Sciences (India) in 1982.
He was a member of the Advisory Board of the *Acta Anatomica* since 1981,
member of the editorial board of *Bionature*, and in addition
member of a number of scientific societies.
He had a large number of research papers to his credit.

Competency Based

Tenth Edition

Volume 1

BD Chaurasia's

Human Anatomy

Regional and Applied **Dissection and Clinical**

As per the latest NMC Guidelines | Competency Based Medical Education (CBME) Curriculum under Graduate Medical Education Regulation

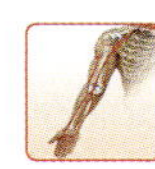

Upper Limb

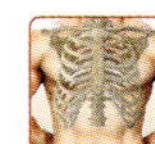

Thorax

Chief Editor

Krishna Garg

MBBS MS PhD FIMSA FIAMS FAMS FASI

Legend of Anatomy; Nation's Who's Who
Fellow, Anatomical Society of India
Lifetime Achievement Awardee
DMA Distinguished Service Awardee
Ex-Professor and Head, Department of Anatomy
Lady Hardinge Medical College, New Delhi

Executive Editor

Yogesh Ashok Sontakke MBBS MD

Additional Professor
Department of Anatomy
Jawaharlal Institute of Postgraduate Medical
Education and Research (JIPMER)
(An Institute of National Importance under the Ministry of Health and Family Welfare, Government of India)
Puducherry

Editors

Pragati Sheel Mittal MBBS MS

Professor, Department of Anatomy
Government Institute of Medical Sciences
Greater Noida, Uttar Pradesh

Mrudula Chandrupatla MBBS MD

Professor and Head, Department of Anatomy
All India Institute of Medical Sciences
Bibinagar, Hyderabad, Telangana

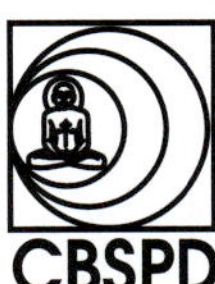

CBS Publishers & Distributors Pvt Ltd

New Delhi • Bengaluru • Chennai • Kochi • Kolkata • Lucknow • Mumbai
Hyderabad • Jharkhand • Nagpur • Patna • Pune • Uttarakhand

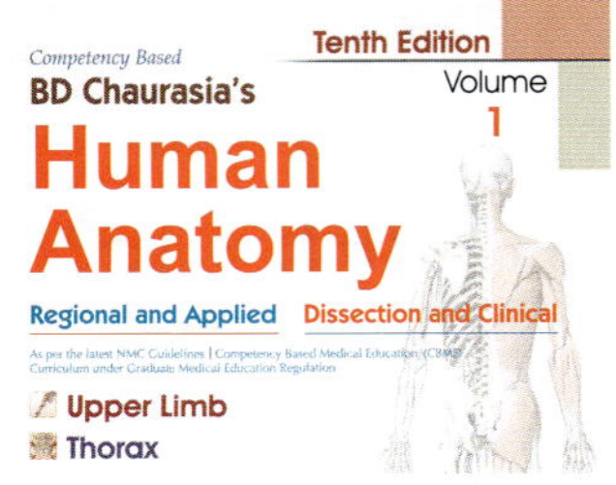

ISBN: 978-93-5466-979-8

Tenth Edition: 2025[1]

First Edition: 1979
Reprint: 1980, 1981, 1982, 1983, 1984, 1985, 1986, 1987, 1988
Second Edition: 1989
Reprint: 1990, 1991, 1992, 1993, 1994
Third Edition: 1995
Reprint: 1996, 1997, 1998, 1999, 2000, 2001, 2002, 2003, 2004
Fourth Edition: 2004
Reprint: 2005, 2006, 2007, 2008, 2009
Fifth Edition: 2010
Reprint: 2011, 2012
Sixth Edition: 2013
Reprint: 2014, 2015
Seventh Edition: 2016
Reprint: 2017, 2018, 2019
Eighth Edition: 2020
Reprint: 2021, 2022
Ninth Edition: 2023
Reprint: 2024

Published by Satish Kumar Jain and produced by Varun Jain for

CBS Publishers & Distributors Pvt Ltd
4819/XI Prahlad Street, 24 Ansari Road, Daryaganj, New Delhi 110 002, India
Ph: 011-23289259, 23266838
Website: www.cbspd.com
e-mail: delhi@cbspd.com

Corporate Office: 204 FIE, Industrial Area, Patparganj, Delhi 110 092, India
Ph: 011-4934 4934 Fax: 011-4934 4935 e-mail: publishing@cbspd.com; publicity@cbspd.com

Branches

- **Bengaluru:** Seema House 2975, 17th Cross, K.R. Road, Banasankari 2nd Stage, Bengaluru 560 070, Karnataka, India
  Ph: +91-80-26771678/79 Fax: +91-80-26771680 e-mail: bangalore@cbspd.com
- **Chennai:** 18/8B, Subbarayan Street, Shenoy Nagar, Chennai 600 030, Tamil Nadu, India
  Ph: +91-44-42032115, 26681266 e-mail: chennai@cbspd.com
- **Kochi:** 42/1325, 1326, Power House Road, Opposite KSEB, Power House, Ernakulum 682 018, Kochi, Kerala, India
  Ph: +91-484-4059061–65, 67 Fax: +91-484-4059065 e-mail: kochi@cbspd.com
- **Kolkata:** 147, Hind Ceramics Compound, 1st Floor, Nilgunj Road, Belghoria, Kolkata 700 056, West Bengal, India
  Ph: +91-33-25633055/56 e-mail: kolkata@cbspd.com
- **Lucknow:** Basement, Khushnuma Complex, 7 Meerabai Marg (behind Jawahar Bhawan), Lucknow 226 001, UP, India
  Ph: +91-522-4000032 e-mail: tiwari.lucknow@cbspd.com
- **Mumbai:** PWD Shed, Gala No. 25/26, Ramchandra Bhatt Marg, Next JJ Hospital Gate No. 2, Opp. Union Bank of India, Noorbaug, Mumbai 400 009, Maharashtra, India
  Ph: +91-22-66661880/89 e-mail: mumbai@cbspd.com

Representatives

- **Hyderabad** 0-9885175004
- **Jharkhand** 0-9811541605
- **Nagpur** 0-8692091830
- **Patna** 0-9334159340
- **Pune** 0-9664372571
- **Uttarakhand** 0-9716462459

Printed at: Thomson Press (India) Ltd., Faridabad, Haryana, India

to

---

my teacher
Shri Uma Shankar Nagayach

— BD Chaurasia

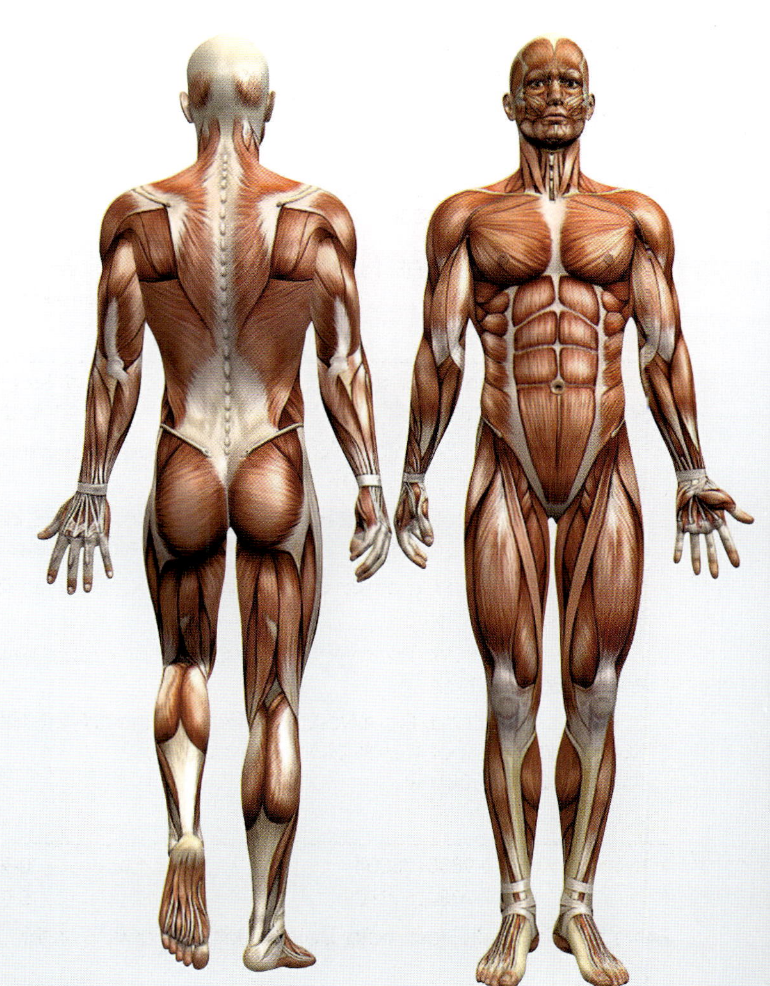

UPPER LIMB and **THORAX**

LOWER LIMB, ABDOMEN and **PELVIS**

Volume 3

HEAD and **NECK**

BRAIN–NEUROANATOMY

Volume 4

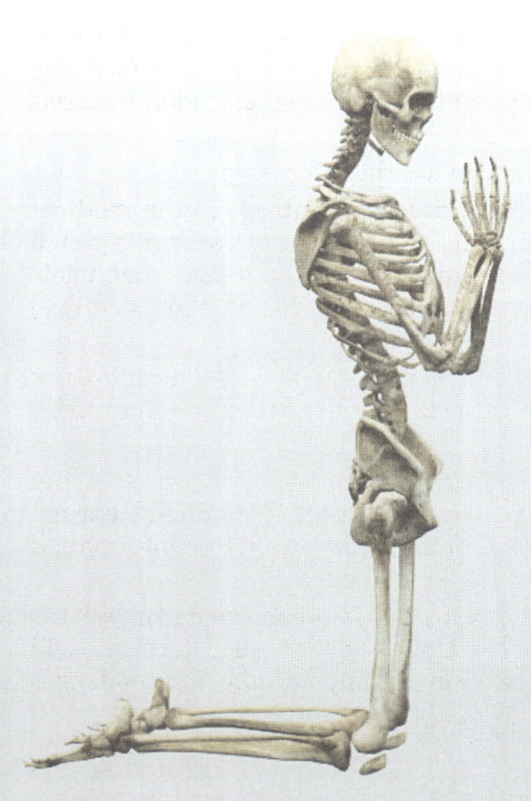

Preface to the Tenth Edition

With the change in time, the needs of the students and curriculum are continuously changing. The science is continuously evolving. To integrate the solutions to common problems faced by the students and to follow the latest NMC guidelines for the CBME curriculum, the most widely accepted and read book has been revised thoroughly to maintain the standards of the last half-century. The primary goal of this book is to help the students for easy understanding and rapid grasping of knowledge for their higher academic achievements, to prepare them for all academic formative, summative and entrance examinations and to make it extremely student-friendly.

Anatomy forms the foundation of the clinical knowledge. This book has been made more clinically oriented with the following salient features:

- **Complete** and **time-tested textbook** boasting unparalleled **quality content** designed to enrich both fundamental and clinical understanding for students.
- **Simple text** is the main feature of the book. It will facilitate easier understanding for students. Small sentences minimize effort, enhancing readability and accessibility. This approach ensures clarity of information, aiding students in grasping complex concepts effortlessly.
- **3D colour illustrated plates** will aid the students in comprehending anatomical structures and their relationships with clarity. These visual aids offer a dynamic perspective, enhancing spatial understanding and facilitating the identification of anatomical features.
- **Simple line diagrams** are incorporated. These diagrams will allow students to easily redraw them during examinations. These diagrams are designed for clarity and simplicity, ensuring that students can accurately reproduce anatomical structures in assessments and examinations efficiently.
- **Flowcharts** will facilitate rapid revision and memorizing of facts, alleviating students' concerns about time constraints during the subject review. These visuals will enhance comprehension and retention. Students can quickly navigate through key concepts, optimizing study time and effectively addressing time limitations in their revision process.
- **Clinical anatomy** sections are integrated at the end of each topic to maintain the purpose towards **early clinical exposure** (ECE). By seamlessly merging theoretical knowledge with practical application, this approach ensures students gain valuable insights into clinical contexts, enhancing their understanding and readiness for real-world clinical scenarios.
- **Dissection boxes** will guide the students in the step-wise dissection of the human cadaver.
- **Tables** are used to summarise essential facts for clear understanding and retention.
- ***QR codes*** for ***eSmartQuiz*** are embedded in the text, which will grant access to online MCQ tests for self-assessment at the end of each chapter. This interactive feature will enhance engagement and facilitate convenient self-evaluation. Students can assess their understanding, reinforce learning, and identify areas for improvement, facilitate a dynamic and effective learning experience.
- *Free* ***Workbook:*** The main textbook is supported with a workbook, which has the following:
  1. **Clinicoanatomical problems** emphasize early clinical exposure and vertical integration in medical education. By integrating anatomical knowledge with clinical practice from the outset, students gain a holistic understanding of medical concepts. This approach fosters practical skills, enhances diagnostic abilities, and promotes a deeper comprehension of the human body's complexities within clinical contexts.
  2. **Practice figures** aid in preparing students for academic examinations by providing hands-on experience with exam-style preparation. It will help to build confidence in tackling the challenges commonly encountered in academic assessments.
  3. **Multiple choice questions (MCQs)** will serve as potent tools for reinforcing learning, assessing comprehension, and enhancing attention and critical thinking skills. Through MCQs, students engage actively with the curriculum, consolidate understanding, and develop the ability to analyse information critically, ultimately fostering deeper comprehension and retention of knowledge.
  4. **Spotters** and **question bank** introduce students to the examination system by familiarising them with the format and types of questions commonly encountered in assessments. These wide ranges of questions will aid the students in preparing for examinations and gaining confidence in tackling examination challenges effectively.

- ***Free access to BDC's Anatomy eBook (digital content through CBSiCentral app)*:** It includes the following:
  a. Additional topics and clinical aspects
  b. *Viva voce* questions, and
  c. Topics for further reference and reading.

  This digital resource will enhance the book's utility, providing students with expanded knowledge and resources for comprehensive learning. Accessible supplementary materials will enhance understanding and facilitate deeper exploration, empowering students to excel in their studies and clinical practice.
- **Free Access to CBSiCentral App:** It includes videos of osteology and soft parts and chapter-wise self-assessment MCQ tests. The videos of the dissection will give three-dimensional image descriptions of tissues and organs, which get effectively registered in the brain for a longer time.
- **Wall charts:** Each volume is provided with meticulously crafted wall charts, elegantly designed and tailored to enhance students' comprehension of anatomy. These visually engaging aids can be easily affixed to walls to grasp the visual impressions of anatomy.

Always remember that success is achieved only through diligent effort and hard work.

Chief Editor
Krishna Garg

Executive Editor
Yogesh Ashok Sontakke

Editors
Pragati Sheel Mittal
Mrudula Chandrupatla

Preface to the First Edition (excerpts)

The necessity of having a simple, systematized and complete book on anatomy has long been felt. The urgency for such a book has become all the more acute due to the shorter time now available for teaching anatomy, and also to the falling standards of English language in the majority of our students in India. The national symposium on 'Anatomy in Medical Education' held at Delhi in 1978 was a call to change the existing system of teaching the unnecessary minute details to the undergraduate students.

This attempt has been made with an object to meet the requirements of a common medical student. The text has been arranged in small classified parts to make it easier for the students to remember and recall it at will. It is adequately illustrated with simple line diagrams which can be reproduced without any difficulty, and which also help in understanding and memorizing the anatomical facts that appear to defy memory of a common student. The monotony of describing the individual muscles separately, one after the other, has been minimised by writing them out in tabular form, which makes the subject interesting for a lasting memory. The relevant radiological and surface anatomy have been treated in separate chapters. A sincere attempt has been made to deal, wherever required, the clinical applications of the subject. The entire approach is such as to attract and inspire the students for a deeper dive in the subject of anatomy.

The book has been intentionally split in three parts for convenience of handling. This also makes a provision for those who cannot afford to have the whole book at a time.

It is quite possible that there are errors of omission and commission in this mostly single-handed attempt. I would be grateful to the readers for their suggestions to improve the book from all angles.

I am very grateful to my teachers and the authors of numerous publications, whose knowledge has been freely utilised in the preparation of this book. I am equally grateful to my professor and colleagues for their encouragement and valuable help. My special thanks are due to my students who made me feel their difficulties, which was a great incentive for writing this book. I have derived maximum inspiration from Prof. Inderbir Singh (Rohtak), and learned the decency of work from Shri SC Gupta (Jiwaji University, Gwalior).

I am deeply indebted to Shri KM Singhal (National Book House, Gwalior) and Mr SK Jain (CBS Publishers & Distributors, Delhi), who have taken unusual pains to get the book printed in its present form. For giving it the desired get-up, Mr VK Jain and Raj Kamal Electric Press are gratefully acknowledged. The cover page was designed by Mr Vasant Paranjpe, the artist and photographer of our college; my sincere thanks are due to him. I acknowledge with affection the domestic assistance of Munne Miyan and the untiring company of my Rani, particularly during the odd hours of this work.

BD Chaurasia

Acknowledgements

We have the blessings and good wishes of Prof NA Faruqi (Aligarh); Dr DC Naik (Rewa); Dr SD Joshi and Dr SS Joshi (Indore); Dr (Brig) Rakesh Gupta (Greater Noida); Dr DR Singh (Lucknow); Dr M Kaul; Dr C Anand and Dr I Bahl (Delhi); Dr Mohsin Azmi (Kanpur); Dr Medha Joshi (Ghaziabad); Dr Surbhi Gupta (Delhi); Dr Nitin Nagarkar (Raipur); Dr CK Shukla (Raipur); Dr Shakuntala Pai (Manipal); Dr Manik Chatterjee (Raipur) and Dr SN Kazi (Pune).

We are thankful to Dr Sangeeta Chouhan, Dr Seema Gupta (Jaipur); Dr Surjit Ghatak (Jodhpur); Dr Vinay Sharma (Muzzafarnagar); Dr Deepu Singh Kataria (UP); Dr Anup Singh Gurjar (Pali); Dr Jagmohan Sharma, Dr Deepak Sharma, Dr Rajesh Arora and Dr Sumit Gupta (Kota); Dr Gopal Sharma and Dr Manoj Sharma (Jhalawar); Dr Rekha Parashar (Dausa); Dr Santosh Kumar (Dholpur); Dr Isha Srivastav, Dr Aprajita Raizada, Dr Sajan Skaria, Dr Hitant Vohra, Dr Anjali Jain, Dr Kalpana Sharma, Dr Praveen Ojha, Dr Prakash KG, Dr Seema Prakash (Udaipur); for giving feedback for various sections of the volumes. We are greatful to Dr K Aravindhan, Dr V Gladwin, Dr Raveendranath V, Dr Suman Verma, Dr Sulochana Sakthivel, Dr Rajasekhar SSSN and Dr Vidhya G (Puducherry) for their support.

We are grateful to Dr Anupma Mahajan (Amritsar); Dr Vanita Gupta (Jammu); Dr Vikas Verma (Lucknow) and Dr Tripta Bhagat (Ghaziabad) for editing chapters to enhance the value of the volumes. We are grateful to Dr Sangeeta and Dr Nusrat Jabeen (Jammu); Dr Gurdeep Singh Kalyan (Gajrola); Dr Rajan Singla (Patiala); Dr Aprajita Sikka (Ludhiana); Dr Bashir (Srinagar) and Dr Ritu (Rajouri); Dr Mubeen (Kathua); Dr RK Srivastava (Kanpur); Dr Punita Manik (Lucknow); Dr Binod Kumar; Dr Sunita Nayak and Dr Shambhu Prasad (Patna); Dr AK Dubey (Ranchi); Dr Satyam Khare, Dr Shilpi Jain and Dr Alok Tripathi (Meerut), for promoting the volumes.

We have been getting constant encouragement and support from Dr Ranjana Verma, Dr Muthukrishnan P, Dr Yogesh Yadav, Dr Pullimi Vineel and Dr Nirupma Gupta (Greater Noida); Dr Nisha Kaul (Ghaziabad); Dr Vinay Singhal (Saharanpur); Dr RK Ashoka (Mathura); Dr Vineet Guhia (Khandwa); Dr Manisha Sinha (Raipur); Dr Jahan Shirin (Kanpur); Dr Damyanti (Manipur) and Dr MK Anand (Bhuj).

Our regards and affection to Dr Rewa Choudhry, Dr Shilpa Paul, Dr Smita Kakar, Dr Anita Tuli, Dr Gayatri Rath, Dr Shashi Raheja, Dr A Shariff, Dr SB Ray, Dr Vandana Mehta, Dr Sabita Mishra, Dr Renu Chauhan, Dr Jyoti Arora, Dr Sneh Agarwal, Dr TS Roy, Dr Ruchi Dhuria, Dr Shaifaly Madan Rustagi (Delhi) and Dr Anjoo Yadav for going through the volumes.

We would like to thank Dr Pritha Bhuiyan (Mumbai); Dr Brijendra Singh (Rishikesh); Retd (Brig) Dr Sushil Kumar (Faridabad); Dr AK Srivastava (Lucknow); Dr MK Pant (Dehradun); Dr Simmi Mehra (Rajkot); Dr Fatima M De Souza (Goa); Dr Mukesh Mittal (Shivpuri); Dr Priti Sinha (Saharanpur); Dr Rashmi Malhotra (Rishikesh); Dr Simmi Soni (Aziznagar); Dr Sunita Gupta (Ahmedabad); Dr Raghunandan Ramanathan (Chennai), Dr BK Aghera (Ahmedabad) and many-many other teachers all over the globe, for giving us good wishes.

We also acknowledge Drs Neetu Sivadasan, Rituraj Majumdar, Nandhini R, Nithya D, Kalaivani K, Jakkula Akhil, Ambiga R, S Nikilesh, Udit Narayan, Jayasree S, Bharathy Mohan P, Nandhini S, Aakriti Mehrotra, Sancy Charly, Madhusingh Thakur, Tarakeshwari RB, Dhivyaa Shree R, Thaiyal Nayagi and Prasanna Raj AV (Puducherry) for their support.

Videos of bones and soft parts of human body, prepared at Kathmandu University School of Medical Sciences, have now been added with the respective chapters and are available at our mobile App CBSiCentral. We are grateful to Dr R Koju, CEO of Kathmandu University School of Medical Sciences (KUSMS) and Dhulikhel Hospital, for his generosity.

The moral support of my (chief editor) family members, Late Dr DP Garg, Dr Suvira Gupta, Dr JP Gupta, Mr Manoj, Ms Rekha, Mr Sanjay, Ms Meenakshi, Dr Manish, Dr Shilpa Garg, Dr Naveen Garg, Dr Manoj, Dr Nalini Shukla, Dr Vikas Verma and Dr Swati Gupta, is appreciated.

The magnanimity shown by Mr SK Jain (Chairman) and Mr Varun Jain (Director), CBS Publishers & Distributors, has been always forthcoming. The unquestionable support of Mr YN Arjuna (Senior Vice President—Publishing, Editorial and Publicity) and his entire team comprising Ms Ritu Chawla (GM—Production), Mr Neeraj Prasad (Graphic Artists), Mr Binay Kumar (Proofreader) and Mr Vikrant Sharma (DTP operator) has made an excellent contribution to bring out this edition. We are really obliged to them and pray for their prosperity.

Editors

Acknowledgements

We extend our heartfelt thanks to the following teachers of anatomy for their consistent academic support, encouragement, and well wishes.

- Dr AB Mishra (Mathura, UP)
- Dr A Hima Bindu (Visakhapatnam, AP)
- Dr Aaditya Madhusudan Tarnekar (Nagpur, Maharashtra)
- Dr Aarushi Jain (Kota, Rajasthan)
- Dr Abhijeet Joshi (Barmer, Rajasthan)
- Dr Abhilasha Priya (Jamshedpur, Jharkhand)
- Dr Abhinav Kumar Mishra (Sitapur, UP)
- Dr Abid Ali (Yenkapally, Telangana)
- Dr Abraham Joseph (Nandyal, AP)
- Dr Aditya Pratap Singh (Prayagraj, UP)
- Dr Ajay Kumar (Ludhiana, Punjab)
- Dr Ajay Nene (Alwar, Rajasthan)
- Dr Ajay Rathva (Vadodara, Gujarat)
- Dr AK Singh (Almora, Uttarakhand)
- Dr AK Srivastava (Lucknow, UP)
- Dr Akhilesh Trivedi (Gwalior, MP)
- Dr Alka Singh (Ayodhya, UP)
- Dr Alka Udainia (Surat, Gujarat)
- Dr Alka V Bhingardeo (Bibinagar, Hyderabad)
- Dr Alka (Kanpur, UP)
- Dr Alok Saxena (Dehradun, Uttarakhand)
- Dr Amar Jayanthi A (Idukki, Kerala)
- Dr Amarappa S Nagalikar (Belagavi, Karnataka)
- Dr Ambica Wadhwa (Jalandhar, Punjab)
- Dr Amit Kumar (Bilaspur, CG)
- Dr Amit Kumar Gupta (Jamshedpur, Jharkhand)
- Dr Amit Kumar Nayak (Varanasi, UP)
- Dr Amit Mehta (Chindwada, MP)
- Dr Amit Srivastava (Datia, MP)
- Dr Amol Durgkar (Chindwada, MP)
- Dr Amol Shinde (Pune, Maharashtra)
- Dr Amrita Kumari (Patna, Bihar)
- Dr Amrut Mahajan (Jalgaon, Maharashtra)
- Dr Amrutha Roopa Ramagalla (Siddipet, Telangana)
- Dr Amudha Mohan Ram (Chilakaluripet, Guntur, AP)
- Dr Anand Mishra (Basti, UP)
- Dr Anant Sachan (Orai, UP)
- Dr Angela A Viswasom (Kollam, Kerala)
- Dr Anil Agrawal (Bilaspur, CG)
- Dr Anil Kumar (Sangareddy, Telangana)
- Dr Anil Kumar Dwivedi (Srinagar, Uttarakhand)
- Dr Anil Rahule (Ramagundam, Telangana)
- Dr Anita (Bharatpur, Rajasthan)
- Dr Anita Fating (Amaravati, Maharashtra)
- Dr Anitha V (Kanyakumari, TN)
- Dr Anjali Aggarwal (Chandigarh)
- Dr Anjali Jain (Ludhiana, Punjab)
- Dr Anjali Jain (Udaipur, Rajasthan)
- Dr Anjali Prasad (Muzaffarpur, Bihar)
- Dr Anjali Sabnis (Navi Mumbai, Maharashtra)
- Dr Anju Partap (Shimla, HP)
- Dr Ankur Kumar (Karauli, Rajasthan)
- Dr Ankur Sharma (Greater Noida, UP)
- Dr Anne George (Kottayam, Kerala)
- Dr Annie Doley (Tezpur, Assam)
- Dr Anshu Gupta (Agra, UP)
- Dr Anshu Sharma (Chandigarh)
- Dr Anshu Soni (Ludhiana, Punjab)
- Dr Anterpreet Arora (Amritsar, Punjab)
- Dr Antima Gupta (Meerut, UP)
- Dr Anu Sharma (Ludhiana, Punjab)
- Dr Anuj Ram Sharma (Muzaffarnagar, UP)
- Dr Anup Singh Gurjar (Pali, Rajasthan)
- Dr Anupama Doddappaiah Panagar (Hosur, TN)
- Dr Anupama Mahajan (Amritsar, Punjab)
- Dr Anuradha (Amritsar, Punjab)
- Dr Anurag (Dehradun, Uttarakhand)
- Dr Anwar Unisa Sabry (Siricilla, Telangana)
- Dr Aparna (Vijayawada, AP)
- Dr Aparna Dixit (Unnao, UP)
- Dr Aparna K Vedapriya (Yadadri, Telangana)
- Dr Aparna Muraleedharan (Puducherry)
- Dr Aprajita Raizada (Udaipur, Rajasthan)
- Dr Aprajita Sikka (Ludhiana, Punjab)
- Dr APS Batra (Sonipat, Haryana)
- Dr Archana Rani (Lucknow, UP)
- Dr Archana Srivastava (Lucknow, UP)
- Dr Archana (Alzapur, Telangana)
- Dr Archana Goel (Shahbad, Haryana)
- Dr Archana Kalyankar (Aurangabad, Maharashtra)
- Dr Archana Kannamwar (Yavatmal, Maharashtra)
- Dr Arindam Banerjee (Durgapur, WB)
- Dr Arun Arya (Muzaffarnagar, UP)
- Dr Arun Kasote (Nagpur, Maharashtra)
- Dr Arun Prasad Singh (Patna, Bihar)
- Dr Arun Pundlikrao Kasote (Jalgaon, Maharashtra)
- Dr Arunabha Tapadar (Uluberia, WB)
- Dr Arvinder Pal Singh Batra (Sonipat, Haryana)
- Dr Arvind Kumar Pankaj (Lucknow, UP)
- Dr Asha Latha (Nellore, AP)
- Dr Ashfaq Ul Hasan (Srinagar, J&K)
- Dr Ashok Kumar Singh (Nalanda, Bihar)
- Dr Ashok Patil (Sangamner, Ahmednagar, Maharashtra)
- Dr Ashima (Nuh, Haryana)
- Dr Ashutosh Mangalagiri (Bhopal, MP)
- Dr Ashwani K Sharma (Jammu, J&K)
- Dr Ashwini Jadhav (Mumbai, Maharashtra)
- Dr AV Kulkarni (Dharwad, Karnataka)
- Dr Avanish Kumar (Patna, Bihar)
- Dr Avinash Abhaya (Chandigarh)
- Dr Avinash Rudrajwar (Durg, CG)
- Dr Azhar Ahmed Siddiqui (Badnapur, Jalna, Maharashtra)
- Dr Azmi Mohsin (Kanpur, UP)
- Dr B Naveen Kumar (Bachupally, Hyderabad, Telangana)
- Dr Babu Rao (Hyderabad, Telangana)
- Dr Badal Singh (Prayagraj, UP)
- Dr Banani Kundu (Uluberia, WB)
- Dr Bandi Sirisha (Telangana)
- Dr Bashir Ahmad Shah (Srinagar, J&K)
- Dr Beena Nambiar (Pariyaram, Kannur, Kerala)
- Dr Berjina Naqshi (Baramulla, J&K)
- Dr Bertha AD Rathinam (Bhopal, MP)
- Dr Bhagyashree (Bilaspur, HP)
- Dr Bharat Patel (Ahmedabad, Gujarat)
- Dr Bhaskar Pal (Haldia, WB)
- Dr Bhaudas Khanderao Jadhav (Mumbai, Maharashtra)
- Dr Bhavana Junagade (Mumbai, Maharashtra)
- Dr Bhavik Doshi (Ahmedabad, Gujarat)
- Dr Bindu Singh (Gorakhpur, UP)
- Dr Binod Kumar (Muzzafarpur, Bihar)
- Dr Bipinchandra Khade (Bhopal, MP)
- Dr Biswabina Ray (Kalyani, WB)
- Dr Bonita Gupte (Jammu)
- Dr Brajesh Ranjan (Banda, UP)
- Dr BR Singh (Nagpur, Maharashtra)
- Dr Brijendra Singh (Rishikesh, Uttarakhand)
- Dr BS Lala (Indore, MP)
- Dr BS Patil (Vijayapura, Karnataka)
- Dr C Kishan Reddy (Karimnagar, Telangana)
- Dr C Lalitha (Bengaluru, Karnataka)
- Dr Chandan Kumar Yadav (Lucknow, UP)
- Dr Charulata A Satpute (Nagpur, Maharashtra)
- Dr Chetan Sahni (Varanasi, UP)
- Dr Chetna Thakur (Agra, UP)
- Dr Chitti Narasamma (Kurnool, AP)
- Dr D Asha Latha (Machlipatnam, AP)
- Dr D Sudhakar Babu (Nizamabad, Telangana)
- Dr Daizy Singh (Ludhiana, Punjab)
- Dr Dalbir Kaur (Agroha, Haryana)
- Dr DAVS Sesi (Kakinada, AP)
- Dr Debjani Roy (Midinapore, WB)
- Dr Deepa Bently (Coimbatore, TN)
- Dr Deepa Deopa (Haldwani, Uttarakhand)
- Dr Deepa Devadas (Varanasi, UP)
- Dr Deepak Joshi (Mumbai, Maharashtra)
- Dr Deepak Sharma (Jaipur, Rajasthan)
- Dr Deepali G Vidhale (Amaravati, Maharashtra)
- Dr Deepali Onkar (Nagpur, Maharashtra)
- Dr Deepanshu Shukla (Lucknow, UP)
- Dr Deepti Shastri (Salem, TN)
- Dr Dhananjay (Bareilly, UP)
- Dr Dhiraj Saxena (Jaipur, Rajasthan)
- Dr DH Gopalan (Chennai, TN)
- Dr Dibyendu Datta (Kolkata, WB)
- Dr Dimpal Patel (Ahmedabad, Gujarat)
- Dr Dinesh Kumar (Delhi)
- Dr Dipali Trivedi (Ahmedabad, Gujarat)
- Dr Dipti Gautam (Mahasamund, CG)
- Dr Dipti Nimje (Nagpur, Maharashtra)
- Dr Divya Mahajan (Chandigarh)
- Dr Durga Paswan (Greater Noida, UP)
- Dr Durgesh Singh (Mirzapur, UP)
- Dr DV Singh (Bareilly, UP)
- Dr Faizal Mohammad (Siddipet, Telangana)
- Dr Fatima M De Souza (Goa)
- Dr Fazal Ur Rehman (Aligarh, UP)
- Dr Feroz Hussain (Guwahati, Assam)
- Dr G Sundar (Vellore, TN)
- Dr GA Jos Hemalatha (Virudhunagar, TN)
- Dr Gajanan L Maske (Yavatmal, Maharashtra)
- Dr Ganesh Khemnar (Kurnool, AP)
- Dr Ganesh Trivedi (Shri Ganganagar, Rajasthan)
- Dr Garima Sharma (Tanda, HP)
- Dr Garima Pardhi (Vidisha, MP)
- Dr Garima Shivhare (Shahbad, Haryana)
- Dr Gaurav Agnihotri (Amritsar, Punjab)

- Dr Gautam A Shroff (Aurangabad, Maharashtra)
- Dr Gayatri Muthiyan (Nagpur, Maharashtra)
- Dr Geetha KN (Mumbai, Maharashtra)
- Dr Ghanshyam Gupta (Jaipur, Rajasthan)
- Dr Ghulam Mohammad Bhat (Srinagar, J&K)
- Dr Gitanjali Arora (Bhubaneswar, Odisha)
- Dr GL Nigam (Banda, UP)
- Dr Gnanavel A (Kanchipuram, TN)
- Dr Gopal Mondal (Barasat, WB)
- Dr Gopal Sharma (Jhalawar, Rajasthan)
- Dr Gouri Shankar Jha (Laheriasarai, Darbhanga, Bihar)
- Dr Gunapriya Raghunath (Chennai, TN)
- Dr Gunwant Chaudhari (Dahod, Gujarat)
- Dr Gursharan S Dhindsa (Faridkot, Punjab)
- Dr Gyan Prakash Mishra (Basti, UP)
- Dr Gyanraj Singh (Jajpur, Odisha)
- Dr Hamid Ansari (Kanpur Dehat, UP)
- Dr Hari Narayan Yadav (Mathura, UP)
- Dr Harish Chaturvedi (Chamba, HP)
- Dr Haritha Nimmagadda (Navi Mumbai, Maharashtra)
- Dr Harpreet Singh Gulati (Jalandhar, Punjab)
- Dr Harsh Chawre (Datia, MP)
- Dr Harsh Mishrikoti P (Belagavi, Karnataka)
- Dr Harsimrajit Kaur (Patiala, Punjab)
- Dr Harsimran Grewal (Patiala, Punjab)
- Dr Hemlata Ambade (Nagpur, Maharashtra)
- Dr Hina Sharma (Udaipur, Rajasthan)
- Dr Hitant Vohra (Ludhiana, Punjab)
- Dr Hrishikesh Jadhav (Sola, Ahmedabad, Gujarat)
- Dr I Gowri (Chevella, Telangana)
- Dr Ila Gujaria (Shivpuri, MP)
- Dr Indra Kumar Patel (Bahraich, UP)
- Dr Indushri (Kannauj, UP)
- Dr Isha Srivastav (Udaipur, Rajasthan)
- Dr Israr Ahmed Khan (Shahdol, MP)
- Dr JP Yadav (Churu, Rajasthan)
- Dr JS Kullar (Amritsar, Punjab)
- Dr J Sreevidya (Chennai, TN)
- Dr Jaba Rajguru (Vadodra, Gujarat)
- Dr Jaedeo Ughade (Parbhani, Maharashtra)
- Dr Jagmohan Sharma (Jaipur, Rajasthan)
- Dr Jagriti Agrawal (Raipur, CG)
- Dr Jaita Chowdhury (Haldia, WB)
- Dr Jami Sagar Prusty (Berhampur, Odisha)
- Dr Jasmeen Shaikh (Hyderabad, Telangana)
- Dr Jasween Kaur (Jalandhar, Punjab)
- Dr Jaswinder Kaur (Ambala, Haryana)
- Dr Javed Ahmad Khan (Srinagar, J&K)
- Dr Javed Akhtar (Patna, Bihar)
- Dr Jaya Prakash (Kamareddy, Telangana)
- Dr Jayasree K (Kozhikode, Kerala)
- Dr Jayasree Reddy (Siddipet, Telangana)
- Dr Jessy Rose George (Kozhikode, Kerala)
- Dr Jeyanthi G (Thirunelveli, TN)
- Dr Jitendra Gupta (Ratlam, MP)
- Dr Jitendra Patel (Ahmedabad, Gujarat)
- Dr Jolly Agarwal (Dehradun, Uttarakhand)
- Dr Joy Ghoshal (Mangalagiri, AP)
- Dr Jwalant Waghmare (Sevagram, Maharashtra)
- Dr Jyoti Gaiwad (Mumbai, Maharashtra)
- Dr Jyoti Ramling Gaikwad (Sanpada, Maharashtra)
- Dr Jyoti Rohilla (Mohali, Punjab)
- Dr Jyotsna Singh (Chandigarh)
- Dr K Manivanan (Kuppam, AP)
- Dr K Shanmuganathan (Puducherry)
- Dr K Udhaya (Tiruchengode, TN)
- Dr Kalpana Ramachandran (Chennai, TN)
- Dr Kalpana Sharma (Udaipur, Rajasthan)
- Dr Kalu Ram Meena (Bikaner, Rajasthan)
- Dr Kalyan Bhattacharya (Kolkata, WB)
- Dr Kamaljeet Kaur (Jalandhar, Punjab)
- Dr Kamil Khan (Lucknow, UP)
- Dr Kanahiya Jee (Barabanki, UP)
- Dr Kanan Shah (Ahmedabad, Gujarat)
- Dr Kanchan Kapoor (Chandigarh)
- Dr Kanika Sachdeva (Amritsar, Punjab)
- Dr Kavita Nanda (Hamirpur, HP)
- Dr Kavita Pahuja (Bikaner, Rajasthan)
- Dr Kiran Kalloor (Palakkad, Kerala)
- Dr Kiran V Padeyappanavar (Belagavi, Karnataka)
- Dr Kirti Nemade (Nagpur, Maharashtra)
- Dr KK Thakur (Doda, J&K)
- Dr KKP Singh (Ranchi, Jharkhand)
- Dr Komala B (Bengaluru)
- Dr Krishnaiah M (Suryapet, Telangana)
- Dr Krishna Gopal (Bareilly, UP)
- Dr Krishna Tiwari (Prayagraj, UP)
- Dr Kulbir Kaur (Amritsar, Punjab)
- Dr Kuldeep (Kannauj, UP)
- Dr Kumar Satish Ravi (Gorakhpur, UP)
- Dr Kunal Chawla (Shimla, HP)
- Dr L Hema (Nellore, AP)
- Dr Lakshmikantha (Meppadi, Wayanad, Kerala)
- Dr Lalatendu Swain (Puri, Odisha)
- Dr Lency Davis (Thrissur, Kerala)
- Dr Lenin S (Kanyakumari, TN)
- Dr Lola Das (Thrissur, Kerala)
- Dr M Chatterjee (Raipur, CG)
- Dr M Prasad (Dhanbad, Jharkhand)
- Dr M Siva Kumar (Thiruvannamalai, TN)
- Dr M Sivakumar (Trichi, TN)
- Dr MA Doshi (Karad, Maharashtra)
- Dr Madasi Pranay Kumar (Karimnagar, Telangana)
- Dr Madhusmita Panda (Balasore, Odisha)
- Dr Mahendra Kumar Pant (Dehradun, Uttarakhand)
- Dr Mahesh GM (Chitradurga, Karnataka)
- Dr Mahesh K Sharma (Chandigarh)
- Dr Mahesh Ugale (Latur, Maharashtra)
- Dr Mahita Bojja (Nagarkurnool, Telangana)
- Dr Malamoni Dutta (Kokrajhar, Assam)
- Dr Mallela Padmavati (Hyderabad, Telangana)
- Dr Mamata Sar (Burla, Odisha)
- Dr Mamta Anand (Prayagraj, UP)
- Dr Mamta Kumari (Pawapuri, Bihar)
- Dr Mamta Sharma (Jalandhar, Punjab)
- Dr Maneesha (Mohali, Punjab)
- Dr Mangesh Lone (Mumbai, Maharashtra)
- Dr Mangesh Selukar (Latur, Maharashtra)
- Dr Mani Kathapillai (Chengalpattu, TN)
- Dr Maninder Kaur (Patiala, Punjab)
- Dr Manish Khanna (Firozabad, UP)
- Dr Manish Patil (Ujjain, MP)
- Dr Manisha Nakhate (Navi Mumbai, Maharashtra)
- Dr Manisha R Gaikwad (Bhubaneswar, Odisha)
- Dr Manisha Upadhyay (Azamgarh, UP)
- Dr Manju Bala (Patiala, Punjab)
- Dr Manjunath V Motagi (Indore, MP)
- Dr Manjusha Tabhane (Nagpur, Maharashtra)
- Dr Manjushree Chakroborty (Nagaon, Assam)
- Dr Manoj Sharma (Jhalawar, Rajasthan)
- Dr Maria Kala (Siddipet, Telangana)
- Dr Martin Lucas A (Bengaluru)
- Dr Md Jawed Akhtar (Patna, Bihar)
- Dr Meenakshi Aggarwal (Ludhiana, Punjab)
- Dr Meenakshi Borkar (Mumbai, Maharashtra)
- Dr Meenakshi Khullar (Faridkot, Punjab)
- Dr Meenakshi Parthsarathy (Bengaluru, Karnataka)
- Dr Meetu Agarwal (Faridabad, Haryana)
- Dr Meghana Mishra (Reva, MP)
- Dr Mehandi V Mahajan (Thiruvallur, TN)
- Dr Mehera Bhoir (Mumbai, Maharashtra)
- Dr MG Puranik (Pune, Maharashtra)
- Dr Mini Kariappa (Thrissur)
- Dr Mini Mol (Mumbai, Maharashtra)
- Dr MM Peerzade (Solapur, Maharashtra)
- Dr Mohammad Mujahid Ansari (Shahdol, MP)
- Dr Mohammad Nazeem Khawaja (Baramulla, J&K)
- Dr Mohd Ajmal (Siddharthnagar, UP)
- Dr Monica Jain (Agroha, Haryana)
- Dr Monika Gupta (Bathinda, Punjab)
- Dr Monika Lalit Piplani (Amritsar, Punjab)
- Dr MP Sultana (Nellore, AP)
- Dr Mrinal Barua (Rishikesh, Uttarakhand)
- Dr Mritunjay Pandey (Deoria, UP)
- Dr MS Arathi (Chennai, TN)
- Dr Mubeen Rashid (Kathua, J&K)
- Dr Mudasir Ahmad Khan (Anantnag, J&K)
- Dr Mukesh Mittal (Shivpuri, MP)
- Dr Mukesh Singhla (Rishikesh, Uttarakhand)
- Dr Muktar Hussain (Badaun, UP)
- Dr Mukul Sarma (Tinsukia, Assam)
- Dr Muthukumaravel Narayanaswamy (Ariyur, Puducherry)
- Dr N Bhanu Sudha Parimala (Mangalagiri, AP)
- Dr Navbir Pasricha (Lucknow, UP)
- Dr Nagraj S (Mahabubnagar, Telangana)
- Dr Naina Wakode (Vidisha, MP)
- Dr Namdeo Y Kamdi (Chandrapur, Maharashtra)
- Dr Nandita Dutta (Jalpaiguri, WB)
- Dr Naresh Thaduri (Bhopal, MP)
- Dr Natwar Agrawal (Jabalpur, MP)
- Dr Nava Kalyani (Hyderabad, Telangana)
- Dr Navita Aggarwal (Bhatinda, Punjab)
- Dr Navneet Kumar (Lucknow, UP)
- Dr Neelam Bala (Amritsar, Punjab)
- Dr Neelam Jit Kaur (Patiala, Punjab)
- Dr Neeraj Pandey (Ghazipur, UP)
- Dr Neeru Goyal (Ludhiana, Punjab)
- Dr Neeta Chhabra (Faridabad, Haryana)
- Dr Neetu Arora (Nalhar, Nuh, Haryana)
- Dr Neha Rai (Bhopal, MP)
- Dr Neha Vijay (Alwar, Rajasthan)
- Dr Nidhi Puri (Bilaspur, HP)
- Dr Nilesh Rakate (Bhopal, MP)
- Dr Nilofer Mulla (Mumbai, Maharashtra)
- Dr Nimisha Madhu (Gaya, Bihar)
- Dr Nirmal Kumar K (Vikarabad, Telangana)
- Dr Nirmaladevi M (Coimbatore, TN)
- Dr Nirmalya Saha (Agartala, Tripura)
- Dr Nirupama Gupta (Greater Noida, UP)

- Dr Nisha Yadav (Etawah, UP)
- Dr Nishigandha Sadamate (Vadodara, Gujarat)
- Dr Nita Gathe (Gondia, Maharashtra)
- Dr Nitin R Mudiraj (Sangali, Maharashtra)
- Dr Nityanand Srivastava (Etawah, UP)
- Dr Nivedita Pandey (Israna, Panipat, Haryana)
- Dr Niyati Airen (Srinagar, Uttarakhand)
- Dr Nusrat Jabeen (Jammu, J&K)
- Dr P Ashok (Hyderabad, Telangana)
- Dr P Bapuji (Eluru, AP)
- Dr P David Anand Kumar (Telangana)
- Dr P Sasikala (Tiruchengode, TN)
- Dr Padamjeet Panchal (Patna, Bihar)
- Dr Padmasini S (Chennai, TN)
- Dr Pankaj Maheria (Valsad, Gujarat)
- Dr Pankaj Singh (Jaipur, Rajasthan)
- Dr Pankaj Soni (Mandi, HP)
- Dr Parveen Akhter (Jammu)
- Dr Praveen Sharma (Sri Ganganagar, Rajasthan)
- Dr Patil Shrish (Chitradurga, Karnataka)
- Dr Payal Kasat (Kharagpur, WB)
- Dr Peter Ericson (Hyderabad, Telangana)
- Dr PG Khanwalkar (Bhopal, MP)
- Dr Phalguni Srimani (Kolkata, WB)
- Dr Piyush Kumar (Dehradun, Uttarakhand)
- Dr PK Ramakrishnan (Palakkad, Kerala)
- Dr PN Panshewdikar (Palghar, Maharashtra)
- Dr Pooja (Rohtak, Haryana)
- Dr Poonam Delmotra (Shahbad, Haryana)
- Dr Poonam Verma (Amritsar, Punjab)
- Dr PP Kulkarni (Islampur, Maharashtra)
- Dr Prabhakaran K (Ahmedabad, Gujarat)
- Dr Prabhjot Kaur (Mandi, HP)
- Dr Pradeep Bokariya (Sevagram, Maharashtra)
- Dr Pradeep Kumar (Gaya, Bihar)
- Dr Pradeep Pawar (Mumbai, Maharashtra)
- Dr Prafulla Pralhadrao Nikam (Wardha, Maharashtra)
- Dr Prajakta Kishve (Hyderabad, Telangana)
- Dr Prajna Paramita Samanta (Bhubaneswar, Odisha)
- Dr Prakash Baburao Hosmani (Solapur, Maharashtra)
- Dr Prakash KG (Udaipur, Rajasthan)
- Dr Pramod (Kanpur, UP)
- Dr Pranab Deb Barma (Tripura)
- Dr Prasanna MB (Ernakulam, Kerala)
- Dr Prashant Chaware (Bhopal, MP)
- Dr Prashant E Natekar (Hyderabad)
- Dr Prashant Munjamkar (Bibinagar, Hyderabad)
- Dr Prateek Singha (Nahan, HP)
- Dr Prathistha Potdar (Greater Noida, UP)
- Dr Pratibha Shakya (Lucknow, UP)
- Dr Pratima Jaiswal (Kota, Rajasthan)
- Dr Praveen B Iyer (Mumbai, Maharashtra)
- Dr Praveen Kurrey (Raipur, CG)
- Dr Praveen Ojha (Udaipur, Rajasthan)
- Dr Praveen Singh (Karamsad, Gujarat)
- Dr Preeti Chaudhary (Bhatinda, Punjab)
- Dr Preeti Goswami (Delhi)
- Dr Prerna Gupta (Amausi, Lucknow, UP)
- Dr Pritha S Bhuiyan (Mumbai, Maharashtra)
- Dr Priti Chaudhary (Bhatinda)
- Dr Priti Nemade (Nagpur, Maharashtra)
- Dr Priti Sinha (Meerut, UP)
- Dr Priya P Roy (Karad, Maharashtra)
- Dr Priya Ranganath (Bengaluru, Karnataka)
- Dr PS Chitra (Ariyalur, TN)
- Dr Pulipati Anil Kumar (Vizianagaram, AP)
- Dr Punita (Lucknow, UP)
- Dr Punita Sharma (Amritsar, Punjab)
- Dr Purushotam Rao (Vikarabad, Telangana)
- Dr PV Satya Kumar (Vijayawada, AP)
- Dr R Azhagiri (Chennai, TN)
- Dr R Manoranjitham (Perambalur, TN)
- Dr R Sarah (Madurai, TN)
- Dr Rachna Agarwal (Bharatpur, Rajasthan)
- Dr Rachna Magotra (Jammu)
- Dr Rachna Rastogi (Greater Noida, UP)
- Dr Rajan Singla (Patiala, Punjab)
- Dr Rajashree Biswal (Cuttack, Odisha)
- Dr Rajashree S Raut (Kolhapur, Maharashtra)
- Dr Rajasri Chunder (Budge, Kolkata, WB)
- Dr Rajat Subhra Das (Raebareli, UP)
- Dr Rajeev Panwar (KK Nagar, Chennai, TN)
- Dr Rajiv Ranjan (Ranchi, Jharkhand)
- Dr Rajendra Prasad (Gaya, Bihar)
- Dr Rajendra Singrolay (Ratlam, MP)
- Dr Rajendrakumar D Virupaxi (Belagavi, Karnataka)
- Dr Rajesh Dehankar (Nagpur, Maharashtra)
- Dr Rajesh Maurya (Dehradun, Uttarakhand)
- Dr Rajkumar KR (Gulbarga, Karnataka)
- Dr Rajlaxmi Panda (Berhampur, Odisha)
- Dr Rajveer Singh Chourasia (Bhawanipatna, Odisha)
- Dr Rakesh Gupta (Bareilly, UP)
- Dr Rakesh Kumar Verma (Lucknow, UP)
- Dr Rakesh Mani (Bikaner, Rajasthan)
- Dr Rakesh Mishra (Lucknow, UP)
- Dr Rakesh Shukla (Mirzapur, UP)
- Dr Ram Kumar Singhal (Bharatpur, Rajasthan)
- Dr Ram Prakash Gupta (Greater Noida, UP)
- Dr Randhir S Chauhan (Solan, HP)
- Dr Randhir Sigh Chauhan (Solan, Himachal Pradesh)
- Dr Rani Raphael M (Alappuzha, Kerala)
- Dr Ranjana Barjatya (Ajmer, Rajasthan)
- Dr Ranjeet Kumar (Deoghar, Jharkhand)
- Dr Ranjneet Guha (Patna, Bihar)
- Dr Rashi Mittal (Jaipur, Rajasthan)
- Dr Rashi Nigam (Kanpur, UP)
- Dr Rashmi Deopujari (Vidisha, MP)
- Dr Rashmi Ghai (Hardoi, UP)
- Dr Rashmi Jaiswal (Bhopal, MP)
- Dr Rashmi Malhotra (Rishikesh, Uttarakhand)
- Dr Rashmi Prasad (Patna, Bihar)
- Dr Rashmi S Sinha (Mumbai, Maharashtra)
- Dr Rashmoni Jana (Delhi)
- Dr Ratesh Kumar (Faridabad, Haryana)
- Dr Raveena Singh (Fatehpur, UP)
- Dr Ravi Kant Sharma (Solan, Himachal Pradesh)
- Dr Raviendra Marathe (Akola, Maharashtra)
- Dr Reeha Mahajan (Vijaypur, Jammu, J&K)
- Dr Reena Singla (Mohali, Punjab)
- Dr Rekha More (Mumbai, Maharashtra)
- Dr Rekha Parashar (Dausa, Rajasthan)
- Dr Renu Kumari (Panipat, Haryana)
- Dr Renuka Ahankari (Pune, Maharashtra)
- Dr Renuka Sharma (Greater Noida, UP)
- Dr Richa Gupta (Chandigarh)
- Dr Richa Niranjan (Srinagar, Uttarakhand)
- Dr Rimpi Gupta (Karnal, Haryana)
- Dr Rimple Bansal (Patiala, Punjab)
- Dr Ritesh Shah (Ahmedabad, Gujarat)
- Dr Ritika Gaddewar (Nagpur, Maharashtra)
- Dr Ritika Sharma (Amritsar, Punjab)
- Dr Ritu Gothwal (Churu, Rajasthan)
- Dr Ritu Saloi (Diphu, Assam)
- Dr Ritu Slathia (Rajouri, J&K)
- Dr RK Diwan (Lucknow, UP)
- Dr RK Shrivtastav (Unnao, UP)
- Dr Rohini Karambelkar (Islampur, Maharashtra)
- Dr Rohini Motwani (Bibinagar, Telangana)
- Dr Roli Joshi (Unnao, UP)
- Dr Romi S (Kollam, Kerala)
- Dr Roonmoni Deka (Guwahati, Assam)
- Dr RS Bulagouda (Vijayapura, Karnataka)
- Dr Rubi Saikia (Jorhat, Assam)
- Dr Ruchi Dhuria (Delhi)
- Dr Ruchi Goyal (Patiala, Punjab)
- Dr Ruchi Jain (Jhansi, UP)
- Dr Ruchi Ratnesh (Deoghar, Jharkhand)
- Dr Rup Sekhar Deka (Nalbari, Assam)
- Dr Rupa Chaparrwal (Indore, MP)
- Dr Rupali Kavitake (Alibagh, Maharashtra)
- Dr Ruta Bapat (Navi Mumbai, Maharashtra)
- Dr S Arrchana (Chengalpattu, TN)
- Dr S Babu Rao (Hyderabad, Telangana)
- Dr S Bharathi Rani (Sivagangai, TN)
- Dr S Diwya Lakshmi (Virudhunagar, TN)
- Dr S Karthick Selvaraj (Kanchipuram, TN)
- Dr S Naveen Kumar (Hyderabad, Telangana)
- Dr S Satish Kumar (Dharmapuri, TN)
- Dr S Satishkumar (Kalakuruchi, TN)
- Dr S Sundarapandian (Chengalpattu, TN)
- Dr Sabin Malik (Ernakulam, Kerala)
- Dr Sabita Mishra (Delhi)
- Dr Sachendra Mittal (Jaipur, Rajasthan)
- Dr Sachin Soni (Bilaspur, HP)
- Dr Sadakat Ali (Dehradun, Uttarakhand)
- Dr Sagun Shukla (Shahjanpur, UP)
- Dr Saif Omar (Bihta, Bihar)
- Dr Saikat Roy (Kalyani, Nadia, WB)
- Dr Sajan Skaria (Udaipur, Rajasthan)
- Dr Sajey PS (Alappuzha, Kerala)
- Dr Saju Binu Cherian (Hyderabad, Telangana)
- Dr Saleena N Ali (Alappuzha, Kerala)
- Dr Samala Niveditha (Nagarkurnool, Telangana)
- Dr Samatha Roshini Padala (Siddipet, Telangana)
- Dr Sambhu Prasad (Sasaram, Bihar)
- Dr Sameer Sathe (Datia, MP)
- Dr Sami Ahmed (Jaipur, Rajasthan)
- Dr Samta Gaur (Pali, Rajasthan)
- Dr Sandeep K Sharma (Ambedkar Nagar, UP)
- Dr Sandeep S Mohite (Karad, Maharashtra)
- Dr Sandhya Kurup (Kolanchery, Kerala)
- Dr Sangeeta Bali (Sitapur, UP)
- Dr Sangeeta Chouhan (Jaipur, Rajasthan)
- Dr Sangeeta Gupta (Jammu, J&K)
- Dr Sangeeta M (Bengaluru)
- Dr Sangeeta Naik (Hyderabad, Telangana)
- Dr Sanjana (Bhatinda, Punjab)
- Dr Sanjay Sharma (Sri Ganganagar, Rajasthan)
- Dr Sanjeev Kolagi (Bagalkot, Karnataka)
- Dr Santhini Arulselvi (Karaikal, Puducherry)
- Dr Santosh Kumar (Dholpur, Rajasthan)
- Dr Santoshkumar A Dope (Latur, Maharashtra)

- Dr Sarada Devi (Moinabad, Telangana)
- Dr Saritha S (Hyderabad, Telangana)
- Dr Saroj Sharma (Faridabad, Haryana)
- Dr Saryu Sen (Sikar, Rajasthan)
- Dr Sashi Bhushan (Kuppam, AP)
- Dr Satheesha KS (Mangaluru, Karnataka)
- Dr Satyashree Ray (Koraput, Odisha)
- Dr Saurabh Kulkarni (Aurangabad, Maharashtra)
- Dr Saurjya Ranjan Das (Bhubaneswar, Odisha)
- Dr Savithri Krishnan (Kollam, Kerala)
- Dr Sayantan Das (Kishanganj, Bihar)
- Dr SD Gupta (Bhopal, MP)
- Dr Seema (Amritsar, Punjab)
- Dr Seema Gupta (Jaipur, Rajasthan)
- Dr Seema Gupta (Ludhiana, Punjab)
- Dr Seema Prakash (Udaipur, Rajasthan)
- Dr Seema Sharma (Rajouri, J&K)
- Dr Seema SR (Bengaluru, Karnataka)
- Dr Shaheen Rizvi (Mumbai, Maharashtra)
- Dr Shaifaly Madan Rustagi (Delhi)
- Dr Shailaja Shetty (Bengaluru, Karnataka)
- Dr Shailendra Singh (Banda, UP)
- Dr Shakuntala Pai (Manipal, Karnataka)
- Dr Shalika Sharma (Vijaypur, J&K)
- Dr Shalini Chaudhary (Sonipat, Haryana)
- Dr Shalni Kumar (Delhi)
- Dr Shantanu Nandy (Bankura, WB)
- Dr Shanthini S (Puducherry)
- Dr Sharad Sawant (Mumbai, Maharashtra)
- Dr Sharmisttha Biswas (Kolkata WB)
- Dr Shashi Munjal (Dehradun, Uttarakhand)
- Dr Shavi Garg (Faridabad, Haryana)
- Dr Sheela Sivan (Perinthalmanna, Malappuram, Kerala)
- Dr Shema Nair (Bhopal, MP)
- Dr Sherry Sharma (Jalandhar, Punjab)
- Dr Shibanee Jena (Jajpur, Odisha)
- Dr Shikha (Delhi)
- Dr Shikha Sharma (Agra, UP)
- Dr Shikky Garg (Firozabad, UP)
- Dr Shilpa Bhimalli (Belagavi, Karnataka)
- Dr Shilpa Sonare (Nagpur, Maharashtra)
- Dr Shirin Jahan (Fatehpur, UP)
- Dr Shivaji B Sukre (Parbhani, Maharashtra)
- Dr Shivani Dhingra (Kannauj, UP)
- Dr Shobha Ramnarayan (Kolenchery, Ernakulum, Kerala)
- Dr Shrikant Verma (Raipur, CG)
- Dr Shruthi BN (Bengaluru, Karnataka)
- Dr Shruti Mamidwar (Chandrapur, Maharashtra)
- Dr Shubhangi Bhagwat Ghule (Jalgaon, Maharashtra)
- Dr Shubhpreet Sodhi (Nahan, HP)
- Dr Shweta Asthana (Udaipur, Rajasthan)
- Dr Shweta Swami (Karnal, Haryana)
- Dr Simmi Mehra (Rajkot, Gujarat)
- Dr Simmi Soni (Aziznagar, Telangana)
- Dr Sindhu Chaudhary (Almora, Uttarakhand)
- Dr Sirikonda Parimala (Mahabubnagar, Telangana)
- Dr SK Chavan (Pune, Maharashtra)
- Dr SM Belsare (Talgaon, Pune, Maharashtra)
- Dr Smruti Rekha Mohanty (Bhubaneswar, Odisha)
- Dr Sohinder Kaur (Jhajjar, Haryana)
- Dr Sonali Thomas (Haldwani, Uttarakhand)
- Dr Sonia Singh (Ludhiana, Punjab)
- Dr Sonu (Greater Noida, UP)
- Dr Soumitra Trivedi (Raipur, CG)
- Dr Soumya Chakraborty Bhattachrya (Kohima, Nagaland)
- Dr Sreevidya J (Chennai, TN)
- Dr SS Saiyad (Nadiad, Gujarat)
- Dr Stuti Srivastava (Udaipur, Rajasthan)
- Dr Shubha Shrivastava (Meerut, UP)
- Dr Subhash Gujar (Vadnagar, Gujarat)
- Dr Subhash K Deshpande (Dharwad, Karnataka)
- Dr Subhash Gupta (Shahjahanpur, UP)
- Dr Subhasis Chakraborty (Kolkata, WB)
- Dr Subodh Kumar (Patna, Bihar)
- Dr Suchetra Chaudhary (Ahmadabad, Gujarat)
- Dr Suchit Kumar (Dehradun, Uttarakhand)
- Dr Sudha R (Salem, TN)
- Dr Sudha Rani (Hazaribagh, Jharkhand)
- Dr Sudhakar Kumar Ray (Mathura, UP)
- Dr Sudhir Saxena (Gwalior, MP)
- Dr Sujata K (Kuppam, AP)
- Dr Sujithaa N (Villupurum, TN)
- Dr Sukhinder Baidwain (Nahan, HP)
- Dr Sumalatha Thimmaraju (Hyderabad, Telangana)
- Dr Suman (Rohtak, Haryana)
- Dr Suman Kumari (Gaya, Bihar)
- Dr Suman Yadav (Tanda, HP)
- Dr Sumedha Anjankar (Raipur, CG)
- Dr Sumit Babuta (Jaipur, Rajasthan)
- Dr Sumit Gupta (Kota, Rajasthan)
- Dr Sumit Patil (Bhopal, MP)
- Dr Sumita Agrawal (Dehradun, Uttarakhand)
- Dr Sumita Shukla (Ayodhya, UP)
- Dr Sundar Lal Jethani (Dehradun, Uttarakhand)
- Dr Sunita Bharti (Navi Mumbai, Maharashtra)
- Dr Sunita Gupta (Ahmedabad, Gujarat)
- Dr Sunita Nayak (Patna, Bihar)
- Dr Suniti Pandey (Kanpur, UP)
- Dr Surajit Ghatak (Jodhpur, Rajasthan)
- Dr Suranjali Sharma (Faridabad, Haryana)
- Dr Surekha Patil (Jaipur, Rajasthan)
- Dr Surekha W Meshram (Gondia, Maharashtra)
- Dr Suresh Kanta Rathee (Rohtak, Haryana)
- Dr Suresh Kumar (Vellore, TN)
- Dr Suresh Sharma (Sri Ganganagar, Rajasthan)
- Dr Susan Varghese (Kollam, Kerala)
- Dr Sushant Swaroop Das (Bilaspur, HP)
- Dr Susheela Rana (Mandi, HP)
- Dr Sushil Jiwane (Bhopal, MP)
- Rt. Brig (Dr) Sushil Kumar (Faridabad, Haryana)
- Dr Sushma Kushal Kataria (Jodhpur, Rajasthan)
- Dr SVV Nagarajamannar (Rajahmundry, AP)
- Dr Swati Bansal (Karnal, Haryana)
- Dr Swati Saxena (Dehradun, Uttarakhand)
- Dr Swati Yadav (Ghaziabad, UP)
- Dr Sweta Singh (Barabanki, UP)
- Dr T Anitha (Villupurum, TN)
- Dr T Rajan (Puducherry)
- Dr T Sreekanth (Peerancheru, Telangana)
- Dr Tapan Kumar Jana (Murshidabad, WB)
- Dr Taqiuddin Mohammed (Hyderabad, Telangana)
- Dr Tarkeshwar Golghate (Nagpur, Maharashtra)
- Dr TC Singel (Dahod, Gujarat)
- Dr Tejaswi HL (Mandya, Karnataka)
- Dr Tejendra Singh (Mathura, UP)
- Dr Teresa Rani (AP)
- Dr Thanuja Kumari (Telangana)
- Dr Thuslima M (Chennai, TN)
- Dr TK Rajashree (Hyderabad, Telangana)
- Dr Tom J Nallikuzhy (Idukki, Kerala)
- Dr Trupti Balwir (Nagpur, Maharashtra)
- Dr Uday Kumar (Telangana)
- Dr Ujwala Bhanarkar (Kalyani, WB)
- Dr UK Gupta (Jaipur, Rajasthan)
- Dr UK Kulkarni (Belagavi, Karnataka)
- Dr Upendra M (Kothagundum, Telangana)
- Dr Usha KK (Manjeri, Kerala)
- Dr V Anandhi (Trichy, TN)
- Dr V Dharani (Villupuram, TN)
- Dr V Rajapriya (Omandurar, TN)
- Dr V Ravi Kumar (Shimoga, Karnataka)
- Dr V Subhashini (Amalapuram, AP)
- Dr Vaishali Inamdar (Nanded, Maharashtra)
- Dr Vandana Mehta (New Delhi)
- Dr Vandana Sidhu (Amritsar, Punjab)
- Dr Vandana Tiwari (Haldwani, Uttarakhand)
- Dr Vanita Gupta (Hapur, UP)
- Dr Vanita Gupta (Udhampur, J&K)
- Dr Varsha Dahiphale (Ambajogai, Maharashtra)
- Dr Varsha Mokhasi (Bengaluru)
- Dr Vasant Vaniya (Vadodra, Gujarat)
- Dr Vashali Kadam (Mumbai, Maharashtra)
- Dr Vasi Padmaja (Telangana)
- Dr Vedula Sailaja (Hyderabad, Telangana)
- Dr Venkateshwar Reddy (Mehboobnagar, Telangana)
- Dr Vijay Anand S Nagdeve (Raipur, CG)
- Dr Vijay Nayak (Bundi, Rajasthan)
- Dr Vijayamma KN (Kerala)
- Dr Vijisha Phalgunan (Puducherry)
- Dr Vikas Saxena (Ajmer, Rajasthan)
- Dr Vikram Ephram (Yadadri, Telangana)
- Dr Vinay Kumar (Saharanpur, UP)
- Dr Vinay Sharma (Muzaffarnagar, UP)
- Dr Vineet Gohiya (Khandwa, MP)
- Dr Vinod Kumar (Turky, Bihar)
- Dr Vinodini (Secunderabad, Telangana)
- Dr Vinoth S (Chennai, TN)
- Dr Vipin Kumar (Varanasi, UP)
- Dr Virendra Bhdhiraja (Karnal, Haryana)
- Dr Vishal Bhadkaria (Sagar, MP)
- Dr Vishnu Gupta (Muzaffarnagar, UP)
- Dr VK Chimurkar (Wardha, Maharashtra)
- Dr VP Rukhmode (Gondia, Maharashtra)
- Dr X Chandra Philip (Puducherry)
- Dr Yogendra Singh (Gorakhpur, UP)
- Dr Yogesh Diwan (Shimla, HP)
- Dr Yogesh Shridhar Ganorkar (Pune, Maharashtra)
- Dr Yogesh Yadav (Hapur, UP)
- Dr Yuvraj Bhosale (Mumbai, Maharashtra)
- Dr Zafar Sultana (Hyderabad, Telangana)
- Dr Zeba Alam (Patna, Bihar)
- Dr Zeba Khan (Mumbai, Maharashtra)
- Dr Zeenat Akhtar (Jammu, J&K)
- Dr Zia Ul Haq (Hyderabad, Telangana)
- Dr Zuberi Hussain Riyaz (Badnapur, Jalna, Maharashtra)
- Pulkit Jain (Ludhiana, Punjab)

Editors

Reviewers

We extend our gratitude to the following anatomy teachers for their unwavering support and for reviewing various topics in the field.

- Dr Aga Ammar Murthuza (Bengaluru, Karnataka)
- Dr Angela (Kollam, Kerala)
- Dr Anjali Jain (Ludhiana, Punjab)
- Dr Anu Sharma (Ludhiana, Punjab)
- Dr Aparna K Vedapriya (Siddipet, Telangana)
- Dr Archana Rani (Lucknow, UP)
- Dr Arvind Kumar Pankaj (Lucknow, UP)
- Dr Ashok KL (Bengaluru, Karnataka)
- Dr Benjamin W (Palakkad, Kerala)
- Dr Dharmaraj Tamgire (Puducherry)
- Dr Dibyendu Datta (Kolkata, WB)
- Dr Dinesh Kumar V (Puducherry)
- Dr Gaurav Agnihotri (Amritsar, Punjab)
- Dr Gitanjali Arora (Bhubaneswar, Odisha)
- Dr Gunapriya Raghunath (Chennai, Tamil Nadu)
- Dr Hitant Vohra (Ludhiana, Punjab)
- Dr Indira CK (Ernakulam, Kerala)
- Dr Jahira Banu T (Puducherry)
- Dr Jaswinder Kaur (Ambala, Haryana)
- Dr Juned Labbai (Mumbai, Maharashtra)
- Dr K Chandra Kumari (Trivandrum, Kerala)
- Dr Komala B (Bengaluru, Karnataka)
- Dr Kumari TK (Kollam, Kerala)
- Dr Maitreyee Mutalik (Sindhudurg, Maharashtra)
- Dr Mubeena Sheikh (Palakkad, Kerala)
- Dr Nagaraja V Pai (Mumbai, Maharashtra)
- Dr Nusrat Jabeen (Jammu, J&K)
- Dr Payal Kasat (Kharagpur, WB)
- Dr PK Ramakrishnan (Palakkad, Kerala)
- Dr Prajna Paramita Samanta (Bhubaneswar, Odisha)
- Dr Pratibha Shakya (Lucknow, UP)
- Dr Pretty Rathnakar (Mangaluru, Karnataka)
- Dr R Gomathi (Puducherry)
- Dr R Sarah (Madurai, Tamil Nadu)
- Dr Rajashree Biswal (Cuttack, Odisha)
- Dr Rakesh Kumar Diwan (Lucknow, UP)
- Dr Rakesh Kumar Verma (Lucknow, UP)
- Dr Rakhi More (Mumbai, Maharashtra)
- Dr Rashmi Sinha (Mumbai, Maharashtra)
- Dr Ravikiran Gole (Mumbai, Maharashtra)
- Dr Rohini K (Bengaluru, Karnataka)
- Dr S Arivu Selvan (Calicut, Kerala)
- Dr S Naveen Kumar (Hyderabad, Telangana)
- Dr Sabin Malik (Guildford, UK)
- Dr Saleena N Ali (Alappuzha, Kerala)
- Dr Sandhya Kurup (Kolanchery, Kerala)
- Dr Sajay PS (Alappuzha, Kerala)
- Dr Saurjya Ranjan Das (Bhubaneswar, Odisha)
- Dr Shantanu Nandy (Kolkata, WB)
- Dr Sharmila Pal (Jadavpur, Kolkata, WB)
- Dr Sheela Sivan (Perimthalmanna, Kerala)
- Dr Smrutirekha Mohanty (Bhubaneswar, Odisha)
- Dr Sneha John (Mumbai, Maharashtra)
- Dr Sreekumar R (Thiruvananthapuram, Kerala)
- Dr Sreevidya J (Chennai, TN)
- Dr Srividya Sreenivasan (Mumbai, Maharashtra)
- Dr Surendra Babu T (Bengaluru, Karnataka)
- Dr Swapna Chavan Thakur (Mumbai, Maharashtra)
- Dr Swetha B (Bengaluru, Karnataka)
- Dr T Rajini (Bengaluru, Karnataka)
- Dr Taquiuddin Mohammed (Canada)
- Dr Ujwala Bhanarkar (Kalyani, WB)
- Dr V Lokanayaki (Chennai, Tamil Nadu)
- Dr Vandana LR (Thiruvananthapuram, Kerala)
- Dr Vasrha R Bhivate (Mumbai, Maharashtra)
- Dr WMS Johnson (Chennai, Tamil Nadu)
- Dr Yogitha R (Bengaluru, Karnataka)

Editors

Contents

eSmartQuiz – Online MCQ Test

After attending the class, students should go through the "*eSmartQuiz* – Online MCQ test" for the following reasons:

- *Reinforcement of Learning*: The "*eSmartQuiz* – Online MCQ test" provide an opportunity to reinforce learning after attending a class or reading a book. It helps to assess understanding and retention of concepts, to solidify knowledge and identify areas that need further revision or clarification.
- *Assessment of Comprehension*: The "*eSmartQuiz* – Online MCQ test" is an effective tool to assess comprehension of the subject matter and to demonstrate the ability to apply the concepts learned in the class.
- *Enhancement of Attention and Critical Thinking*: The "*eSmartQuiz* – Online MCQ test" will help to make students attentive for the class and to enhance critical thinking skills by selecting the most appropriate answer among the given options.

Each *eSmartQuiz* test consists of 10 MCQs, mostly image-based, and the students can see their scores at the end of each test. These questions will be modified after a certain interval. Use the given links or scan the QR code (given in each chapter) for the test. One student can solve each test only one time.

Chapter	***Links eSmartQuiz***
Upper Limb	
1. Introduction	https://forms.gle/cbNoHpx1AZ1Cci3WA
2. Bones	https://forms.gle/BNwB1uVpZ3QkKH3LA
3. Pectoral Region	https://forms.gle/2uvWyFGqwH58Aqgc9
4. Axilla	https://forms.gle/tn4WgHoLYpHZMkGp9
5. Back	https://forms.gle/eV9AjxwFU8bvDVRp6
6. Scapular Region	https://forms.gle/LHZ9MCB8r8pwJjfM6
7. Cutaneous Nerves, Superficial Veins and Lymphatic Drainage	https://forms.gle/nvVW9dhwfkLpNmHA8
8. Arm	https://forms.gle/q9G441mXn6e7D5YA9
9. Forearm and Hand	https://forms.gle/TD47GgMsajUsaKbP7
10. Joints of Upper Limb	https://forms.gle/Uz58AQZEBoV8jC2V6
11. Surface Marking and Radiological Anatomy of Upper Limb	https://forms.gle/pFqy9AdXNZU9WnJa6
Thorax	
12. Introduction	https://forms.gle/JmnZB66BgAFrQGgz5
13. Bones and Joints of Thorax	https://forms.gle/dsP6Ps5dw7sk3xYw5
14. Walls of Thorax	https://forms.gle/YZUu7n85AzWVqKEt6
15. Thoracic Cavity and Pleurae	https://forms.gle/uqdyCGyqE765sxFK6
16. Lungs	https://forms.gle/n7zigPn8smjNhTbD7
17. Mediastinum	https://forms.gle/RbeqSJKtANvFu6ay9
18. Pericardium and Heart	https://forms.gle/qys5zAdbsMTrNNSs8
19. Superior Vena Cava, Aorta and Pulmonary Trunk	https://forms.gle/ZDEkSQRMBM2H7mPf8
20. Trachea, Oesophagus and Thoracic Duct	https://forms.gle/CYwJap1ASNUaQpkQ9
21. Surface Marking and Radiological Anatomy of Thorax	https://forms.gle/PmCLumZeqdWXiPWx5

Index of Competencies

As per the latest NMC Guidelines | Competency Based Medical Education (CBME) Curriculum under Graduate Medical Education Regulation

Code	Competency	Chapter	Page no.
AN8.1	Identify the given bone, its side, anatomical position, joint formation, important features and clinical anatomy (clavicle, scapula, humerus, radius, ulna, carpal bones)	2	6, 9
AN8.2	Demonstrate important muscle attachments on the given bone	2	6, 9
AN8.3	Identify and name various bones in articulated hand, specify the parts of metacarpals and phalanges and enumerate the peculiarities of pisiform	2	23
AN8.4	Describe scaphoid fracture and explain the anatomical basis of avascular necrosis	2	25
AN9.1	Describe attachment, nerve supply and action of pectoralis major and pectoralis minor and describe clavipectoral fascia	3	37
AN9.2	Describe the location, extent, deep relations, structure, age changes, blood supply, lymphatic drainage, microanatomy and applied anatomy of breast	3	32
AN9.3	Describe development of breast, associated age changes and congenital anomalies	3	35
AN10.1	Identify and describe boundaries and contents of axilla	4	43
AN10.2	Identify, describe and demonstrate the origin, extent, course, parts, relations and branches of axillary artery and tributaries of vein	4	46
AN10.3	Describe, identify and demonstrate formation, branches, relations, area of supply of branches, course and relations of terminal branches of brachial plexus	4	52
AN10.4	Describe the anatomical groups of axillary lymph nodes and specify their areas of drainage	3, 4	34, 51
AN10.5	Explain variations in formation of brachial plexus	4	52
AN10.6	Explain the anatomical basis of clinical features of Erb's palsy and Klumpke's paralysis	4	55
AN10.7	Describe axillary lymph nodes, areas of drainage and anatomical basis of their enlargement	3, 4	34, 51
AN10.8	Describe, identify, and demonstrate the position, attachment, nerve supply, and actions of the trapezius and latissimus dorsi	5	58
AN10.9	Describe the arterial anastomosis around the scapula and mention the boundaries of triangle of auscultation	5, 6	60, 72
AN10.10	Describe and identify the deltoid and rotator cuff muscles	6	64, 68
AN10.11	Describe and demonstrate attachment, action and clinical anatomy of serratus anterior muscle	3, 6	41, 68
AN10.12	Describe and demonstrate shoulder joint for—type, articular surfaces capsule, synovial membrane, ligaments, relations, movements, muscles involved, blood supply, nerve supply and applied anatomy	10	143
AN10.13	Explain anatomical basis of injury to axillary nerve during intramuscular injections	6	68, 71
AN11.1	Describe and demonstrate muscle groups of upper arm with emphasis on biceps and triceps brachii	8	84, 95
AN11.2	Identify and describe origin, course, relations, branches (or tributaries), termination of important nerves and vessels in arm	8	87
AN11.3	Describe the anatomical basis of venepuncture of cubital veins	7	79
AN11.4	Describe the anatomical basis of Saturday night paralysis	8	98
AN11.5	Identify and describe boundaries and contents of cubital fossa	8	92
AN11.6	Describe the anastomoses around the elbow joint	8	91
AN12.1	Describe and demonstrate important muscle groups of ventral forearm with attachments, nerve supply and actions	9	101
AN12.2	Identify and describe origin, course, relations, branches (or tributaries), termination of important nerves and vessels of forearm	9	107
AN12.3	Identify and describe flexor retinaculum with its attachments	9	113
AN12.4	Explain anatomical basis of carpal tunnel syndrome	9	127
AN12.5	Identify and describe small muscles of hand. Also describe movements of thumb and muscles involved	9	115
AN12.6	Describe and demonstrate movements of thumb and muscles involved	10	158
AN12.7	Identify and describe course and branches of important blood vessels and nerves in hand	9	122
AN12.8	Describe anatomical basis of claw hand	9	127
AN12.9	Identify and describe fibrous flexor sheaths, ulnar bursa, radial bursa and digital synovial sheaths	9	105
AN12.10	Explain infection of fascial spaces of palm	9	129
AN12.11	Identify, describe and demonstrate important muscle groups of dorsal forearm with attachments, nerve supply and actions	9	134
AN12.12	Identify and describe origin, course, relations, branches (or tributaries), termination of important nerves and vessels of back of forearm	9	138
AN12.13	Describe the anatomical basis of wrist drop	8	98
AN12.14	Identify and describe compartments deep to extensor retinaculum and describe the boundaries and contents of anatomical snuff box	9	133
AN12.15	Identify and describe extensor expansion formation	9	136
AN13.1	Describe and explain fascia of upper limb and compartments, veins of upper limb and its lymphatic drainage	7	77
AN13.2	Describe dermatomes of upper limb	7	75

(Contd.)

(*Contd.*)

Code	Competency	Chapter	Page no.
AN13.3	Identify and describe the type, articular surfaces, capsule, synovial membrane, ligaments, relations, movements, blood and nerve supply of elbow joint, proximal and distal radioulnar joints, wrist joint and first carpometacarpal joint	10	148
AN13.4	Describe sternoclavicular joint, acromioclavicular joint, carpometacarpal joints, and metacarpophalangeal joint	10	141, 158
AN13.5	Identify the bones and joints of upper limb seen in anteroposterior and lateral view radiographs of shoulder region, arm, elbow, forearm, and hand	11	167
AN13.6	Identify and demonstrate important bony landmarks of upper limb: Jugular notch, sternal angle, acromial angle, spine of the scapula, vertebral level of the medial end and inferior angle of the scapula	3	30
AN13.7	Identify and demonstrate surface projection of—cephalic and basilic vein, palpation of brachial artery, radial artery; testing of muscles—trapezius, pectoralis major, serratus anterior, latissimus dorsi, deltoid, biceps brachii, brachioradialis	11	163
AN21.1	Identify and describe the salient features of sternum, typical rib and typical thoracic vertebra	13	189
AN21.2	Identify and describe the features of atypical ribs and atypical thoracic vertebrae	13	195
AN21.3	Describe and demonstrate the boundaries of thoracic inlet, cavity, and outlet	12	183
AN21.4	Describe and demonstrate extent, attachments, direction of fibres, nerve supply, and actions of intercostal muscles	14	206
AN21.5	Describe and demonstrate origin, course, relations and branches of a typical intercostal nerve	14	208
AN21.6	Mention origin, course and branches/tributaries of: 1. Anterior and posterior intercostal vessels 2. Internal thoracic vessels	14	212
AN21.7	Mention the origin, course, relations and branches of: 1. Atypical intercostal nerve 2. Superior intercostal artery, subcostal artery	14	208, 212
AN21.8	Describe and demonstrate type, articular surfaces and movements of manubriosternal, costovertebral, costotransverse and xiphisternal joints	13	202
AN21.9	Describe and demonstrate mechanics and types of respiration	14	219
AN21.10	Describe costochondral and interchondral joints	13	202
AN21.11	Mention boundaries and contents of the superior, anterior, middle, and posterior mediastinum	17	244
AN22.1	Describe and demonstrate subdivisions, sinuses in pericardium, blood supply, and nerve supply of pericardium	18	249
AN22.2	Describe and demonstrate external and internal features of each chamber of heart	18	258
AN22.3	Describe and demonstrate origin, course and branches of coronary arteries	18	269
AN22.4	Describe anatomical basis of ischaemic heart disease	18	272
AN22.5	Describe and demonstrate the formation, course, tributaries and termination of coronary sinus	18	274
AN22.7	Mention the parts, position and arterial supply of the conducting system of heart	18	266
AN23.1	Describe and demonstrate the external appearance, relations, blood supply, nerve supply, lymphatic drainage and applied anatomy of oesophagus	20	292
AN23.2	Describe and demonstrate the extent, relations, tributaries of thoracic duct and enumerate its applied anatomy	20	296
AN23.3	Describe and demonstrate origin, course, relations, tributaries, and termination of superior vena cava, azygos, hemiazygos and accessory hemiazygos veins. For superior vena cava *see* Chapter 19	14, 19	214, 278
AN23.4	Mention the extent, branches and relations of arch of aorta and descending thoracic aorta	19	281
AN23.5	Identify and mention the location and extent of thoracic sympathetic chain	14	217
AN23.6	Describe the splanchnic nerves	14	217
AN24.1	Mention the blood supply, lymphatic drainage and nerve supply of pleura, extent of pleura and describe the pleural recesses and their applied anatomy	15	225
AN24.2	Identify side, external features, and relations of structures which form root of lung and bronchial tree and their clinical correlate	16	233
AN24.3	Describe a bronchopulmonary segment with its clinical anatomy	16	238
AN24.4	Identify phrenic nerve and describe its formation and distribution	19	286
AN24.5	Mention the blood supply, lymphatic drainage and nerve supply of lungs	16	235
AN24.6	Describe the extent, length, relations, blood supply, lymphatic drainage and nerve supply of trachea	20	289
AN25.1	Identify, draw, and label a slide of trachea and lung	20	291
AN25.2	Describe development of pleura, lung and heart	16, 18	239, 276
AN25.4	Describe embryological basis of: (1) Atrial septal defect, (2) Ventricular septal defect, (3) Fallot's tetralogy	18	277
AN25.5	Describe developmental basis of congenital anomalies, transposition of great vessels, dextrocardia, patent ductus arteriosus and coarctation of aorta	19	281
AN25.6	Mention development of aortic arch arteries, SVC, IVC and coronary sinus	19	287
AN25.7	Identify structures seen on a plain X-ray chest (PA view)	21	304
AN25.8	Identify and describe in brief a barium swallow	21	306
AN25.9	Demonstrate surface marking of lines of pleural reflection, lung borders and fissures, trachea, heart borders, apex beat and surface projection of valves of heart	21	299

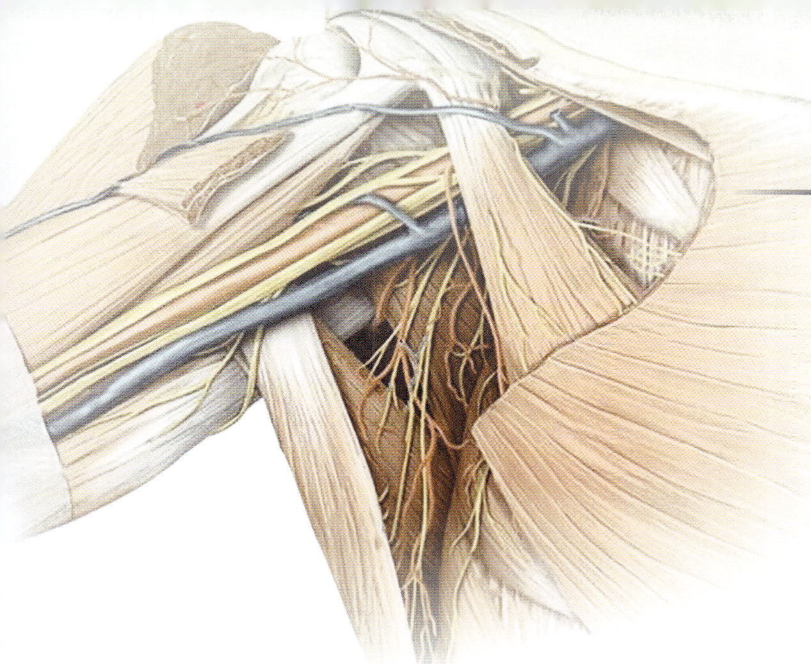

Section 1

Upper Limb

1. Introduction
2. Bones
3. Pectoral Region
4. Axilla
5. Back
6. Scapular Region
7. Cutaneous Nerves, Superficial Veins and Lymphatic Drainage
8. Arm
9. Forearm and Hand
10. Joints of Upper Limb
11. Surface Marking and Radiological Anatomy of Upper Limb

Appendix 1: Major Nerves and Arteries of Upper Limb

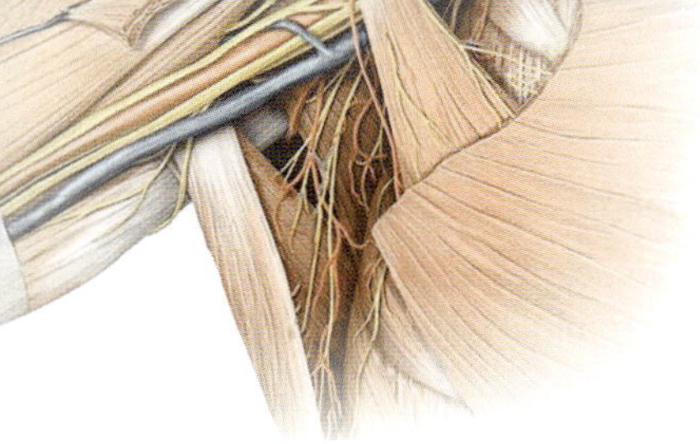

Chapter

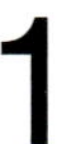

1

Introduction

Knowledge of anatomy is essential to create a strong foundation for clinical expertise and patient care proficiency. Anatomy is about knowing the nomenclature of the human body structure and its functioning mechanism. Cadaveric dissection is a major attraction for all the students of medicine.

With the evolution of the erect posture in man, the function of weight-bearing was taken over by the lower limbs. Thus, the upper limbs, especially the hands, became free and gradually evolved with great manipulative skills. This has become possible because of a wide range of mobility at the shoulder. The whole upper limb works as a jointed lever. The human hand is a grasping tool. It is exquisitely adaptable to perform various complex functions under the control of a large area of the brain. The unique positions of humans as master mechanics of the animal world is because of the skilled movements of their hands.

PARTS OF THE UPPER LIMB

It has been seen that the upper limb is made up of four parts (Plate 1.1, Table 1.1):

1. Shoulder region
2. Arm or brachium
3. Forearm or antebrachium
4. Hand or manus.

1. *Shoulder region*: It includes:

a. *Pectoral* or *breast region* on the front of the chest
b. *Axilla* or *armpit*
c. *Scapular region* on the back, comprising parts around the scapula
d. *Bones and joints*: The bones of the shoulder girdle are the *clavicle* and the *scapula*. Of these, only the clavicle articulates with the axial skeleton at the *sternoclavicular joint*. The scapula is mobile and is held in position by muscles. The clavicle and scapula articulate with each other at the *acromioclavicular joint*.

2. *Arm* (*upper arm or brachium*): It extends from the shoulder to the elbow (cubitus). The bone of the arm is the *humerus*. Its upper end meets the scapula and forms the *shoulder joint*. The shoulder joint permits movements of the arm.

Plate 1.1: Parts and bones of upper limb

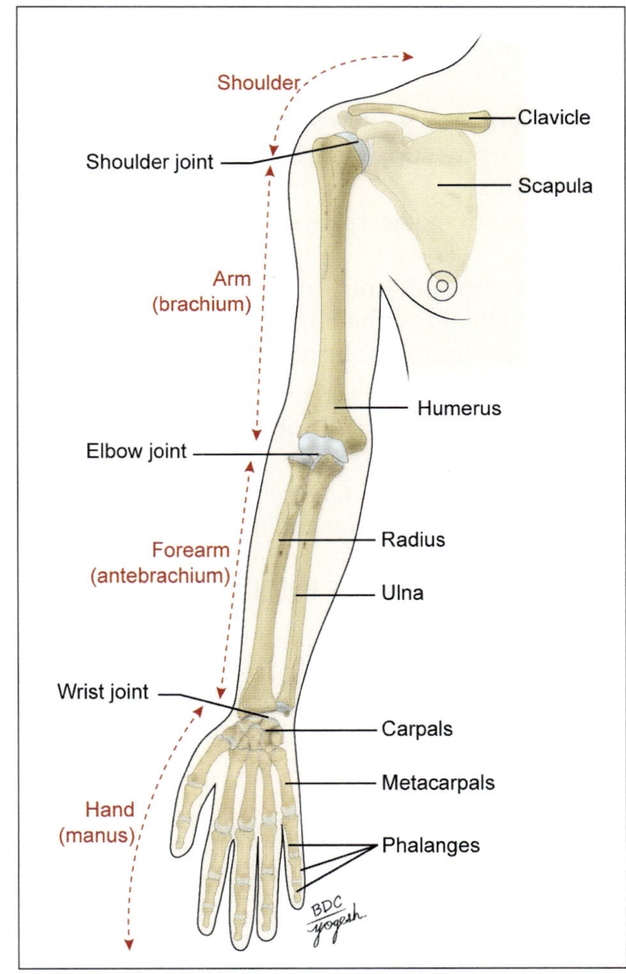

3. *Forearm* (*antebrachium*): It extends from the elbow to the wrist. The bones of the forearm are the *radius* and *ulna*. At their upper ends, they meet the lower end of the humerus to form the *elbow joint*. Their lower ends meet the carpal bones to form the *wrist joint*. The radius and ulna meet each other at the *radioulnar joints*. The elbow joint permits movements of the forearm, namely *flexion* and *extension*. The radioulnar joints permit rotatory movements of the forearm called *pronation* and *supination*. In a mid-flexed elbow, the palm faces upwards in supination and downwards in pronation.

TABLE 1.1: Parts of the upper limb

Parts	*Subdivisions*	*Bones*	*Joints*
Shoulder region	a. Pectoral region b. Axilla or armpit c. Scapular region	Clavicle Scapula	Sternoclavicular joint Acromioclavicular joint
Upper arm (arm or brachium)	—	Humerus	Shoulder joint
Forearm (antebrachium)	—	Radius Ulna	Elbow joint Radioulnar joints
Hand	Wrist (carpus) Hand proper (metacarpus) 5 digits (lateral to medial): 1st – thumb or pollex 2nd – index or forefinger 3rd – middle finger 4th – ring finger 5th – little finger	8 carpal bones 5 metacarpal bones 14 phalanges: two for the thumb, and three for each of the four fingers	Wrist joint (radiocarpal joint) Intercarpal joints Carpometacarpal joints Intermetacarpal joints Metacarpophalangeal joints Proximal and distal interphalangeal joints

During the movement of pronation, the radius rotates around the ulna.

4. *Hand (manus)*: It includes:

a. *Wrist* or carpus, supported by 8 carpal bones arranged in two rows.
b. *Hand proper* or metacarpus, supported by 5 metacarpal bones.
c. *Five digits* (thumb and four fingers). Each finger is supported by three phalanges, but the thumb has only 2 phalanges (in total 14 phalanges).

The *carpal bones* form the wrist joint with the radius, *intercarpal joints* with one another, and *carpometacarpal joints* with the metacarpals.

The phalanges form *metacarpophalangeal joints* with the metacarpals and *interphalangeal joints* with one another.

FUNCTIONAL ANATOMY OF UPPER LIMB

In human beings, the upper limb is highly evolved. The upper limb has its own peculiarities that make it different from the lower limb. Table 1.2 shows homologous parts of upper and lower limbs.

Peculiarities of the Upper Limb

- The skillful activities performed by human beings are due to the following peculiarities of the upper limb:
  1. Smaller and shorter upper limb than lower limb
  2. Freely moveable shoulder joint
  3. Long arm and forearm bones
  4. Presence of a carrying angle (angle between long axis of arm and forearm)
  5. Supination and pronation movements as adaptability to pick the food and eat using upper limb
  6. Arrangements of carpal bones in two rows
  7. Laterally placed thumb
  8. Separated long, slender digits
  9. Nail and nail bed protecting the terminal phalanx
  10. Grasping and skill movements of hand
  11. Opposition actions of thumb and little finger.

TABLE 1.2: Homologous parts of the limbs

Upper limb	*Lower limb*
Shoulder girdle	Hip girdle
Shoulder joint	Hip joint
Arm with humerus	Thigh with femur
Elbow joint	Knee joint
Forearm with radius and ulna	Leg with tibia and fibula
Wrist joint	Ankle joint
Hand with a. Carpus b. Metacarpus c. 5 digits	Foot with a. Tarsus b. Metatarsus c. 5 digits

Transmission of Force in Upper Limb

The weight transmission in upper limb occurs in the following manner (Flowchart 1.1, Plate 1.2):
Weight → hand → wrist joint → radius → interosseous membrane → ulna → elbow joint → humerus → shoulder joint → scapula → coracoclavicular ligament → clavicle → sternoclavicular joint and costoclavicular ligament → axial skeleton.

Flowchart 1.1: Lines of force transmission

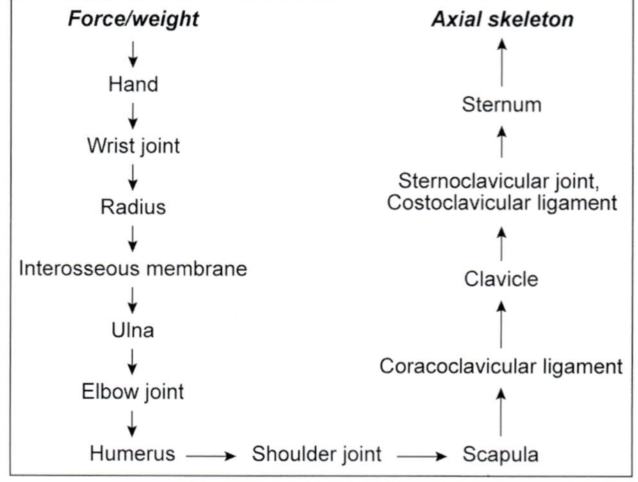

Plate 1.2: Line of force transmission in the upper limb

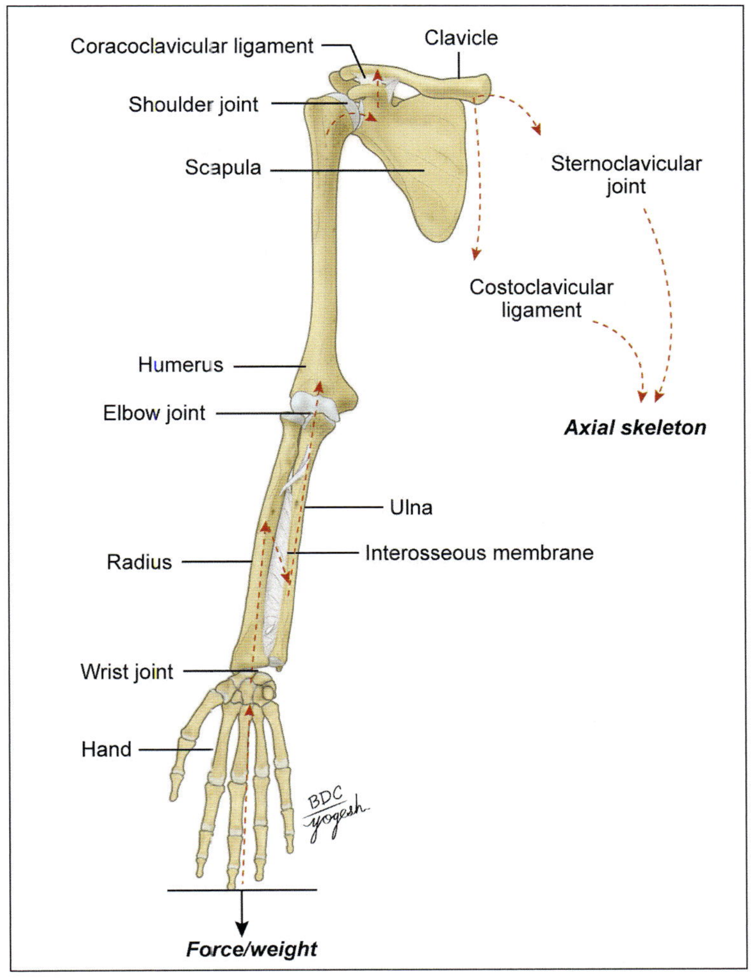

BDC's Anatomy *e*-book

1. Evolution of upper limb
2. Study of Anatomy
3. How to identify structures in cadaver?
4. Instruments required for the dissection
5. Viva voce questions

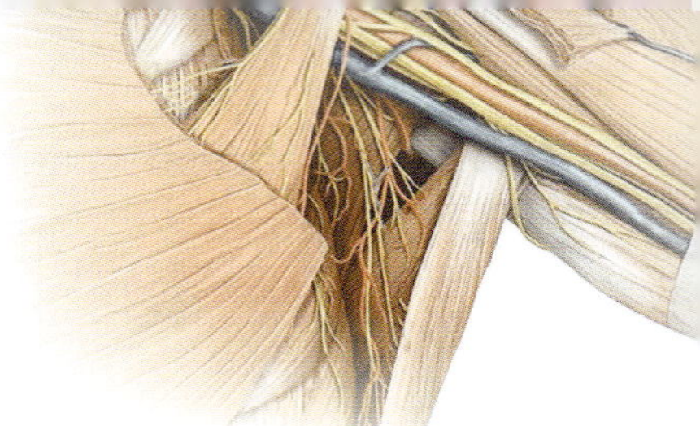

Chapter

2

Bones

Competencies:

AN8.1 Identify the given bone, its side, important features and keep it in anatomical position.

AN8.2 Identify and describe joints formed by the given bone.

- The study of bones of the upper limb has a clinical significance. It helps to understand the attachment of various muscles and ligaments, various joints, their movements and their applied aspects, such as bone fractures and anomalies.
- Each upper limb is supported with 32 bones as follows:

Clavicle	1
Scapula	1
Humerus	1
Radius	1
Ulna	1
Carpals	8
Metacarpals	5
Phalanges	14
Total	**32 bones**

Competencies:

AN8.1 Identify the given bone, its side, anatomical position, joint formation, important features and clinical anatomy (clavicle, scapula, humerus, radius, ulna, carpal bones).

AN8.2 Demonstrate important muscle attachments on the given bone.

CLAVICLE

The clavicle (Latin *a small key*) is a long bone. It supports the shoulder so that the arm can swing clearly away from the trunk. The clavicle transmits the weight of the limb to the sternum. The bone has a curved part called the shaft and two ends, lateral and medial.

Side Determination and Anatomical Position

For the side determination, hold the clavicle horizontally in such a way that:

1. Its lateral end is flat, and the medial end is large and quadrilateral.
2. The shaft is slightly curved so that it is convex forwards in its medial 2/3rd, and concave forwards in its lateral 1/3rd.
3. The inferior surface is grooved longitudinally in its middle 1/3rd.

Peculiarities of the Clavicle

1. It is the only long bone that lies horizontally.
2. It is subcutaneous throughout.
3. It is the first bone to start ossifying.
4. It is the only long bone that ossifies in membrane.
5. It is the only long bone that has two primary centres of ossification.
6. There is medullary cavity in its medial 2/3rd.
7. It is occasionally pierced by the middle supraclavicular nerve.

Features

Shaft

The shaft (Plate 2.1a, Figs 2.1a and b, Flowchart 2.1) is divisible into the lateral one-third and the medial two-thirds.

1. *Lateral one-third*

The lateral one-third of the shaft is flattened from above downwards. It has two borders – anterior and posterior; and two surfaces – superior and inferior.

Borders: The *anterior border* is concave forwards. The *posterior border* is convex backwards.

Surfaces: The *superior surface* is subcutaneous, and the *inferior surface* presents an elevation called the *conoid tubercle* (Greek cone) and a ridge called the *trapezoid ridge*.

2. *Medial two-thirds*

The medial two-thirds of the shaft is rounded and is said to have four surfaces: anterior, posterior, superior and inferior. The *anterior surface* is convex forwards. The *posterior surface* is smooth. The *superior surface* is rough in its medial part. The *inferior surface* has a rough oval impression at the medial end. The lateral half of this surface has a longitudinal *subclavian groove*. The *nutrient foramen* lies at the lateral end of the groove.

Plate 2.1: Clavicle and Scapula (a) Features of right clavicle (superior and inferior views). (b) Features of right scapula (anterior and posterior views)

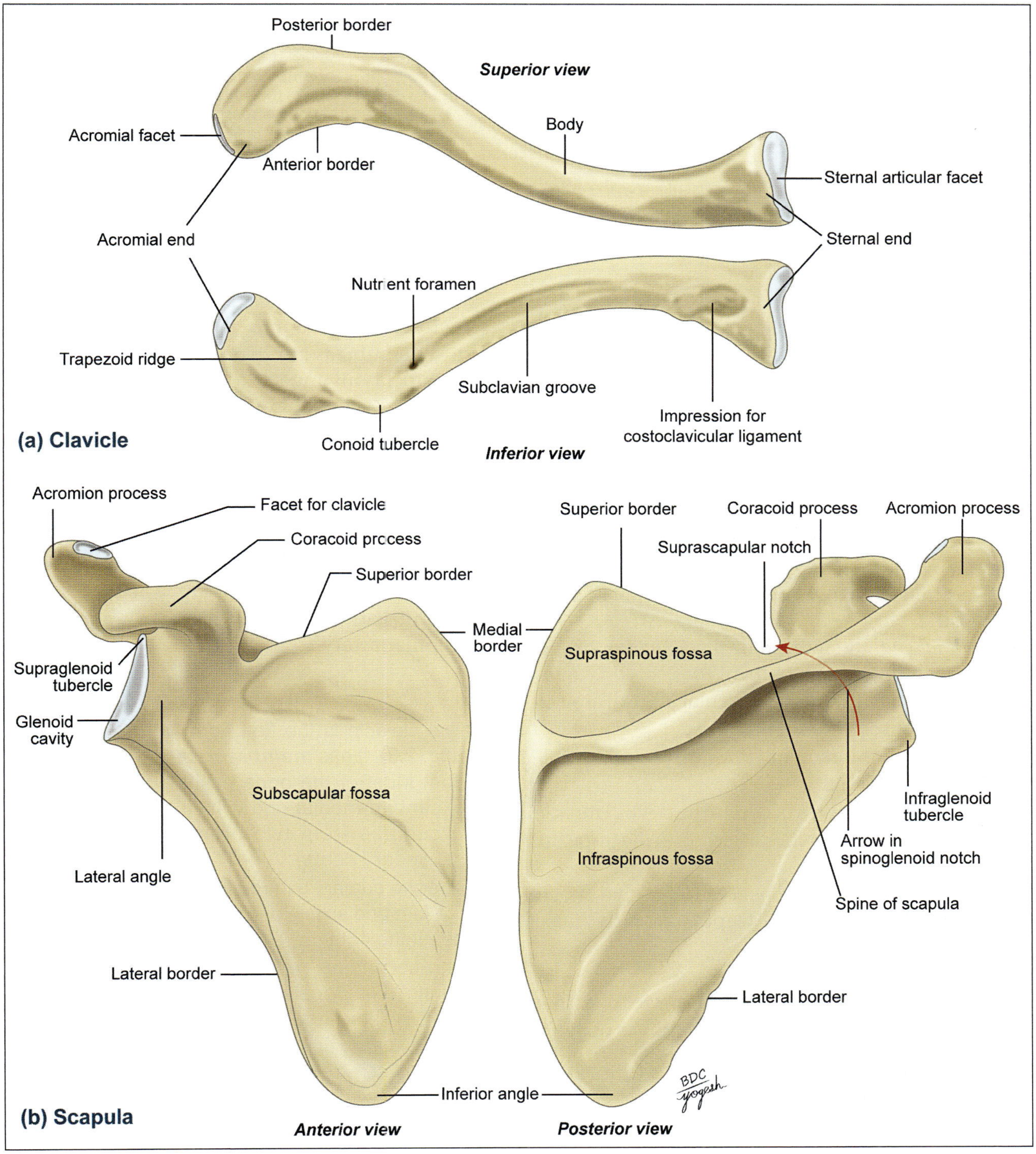

Posterior border
Superior view
Acromial facet
Body
Anterior border
Sternal articular facet
Acromial end
Sternal end
Nutrient foramen
Trapezoid ridge
Subclavian groove
Impression for costoclavicular ligament
(a) Clavicle
Conoid tubercle
Inferior view
Acromion process
Facet for clavicle
Coracoid process
Superior border
Superior border
Coracoid process
Acromion process
Suprascapular notch
Medial border
Supraspinous fossa
Supraglenoid tubercle
Glenoid cavity
Subscapular fossa
Infraglenoid tubercle
Arrow in spinoglenoid notch
Infraspinous fossa
Lateral angle
Spine of scapula
Lateral border
Lateral border
Inferior angle
(b) Scapula
Anterior view
Posterior view

Acromial end
Lateral 1/3rd
Sternal end
Medial 2/3rd
Lateral 1/3rd
Medial 2/3rd
(a) Superior view
Trapezoid ridge
Subclavian groove
Impression for costoclavicular ligament
Nutrient foramen
Conoid tubercle
(b) Inferior view

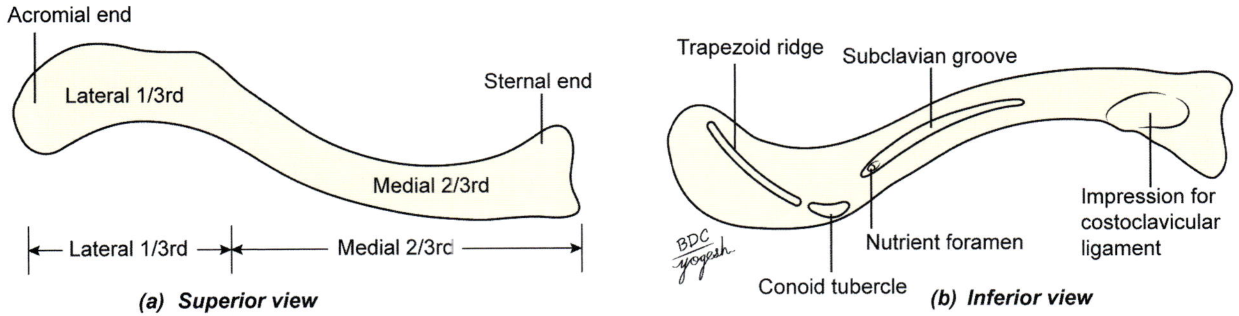

Figs 2.1a and b: General features of right clavicle: (a) Superior aspect and (b) inferior aspect

Flowchart 2.1: Features of clavicle

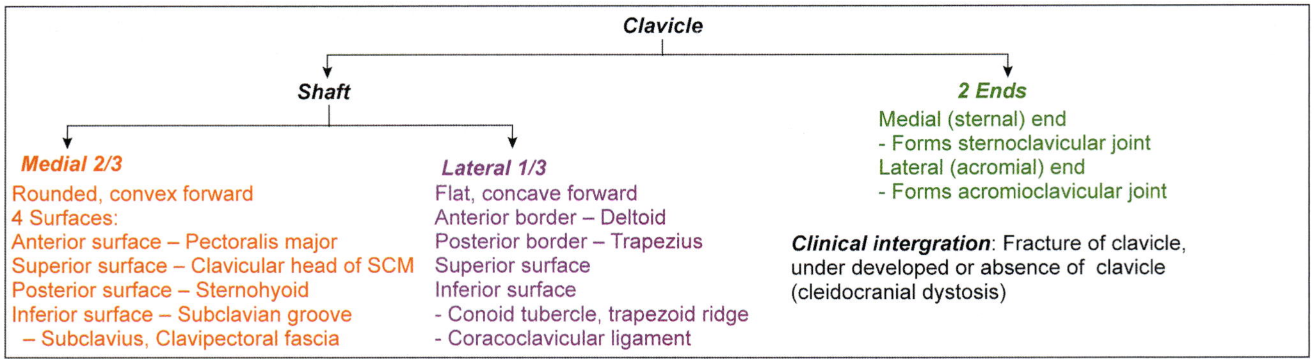

Ends of Clavicle

1. ***Lateral or acromial end*** (*Greek peak of shoulder*) is flattened from above downwards. It bears a facet that articulates with the acromion process of the scapula to form the *acromioclavicular joint*.
2. ***Medial or sternal end*** is quadrangular and articulates with the clavicular notch of the manubrium sterni to form the *sternoclavicular joint*.

Attachments (Figs 2.2a and b)

1. *At the lateral end,* the margin of the articular surface for its acromioclavicular joint gives attachment to the joint capsule.
2. *At the medial end,* the margin of the articular surface for the sternum gives attachment to:
   a. Fibrous capsule of sternoclavicular joint all around.
   b. Articular disc posterosuperiorly.
   c. Interclavicular ligament superiorly.
3. *Lateral one-third of shaft*
   a. Anterior border gives origin to the deltoid muscle.
   b. Posterior border provides insertion to the trapezius muscle.
   c. Conoid tubercle and trapezoid ridge give attachment to the conoid and trapezoid parts of the coracoclavicular ligament.
4. *Medial two-thirds of the shaft*
   a. Anterior surface gives origin to the pectoralis major.
   b. Medial half of the superior surface gives origin to the clavicular head of the sternocleidomastoid.
   c. Posterior surface close to medial end gives origin to sternohyoid muscle.
   d. The subclavian groove gives insertion to the subclavius muscle. The margins of the groove give attachment to the clavipectoral fascia.
   e. The oval impression on the inferior surface at the medial end gives attachment to the costoclavicular ligament.
   f. The *subclavian* vessels and *divisions of trunks of brachial plexus* pass towards the axilla lying between the inferior surface of the clavicle and upper surface of first rib. Subclavius muscle acts as a cushion.

The nutrient foramen transmits a branch of the suprascapular artery.

OSSIFICATION

- The clavicle is the first bone in the body to ossify (Fig. 2.3). It has ***membranocartilaginous*** ossification: Most of the bone ossifies in the membrane, except its medial end, which ossifies in cartilage. It ossifies from two primary centres and one secondary centre.
- The two primary centres appear in the shaft between the fifth and sixth weeks of intrauterine life, and fuse about the 45th day.
- The secondary centre for the medial end appears during 15–17 years, and fuses with the shaft during 21–22 years. Occasionally, there may be a secondary centre for the acromial end.

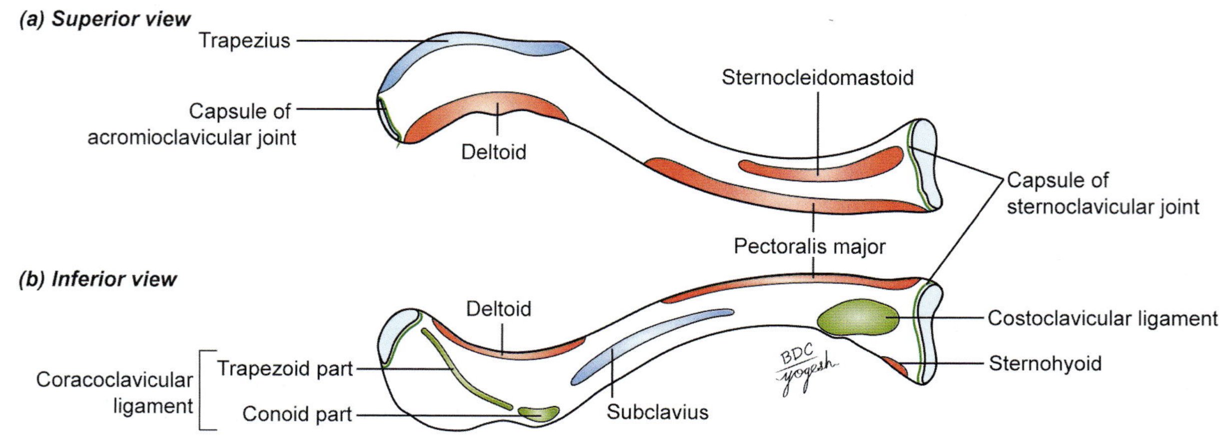

Figs 2.2a and b: Attachments of right clavicle: (a) Superior aspect and (b) inferior aspect

The sternal end of the clavicle is the growing end of the clavicle because secondary centre epiphysis at this end appears in the late teens and fuses by the age of 21–22 years. Hence, nutrient foramen is directed away from sternal end.

CLINICAL ANATOMY

- The clavicle is commonly fractured by falling on the outstretched hand (indirect violence). The most common site of fracture is the junction between the two curvatures of the bone, which is the weakest point. The lateral fragment may be displaced downwards by the weight of the limb as trapezius muscle alone is unable to support the weight of upper limb (Fig. 2.4a). The *medial fragment* is elevated due to sternocleidomastoid muscle. Fracture of clavicle is treated by immobilisation with figure-of-eight bandage (Fig. 2.4b).
- The clavicles may be congenitally absent, or imperfectly developed with defective ossification of the skull bones in a disease called *cleidocranial dysostosis*. In this condition, the shoulders can be approximated anteriorly in front of the chest (Fig. 2.5).

A nonunion of two primary centres of ossification results in ***clavicular dysostosis***. In this condition, the medial and lateral parts of clavicle remain separate.

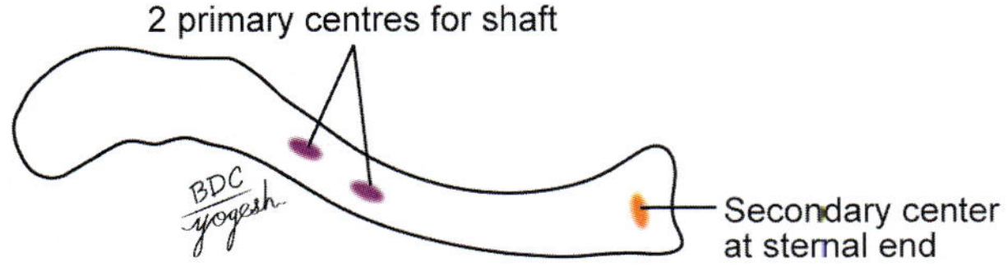

Fig. 2.3: Ossification of clavicle

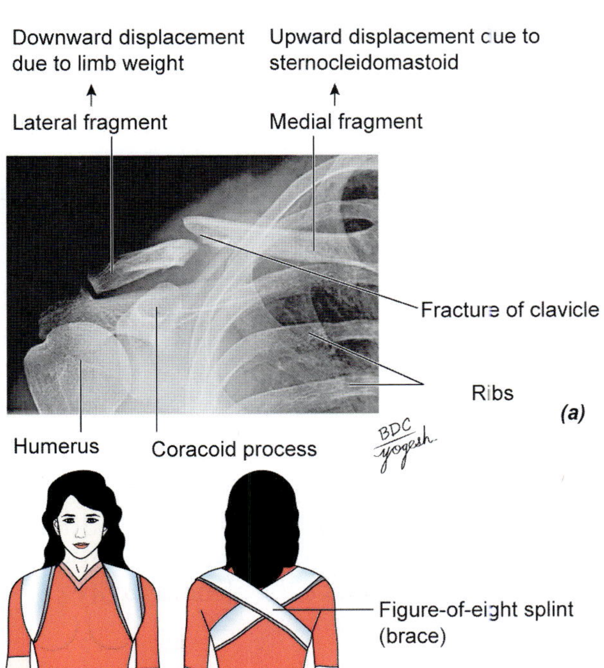

Figs 2.4a and b: Fracture of clavicle: (a) Radiological findings and (b) figure-of-eight splint

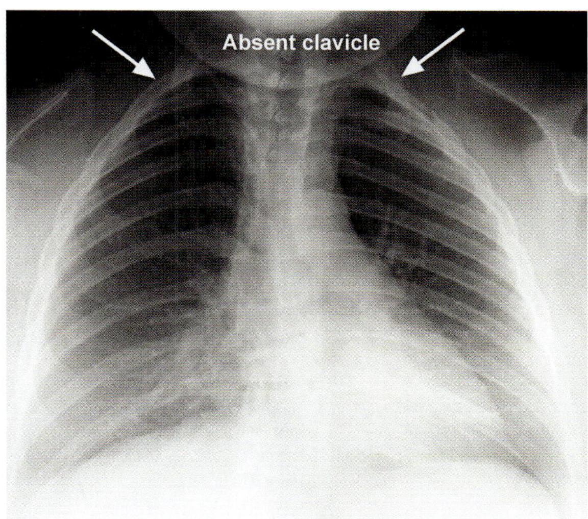

Fig. 2.5: Absence of clavicles in cleidocranial dysostosis

Competencies:

AN8.1 Identify the given bone, its side, anatomical position, joint formation, important features and clinical anatomy (clavicle, scapula, humerus, radius, ulna, carpal bones).

AN8.2 Demonstrate important muscle attachments on the given bone.

SCAPULA

The scapula (Latin *shoulder blade*) is a thin bone placed on the posterolateral aspect of the thoracic cage. The scapula has two surfaces, three borders, three angles and three processes (Plate 2.1b, Fig. 2.6, Flowchart 2.2).

Side Determination and Anatomical Position

For the side determination, hold the scapula in such a way that:

1. Its lateral or glenoid (Greek *socket*) angle is large and bears the glenoid cavity.
2. The dorsal surface is divided by the triangular spine into the supraspinous and infraspinous fossae (Figs 2.6 and 2.7).
3. Its acute inferior angle is directed downwards.

Features

Scapula has (Figs 2.6a and b):

- *Two surfaces*: Costal and dorsal
- *Three borders*: Superior, medial and lateral
- *Three angles*: Superior, inferior and lateral
- *Three processes*: Spinous, acromion and coracoid.

Surfaces

1. **Costal surface** or subscapular fossa: It is concave and is directed medially and forwards. It is marked by three longitudinal ridges. Another thick ridge adjoins the lateral border. This part of the bone is almost rod-like.
2. **Dorsal surface:** It gives attachment to the *spine of the scapula*, which divides the surface into a smaller *supraspinous fossa* and a larger *infraspinous fossa*. The two fossae are connected by the *spinoglenoid notch* situated lateral to the root of the spine.

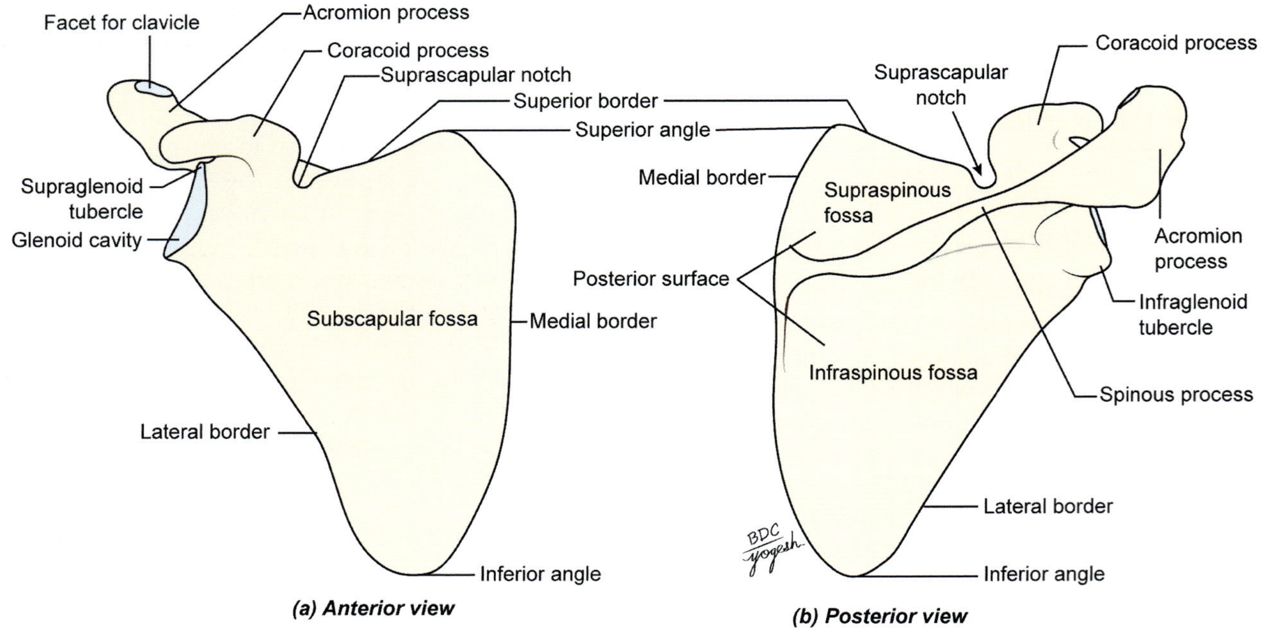

Figs 2.6a and b: General features of right scapula: (a) Costal surface and (b) dorsal surface

Flowchart 2.2: Features of scapula

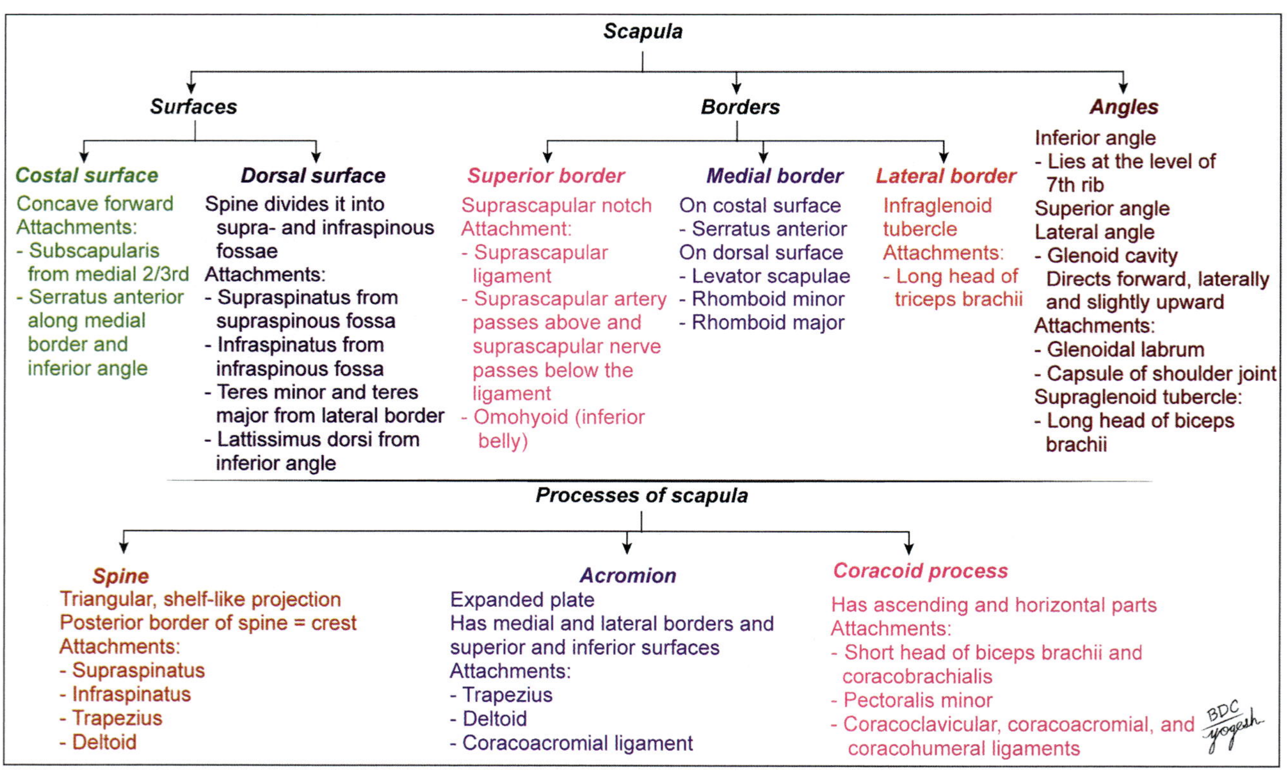

Borders

1. **Superior border:** It is shortest. Near the root of the coracoid process, it presents the *suprascapular notch.*
2. **Lateral border:** It is thick. At the upper end, it presents the *infraglenoid tubercle.*
3. **Medial border:** It is thin. It extends from the superior angle to the inferior angle.

Angles

1. **Superior angle:** It lies at the junction of superior and medial borders of scapula.
2. **Inferior angle:** It is more pointed and directed downwards. It covers the 7th rib or 7th intercostal space.
3. **Lateral** or **glenoid angle:** It is broad and bears the glenoid cavity or fossa, which is directed forward, laterally and slightly upwards. A supraglenoid tubercle is present above the glenoid cavity.

Processes

1. **Spine** or spinous process is a triangular plate of bone with three borders (anterior, lateral and posterior) and two surfaces. The posterior border of spine is called

the *crest of the spine.* The crest has upper and lower lips. The spine divides the dorsal surface of scapula into the supraspinous and infraspinous fossae.

2. **Acromion** process, an expanded plate, has two borders, medial and lateral; two surfaces, superior and inferior; and a facet for the clavicle.
3. **Coracoid process** (Greek *like a crow's beak*) is directed forwards and slightly laterally. It is bent and finger-like. It comprises a root; lateral and medial borders, superior aspect an a tip.

Attachments (Figs 2.7 to 2.9)

Surfaces

1. Subscapularis muscle arises from the medial two-thirds of the subscapular fossa.
2. Supraspinatus arises from the medial two-thirds of the supraspinous fossa, including the upper surface of the spine.
3. Infraspinatus arises from the medial two-thirds of the infraspinous fossa, including the lower surface of the spine.

Borders

4. Inferior belly of the omohyoid arises from the upper border near the suprascapular notch.
5. Transverse scapular or suprascapular ligament bridges across the suprascapular notch and converts it into a foramen, which transmits the suprascapular nerve. The suprascapular vessels lie above the ligament.
6. Long head of the triceps brachii arises from the infraglenoid tubercle.
7. Teres minor arises by two slips from the upper two-thirds of the rough strip on the dorsal surface along the lateral border. Circumflex scapular artery lies between the two slips.
8. Teres major arises from the lower one-third of the rough strip on the dorsal aspect of the lateral border.
9. Levator scapulae is inserted along the dorsal aspect of the medial border, from the superior angle up to the root of the spine.
10. Rhomboid minor is inserted into dorsal aspect of the medial border opposite the root of the spine.
11. Rhomboid major is inserted into dorsal aspect of the medial border between the root of the spine and the inferior angle.

Angles

12. Serratus anterior is inserted along the medial border of the costal surface: One digitation from the superior angle to the root of spine, two digitations to the medial border and five digitations to the inferior angle.
13. Latissimus dorsi arises from inferior angle.
14. The margin of the glenoid cavity gives attachment to the capsule of the shoulder joint and to the glenoidal labrum (Latin *lip*). The long head of the biceps brachii arises from the supraglenoid tubercle.
15. Long head of biceps brachii arises from the supraglenoid tubercle.

Spine, acromion and coracoid process

16. Trapezius is inserted into the upper border of the crest of the spine and into the medial border of the acromion process.
17. Deltoid arises from the lower border of the crest of the spine and from the lateral border of the acromion. The acromial fibres are *multipennate.*
18. The margin of the facet for clavicle on the medial aspect of the acromion process gives attachment to the *capsule of the* acromioclavicular joint (Fig. 2.10).
19. Pectoralis minor is inserted into the medial border and superior surface of the coracoid process.
20. Short head of biceps brachii arises from lateral part of the tip of coracoid process. The coracobrachialis arises from medial part of the tip of coracoid process.
21. Coracohumeral ligament is attached to the root of the coracoid process.
22. Coracoclavicular ligament is attached to the coracoid process: The trapezoid part on the superior aspect and the conoid part near the root.
23. Coracoacromial ligament is attached (a) to the lateral border of the coracoid process and (b) to the medial side of the tip of the acromion process.

OSSIFICATION

- The scapula ossifies **eight centres:** from one primary centre and seven secondary centres.
- The primary centre appears near the glenoid cavity during the eighth week of development.
- The first secondary centre appears in the middle of the coracoid process during the first year and fuses by the 15th year. The subcoracoid centre appears in the root of the coracoid process during the 10th year and fuses by the 14th to 17th years (Fig. 2.10).
- The other centres, including two for the acromion process, one for the lower part of rim of the glenoid cavity, one for the medial border and one for the inferior angle, appear at puberty and fuse by the 20th year.

CLINICAL ANATOMY

- Paralysis of the serratus anterior causes 'winging' of the scapula. The medial border of the bone becomes unduly prominent, and the arm cannot be abducted beyond 90° (Fig. 2.11).
- The *scaphoid* scapula is a developmental anomaly, in which the medial border is concave.

Sprengel's deformity is a congenital anomaly in which scapula is situated higher in the back (Otto GK Sprengel, German Surgeon, 1852–1915). It occurs due to the developmental failure of descent of scapula and shoulder from the neck to its adult position.

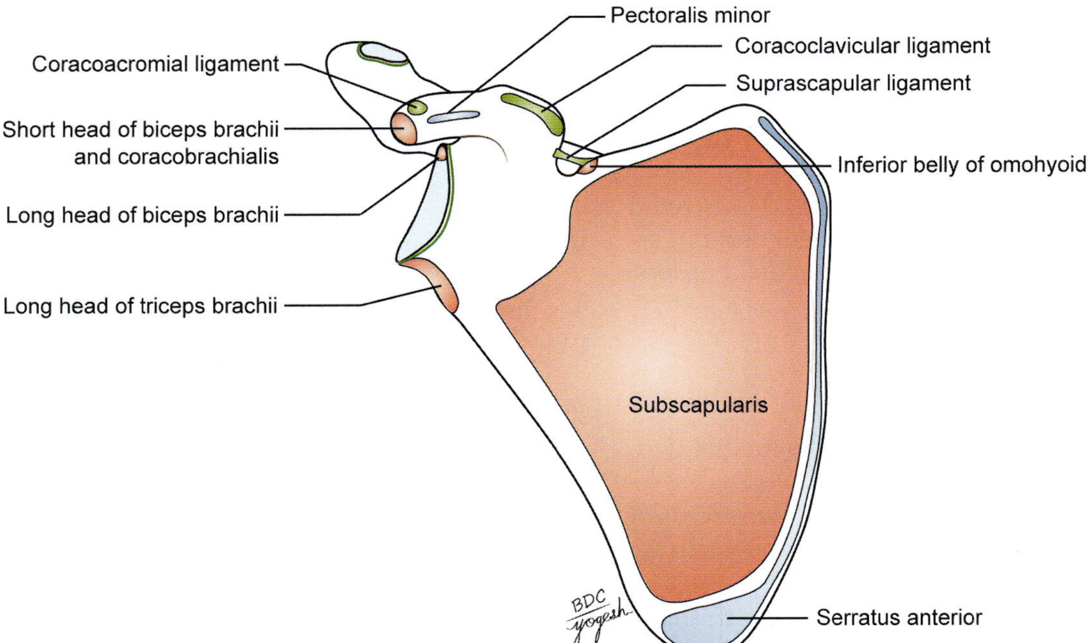

Fig. 2.7: Attachments of right scapula: Costal aspect

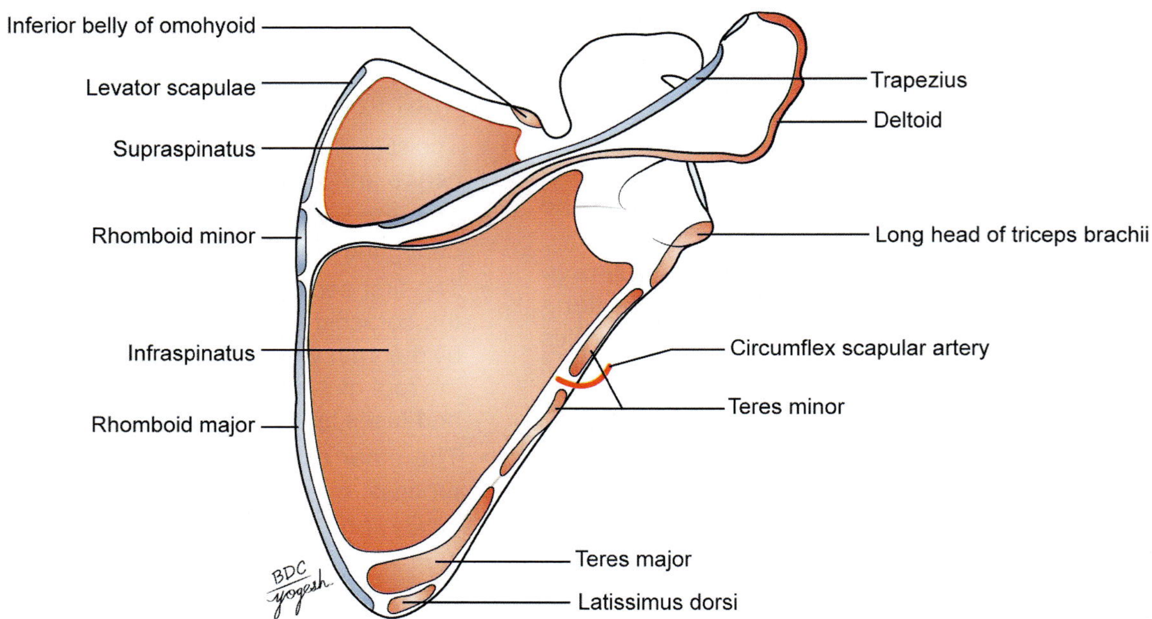

Fig. 2.8: Attachments of right scapula: Dorsal aspect

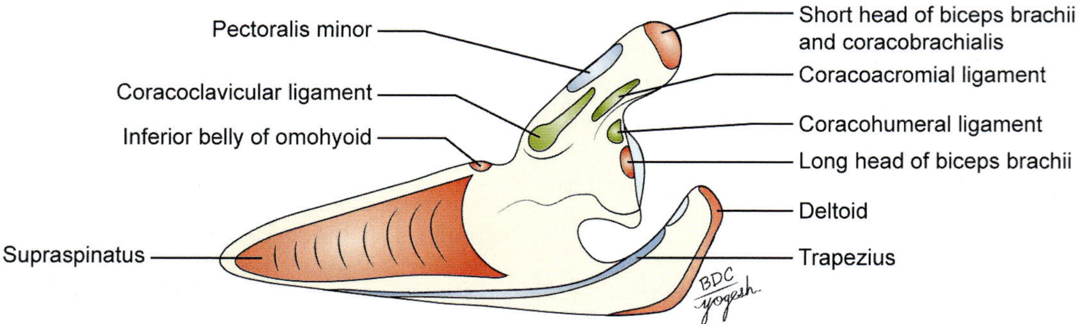

Fig. 2.9: Right scapula: Superior aspect

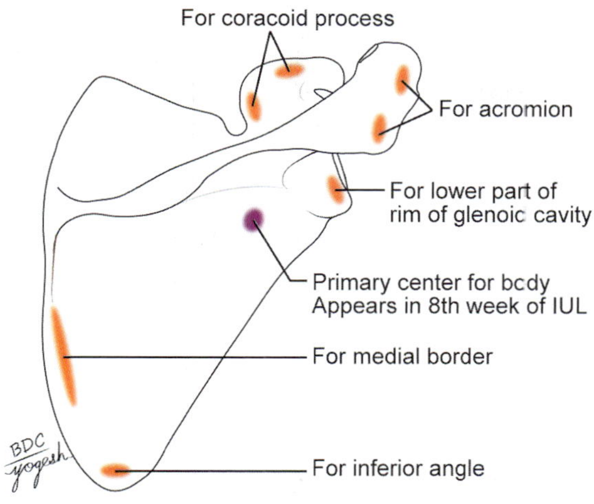

Fig. 2.10: Ossification of scapula

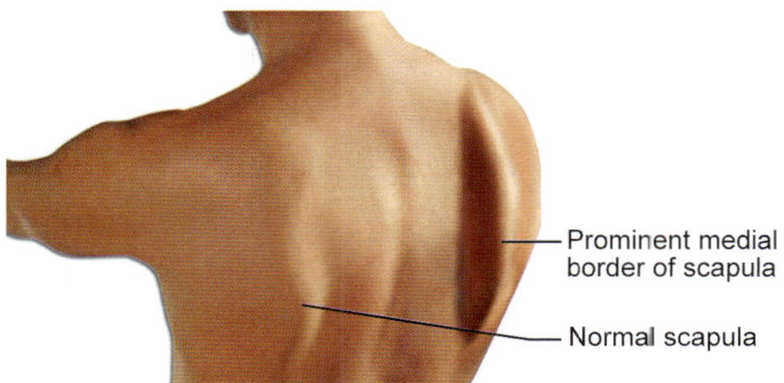

Fig. 2.11: Winging of right scapula

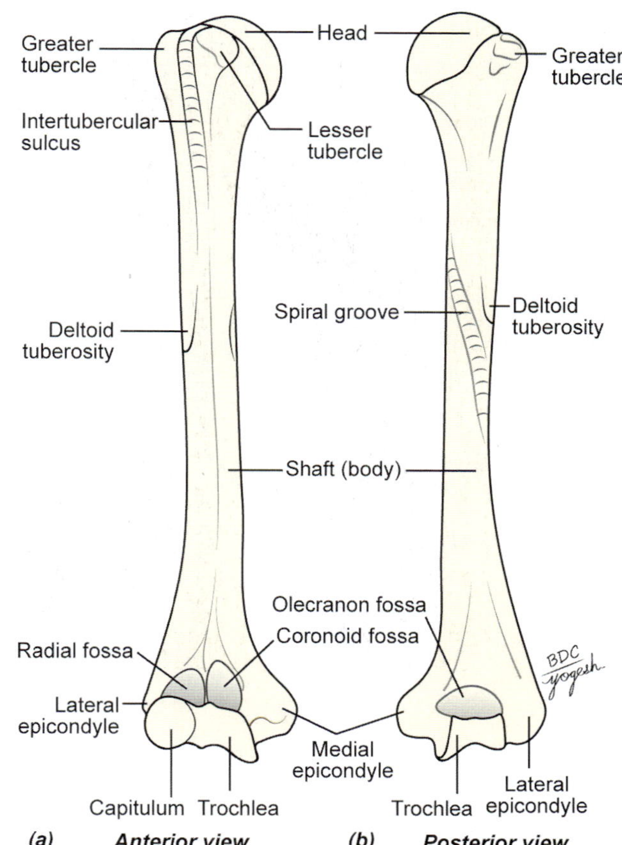

Figs 2.12a and b: General features of right humerus: (a) Seen from front and (b) seen from back

HUMERUS

The humerus is the bone of the arm. It is the longest bone of the upper limb (Fig. 2.12, Plate 2.2, Flowchart 2.3).

Side Determination and Anatomical Position

For the side determination, hold the humerus vertically in such a way that:

1. The upper end is rounded to form the head.
2. The lesser tubercle projects from the front of the upper end and is limited laterally by the intertubercular sulcus or bicipital groove.
3. The lower end is expanded from side-to-side and has a prominent medial epicondyle.

Features

Upper End

1. ***Head***: It is directed medially, backwards and upwards. It articulates with the glenoid cavity of the scapula to form the shoulder joint. The head forms about one-third of a sphere and is much larger than the glenoid cavity (Fig. 2.12).
2. ***Neck***: Humerus has three necks:
   a. *Anatomical neck* is the line separating the head from the rest of the upper end.
   b. *Morphological neck* lies at junction of upper end of diaphysis with upper epiphysis. It disappears in adults.
   c. *Surgical neck* is the narrow line separating the upper end of humerus from the shaft. It lies 0.5 cm below morphological neck.
3. ***Lesser tubercle*** (Latin *lump*) is an elevation on the anterior aspect of the upper end.
4. ***Greater tubercle*** is an elevation that forms the lateral part of the upper end. Its upper and posterior aspect is marked by three smooth impressions: upper, middle and lower.
5. ***Intertubercular sulcus*** or *bicipital groove* separates the lesser tubercle medially from the anterior part of the greater tubercle. The sulcus has medial and lateral lips that represent downward prolongations of the lesser and greater tubercles.

Shaft

The shaft is rounded in the upper half and triangular in the lower half. It has three borders and three surfaces.

Borders

1. ***Anterior border:*** Upper one-third of the *anterior border* forms the lateral lip of the intertubercular centre's sulcus. In its middle part, it forms the anterior margin of the *deltoid tuberosity*. The lower half of the anterior border is smooth and rounded.
2. ***Lateral border:*** It is prominent only at the lower end, where it forms the *lateral supracondylar ridge*. In the upper part, it is barely traceable up to the posterior surface of the greater tubercle. In the middle part, it is interrupted by the *radial* or *spiral groove*.

Plate 2.2: Humerus

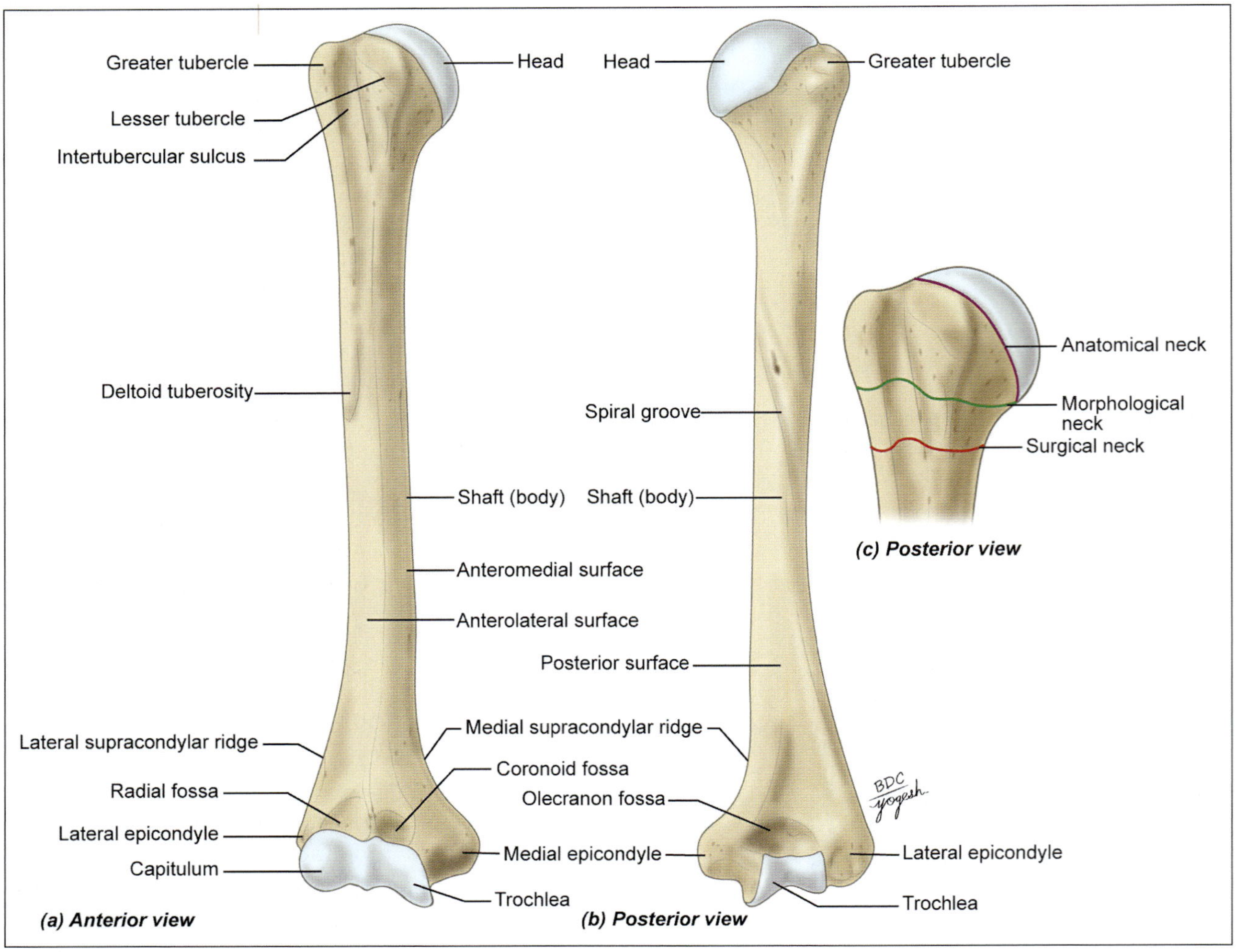

Greater tubercle
Lesser tubercle
Intertubercular sulcus
Head
Deltoid tuberosity
Shaft (body)
Anteromedial surface
Anterolateral surface
Lateral supracondylar ridge
Medial supracondylar ridge
Radial fossa
Coronoid fossa
Lateral epicondyle
Capitulum
Medial epicondyle
Trochlea

(a) Anterior view

Head
Greater tubercle
Spiral groove
Shaft (body)
Posterior surface
Medial supracondylar ridge
Olecranon fossa
Medial epicondyle
Lateral epicondyle
Trochlea

(b) Posterior view

Anatomical neck
Morphological neck
Surgical neck

(c) Posterior view

BDC yogesh

Flowchart 2.3: Features and attachments of humerus

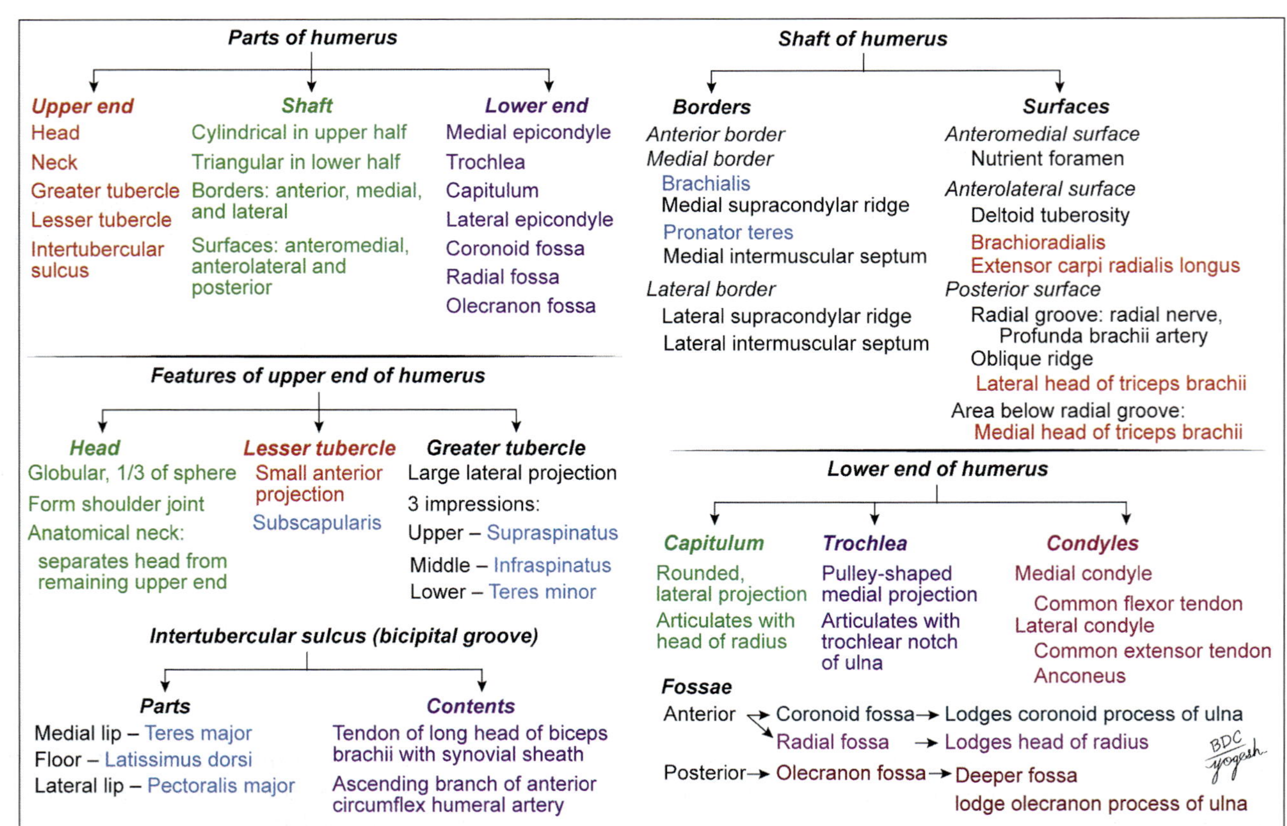

3. ***Medial border:*** Upper part of the *medial border* forms the medial lip of the intertubercular sulcus. About its middle, it presents a rough strip. It is continuous below with the *medial supracondylar ridge*.

Surfaces

1. ***Anterolateral surface:*** It lies between the anterior and lateral borders. A little above the middle, it is marked by a V-shaped *deltoid tuberosity (Greek triangular-shaped).*
2. ***Anteromedial surface:*** It lies between the anterior and medial borders. Its upper one-third is narrow and forms the floor of the intertubercular sulcus. A nutrient foramen is present near the medial border below its middle part.
3. ***Posterior surface:*** It lies between the medial and lateral borders. Its upper part is marked by an oblique ridge. The middle one-third is crossed by the *radial groove*.

Lower End

The lower end of the humerus is expanded from side-to-side, and has articular and non-articular parts. The *articular part* includes the following:

1. **Capitulum** (Latin *little head*): It is a rounded projection that articulates with the head of the radius.
2. **Trochlea** (Greek *pulley*): It is a pulley-shaped surface. It articulates with the trochlear notch of the ulna. The medial edge of the trochlea projects down 6 mm more than the lateral edge – this results in the formation of the *carrying angle* (*see* Fig. 10.14).

The *non-articular part* includes the following:

1. **Medial epicondyle:** It is a prominent bony projection on the medial side of the lower end. It is subcutaneous and is easily felt on the medial side of the elbow.
2. *Medial supracondylar ridge* is a sharp ridge just above the medial epicondyle.
3. **Lateral epicondyle:** It is smaller than the medial epicondyle. Its anterolateral part has a muscular impression.
4. The sharp lateral margin just above the lower end is called the *lateral supracondylar ridge.*
5. **Coronoid fossa:** It is a depression just above the anterior aspect of the trochlea. It accommodates the coronoid process of the ulna when the elbow is flexed.
6. **Radial fossa:** It is a depression present just above the anterior aspect of the capitulum. It accommodates the head of the radius when the elbow is flexed.
7. **Olecranon fossa** *(Greek ulna head)*: It lies just above the posterior aspect of the trochlea. It accommodates the olecranon process of the ulna when the elbow is extended.

Attachments (Figs 2.13 a and b)

Upper end

1. Capsular ligament of the shoulder joint is attached to the anatomical neck except on the medial side, where the line of attachment extends down by about 1–2 cm on the shaft. The capsular attachment is interrupted at the intertubercular sulcus to provide passage to the tendon of the long head of the biceps brachii.
2. Subscapularis is inserted into the lesser tubercle.
3. Supraspinatus is inserted into the uppermost impression on the greater tubercle.
4. Infraspinatus is inserted into the middle impression on the greater tubercle.
5. Teres minor is inserted into the lower impression on the greater tubercle.
6. Pectoralis major is inserted into the lateral lip of the intertubercular sulcus.
7. Latissimus dorsi is inserted into the floor of the intertubercular sulcus.
8. Teres major is inserted into the medial lip of the intertubercular sulcus.
9. The contents of the intertubercular sulcus are:
   a. *Tendon of the long head of the biceps brachii* and its synovial sheath.
   b. Ascending branch of the anterior circumflex humeral artery.

(*Mnemonic*: for the Attachments of bicipital groove: "*Lady between 2 majors*": Lateral lip – pectoralis major, Medial lip – teres major, Floor – latissimus dorsi).

Shaft

10. Coracobrachialis is inserted into the rough area on the middle of the medial border.
11. Deltoid is inserted into the deltoid tuberosity.
12. Brachialis arises from the lower halves of the anteromedial and anterolateral surfaces of the shaft. Part of the area extends onto the posterior aspect.
13. Lateral head of triceps brachii arises from oblique ridge on the upper part of posterior surface above the radial groove, while its *medial head* arises from posterior surface below the radial groove.

Lower end

14. *Common flexor origin*: The superficial flexor muscles of the forearm arise by a common origin from the anterior aspect of the medial epicondyle as the common flexor origin.
15. Pronator teres (humeral head) arises from the lower one-third of the medial supracondylar ridge.
16. *Common extensor origin*: The superficial extensor muscles of the forearm and supinator arise from the lateral epicondyle as *common extensor origin*.
17. Anconeus arises from the posterior surface of the lateral epicondyle.
18. Brachioradialis arises from the upper two-thirds of the lateral supracondylar ridge.
19. Extensor carpi radialis longus arises from the lower one-third of the lateral supracondylar ridge.
20. Capsular ligament of the elbow joint is attached to the lower end along a line that reaches the upper limits of the radial and coronoid fossae anteriorly and of the olecranon fossa posteriorly.

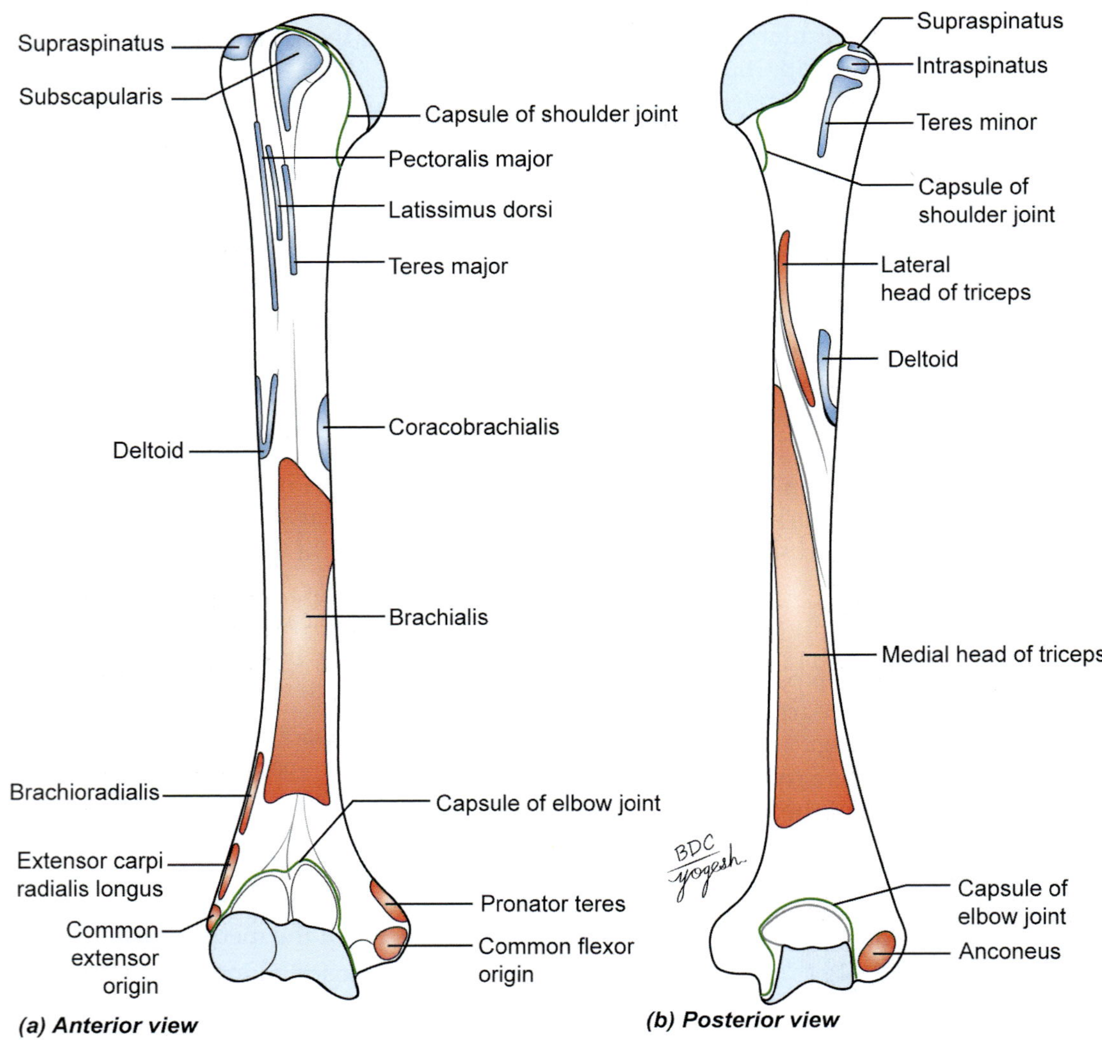

Figs 2.13a and b: Attachments of right humerus: (a) Anterior view and (b) posterior view

OSSIFICATION

The humerus ossifies from one primary and seven secondary centres as follows:

One primary centre for shaft appears in 8th week of intrauterine life.

Three secondary centres for upper end:

- One for head – appears by 1st year.
- One for greater tubercle – appears by 2nd year.
- One for lesser tubercle – appears by 5th year.

  These centres fuse with each other to form a single upper end by 6th year and fuse with shaft by 20th year.

Four secondary centres for lower end

- One for capitulum and lateral part of trochlea – appears by 1st year.
- One for medial part of trochlea – appears by 10th year
- One for lateral epicondyle – appears by 12th year
- These centres fuse by 14th year and with the rest of shaft by 16th year.
- One for medial epicondyle – appears by the 6th year and fuses with rest of the bone by 20th year.

CLINICAL ANATOMY

- *Nerves related to humerus*: It is related to the following three nerves (Fig. 2.14):
  1. Axillary nerve around the surgical neck
  2. Radial nerve in radial groove
  3. Ulnar nerve posterior to the medial epicondyle.
- The common sites of fracture of humerus are the surgical neck, shaft and supracondylar region. Fracture of surgical neck may involve axillary nerve.
- *Supracondylar fracture* is common in young age. It is produced by a fall on the outstretched hand. The lower fragment is mostly displaced backwards, so that the elbow is unduly prominent, as in dislocation of the elbow joint. This fracture may cause injury to the median nerve. It may also lead to *Volkmann's ischaemic contracture* caused by occlusion of the brachial artery (Figs 2.15a and b).
- The humerus has a poor blood supply at the junction of its upper one-third and lower two- thirds. Fractures at this site show delayed union or non-union.
- The head of the humerus commonly dislocates inferiorly (subglenoid). It may be anterior (commonest) or posterior to the infraglenoid tubercle (Fig. 2.16).

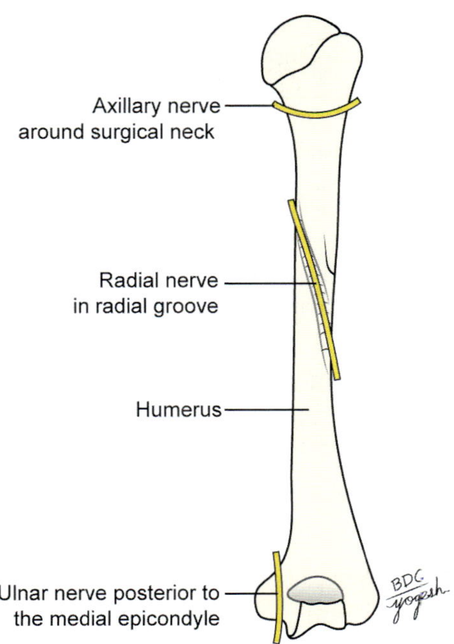

Fig. 2.14: Relation of axillary, radial and ulnar nerves to the back of humerus

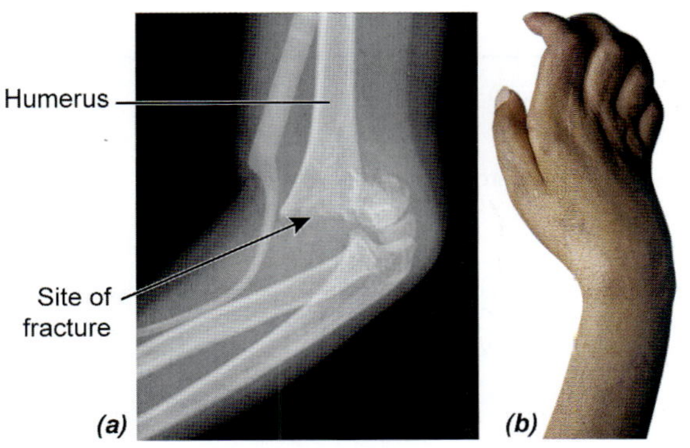

Figs 2.15a and b: (a) X-ray of supracondylar fracture of humerus, position of brachial artery shown and (b) Volkmann's ischaemic contracture

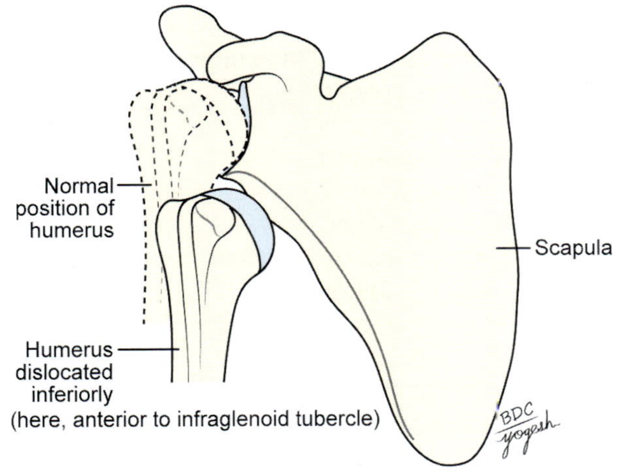

Fig. 2.16: Inferior dislocation of humerus

RADIUS

The radius is the lateral bone of the forearm, and is homologous with the tibia of the lower limb (Latin *radius* = ray) (Fig. 2.17, Plate 2.3, Flowchart 2.4).

Side Determination and Anatomical Position

For the side determination, hold the radius vertically in such a way that:

1. Upper end has a disc-shaped head and a narrow neck, while lower end is expanded with a styloid process. Close to neck, it presents a radial tuberosity.
2. Lower end presents a tubercle on the posterior surface called dorsal tubercle of Lister.
3. The medial border of the shaft is the sharpest border.

Features

Upper End

1. **Head:** It is disc-shaped and is covered with hyaline cartilage (Fig. 2.17). It has a superior concave surface, that articulates with the capitulum of the humerus at the elbow joint. The circumference of the head is also articular. It fits into a socket formed by the radial notch of the ulna and the *annular ligament*, thus forming the *superior radioulnar joint*.
2. **Neck:** It is enclosed by the narrow lower margin of the annular ligament.
3. **Radial tuberosity:** It lies just below the medial part of the neck. It has a rough posterior part and a smooth anterior part.

Shaft

It has three borders and three surfaces (Plate 2.3c, Fig. 2.17).

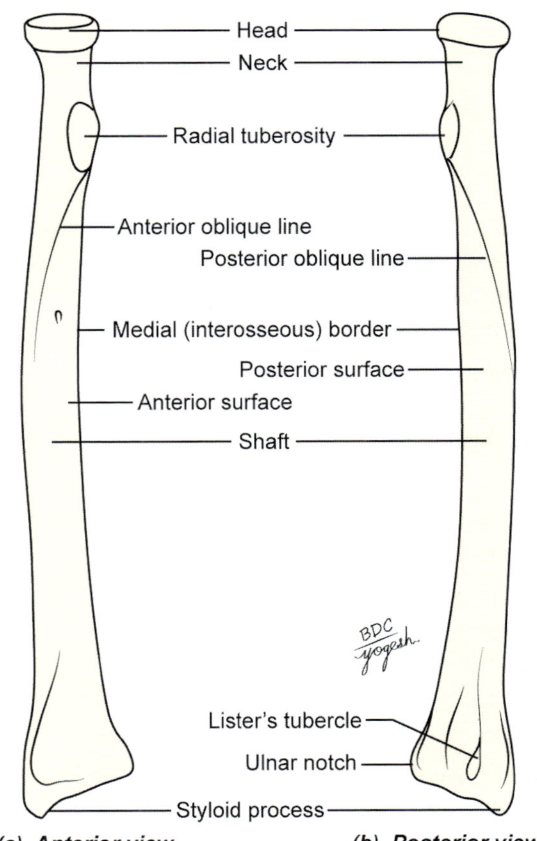

Figs 2.17a and b: Features of (a) anterior and (b) posterior views of radius

Plate 2.3: Radius and Ulna: (a) Features of right radius (anterior and posterior views), (b) features of right ulna (anterior and posterior views), (c) transverse section of radius and ulna (inferior view), (d) proximal end of right ulna (medial and lateral views)

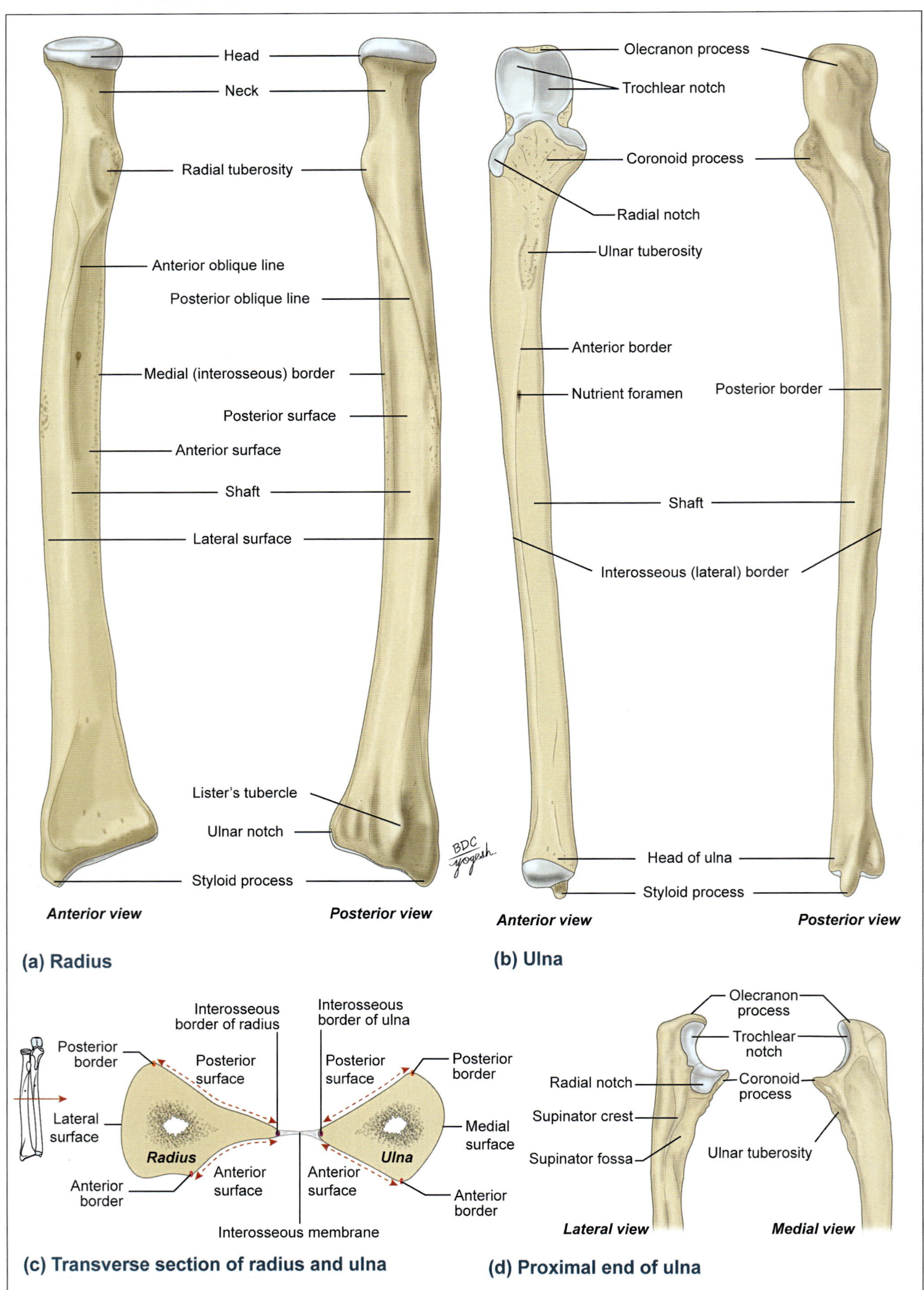

Flowchart 2.4: Fectures of radius

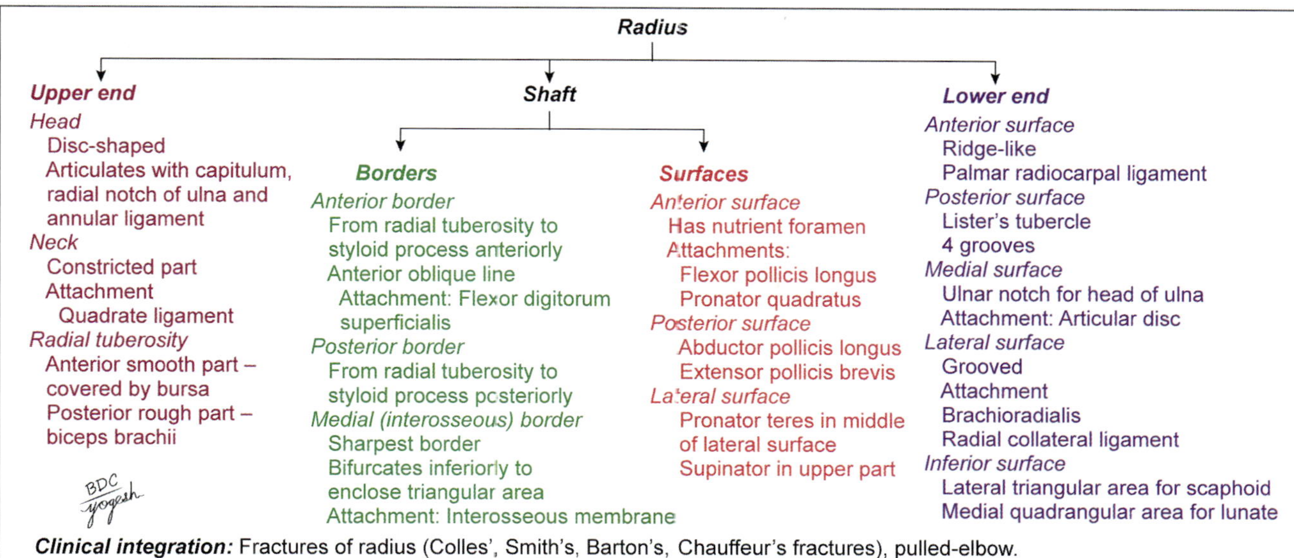

Borders

1. **Anterior border:** It extends from the anterolateral part of the radial tuberosity to the styloid process. It is oblique in the upper half of the shaft and vertical in the lower half. The lowest part is sharp and crest-like. The oblique part is called the *anterior oblique line*.
2. **Posterior border:** It is clearly defined only in its middle one-third. Its upper oblique part is known as the *posterior oblique line*.
3. **Medial** or **interosseous border:** It is the sharpest border. It extends from the radial tuberosity above to the posterior margin of the ulnar notch below. The interosseous membrane is attached to its lower three-fourths. In its lower part, it forms the posterior margin of an elongated triangular area.

Surfaces

1. **Anterior surface:** It lies between the anterior and interosseous borders. A nutrient foramen opens in its upper part and is directed upwards. The nutrient artery is a branch of the anterior interosseous artery.
2. **Posterior surface:** It lies between the posterior and interosseous borders.
3. **Lateral surface:** It lies between the anterior and posterior borders. It shows a roughened area in its middle part.

Lower End

The lower end is expanded. It has five surfaces.

1. The anterior surface is in the form of a thick, prominent ridge. The *radial artery* is palpated against this surface.
2. The posterior surface presents four grooves for the extensor tendons. The dorsal tubercle of Lister lies lateral to an oblique groove.
3. The medial surface is occupied by the *ulnar notch* for the head of the ulna.
4. The lateral surface is prolonged downwards to form the styloid (Greek *pillar*) process.
5. The inferior surface bears a triangular area for the scaphoid bone and a medial quadrangular area for the lunate bone. This surface takes part in forming the wrist joint (*see* Fig. 10.24).

Attachments (Figs 2.18 and 2.19)

1. The quadrate ligament is attached to the medial part of the neck.
2. The biceps brachii is inserted into the rough posterior part of the radial tuberosity. The anterior part of the radial tuberosity is covered by a bursa.
3. The oblique cord is attached on the medial side just below the radial tuberosity.
4. The radial head of the flexor digitorum superficialis takes origin from the anterior oblique line.
5. The extensor retinaculum is attached to the lower part of the sharp anterior border.
6. The interosseous membrane is attached to the lower three-fourths of the interosseous border.
7. The flexor pollicis longus takes origin from the upper two-thirds of the anterior surface.
8. The pronator quadratus is inserted into the lower part of the anterior surface and into the triangular area on the medial side of the lower end. The radial artery is palpated for 'radial pulse', as it lies on the pronator quadratus, lateral to the tendon of flexor carpi radialis (*see* Fig. 9.4).
9. The abductor pollicis longus and the extensor pollicis brevis arise from the posterior surface.
10. The supinator is inserted into the upper part of the lateral surface.
11. The pronator teres is inserted into the middle of the lateral surface.
12. The brachioradialis is inserted into the lowest part of the lateral surface just above the styloid process.
13. The articular disc of the inferior radioulnar joint is attached to the lower border of the ulnar notch (*see* Fig. 10.25).
14. The articular capsule of the wrist joint is attached to the anterior and posterior margins of the inferior articular surface.

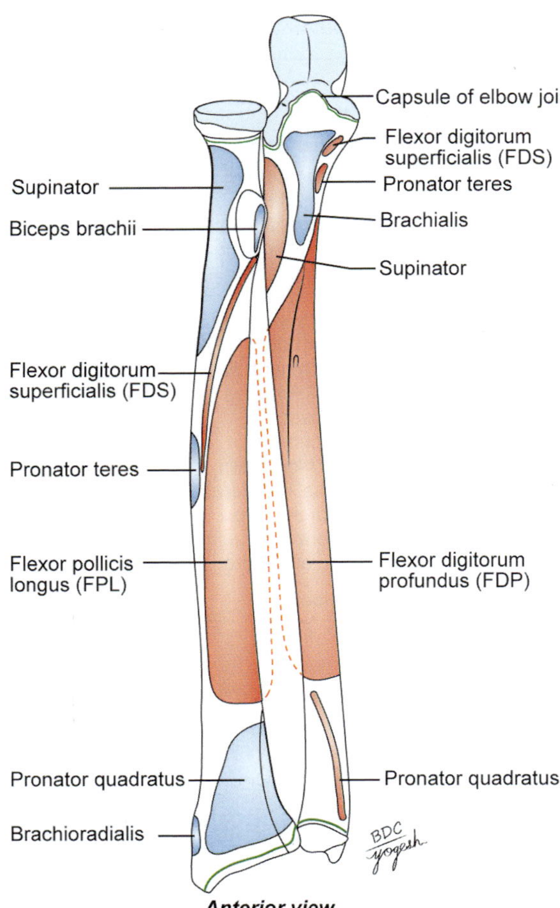

Fig. 2.18: Attachments of right radius and ulna: Anterior aspect

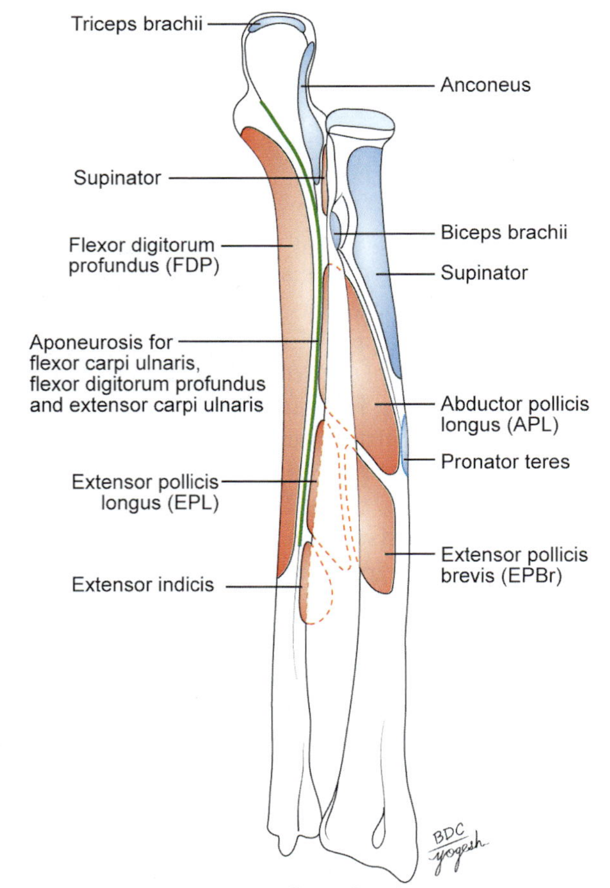

Fig. 2.19: Attachments of right radius and ulna: Posterior aspect

Structures related to the grooves are:

1st groove – between sharp (crest-like) lowest part of anterior border and styloid process gives passage to *abductor pollicis longus and extensor pollicis brevis.*

2nd groove – between styloid process and dorsal tubercle gives way to *extensor carpi radialis longus* and *extensor carpi radialis brevis* tendons.

3rd oblique groove – medial to dorsal tubercle gives passage to *extensor pollicis longus* tendon.

4th groove – on the medial aspect gives passage to tendons of *extensor digitorum, extensor indicis, posterior interosseous nerve* and *anterior interosseous artery*.

OSSIFICATION

- The radius ossifies from one primary and two secondary centres as follows:
  1. One primary centre appears in 8th week of IUL – for shaft.
  2. One secondary centre appears in 1st year – for lower end and fuses with shaft by 17th–19th years.
  3. One secondary centre appears in 5th year – for upper end and fuses with shaft by 14th–17th years. Thus, lower end of radius is growing end.

CLINICAL ANATOMY

- *Colles' fracture*: The radius commonly gets fractured about 2 cm above its lower end, and it is called Colles' fracture (Fig. 2.20a). The distal fragment is displaced upwards and backwards, which creates the dinner-fork (bayonet-like) deformity.
- *Smith's fracture*: In this fracture, the distal fragment gets displaced anteriorly (reverse of Colles' fracture) (Fig. 2.20b).
- *Pulled elbow* (subluxation of head of radius): It occurs due to the sudden powerful jerk on the hand of a child with dislodgement of the head of the radius from the annular ligament (Figs 2.21a and b).

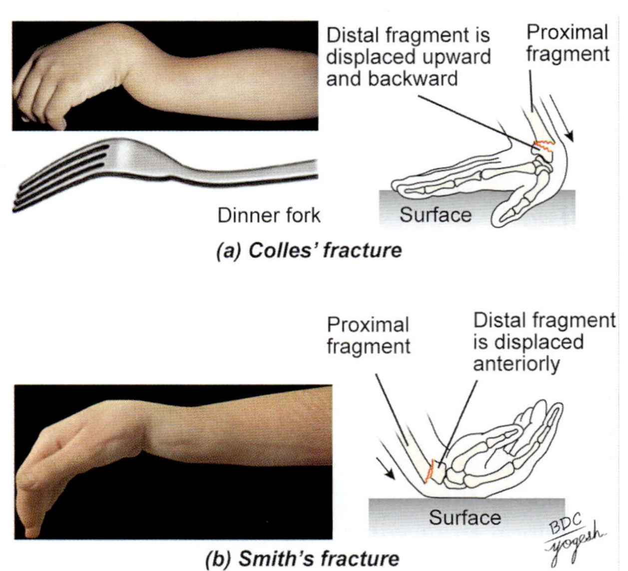

Figs 2.20a and b: (a) Colles' fracture with dinner fork deformity and (b) Smith's fracture

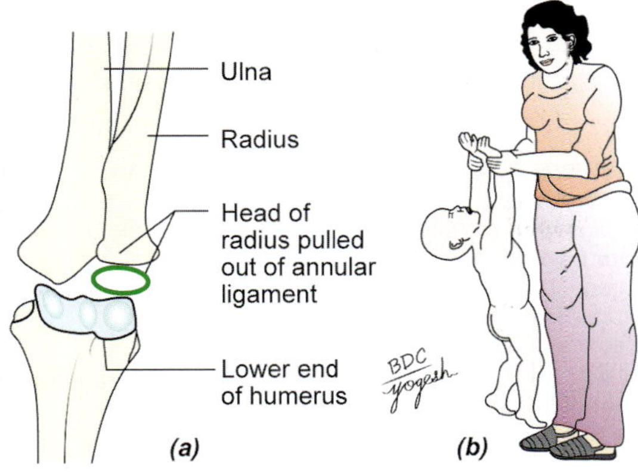

Figs 2.21a and b: (a) Position of bones and (b) pulled elbow

ULNA

The ulna is the medial bone of the forearm and is homologous with the fibula of the lower limb (Figs 2.22a and b, Flowchart 2.5).

Side Determination and Anatomical Position

For the side determination, hold the ulna vertically in such a way that:

1. The upper end is hook-like, with its concavity directed forwards.
2. The lateral border of the shaft is sharp and crest-like.
3. Pointed styloid process lies posteromedial to the rounded head of ulna at its lower end.

Features

Upper End

The upper end presents the olecranon and coronoid processes, and the trochlear and radial notches (Plate 2.3, Fig. 2.22).

1. **Olecranon process:** It projects upwards from the shaft. It has superior, anterior, posterior, medial and lateral surfaces.
   - The *superior surface* in its posterior part shows a roughened area.
   - The *anterior surface* is articular; it forms the upper part of the trochlear notch.
   - The *posterior surface* forms a triangular subcutaneous area, which is separated from the skin by a *bursa*.
   - The *medial surface* is continuous inferiorly with the medial surface of the shaft.
   - The *lateral surface* is smooth, continues as posterior surface of shaft.
2. **Coronoid process** (Greek *like crow's beak*): It projects forwards from the shaft just below the olecranon process. It has four surfaces: superior, anterior, medial and lateral.
   - The *superior surface* forms the lower part of the trochlear notch.
   - The *anterior surface* is triangular and rough. Its lower corner forms the *ulnar tuberosity*.

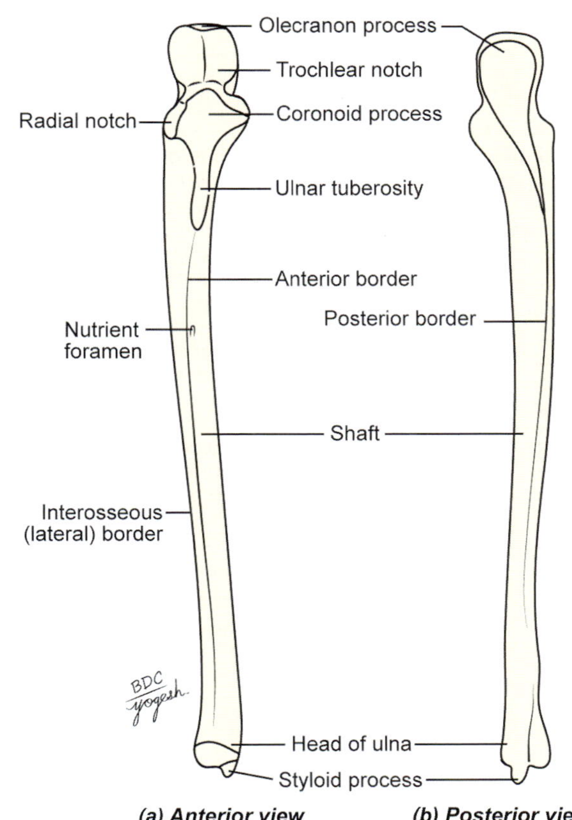

Figs 2.22a and b: Features of (a) anterior surface and (b) posterior surface of ulna

   - The upper part of its *lateral surface* is marked by the *radial notch* for the head of the radius. The annular ligament is attached to the anterior and posterior margins of the notch. The lower part of the lateral surface forms a depressed area (supinator fossa) to accommodate the radial tuberosity. It is limited behind by a ridge called the *supinator crest*.
   - *Medial surface* is continuous with medial surface of the shaft.
3. **Trochlear notch:** It forms a C-shaped articular surface that articulates with the trochlea of the humerus to form the elbow joint.
4. **Radial notch:** It articulates with the head of the radius to form the superior radioulnar joint.

Shaft

The shaft has three borders and three surfaces (Plate 2.3c, Figs 2.22a and b).

Borders

1. **Interosseous** or **lateral border:** It is the sharpest in its middle two-fourths. Inferiorly, it is ill-defined. Superiorly, it is continuous with the supinator crest.
2. **Anterior border:** It is thick and rounded. It begins above on the medial side of the ulnar tuberosity and terminates at the medial side of the styloid process.
3. **Posterior border:** It is subcutaneous. It begins above, at the apex of the triangular subcutaneous area at the back of the olecranon process, and terminates at the base of the styloid process.

Flowchart 2.5: Features of ulna

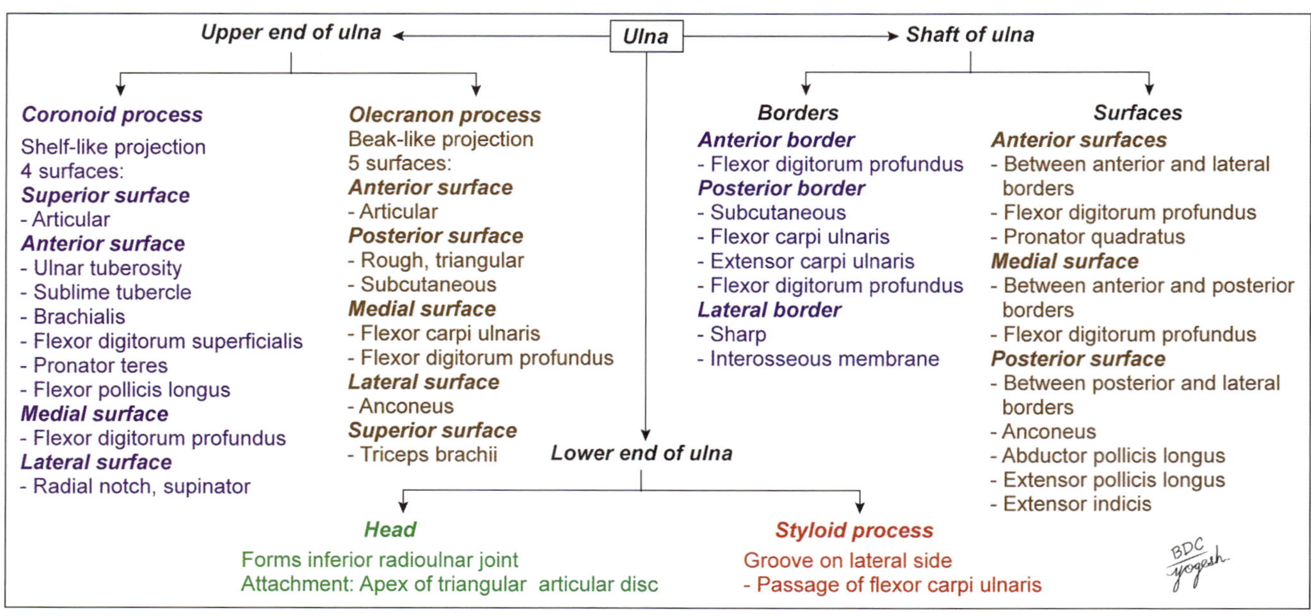

Surfaces

1. **Anterior surface:** It lies between the anterior and interosseous borders. A nutrient foramen is present on the upper part of this surface. It is directed upwards. The nutrient artery is derived from the anterior interosseous artery.
2. **Medial surface:** It lies between the anterior and posterior borders.
3. **Posterior surface:** It lies between the posterior and interosseous lateral borders. It is subdivided into three areas by two lines. An oblique line divides it into upper and lower parts. The lower part is further divided by a vertical line into a medial and a lateral area.

Lower End

The lower end has head and a styloid process.

- **Head:** Laterally, it articulates with the ulnar notch of the radius to form the *inferior radioulnar joint*. Its inferior surface is smooth.
- **Styloid process:** It projects downwards from postero-medial side of lower end of the ulna. Posteriorly, between the head and the styloid process, there is a groove for the tendon of the extensor carpi ulnaris (Fig. 2.25b).

Attachments (Figs 2.18 and 2.19)

1. Triceps brachii is inserted into the rough posterior part of the superior surface of the olecranon process. The anterior part of the surface is covered by a bursa.
2. Anconeus is inserted into the lateral aspect of the olecranon process and the upper one-fourth of the posterior surface of the shaft.
3. Capsular ligament of the elbow joint is attached to the margins of the trochlear notch.
4. Annular ligament of the superior radioulnar joint is attached to the anterior and posterior margins of radial notch of ulna.
5. Anterior band and oblique band of ulnar collateral ligament are attached to medial margin of anterior surface of coronoid process.
6. Posterior band and oblique band of ulnar collateral ligament are attached to medial surface of olecranon process (*see* Fig. 10.12).
7. Brachialis is inserted into the anterior surface of the coronoid process, including the ulnar tuberosity.
8. Supinator arises from the supinator crest and from the triangular area in front of the crest.
9. Flexor digitorum superficialis (ulnar head) arises from a tubercle at the upper end of the medial margin of the coronoid process.
10. Pronator teres (ulnar head) arises from the medial margin of the coronoid process.
11. Oblique cord is attached to the ulnar tuberosity.
12. Interosseous membrane is attached to the interosseous border.
13. Flexor carpi ulnaris (ulnar head) arises from the medial surface of the olecranon process and from the posterior border.
14. Extensor carpi ulnaris arises from the posterior border.
15. Flexor digitorum profundus (Latin *deep*) arises from:
    a. Upper three-fourths of the anterior and medial surfaces of the shaft.
    b. Medial surfaces of the coronoid and olecranon processes.
    c. Posterior border of the shaft through an aponeurosis, which also gives origin to the flexor carpi ulnaris and the extensor carpi ulnaris.
16. Pronator quadratus takes origin from the oblique ridge on the lower part of the anterior surface.

17. The lateral part of the posterior surface gives origin from above downwards to the abductor pollicis longus, the extensor pollicis longus and the extensor indicis.
18. Ulnar collateral ligament of the wrist is attached to the styloid process.
19. Articular disc of the inferior radioulnar joint is attached by its apex to a small rough area just lateral to the styloid process (*see* Fig. 10.25).

OSSIFICATION

The ulna ossifies from one primary and two secondary centres as follows:

- The primary centre – For shaft appears during 8th week of intrauterine life.
- The secondary centre

  One for upper end (at olecranon process) appears during 11th year – fuses with shaft by the 16th year.

  One for lower end appears by 6th year and fuses with shaft by shaft by the 18th year.

  Thus, the lower end of ulna is the growing end.

CLINICAL ANATOMY

- The ulna is the stabilising bone of the forearm, with its trochlear notch gripping the lower end of the humerus. On this foundation, the radius can pronate and supinate for efficient working of the upper limb.
- The shaft of the ulna may fracture either alone or along with that of the radius. Cross-union between the radius and ulna must be prevented to preserve pronation and supination of the hand.
- *Nightstick fracture* is the fractured shaft of ulna without any other fracture. It occurs due to direct hit on shaft of ulna, may occur when watchman raises his arm against trauma.
- *Monteggia fracture* is the fracture of upper one-third of ulna with dislocation of the head of radius.
- *Hume fracture* is a fracture of olecranon with anterior dislocation of head of radius.
- *Madelung's deformity* is dorsal subluxation (displacement) of the lower end of the ulna, due to retarded growth of the lower end of the radius (Fig. 2.23).

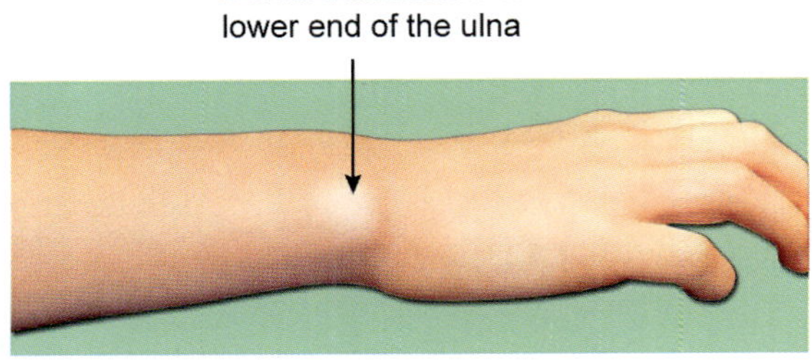

Fig. 2.23: Madelung's deformity

Competency:

AN8.3 Identify and name various bones in articulated hand, specify the parts of metacarpals and phalanges and enumerate the peculiarities of pisiform.

CARPAL BONES

The carpus is (Greek *Karpos, wrist*) made up of 8 carpal bones, which are arranged in two rows (Figs 2.24 and 2.25a and b, Plate 2.4, Flowchart 2.6).

A. The proximal row (from lateral to medial side):
   1. Scaphoid (Greek *boat, wrist*)
   2. Lunate (Latin *moon-shaped*)
   3. Triquetral (Latin *three-cornered*)
   4. Pisiform (Greek *pea*).

B. The distal row (from lateral to medial):
   1. Trapezium (Greek *four-sided geometric figure*)
   2. Trapezoid (Greek *baby's shoe*)
   3. Capitate (Latin *head*)
   4. Hamate (Latin *hook*).

(*Mnemonic*: She looks too pretty, try to catch her).

Identification

The individual carpal bones can be identified by their shape and the side can be determined based on their articular surfaces. For details, *refer* Table 2.1 (Figs 2.24 and 2.25 a and b, Plate 2.4).

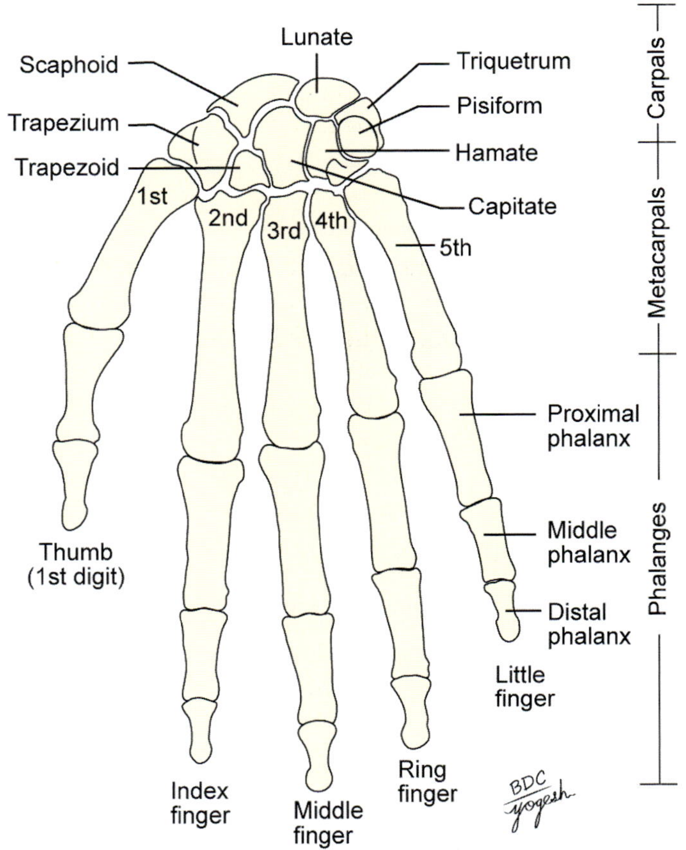

Fig. 2.24: Skeleton of the right hand: Palmar aspect

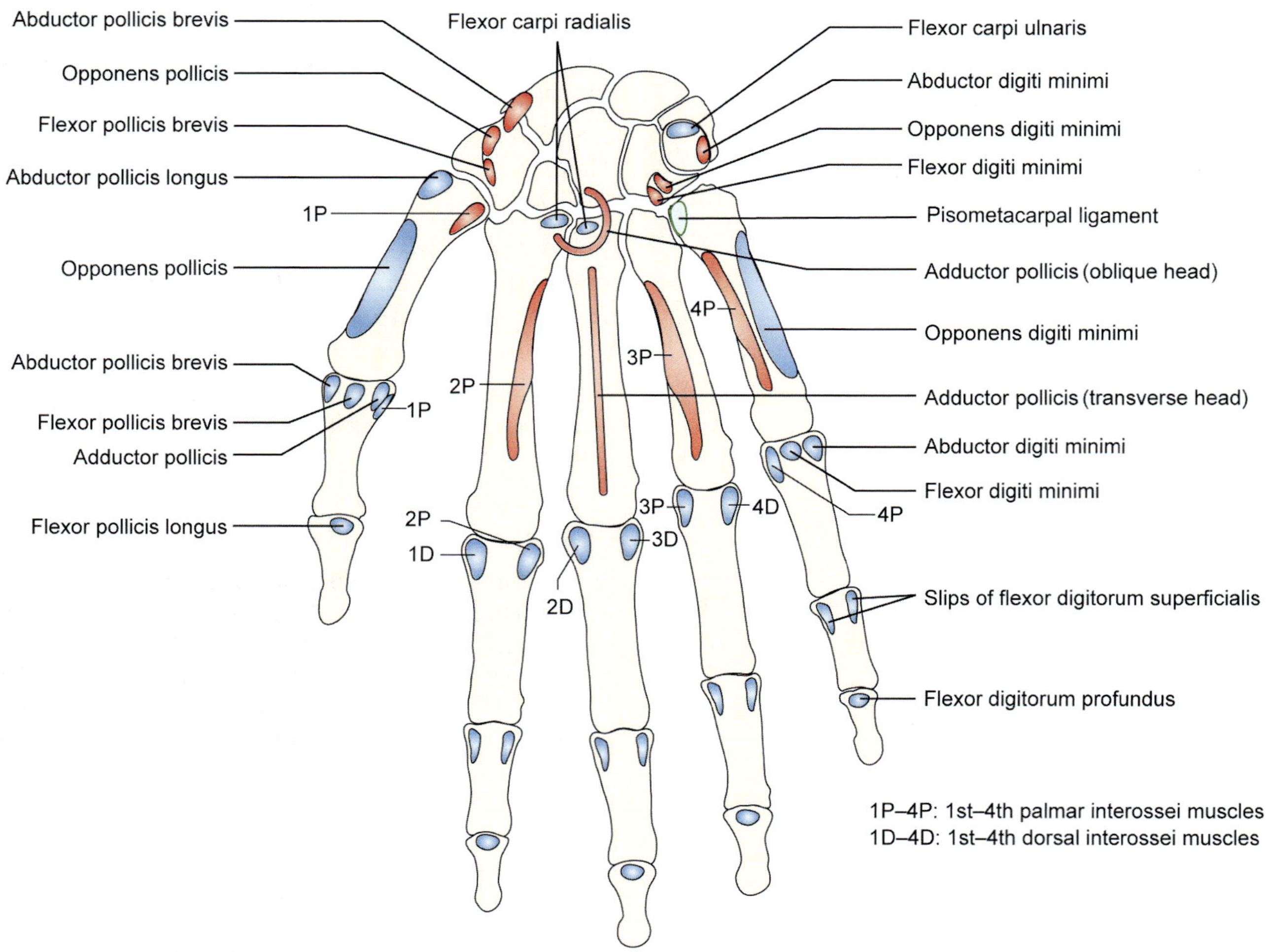

Figs 2.25a and b: Attachments on the skeleton of hand: (a) Anterior aspect and (b) posterior aspect

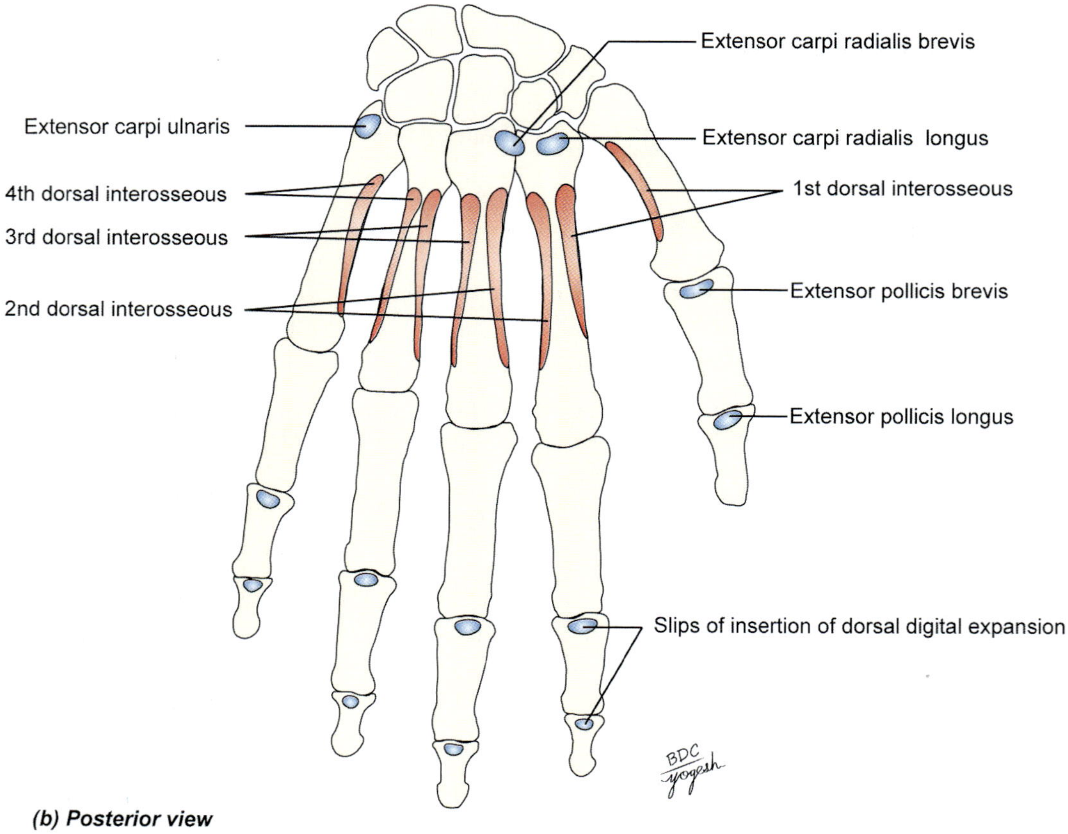

Plate 2.4: Bones of the hand

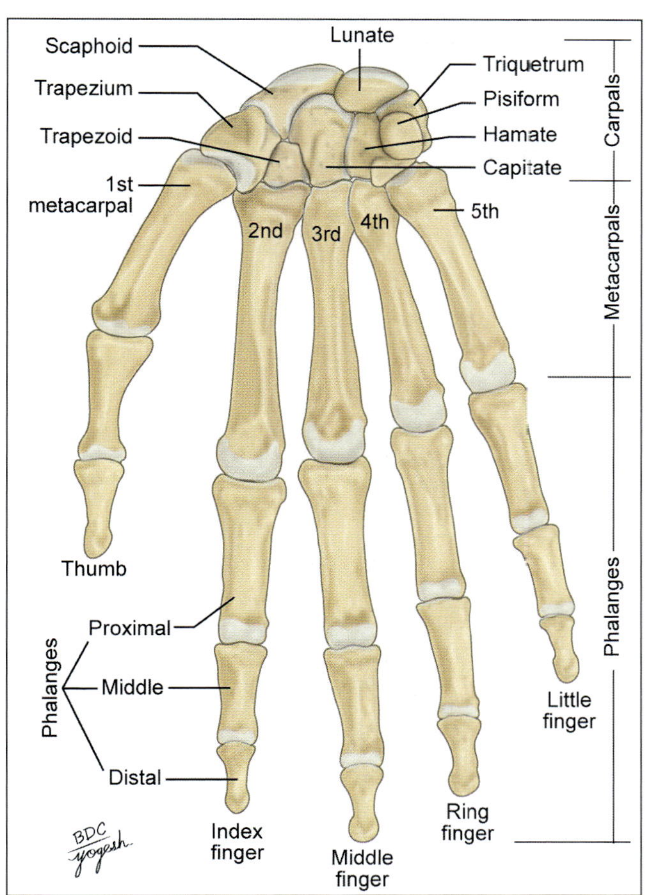

OSSIFICATION

The carpal bones ossify from secondary centres except for capitate and hamate, as follows:

Capitate – 2nd month of IUL

Hamate – 3rd month of IUL

Triquetrum – 3rd year

Lunate – 4th year

Scaphoid, trapezium, trapezoid – 5th year

Pisiform – 12th year (9–12 years).

Competency:

AN8.4 Describe scaphoid fracture and explain the anatomical basis of avascular necrosis.

CLINICAL ANATOMY

- *Fracture of the scaphoid* is quite common in a fall on the outstretched hand. Normally, the scaphoid has two nutrient arteries from the radial artery, one entering the palmar surface and the other the dorsal surface. Occasionally (13% of cases), the proximal part of scaphoid receives supply from its distal part. In these cases, the fracture of proximal part of scaphoid may result in a lack of blood supply, and it may result in avascular necrosis or nonunion (Fig. 2.26).
- Anterior dislocation of the lunate may produce *carpal tunnel syndrome* like features (Figs 2.27a to c).

TABLE 2.1: Identification of the individual carpal bones (Figs 2.24 and 2.25 a and b, Plate 2.4)

Carpal bone	*Identification features*	*Attachments*
1. Scaphoid	Boat-shaped. Has tubercle on lateral part of its anterior surface. Has constricted neck.	Tubercle of scaphoid: Abductor pollicis Brevis. Flexor retinaculum.
2. Lunate	Moon-shaped. Small semilunar articular surface for the scaphoid is on the lateral side. Quadrilateral articular surface for the triquetral is on the medial side.	–
3. Triquetral	Pyramidal-shaped. Oval facet on the distal part of its anterior surface for articulation with pisiform.	–
4. Pisiform	Pea-shaped and smallest carpal bone Oval facet for the triquetral lies on the proximal part of the dorsal surface. Lateral surface is grooved by the ulnar nerve. Sesamoid bone in the tendon of flexor carpi ulnaris.	Insertion to flexor carpi ulnaris, and abductor digiti minimi. Flexor and extensor retinaculae
5. Trapezium	Quadrilateral in shape. Groove (for the tendon of the flexor carpi radialis) and crest on its anterior surface.	Crest: Origin to the abductor pollicis brevis, flexor pollicis brevis, opponens pollicis. Flexor retinaculum.
6. Trapezoid	Shoe-shaped. Posterior surface is larger than anterior.	Anterior surfaces: Some fibers of oblique head of adductor pollicis arise.
7. Capitate	Largest carpal bone. Rounded head on its proximal surface.	
8. Hamate	Wedge-shaped. Hook-like process projects from distal part of its anterior surface.	Hook: Flexor retinaculum, origin of flexor digiti minimi and opponens digiti minimi.

Flowchart 2.6: Features of carpals

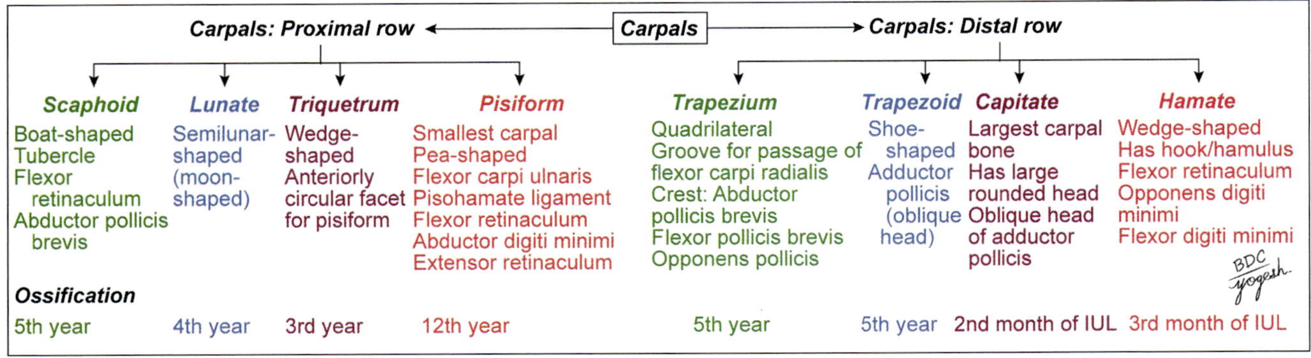

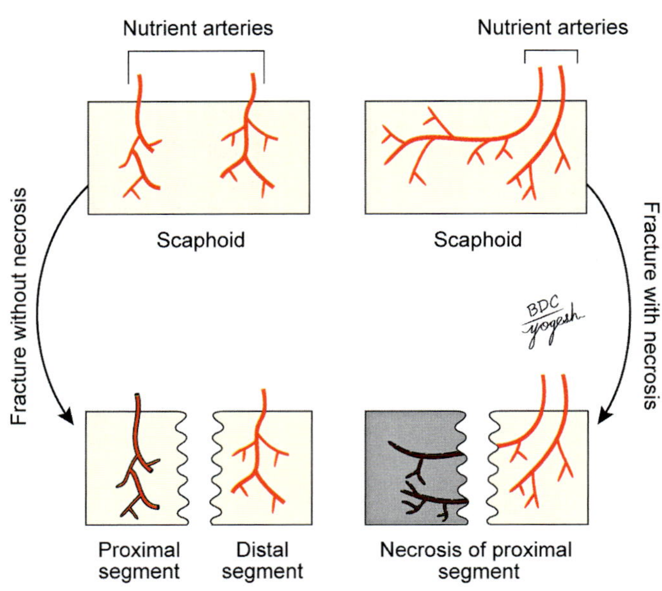

Fig. 2.26: Fracture of the scaphoid

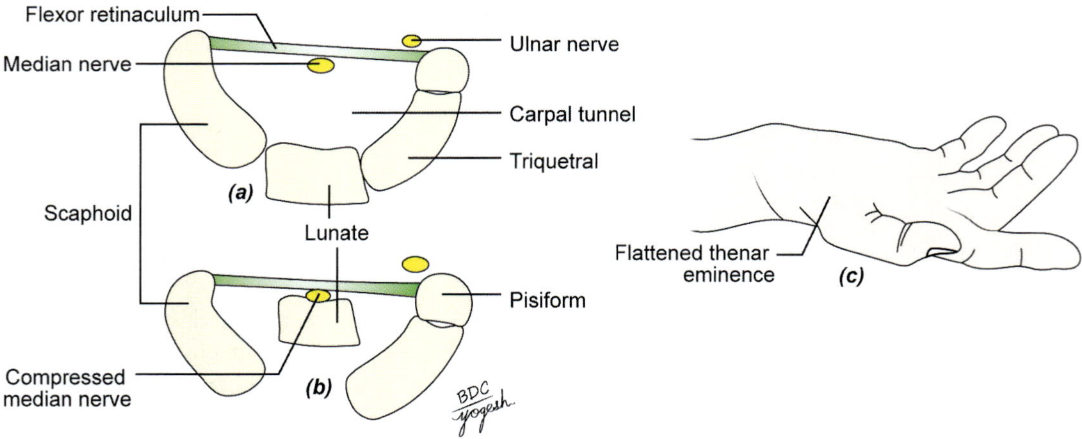

Figs 2.27a to c: (a) Normal position of nerves, (b) dislocation of lunate leading to carpal tunnel syndrome and (c) ape-like deformity of the hand (flattened thenar eminence)

METACARPAL BONES

1. The metacarpal bones are 5 miniature long bones, which are numbered from lateral to the medial side (Figs 2.24 and 2.25 a and b, Plate 2.4).
2. Each bone has a head, shaft and base.
   a. The head is round and placed distally.
   b. The shaft is concave on the palmar surface. Its dorsal surface bears a flat triangular area in its distal part.
   c. The base lies proximally and smaller than the head.

The features and attachments of the individual metacarpals are given in Table 2.2.

TABLE 2.2: Features of the individual metacarpal bones

Metacarpal	*Identification features*	*Attachments*
1st	Shortest and stoutest of all metacarpals. Base has a concavoconvex articular surface for the trapezium. Head is less convex and broader than other metacarpals. The anterolateral surface is larger than the anteromedial.	*Base*: Insertion of abductor pollicis longus on the lateral side of its base, and origin of 1st palmar interossei *Shaft*: Insertion of opponens pollicis on its anterolateral surface, origin of lateral head of 1st dorsal interossei.
2nd	Its base is grooved. The medial edge of the groove is larger. The medial side of the base bears an articular strip, which is constricted in the middle.	*Base*: Insertion of flexor carpi radialis on its palmar surface, extensor carpi radialis longus on its dorsal surface, and origin of oblique head of the adductor pollicis from its palmar surface. *Shaft*: Origin of medial head of the 1st dorsal interosseous muscle.
3rd	Its base has a styloid process on its dorsolateral side. The lateral side of the base bears an articular strip, which is constricted in the middle. The medial side of the base has two small oval facets for the 4th metacarpal.	*Base*: Insertion of flexor carpi radialis on its palmar surface and extensor carpi radialis brevis on its dorsal surface, origin of oblique head of the adductor pollicis from its palmar surface. *Shaft*: Origin of transverse head of the adductor pollicis from the ridge on its palmar surface, origin of lateral head of 3rd dorsal interosseous muscle.
4th	Its base has two small oval facets on its lateral side for the 3rd metacarpal and a single facet on its medial side for the 5th metacarpal.	*Shaft*: Origin of 3rd palmar, 3rd dorsal and lateral head of the 4th dorsal interossei muscles. *Base*: Insertion of extensor carpi ulnaris.
5th	Its base has strip-like facet on the lateral side for the 4th metacarpal. The medial side of the base is non-articular and has a tubercle.	*Shaft*: Insertion of opponens digiti minimi. Origin of 4th palmar and medial head of 4th dorsal interossei muscle.

Note: The 1st metacarpal is rotated medially through 90°. Hence, its movements take place at right angles to those of other digits. Palmar surface is divided into larger anterolateral and smaller anteromedial areas by a ridge.

OSSIFICATION

- The shafts ossify from one primary centre each, which appears during the 9th week of development.
- A secondary centre for the head appears in the 2nd–5th metacarpals, and for the *base* in the 1st metacarpal. It appears during the 2nd–3rd year and fuses with the shaft at about 16–18 years (Fig. 2.28).

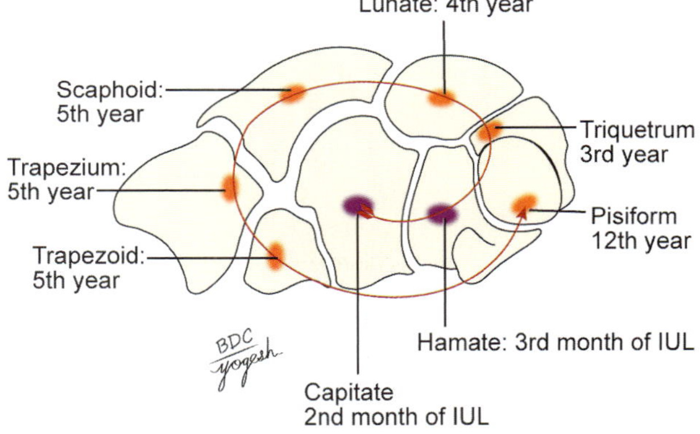

Fig. 2.28: Ossification of carpal bones

CLINICAL ANATOMY

- *Bennett's fracture* is a fracture of the base of the 1st metacarpal (Fig. 2.29).
- *Boxer's fracture*: It is a fracture of neck of metacarpals due to violent trauma, with anterior displacement of distal fragment. It commonly involves the 5th metacarpal (Fig. 2.30).
- Tubercular or syphilitic disease of the metacarpals or phalanges in a child is located in the middle of the diaphysis rather than in the metaphysis because the nutrient artery breaks up into a plexus immediately upon reaching the medullary cavity. In adults, however, the chances of infection are minimised because the nutrient artery is replaced (as the major source of supply) by periosteal vessels.
- ***Polydactyly:*** It is an abnormality of fingers or toes. There are extra digits which are not formed fully. These have poor muscular development and are useless. The extra digit is either medial or lateral to the hand or foot. It is inherited as a dominant characteristic (Fig. 2.31).

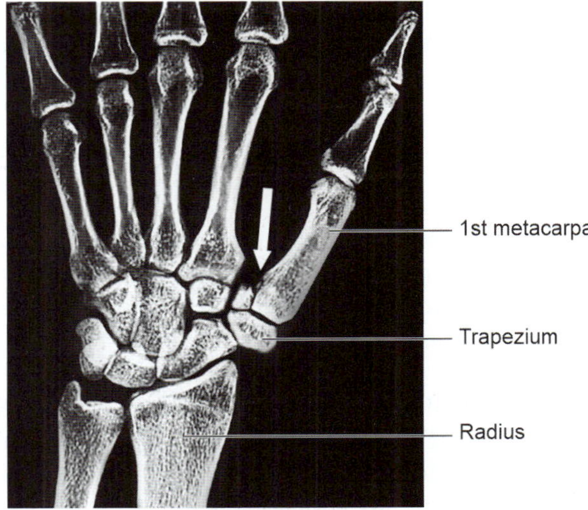

Fig. 2.29: Bennett's fracture

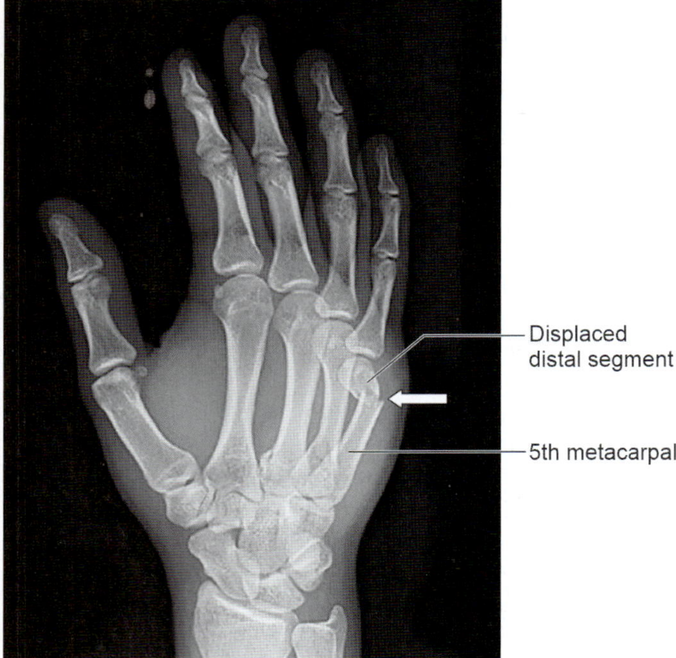

Fig. 2.30: Boxer's fracture

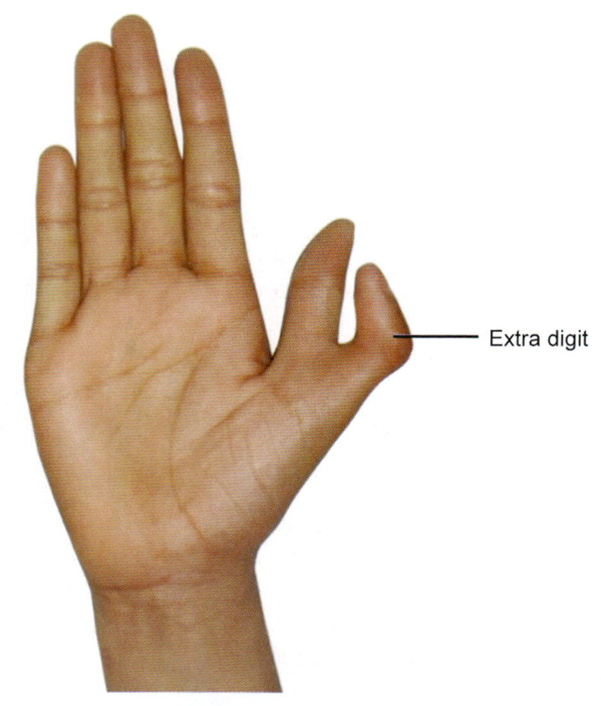

Fig. 2.31: Six digits (polydactyly)

PHALANGES

There are 14 phalanges in each hand, three for each finger and two for the thumb. Each phalanx has a base, a shaft and a head (Figs 2.24 and 2.25a and b, Plate 2.4).

Base

In the proximal phalanx, the base is marked by a concave oval facet for articulation with the head of the metacarpal bone. In the middle phalanx, or a distal phalanx, it is marked by two small concave facets separated by a smooth ridge.

Shaft

The shaft tapers towards the head. The dorsal surface is convex from side-to-side. The palmar surface is flattened from side-to-side, but is gently concave in its long axis.

Head

In the proximal and middle phalanges, the head has a pulley-shaped articular surface. In the distal phalanges, the head is non-articular and is marked anteriorly by a rough horseshoe-shaped tuberosity, which supports the sensitive pulp of the finger/tip.

Attachments

1. *Base of the distal phalanx:*
   a. Flexor digitorum profundus is inserted on the palmar surface.
   b. Two-sided slips of digital expansion fuse to be inserted on the dorsal surface. These also extend the insertion of lumbrical and interossei muscles.
2. *Middle phalanx:*
   a. Two slips of flexor digitorum superficialis are inserted on each side of the shaft.
   b. Extensor digitorum is inserted on the dorsal surface of the base through dorsal digital expansion.
3. *Proximal phalanx:*
   a. On each side of the base, parts of the *lumbricals* and interossei are inserted.
4. *Base of proximal phalanx of thumb:*
   a. Abductor pollicis brevis and flexor pollicis brevis are inserted on the lateral side.
   b. Adductor pollicis and the 1st palmar interosseous are inserted on the medial side.
   c. Extensor pollicis brevis is inserted on the dorsal surface.
5. *Base of distal phalanx of thumb:*
   a. Flexor pollicis longus is inserted on its palmar side.
   b. Extensor pollicis longus is inserted on its dorsal side.
6. *Base of proximal phalanx of little finger:* Abductor digiti minimi and flexor digiti minimi are inserted on its medial side.

OSSIFICATION

- The shaft of each phalanx ossifies from a primary centre which appears during the 8th week of development in the distal phalanx, 10th week in the proximal phalanx and 12th week in the middle phalanx.
- The secondary centre appears for the base during 2–4 years and fuses with the shaft during 16–18 years (Fig. 2.29).

CLINICAL ANATOMY

Fracture of distal phalanx of middle finger is commonest. It is treated by splinting the injured phalanx to the adjacent normal finger. This is called 'buddy splint' (Fig. 2.32).

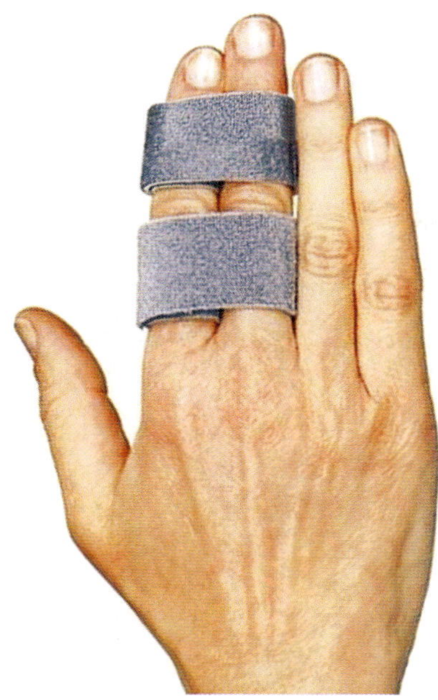

Fig. 2.32: Buddy splint of the fingers

VIDEO

Video 1.2.1 Clavicle ▶ Introduction and general features ▶ Attachments
Video 1.2.2 Scapula ▶ General features and side determination ▶ Attachments, relations and joints of scapula ▶ Movements of shoulder girdle
Video 1.2.3 Humerus ▶ Introduction, general features and side identification ▶ Attachments and relations
Video 1.2.4 Radius ▶ Introduction, general features and side identification ▶ Attachments and relations ▶ Attachments of muscles
Video 1.2.5 Ulna ▶ General features and side identification ▶ Attachments and relations
Video 1.2.6 Hand ▶ General features ▶ Attachments and relations ▶ Extensor retinaculum

Facts to Remember

- Clavicle is the most commonly fractured bone in the body.
- Commonest site of fracture clavicle is the junction of its lateral 1/3rd and medial 2/3rd.
- The strongest ligament of the upper limb is coracoclavicular ligament.
- The commonest fracture of the humerus is supracondylar fracture.
- The most commonly injured nerve in supracondylar fracture of humerus is the median nerve.
- Axillary, radial and ulnar nerves are intimately related to humerus and are liable to be injured.
- The most common site of the fracture of radius is distal end of radius 2.5 cm proximal to the wrist.
- Radial pulse is felt close to the lower end of anterior surface of shaft of radius.
- The most commonly fractured carpal bone is scaphoid.
- The most commonly dislocated carpal bone is lunate.
- The largest carpal bone and the first carpal bone to ossify is capitate.
- Pisiform bone is a sesamoid bone in the tendon of flexor carpi ulnaris muscle.
- The first metacarpal is the shortest and stoutest metacarpal.
- Bennett' fracture – fracture of base of the 1st metacarpal.
- Boxer's fracture – fracture of neck of metacarpals, commonly involves 5th metacarpal.
- All metacarpals have epiphysis at their distal end or head, except the first metacarpal, which has epiphysis at its proximal end or base.
- The third metacarpal is the longest, and the axis of abduction and adduction passes through its centre.

BDC's Anatomy *e*-book

Digital Content available with the BDC's Anatomy ebook:

1. Functions of the clavicle
2. Ossification of humerus, radius and ulna
3. Table e2.1: Ossification of humerus, radius and ulna
4. Importance of capsular attachments and epiphyseal lines
5. Table e2.2: Relation of capsular attachments and epiphyseal lines
6. Table e2.3: Differences between metacarpals and metatarsals
7. Features of the individual carpal bones
8. Sesamoid bones in upper limb
9. Further reading
10. Viva voce questions

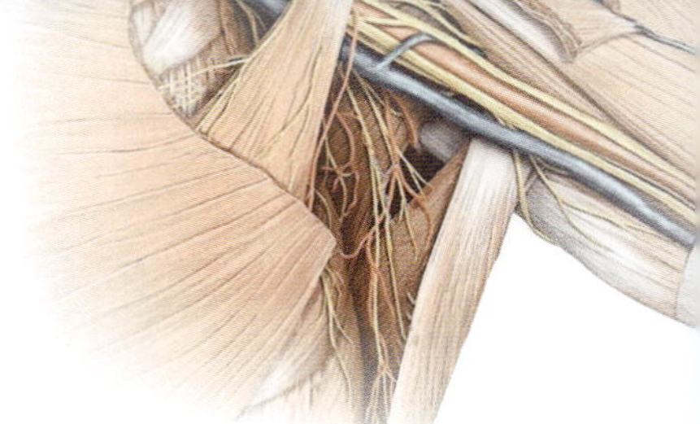

Chapter

3

Pectoral Region

The pectoral region (Latin *pectus* = chest) lies on the front of the chest. It essentially consists of structures that connect the upper limb to the anterolateral chest wall. Breast lies in this region.

Competency:

AN13.6 Identify and demonstrate important bony landmarks of upper limb: Jugular notch, sternal angle, acromial angle, spine of the scapula, vertebral level of the medial end and inferior angle of the scapula.

SURFACE LANDMARKS

Surface landmarks are useful for clinical integration of the gross anatomy. The following features of the pectoral region can be seen or felt on the surface of body (Fig. 3.1).

1. **Clavicle:** It lies horizontally at the root of the neck, separating it from the front of the chest. The bone is subcutaneous, therefore, palpable throughout its length.
2. **Jugular notch** (interclavicular or suprasternal notch): It lies between the medial ends of the clavicles, at the superior border of the manubrium sterni.
3. **Sternal angle** (angle of Louis): It is felt as a transverse ridge about 5 cm below the jugular notch. Importance of sternal angle.
   - *Rib identification*: Second costal cartilage articulates on either side, opposite the sternal angle. It helps in counting ribs.
   - *Vertebral level*: Sternal angle lies at the level of lower border of the fourth thoracic vertebra.
4. **Epigastric fossa** (pit of the stomach): It is the depression in the infrasternal angle. The fossa overlies the xiphoid process and is bounded on each side by the seventh costal cartilage.
5. **Nipple:** It is markedly variable in position in females. In males and immature females, it usually lies in the fourth intercostal space just medial to the midclavicular line; or 10 cm from the midsternal line. Nipple is surrounded by a pigmented circular area called *areola*.

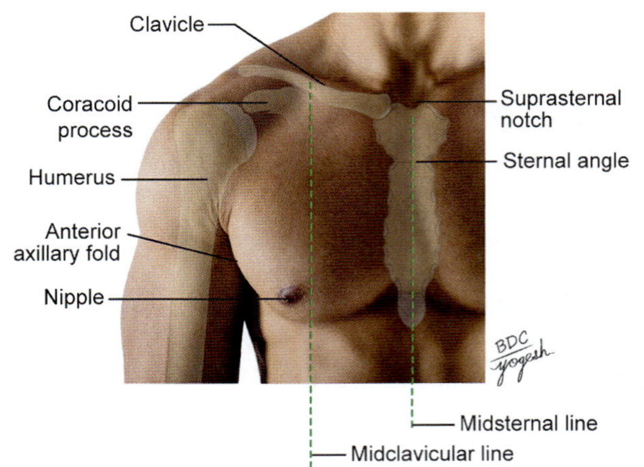

Fig. 3.1: Surface landmarks of pectoral region

6. **Infraclavicular fossa:** It is the junction of the clavicle. It is medially by the pectoralis major, laterally by the anterior fibres of the deltoid, and superiorly by the clavicle.
7. Coracoid process of scapula lies 2.5 cm below the clavicle in the infraclavicular fossa.
8. Acromion process of the scapula (*acron* = summit; *omos* = shoulder) lies subcutaneously forming the top of the shoulder.
9. **Axilla** (Latin armpit): It is a pyramidal space between the arm and chest.

Anatomical Lines

- The following anatomical lines are useful for clinical description of structures (Figs 3.1 and 3.2).
- *Midsternal line*: It is the middle line of sternum, and it passes through the midsagittal plane.
- *Parasternal line*: It lies along the lateral edge of sternum.
- *Midclavicular line*: It is an imaginary line passing through the middle of clavicle, tip of 9th costal cartilage and midinguinal point.
- *Anterior axillary line*: It lies along the anterior axillary fold.
- *Posterior axillary line*: It lies along the posterior axillary fold.
- *Midaxillary line*: It lies midway between anterior and posterior axillary folds.

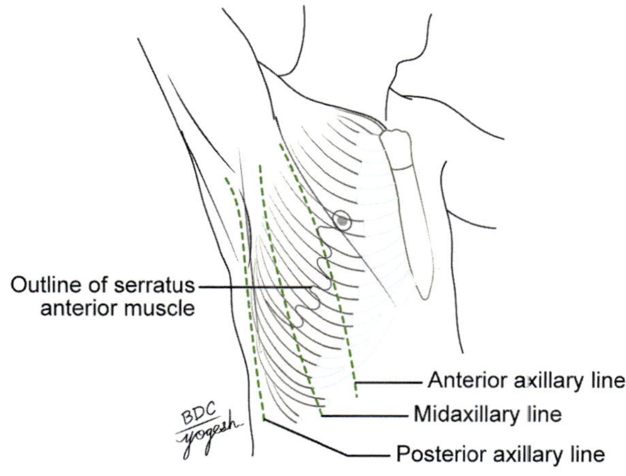

Fig. 3.2: Anatomic reference lines of lateral chest wall

DISSECTION

Mark the following points:

i. Centre of the suprasternal notch
ii. Xiphoid process
iii. 7 o'clock position at the margin of areola (left side), and 5 o'clock position at the margin of areola (right side)
iv. Lateral end of clavicle (Fig. 3.3).

Give an incision vertically down from the first point to the second, which joins the centre of the suprasternal notch to the xiphoid process in the midsagittal plane. From the lower end of this line, extend the incision upward and laterally till you reach to the third point on the areolar margin.

Encircle the areola and carry the incision upwards and laterally till the anterior axillary fold is reached.

Continue the line of incision downwards along the medial border of the upper arm till its junction of upper one-third and lower two-thirds. Extend this incision transversely across the arm.

Make another incision horizontally from the xiphoid process across the chest wall till the posterior axillary fold.

Lastly, give horizontal incision from the centre of suprasternal notch to the lateral (acromial) end of the clavicle.

Reflect the two flaps of skin towards the upper limb.

SUPERFICIAL FASCIA

The superficial fascia of the pectoral region contains moderate amount of fat.

Contents

1. Fat
2. Loose connective tissue
3. Cutaneous nerves
4. Cutaneous blood vessels
5. Platysma
6. Breast (mammary gland).

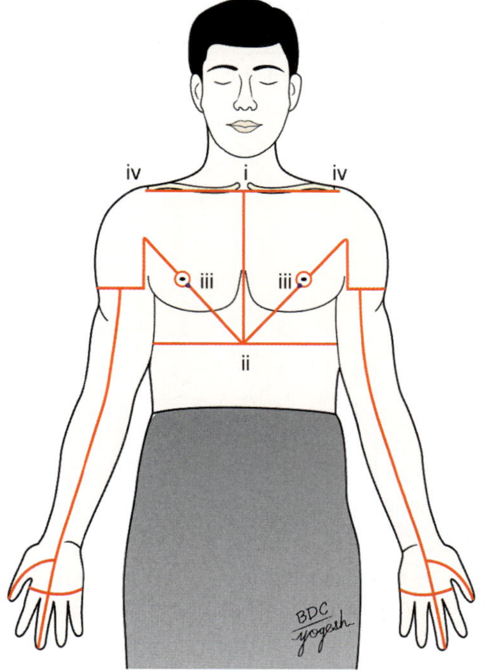

Fig. 3.3: Points and lines of incision

Cutaneous Nerves of the Pectoral Region

1. **Medial, intermediate and lateral supraclavicular nerves:** They are branches of the cervical plexus (C3, C4). They supply the skin over the upper half of the deltoid and from the clavicle down to the second rib.
2. **Second to sixth intercostal nerves:** The *anterior* and *lateral cutaneous* branches of the 2nd to 6th intercostal nerves supply the skin below the level of the second rib. The intercostobrachial nerve of T2 supplies the skin of the floor of the axilla and the upper half of the medial side of the arm (Fig. 3.4).

It is of interest to note that the area supplied by spinal nerves C3 and C4 directly meets the area supplied by spinal nerves T2 and T3. This is because of the fact that the intervening nerves (C5–C8 and T1) have been 'pulled away' to supply the upper limb (Fig. 3.5).

Cutaneous Vessels

The anterior cutaneous nerves are accompanied by the *perforating branches of the internal thoracic artery*. The 2nd, 3rd and 4th of these branches are large in females for supplying the breast. The lateral cutaneous nerves are accompanied by the *lateral cutaneous branches of the posterior intercostal arteries*.

Platysma

The platysma (Greek *broad*) is a thin, broad sheet of subcutaneous muscle. The fibres of the muscle arise from the deep fascia covering the pectoralis major; run upwards and medially, crossing the clavicle and the side of the neck, and are inserted into the base of the mandible and into skin over the posterior and lower part of the face. The platysma is supplied by a branch of the *facial nerve*. When the angle of the mouth is pulled down, the muscle contracts and wrinkles the skin of the neck. The platysma may protect the external jugular vein (which underlies the muscle) from external pressure.

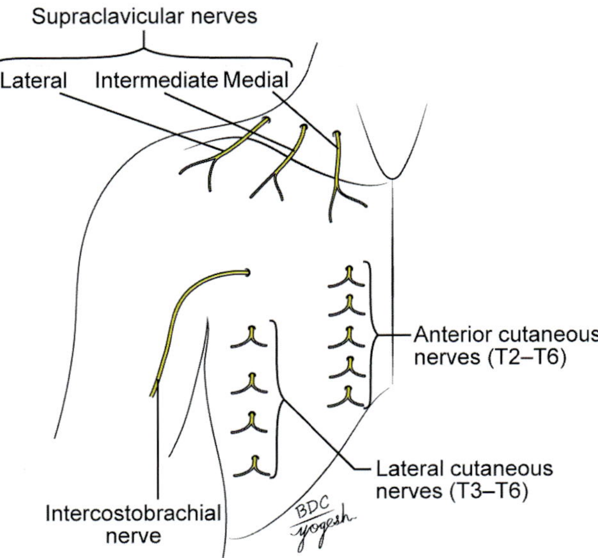

Fig. 3.4: Cutaneous nerves of the pectoral region

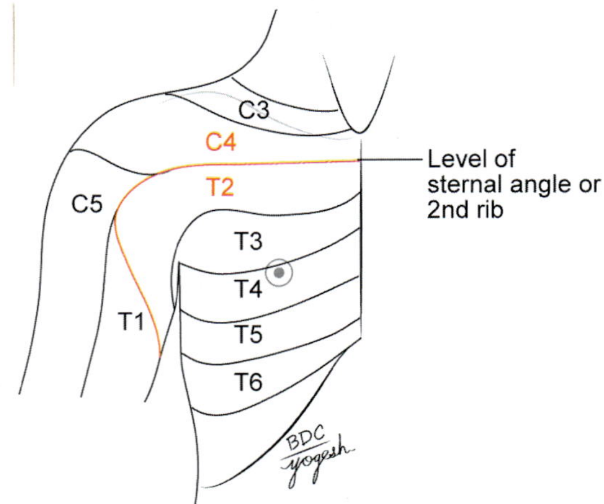

Fig. 3.5: Areas supplied by cutaneous nerves of the pectoral region

Competency:
AN9.2 Describe the location, extent, deep relations, structure, age changes, blood supply, lymphatic drainage, microanatomy and applied anatomy of breast.

MAMMARY GLAND/BREAST

Mammary gland is a modified sweat gland located in the superficial fascia of the pectoral region (Latin *mamma* = breast) (Plate 3.1, Flowchart 3.1).

The glandular tissue is found in both sexes, but is rudimentary in the male. It is well developed in the female after puberty. It forms an important accessory organ of the female reproductive system, and provides nutrition to the newborn in the form of milk.

Location

The breast lies in the superficial fascia of the pectoral region. A small extension of the superolateral part, called the *axillary tail of Spence*, passes through an opening in the deep fascia and lies in the axilla (Fig. 3.6). The opening is called *foramen of Langer*.

Shape

The shape of breast is variable. It may be hemispherical, conical, pyriform, pendulous or flat.

Extent of the Base

1. Vertically, it extends from the 2nd to the 6th ribs.
2. Horizontally, it extends from the lateral border of the sternum to the midaxillary line (Fig. 3.5).

Deep Relations

The deep surface of the breast is related to the following structures from superficial to deep (Figs 3.7 and 3.8).

1. Deep fascia (pectoral fascia) covering the pectoralis major.
2. Three muscles: *Pectoralis major, the serratus anterior and the external oblique muscle of the abdomen.*
3. **Retromammary space:** The breast is separated from the pectoral fascia by loose areolar tissue, called the *retromammary space*. Because of the presence of this loose tissue, the normal breast can be moved freely over the pectoralis major.

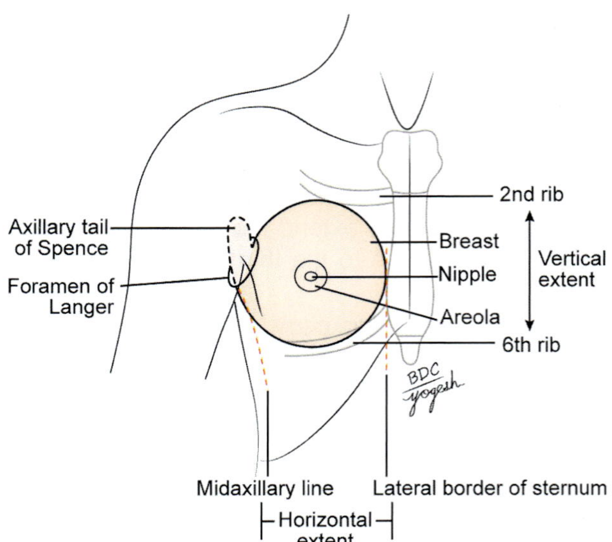

Fig. 3.6: Location and extent of right breast

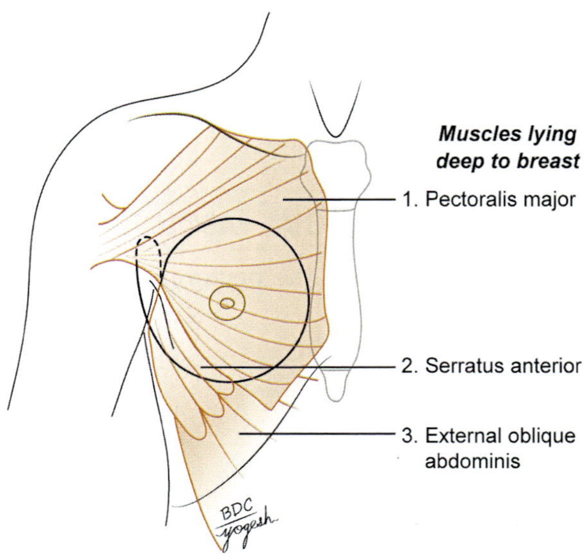

Fig. 3.7: Muscles lying deep to the breast

Plate 3.1: Female breast

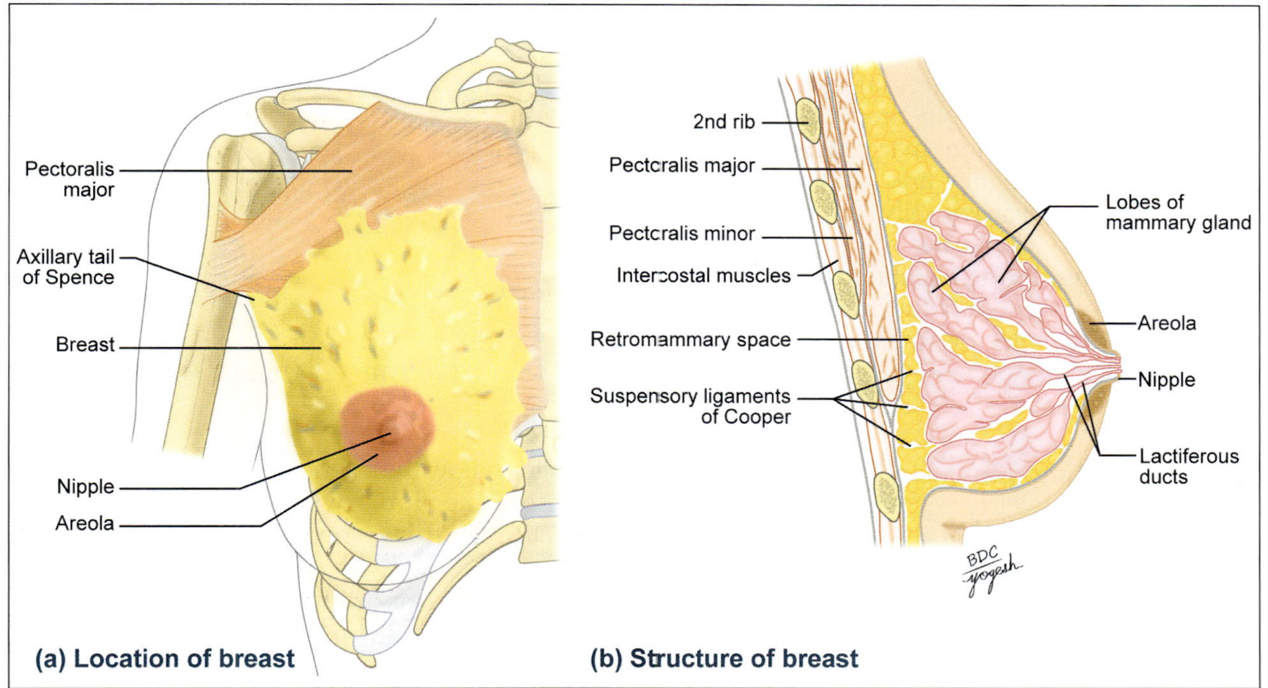

Flowchart 3.1: Breast

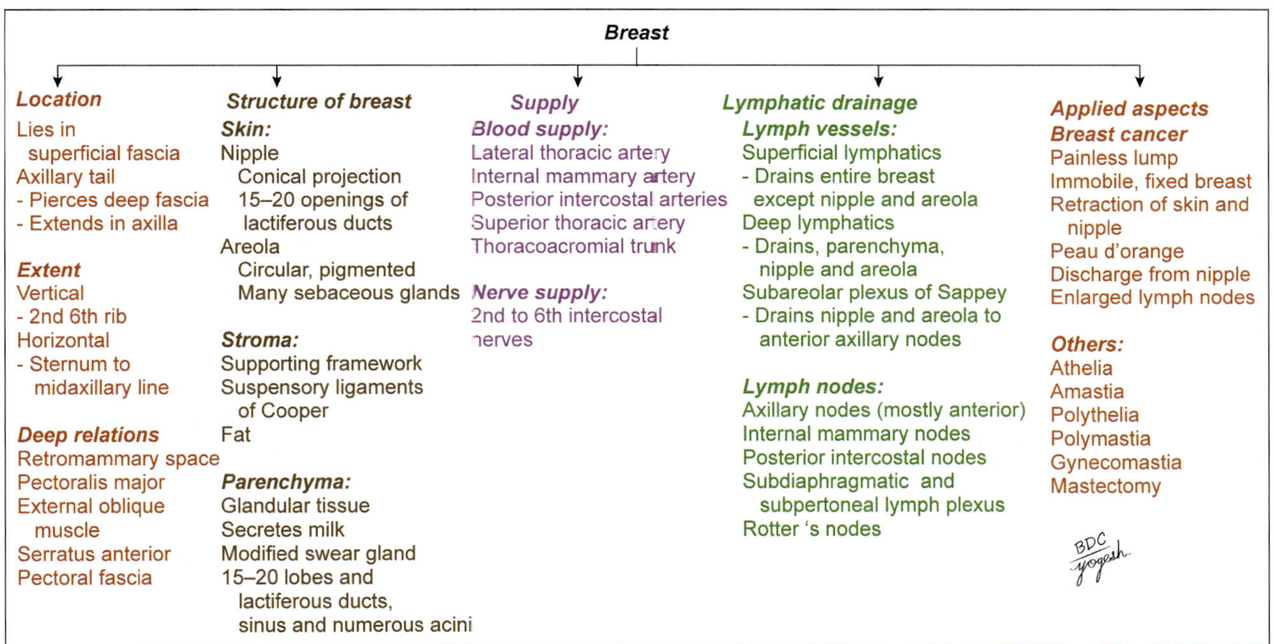

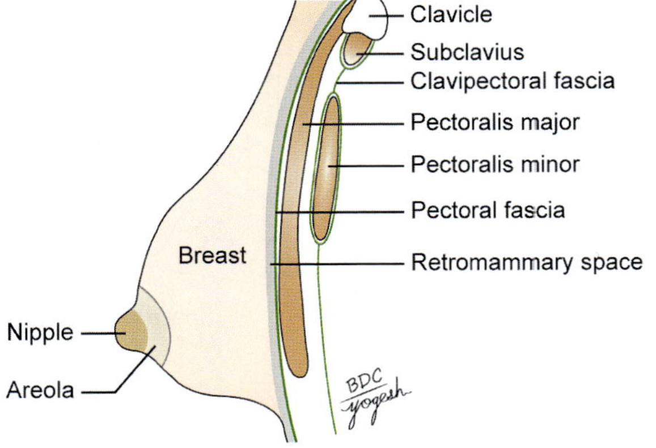

Fig. 3.8: Deep relations of breast

Structure of the Breast

The breast consists of the following three components:

1. Skin
2. Stroma
3. Parenchyma: Parenchyma is the mammary gland proper.

Skin

It covers the gland and presents the following features:

1. **Nipple:** A conical projection, called the *nipple*, is present just below the centre of the breast at the level of the 4th intercostal space, 10 cm from the midline. The nipple is pierced by 15 to 20 lactiferous ducts.

It contains circular and longitudinal smooth muscle fibres and a rich nerve supply. It can make the nipple stiff or flatten on stimulation.

2. **Areola:** The skin surrounding the base of the nipple is pigmented and forms a circular area called the *areola*. This region is rich in modified *sebaceous glands*, particularly at its outer margin. These become enlarged during pregnancy and lactation to form raised *tubercles of Montgomery*. Oily secretions of these glands lubricate the nipple and areola, and prevent them from cracking during lactation. The skin of the areola and nipple is devoid of hair and there is no fat subjacent to it. The color of areola becomes darker during pregnancy.

Stroma

It forms the supporting framework of the gland. It is partly fibrous and partly fatty.

The fibrous stroma forms septa, known as the *suspensory ligaments of Cooper*, which anchor the skin and gland to the pectoral fascia and maintain the normal shape of the breast (Figs 3.9a and b).

The fatty stroma forms the main bulk of the gland. It is distributed all over the breast except beneath the areola and nipple.

Parenchyma (Mammary Gland)

Mammary gland is a compound tubuloalveolar gland that secretes milk. It is a modified sweat gland and consists of 15 to 20 lobes. Each lobe is a cluster of alveoli and is drained by a *lactiferous duct*. The lactiferous ducts converge towards the nipple and open on it. Near its termination, each duct has a dilatation called a *lactiferous sinus* (Figs 3.9a and b).

Arterial Supply

The breast is highly vascular. It is supplied by branches of the following arteries (Fig. 3.10).

1. Internal thoracic (mammary) artery, a branch of the subclavian artery, through its perforating branches.
2. The lateral thoracic, superior thoracic and acromiothoracic (thoracoacromial) branches of the axillary artery.
3. Lateral branches of the posterior intercostal arteries.

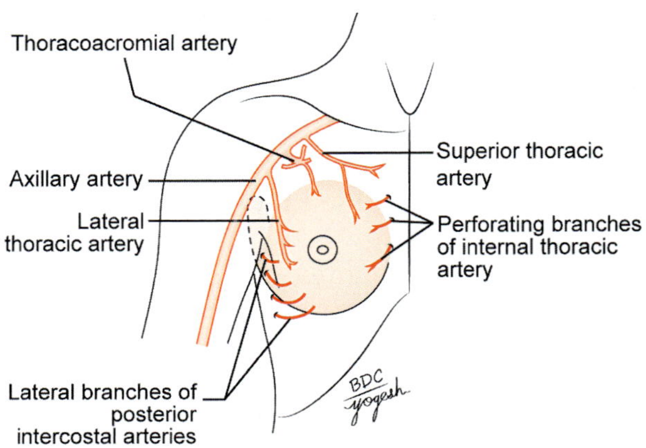

Fig. 3.10: Blood supply of breast

Venous Drainage

The veins follow the arteries. They first converge towards the base of the nipple, where they form an anastomotic venous circle, from where veins run in superficial and deep sets.

1. Superficial veins drain into the internal thoracic vein.
2. Deep veins drain into the axillary and posterior intercostal veins.

Nerve Supply

The breast is supplied by the anterior and lateral cutaneous branches of the 2nd to 6th intercostal nerves (4th to 6th intercostal nerves, as per 42nd Edn. Gray's Anatomy). The nerves convey sensory fibres to the skin and autonomic fibres to smooth muscle and to blood vessels. The nerves do not control the secretion of milk. Secretion is controlled by the hormone prolactin, secreted by the *pars anterior* of the *hypophysis cerebri*. The diagnosis and management of breast disease should be done carefully.

Competencies:

AN10.4 Describe the anatomical groups of axillary lymph nodes and specify their areas of drainage.

AN10.7 Describe axillary lymph nodes, areas of drainage and anatomical basis of their enlargement.

Lymphatic Drainage

Lymphatic drainage of the breast assumes great importance to the surgeon because carcinoma of the

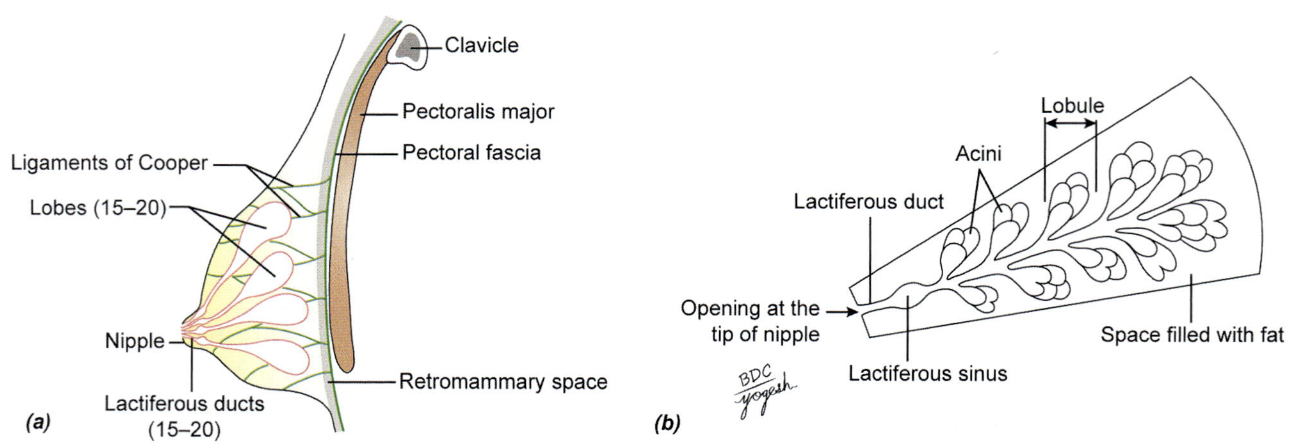

Figs 3.9a and b: Structure of breast: (a) Sagittal section; (b) Structure of lobe

breast spreads mostly along lymphatics to the regional lymph nodes. The subject can be described under two heads—the lymph nodes and the lymphatic vessels.

Lymph Nodes

Lymph from the breast drains into the following lymph nodes (Fig. 3.11).

1. The axillary lymph nodes, chiefly the anterior (or pectoral) group. The posterior, lateral, central and apical groups of nodes also receive lymph from the breast either directly or indirectly.
2. The anterior thoracic (parasternal) nodes lie along the internal mammary (thoracic) vessels.
3. Some lymph from the breast also reaches the supraclavicular nodes, the cephalic (deltopectoral) node, the posterior intercostal nodes (lying in front of the heads of the ribs), the subdiaphragmatic and subperitoneal lymph plexuses.

Lymphatic Vessels

The lymphatic vessels draining breast are divided into two groups:

1. **Superficial lymphatics** drain the skin over the breast except for the nipple and areola. The lymphatics pass radially to the surrounding lymph nodes (axillary, anterior thoracic, supraclavicular and cephalic) (Fig. 3.11).
2. **Deep lymphatics** drain the parenchyma of the breast. They also drain the nipple and areola.

Important Points

1. About 75% of the lymph from the breast drains into the axillary nodes, 20% into the anterior thoracic nodes, and 5% into the posterior intercostal nodes. Among the axillary nodes, the lymphatics end mostly in the anterior group (closely related to the axillary tail) and partly in the posterior and apical groups. Lymph from the anterior and posterior groups passes to the central and lateral groups and through them to the apical group. Finally, it reaches the supraclavicular nodes.

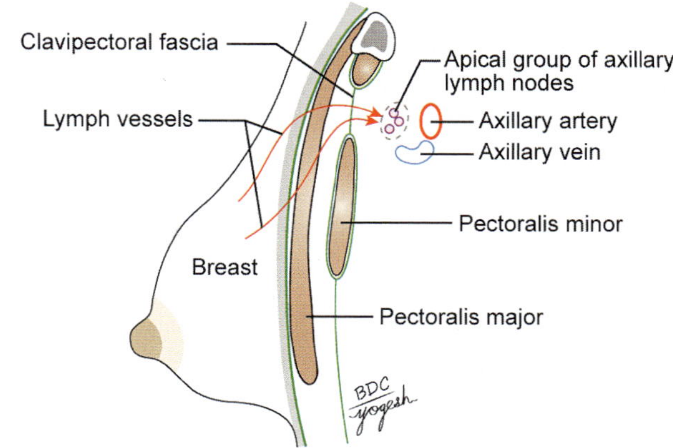

Fig. 3.12: Direct pathway of deep lymphatics of the breast through pectoralis major and clavipectoral fascia to apical group of axillary lymph nodes

2. **Subareolar plexus of Sappey:** It is a plexus of lymph vessels that is present deep to the areola. It drains into the anterior or pectoral group of lymph nodes.
3. The lymphatics from the deep surface of the gland pass through the pectoralis major muscle and the clavipectoral fascia to reach the apical nodes (Fig. 3.12).
4. Lymphatics from the lower and inner quadrants of the breast may communicate with the subdiaphragmatic and subperitoneal lymph plexuses after crossing the costal margin and then piercing the anterior abdominal wall through the upper part of the linea alba.
5. Anterior and central groups of nodes are commonly involved in carcinoma breast.

Competency:
AN9.3 Describe development of breast, associated age changes and congenital anomalies.

Development of the Breast and Age Changes

Embryonic Development

1. The parenchyma (glandular tissue) of breast develops from ectoderm, whereas the fibrous stroma, suspensory ligaments, fat and myoepithelial cells develop from the surrounding mesoderm.

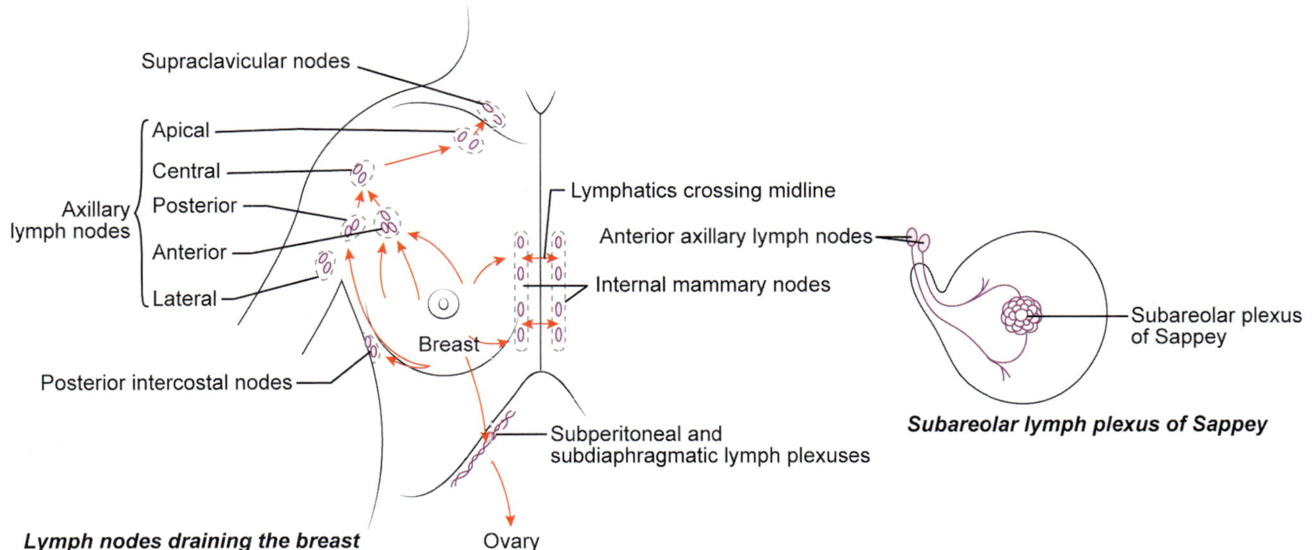

Fig. 3.11: Lymphatic drainage of right breast

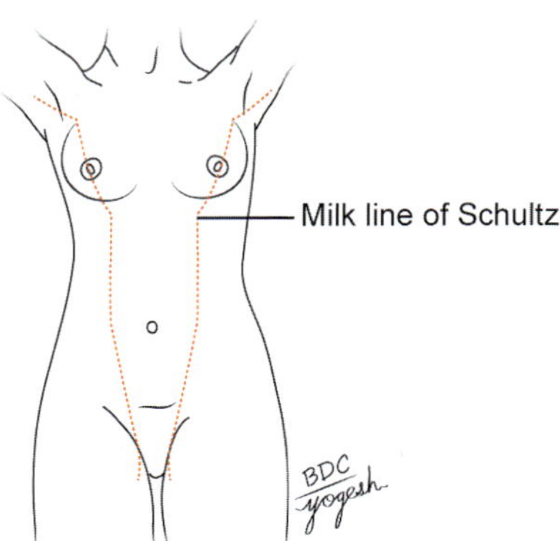

Fig. 3.13: Mammary ridge

2. An ectodermal thickening, called the *mammary ridge*, milk line or ***line of Schultz,*** forms parenchyma (Fig. 3.13). This ridge extends from the axilla to the groin. It appears during the 6th week of intrauterine life, but in human beings, it disappears over most of its extent, persisting only in the thoracic region.
3. The persisting part of the mammary ridge is converted into a mammary pit. Secondary buds (15–20) grow down from the floor of the pit. These buds divide and subdivide to form the lobes of the gland. The entire system is first solid but is later canalised. At birth or later, the nipple is everted at the site of the original pit.

Development at Puberty

1. At puberty, owing to the deposition of fat and connective tissue, female mammary glands enlarge rapidly. Under the influence of estrogen and progesterone, duct system grows.

Development during Pregnancy

1. During pregnancy, the glandular tissue rapidly develops and forms buds and alveoli.

Development Anomalies

a. Amastia – absence of the breast
b. Athelia – absence of nipple
c. Polymastia – supernumerary breasts
d. Polythelia – supernumerary nipples
e. Gynaecomastia – development of breasts in a male (occurs in Klinefelter's syndrome).

Histology of Breast

- Mammary gland is a *modified apocrine sweat gland*. It is composed of ducts, parenchyma and stroma (Plate 3.2).
- *Ducts*: Mammary gland has the following order of ducts:
  - *Lactiferous duct*: Lined by columnar epithelium (terminal part shows transformation from columnar to stratified squamous epithelium).
  - *Interlobular ducts*: Lined by cuboidal to low columnar epithelium.
  - *Intralobular ducts*: Lined by cuboidal epithelium.
  - *Alveolar ducts*: Lined by low cuboidal epithelium.
- Parenchyma
  - Each gland shows 15–20 lobes of compound tubuloalveolar gland.
  - ***Nonlactating inactive glands:*** Shows spherical masses or cords of alveolar cells.
  - ***Lactating active glands:*** Shows numerous branched ducts with clusters of alveoli that are lined by simple columnar epithelium.
- *Stroma*: Consists of interlobular, intralobar, and interlobar connective tissue.

CLINICAL ANATOMY

Breast cancer (carcinoma of breast): The upper and outer quadrants of breast are a frequent site of carcinoma (cancer). The first lymph node draining the tumour-bearing area is called 'sentinel node.'

- Incisions of breast for removal of carcinoma or drainage of abscess are usually made radially to avoid cutting the lactiferous ducts (Fig. 3.9).
- Cancer cells may infiltrate the suspensory ligaments. The breast then becomes fixed. Contraction of the ligaments can cause retraction or puckering (folding) of the skin.
- Infiltration of lactiferous ducts and their consequent fibrosis can cause *retraction of the nipple*.
- Obstruction of superficial lymph vessels by cancer cells may produce oedema of the skin giving rise to an appearance like that of the skin of an orange (***peau d'orange*** appearance) (Fig. 3.14).
- Because of communications of the superficial lymphatics of the breast across the midline, cancer may spread from one breast to the other.
- Because of communications of the lymph vessels with those in the abdomen, cancer of the breast may spread to the liver, and cancer cells may 'drop' into the pelvis producing secondaries (Fig. 3.11). Some cancer cells may deposit on the ovary and form a secondary tumor called ***Krukenberg's tumour***.
- Breast cancer may spread through venous channels to the vertebrae and to the brain.
- Carcinoma usually arises from epithelium of large ducts.
- Self-examination of breasts helps in early detection of breast cancers. It includes examination for symmetry of breasts and nipples, change in colour of skin, retraction of nipple, discharge from nipple on squeezing it, palpation with palm of hand for lump and to raise the arm to feel lymph nodes in axilla.
- **Mammogram** may reveal cancerous mass (Fig. 3.15).
- **Fine needle aspiration cytology** is safe and quick method of diagnosis of lesion of breast.
- Retracted nipple is a sign of tumour in the breast.
- Size of mammary gland can be increased by putting an implant inside the gland. The size can be reduced by breast reduction surgery.
- Cancer of the mammary glands is the most common cancer in females of all ages. It is more frequently seen in postmenopausal females due to lack of oestrogen hormones.
- *Mastectomy* is the medical term for the surgical removal of one or both breasts, partially or completely.
- *Radical mastectomy* is a surgical procedure involving the removal of breast, underlying pectoral muscles and lymph nodes of the axilla.

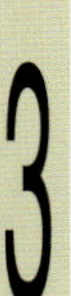

Plate 3.2: Histology of mammary gland

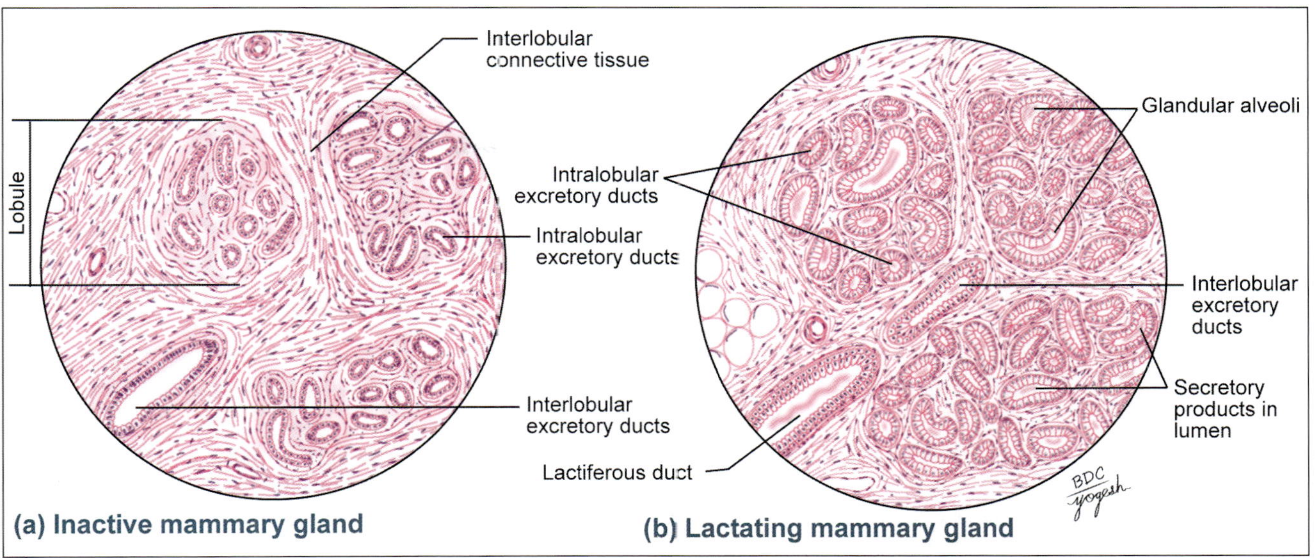

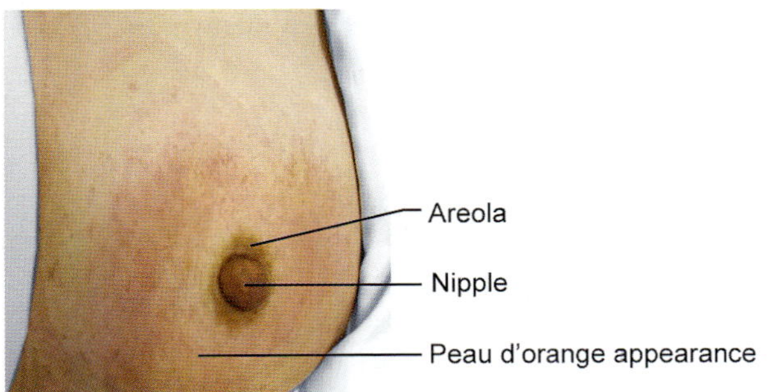

Fig. 3.14: Peau d'orange appearance

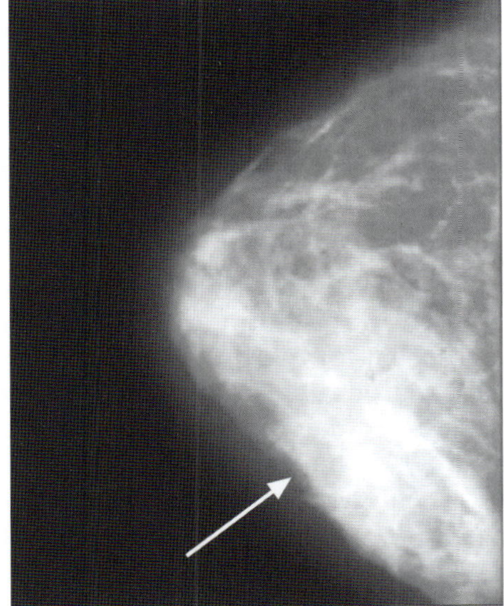

Fig. 3.15: Mammogram showing cancerous lesion

DEEP FASCIA

The deep fascia covering the pectoralis major muscle is called the pectoral fascia.

- *Extension*:
  - Superiorly: Attaches to the clavicle
  - Medially: Attaches to the sternum
  - Superolaterally: Continues as deep fascia over deltoid muscle
  - Inferolaterally: Turns to continue as axillary fascia.

Inferiorly: Continue as fascia covering the lower part of thoracic range.

Competency:
AN9.1 Describe attachment, nerve supply and action of pectoralis major and pectoralis minor and describe clavipectoral fascia.

MUSCLES OF THE PECTORAL REGION

Pectoral region has three muscles (Figs 3.16 to 3.18, Tables 3.1 and 3.2, Flowchart 3.2, Plates 3.3 and 3.4):

1. Pectoralis major
2. Pectoralis minor
3. Subclavius.

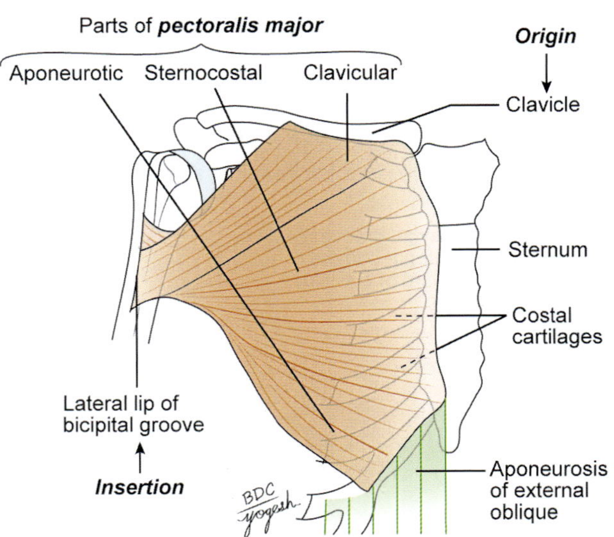

Fig. 3.16: Pectoralis major muscle

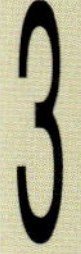

TABLE 3.1: Muscles of the pectoral region

Muscle	*Origin*	*Insertion*
Pectoralis major Thick, bulky, fan-shaped muscle	**Clavicular head:** Anterior surface of medial two-thirds of clavicle **Sternocostal head:** • Lateral half of anterior surface of manubrium and sternum up to 6th costal cartilage • 2nd to 6th costal cartilages, sternal end of 6th rib • Aponeurosis of the external oblique muscle of abdomen	It is inserted by a bilaminar tendon on the lateral lip of the bicipital groove in form of U-shaped bilaminar tendon The two laminae are continuous with each other inferiorly Its anterior lamina is thicker and shorter than the thinner and longer posterior lamina. Anterior lamina receives superficial clavicular and deep manubrial fibres; posterior lamina gets costal, sternal and aponeurotic fibres
Pectoralis minor	• 3, 4, 5 ribs near the costochondral junction • Intervening fascia covering external intercostal muscles	Medial border and upper surface of the coracoid process of scapula
Subclavius	First rib at the costochondral junction	Subclavian groove (on the inferior surface of middle-third of clavicle)

TABLE 3.2: Nerve supply and actions of muscles

Muscle	*Nerve supply*	*Actions*
Pectoralis major	Medial and lateral pectoral nerves	• As a whole the muscle: Adduction and medial rotation of the shoulder joint (arm) • Clavicular part: Flexion of the arm • Sternocostal part: Extension of flexed arm against resistance
Pectoralis minor	Medial and lateral pectoral nerves	• Draws the scapula forward (with serratus anterior) • Depresses the shoulder. Accessory muscle of respiration in forced inspiration
Subclavius	Nerve to subclavius (branch of upper trunk of brachial plexus)	Stabilises the clavicle during movements of the shoulder joint Forms a cushion for axillary vessels and brachial plexus

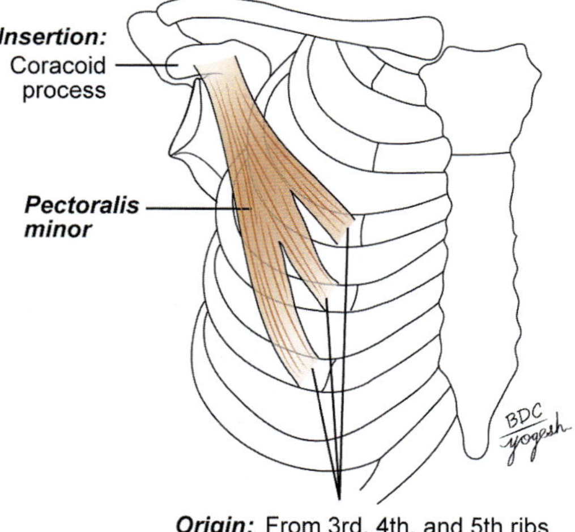

Fig. 3.17: Pectoralis minor muscle

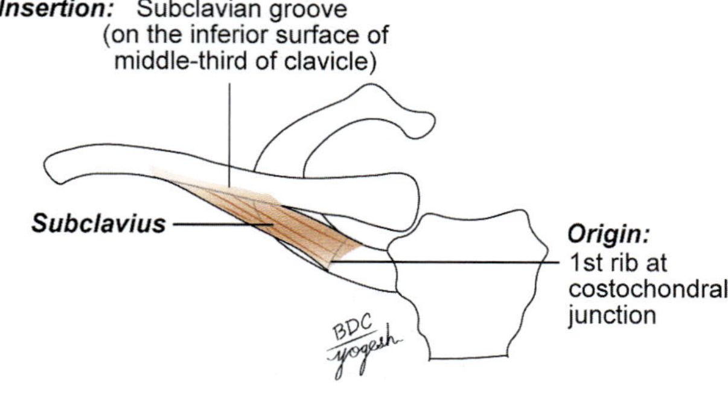

Fig. 3.18: Subclavius muscle

Pectoralis Major

Bilaminar Tendon of Pectoralis Major

The muscle is inserted by a U-shaped bilaminar tendon into the lateral lip of the intertubercular sulcus of the humerus. The two laminae are continuous with each other inferiorly.

Anterior lamina is thicker and shorter than the posterior. It receives two strata of muscle fibres: Superficial fibres arising from the clavicle and deep fibres arising from the manubrium (Plate 3.3b).

Posterior lamina is thinner and longer than the anterior lamina. It is formed by remaining sternal fibers, costal and aponeurotic fibres. Out of these, only the fibres from the sternum and aponeurosis are twisted around the lower border of the rest of the muscle. The twisted fibres form the anterior axillary fold.

The twisted fibres pass upwards and laterally to get inserted successively higher into the posterior lamina of the tendon. Fibres arising lowest are inserted the highest.

Clinical Testing

1. The clavicular head is made prominent by flexing the arm to a right angle. The sternocostal head can be tested by extending the flexed arm against resistance (Fig. 3.19a).
2. Sternocostal head is made prominent by abducting arm to 60° and then touching the opposite hip.

Plate 3.3: Pectoralis major muscle: (a) Gross features and parts of muscle, (b) bilaminar insertion

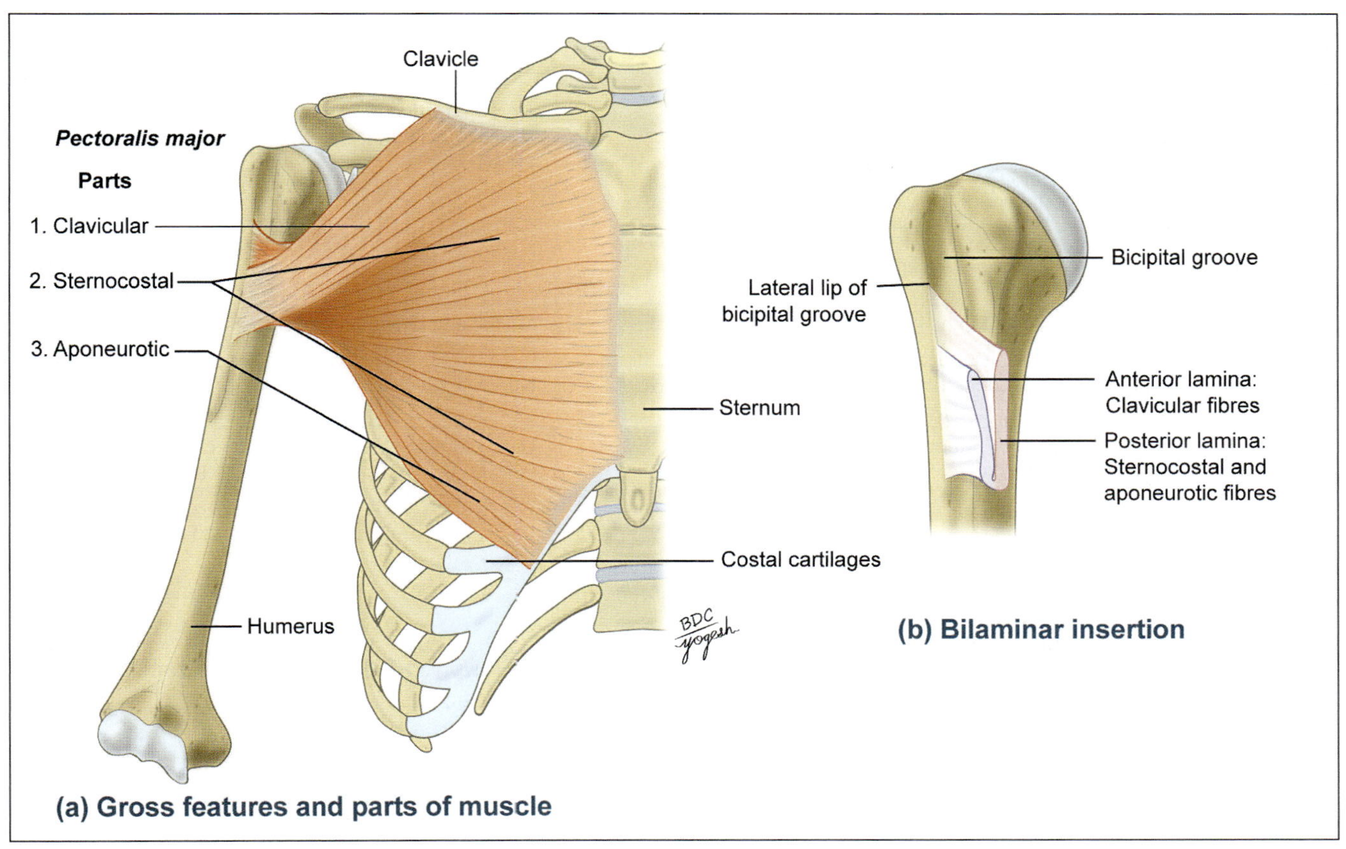

Plate 3.4: Pectoralis minor and subclavius muscles

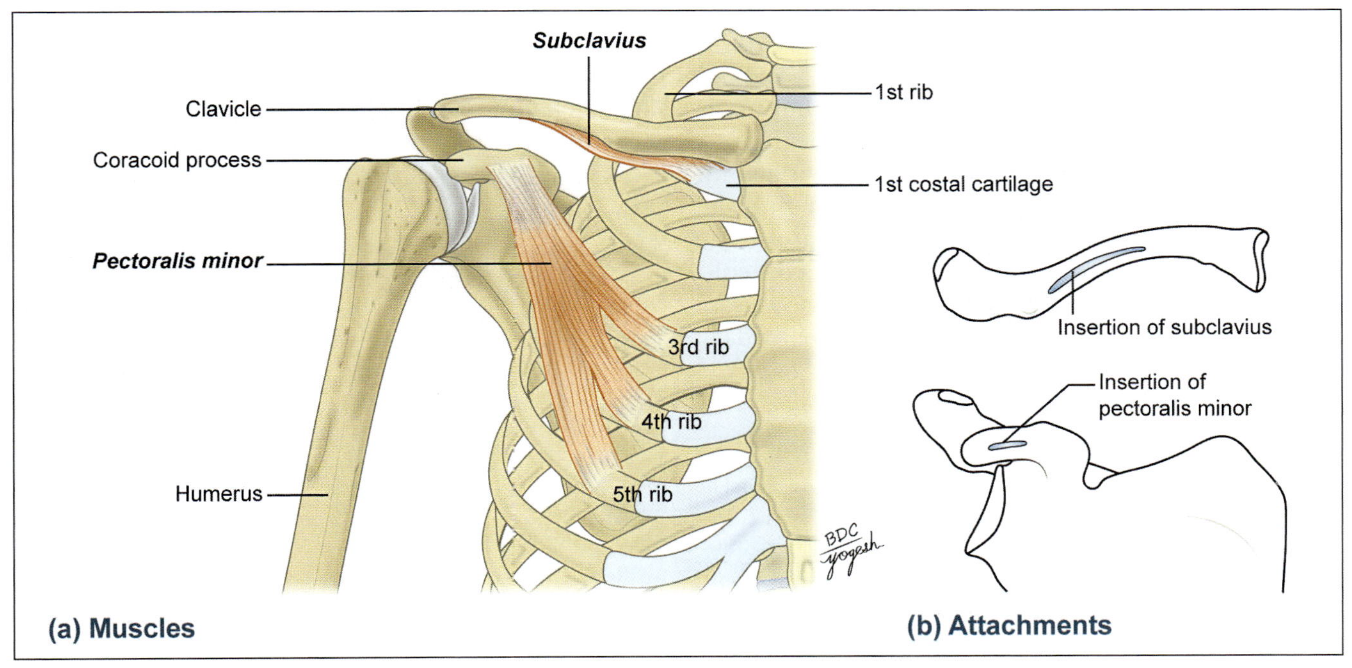

3. Lifting a heavy rod makes clavicular part prominent (right arm). Depressing a heavy rod shows sternocostal part as prominent (left arm) (Fig. 3.19a).
4. Pressing the fists against each other makes the whole muscle prominent (Fig. 3.19b).

Clavipectoral Fascia

Clavipectoral fascia is a fibrous sheet situated deep to the clavicular portion of the pectoralis major muscle. It extends from the clavicle above to the axillary fascia below (Fig. 3.20, Flowchart 3.3). Its upper part splits to

Flowchart 3.2: Pectoral muscles and serratus anterior muscle

Muscles	Origin	Insertion	Nerve supply	Actions
Pectoralis major Large bulky fan-shaped muscle	Clavicular head: Anterior surface of medial half of clavicle Sternocostal head: - Lateral half of anterior surface sternum upto 6th costal cartilage - 2nd to 6th costal cartilage - External oblique aponeurosis	Lateral lip of bicipital groove by bilaminar tendon: Anterior lamina Clavicular fibers Posterior lamina Sternocostal fibres (lowest fibres inserts highest)	Medial and lateral pectoral nerve	Adduction and medial rotation of arm - Clavicular head: Flexion of arm - Sternocostal head: Extension of flexed arm
Pectoralis minor	From 3rd, 4th, 5th ribs near costal cartilages	Coracoid process	Medial and lateral pectoral nerves	Protraction of scapula
Subclavius	First rib at costochondral junction	Subclavian groove	Nerve to subclavius	Protection of brachial plexus and subclavian vessels
Serratus anterior	8 digitation from lateral surface of upper 8 ribs and fascia covering intercostal muscles	Medial border of scapula (costal surface) 1st digitation: Superior angle Next 2–3 digitations: -Medial border Last 4–5 digitations: - At inferior angle	Long thoracic nerve (C5–7)	Stabilization of clavicle Pushing and punching (with pectoralis minor) Overhead abduction at shoulder (with trapezius)

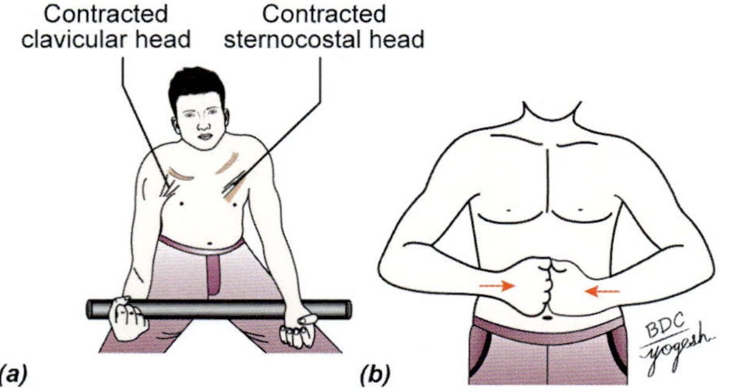

Figs 3.19a and b: Clinical testing of pectoralis major: (a) Testing of clavicular and sternocostal heads and (b) testing of whole muscle

Flowchart 3.3: Clavipectoral fascia

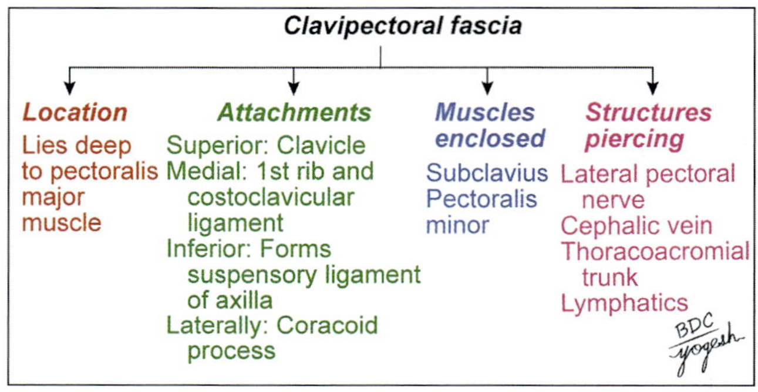

enclose the *subclavius muscle*. The posterior lamina is fused to the investing layer of the deep cervical fascia and to the *axillary sheath*. Inferiorly, the clavipectoral fascia splits to enclose the pectoralis minor muscle. Medially, it is attached to external intercostal muscle of upper intercostal spaces and laterally to coracoid process. Below this muscle, it continues as the *suspensory ligament*, which is attached to the dome of the axillary fascia and helps to maintain it.

The clavipectoral fascia is pierced by the following structures (Fig. 3.21):

1. Lateral pectoral nerve
2. Cephalic vein
3. Thoracoacromial artery
4. Lymphatics passing from the breast and pectoral region to the apical group of axillary lymph nodes.

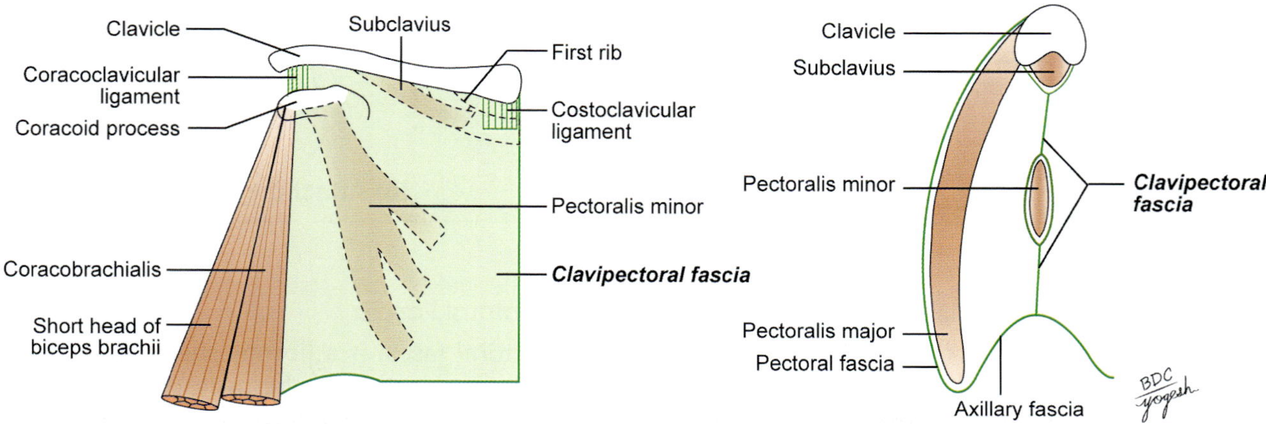

Figs 3.20a and b: Clavipectoral fascia: (a) Attachments in anterior view and (b) attachments in sagittal section

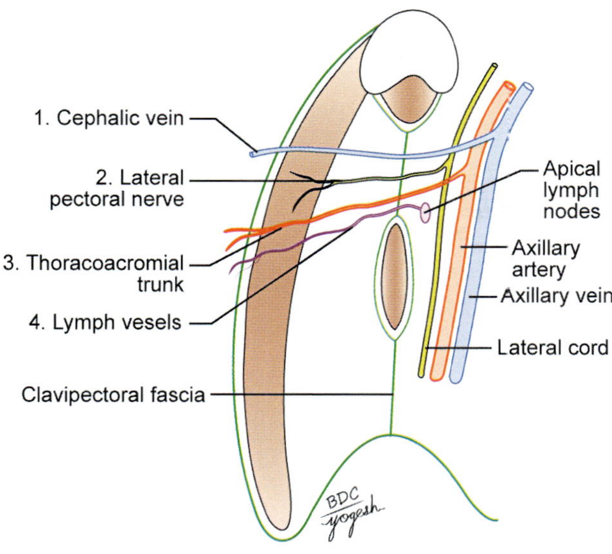

Fig. 3.21: Structures piercing clavipectoral fascia

Competency:

AN10.11 Describe and demonstrate attachment, action and clinical anatomy of serratus anterior muscle.

Serratus Anterior

Serratus anterior muscle is not strictly muscle of the pectoral region, but it is convenient to consider it here (Latin, *serrate* = to saw) (Plate 3.5, Fig. 3.22). It is also called **boxer's muscle/swimmer's muscle** (Flowchart 3.2).

Origin

Serratus anterior muscle arises by eight digitations from the upper 8 ribs in the midaxillary plane and from the fascia covering the intervening intercostal muscles. The first digitation arises from the 1st and 2nd ribs, whereas all other digitations arise from their corresponding ribs.

Insertion

All 8 digitations pass backwards around the chest wall. The muscle is inserted into the *costal surface* of the scapula along its medial border as follows (Figs 3.22a, b):

- 1st digitation at the superior angle
- 2nd and 3rd digitations along the entire medial border
- Remaining digitations on the triangular area at the costal surface of inferior angle of scapula.

Nerve Supply

Long thoracic nerve (branch of C5, C6, C7 roots of brachial plexus) (Fig. 3.22a).

Actions

1. **Pushing and punching action (boxer's muscle):** Along with the pectoralis minor, the muscle pulls the scapula forwards around the chest wall to protract the upper limb.
2. **Overhead abduction of arm:** The fibres inserted into the inferior angle of the scapula pull it forwards and rotate the scapula so that the glenoid cavity is turned upwards. In this action, the serratus anterior is helped by the trapezius, which pulls the acromion process upwards and backwards.
3. Steadies the scapula during weight carrying.
4. Helps in forced inspiration.

CLINICAL ANATOMY

1. **Winging of scapula:** Paralysis of the serratus anterior produces 'winging of scapula' in which the inferior angle and the medial border of the scapula are unduly prominent. It occurs due to injury to *long thoracic nerve*. The patient is unable to do any pushing action, nor can he raise his arm above the head. Any attempt to do these movements makes the inferior angle of the scapula still more prominent.

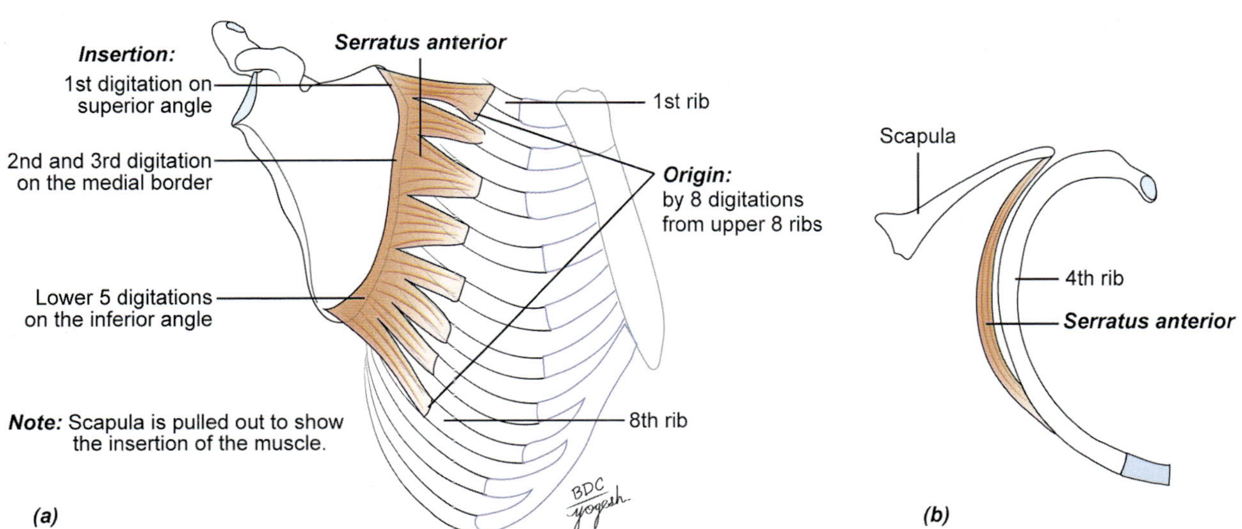

Figs 3.22a and b: Serratus anterior muscle: (a) Origin and insertion and (b) horizontal section through axilla showing relationship to the thoracic wall

Plate 3.5: Serratus anterior muscle and long thoracic nerve

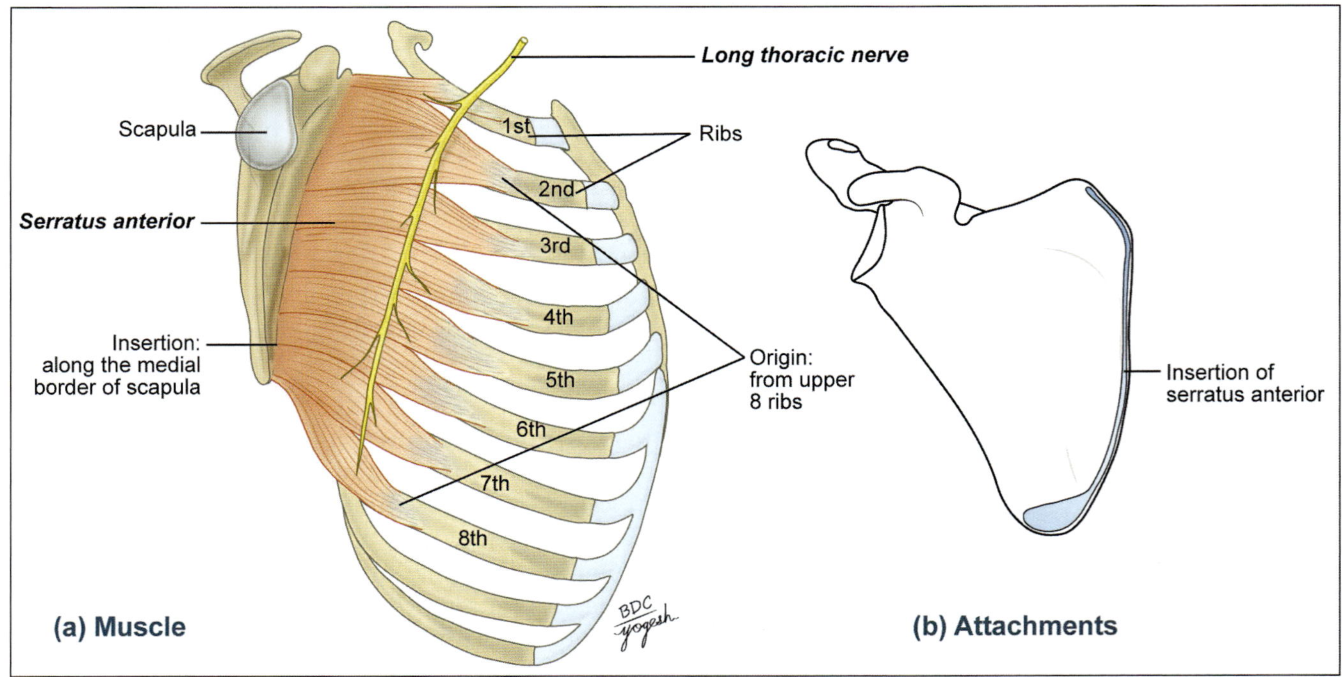

2. **Clinical testing:** Forward pressure with the hands against a wall, or against resistance offered by the examiner, makes the medial border and the inferior angle of the scapula prominent (winging of scapula), if the serratus anterior is paralysed.

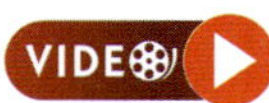

Video 1.3 Pectoral Region ▶ Mammary gland and muscles of pectoral region.

DISSECTION

Identify the extensive pectoralis major muscle in the pectoral region and the prominent deltoid muscle on the lateral aspect of the shoulder joint and upper arm.

Demarcate the deltopectoral groove by removing the deep fascia. Now identify the cephalic vein, a small artery and a few lymph nodes in the groove.

Clean the fascia over the pectoralis major muscle and look for its attachments. Divide the clavicular head of the muscle and reflect it laterally. Medial and lateral pectoral nerves will be seen supplying the muscle.

Make a vertical incision 5 to 6 cm from the lateral border of sternum and reflect its sternocostal head laterally.

Identify the pectoralis minor muscle under the central part of the pectoralis major. Note clavipectoral fascia extending between pectoralis minor muscle and the clavicle bone.

Identify the structures piercing the clavipectoral fascia: These are cephalic vein, thoracoacromial artery and lateral pectoral nerve. If some fine vessels are also seen, these are the lymphatic channels.

Also, identify the serratus anterior muscle showing serrated digitations on the side of the chest wall.

Facts to Remember

- The mammary gland is a modified apocrine sweat gland. It lies in the superficial fascia.
- Most of the lymph from breast is drained into the anterior axillary lymph nodes.
- The subareolar plexus of Sappey is a plexus of lymph vessels deep to the areola, which drain into anterior axillary lymph nodes.
- Rotter's lymph nodes lie between pectoralis major and pectoralis minor (hence called interpectoral nodes).
- The upper and outer quadrants of the breast are the most common site of breast cancer.
- 75% of lymph from mammary gland drains into axillary; 20% into anterior thoracic and 5% into posterior intercostal lymph nodes.
- Pectoralis major is the largest muscle of the pectoral region.
- Pectoralis minor is the key muscle of the pectoral region, as it divides the axillary artery into three parts.

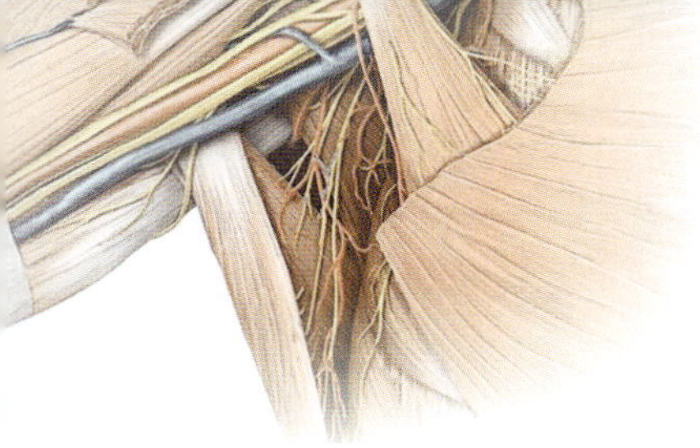

Chapter

4

Axilla

Competency:
AN10.1 Identify and describe boundaries and contents of axilla.

Axilla (Latin *armpit*) is a pyramidal space situated between the upper part of the arm and the chest wall (Figs 4.1a–c, Flowchart 4.1, Plate 4.1). It contains the brachial plexus, axillary vessels and axillary lymph nodes. It gives passage to the neurovascular structures from the root of the neck to the upper limb and vice versa.

DISSECTION

Place a rectangular wooden block under the neck and shoulder region of cadaver (Figs 4.1a–c). Ensure that the block supports the body firmly. Abduct the limb at right angles to the trunk, and strap the wrist firmly on block projecting towards your side. In continuation with earlier dissection, reflect the lower skin flap till the posterior axillary fold, made up by the subscapularis, teres major and latissimus dorsi muscles, is seen. Clean the fat and remove the lymph nodes and superficial veins to reach depth of the armpit. Identify two muscles arising from the tip of the coracoid process of scapula; out of these, the short head of biceps brachii muscle lies on the lateral side and the coracobrachialis on the medial side.

The pectoral muscles with the clavipectoral fascia form anterior boundary of the region.

Look for upper three intercostal muscles and serratus anterior muscle, which make the medial wall of axilla.

Clean the fat in the axilla carefully and identify the branches of the axillary artery, the axillary lymph nodes and the brachial plexus (Table 4.1).

BOUNDARIES

It resembles a four-sided pyramid. It has the following boundaries (Figs 4.2 and 4.3a and b):

- Apex
- Base
- *Four walls*: Anterior, posterior, medial and lateral.

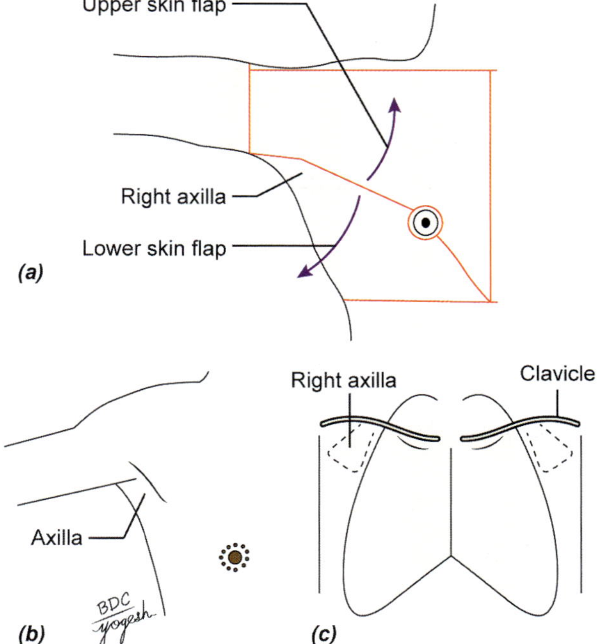

Figs 4.1a to c: (a) Dissection of axilla, (b) axilla in living body, and (c) relations to the skeleton

Flowchart 4.1: Axilla

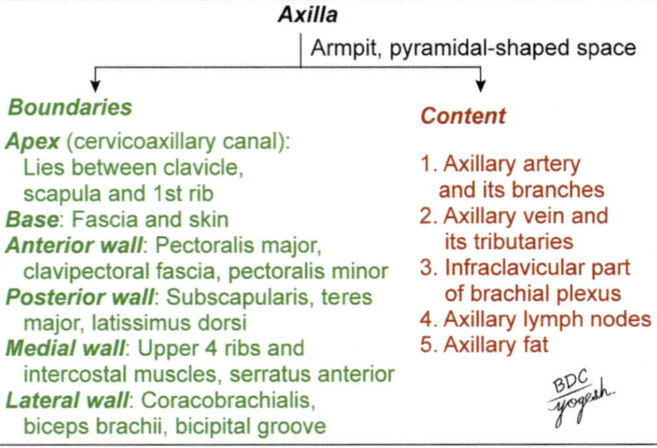

The axilla is disposed obliquely in such a way that the apex is directed upwards and medially towards the root of the neck, and the base is directed downwards.

Plate 4.1: Axilla: (a) Location and (b) walls of axilla

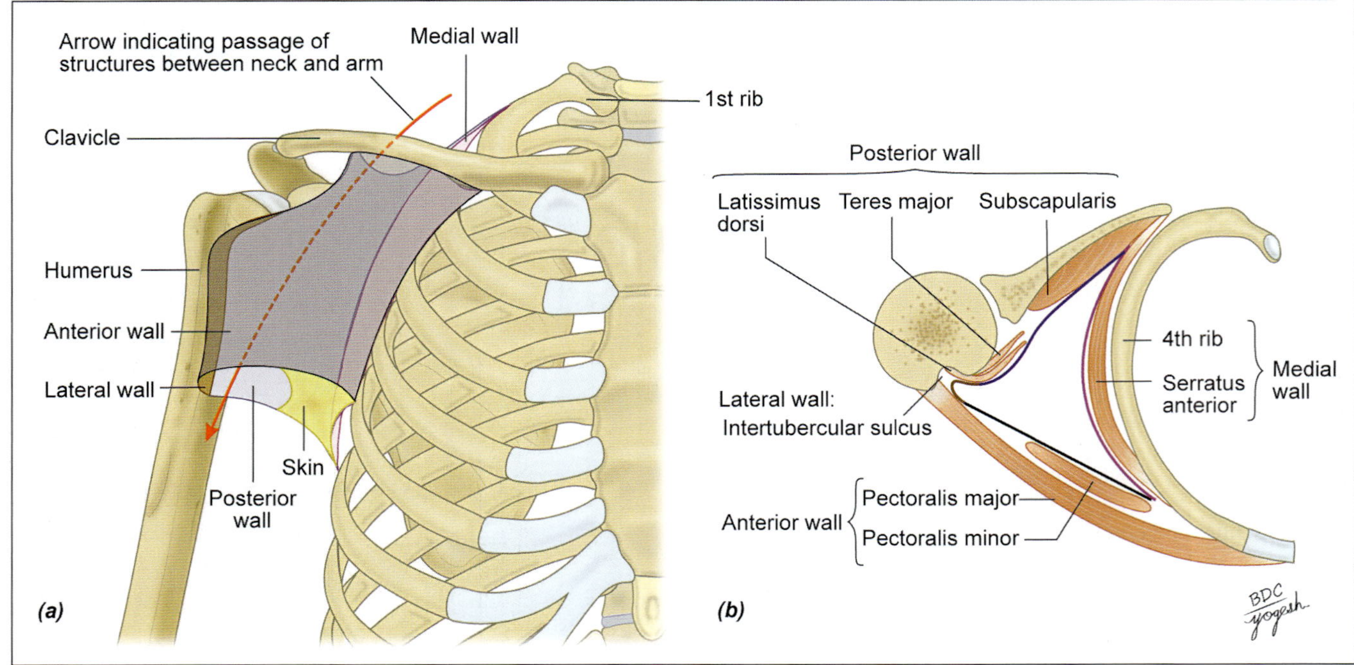

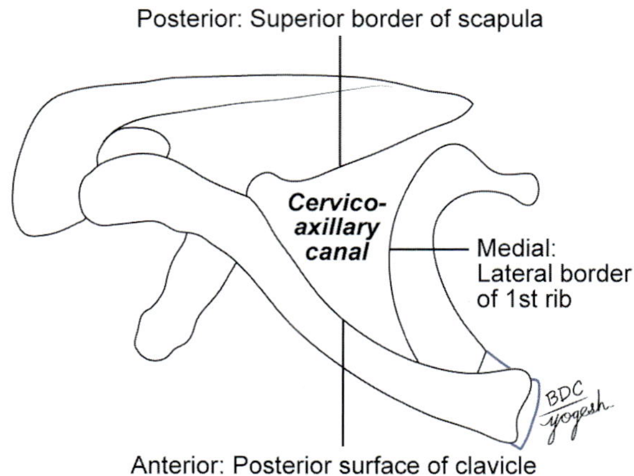

Fig. 4.2: Boundaries of apex of axilla or cervicoaxillary canal (superior view)

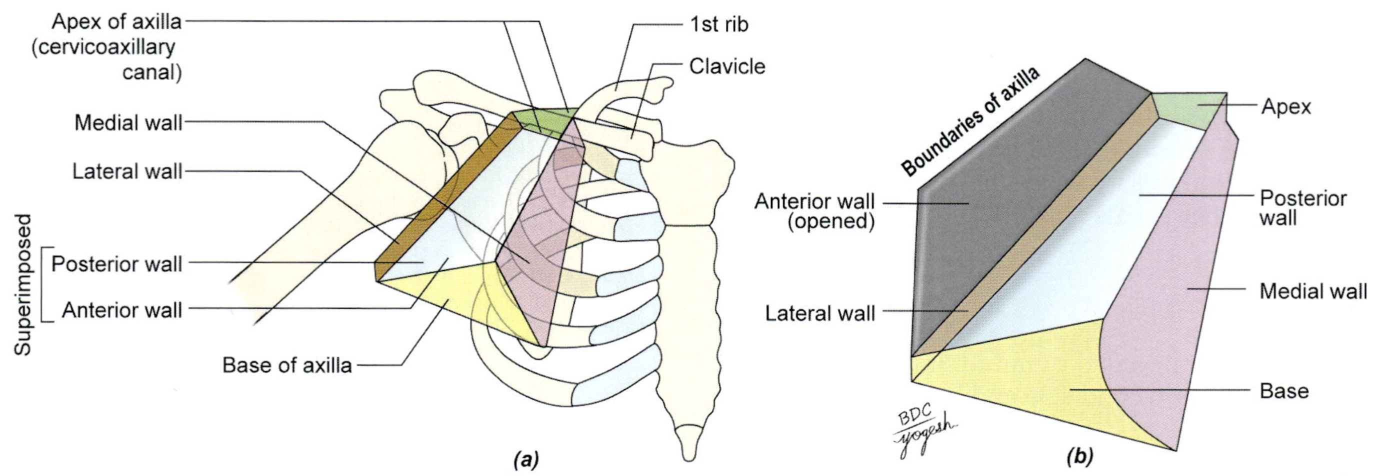

Figs 4.3a and b: (a) Walls of the axilla and (b) opened-up axilla

TABLE 4.1: Identification and locations of the structures in the axilla

Name of structure	*Identification*
Branches of axillary artery	
Superior thoracic artery	Runs along the superior border of pectoralis minor muscle.
Thoracoacromial trunk	Emerges at the superior border of pectoralis minor muscle. It pierces clavipectoral fascia and divides into four branches.
Lateral thoracic artery	Runs along the lateral border of pectoralis minor.
Subscapular artery	Runs along the lower border of subscapularis.
Anterior circumflex humeral artery	Passes in front of surgical neck of humerus.
Posterior circumflex humeral artery	Leaves axilla along with axillary nerve through quadrangular intermuscular space.
Axillary lymph nodes	
Anterior group	Lies along the lower border of the pectoralis minor along the lateral thoracic vessels.
Posterior group	Lies along the lower margin of the posterior wall of axilla along the subscapular vessels.
Lateral group	Lies posteromedial to the axillary vein.
Central group	Lies in the fat of the axilla.
Apical group	Lies behind and above the pectoralis minor, medial to the axillary vein.
Brachial plexus and its branches Cords	The 2nd part of the axillary artery is related laterally to the lateral cord, medially to the medial cord and posteriorly to the posterior cord.
Lateral pectoral nerve	Carefully reflect the pectoralis major upward to visualise the lateral pectoral nerve.
Musculocutaneous nerve	Musculocutaneous nerve pierces coracobrachialis muscle.
Median nerve	Lateral root of median nerve joins with medial root in front of 3rd part of axillary artery. Together, they form a 'Y'-shaped structure.
Medial pectoral nerve	Reflect pectoralis major laterally to visualise medial pectoral nerve, which pierces the pectoralis minor muscle.
Medial cutaneous nerve	Is a very thin nerve that runs on the medial side of axillary vein.
Medial cutaneous nerve of forearm	Is a thin nerve and runs downward between axillary artery and vein, anterior to the thicker ulnar nerve.
Axillary nerve	Lies posterolateral to the axillary artery and leaves the axilla through the quadrangular muscular space.
Radial nerve	Lies hidden behind the axillary artery.
Upper and lower subscapular nerves and nerve to latissimus dorsi	Run downwards posterior to the axillary artery and vein on the anterior surface of subscapularis muscle. Nerve to latissimus dorsi is larger and lies in between upper and lower subscapular nerves.
Long thoracic nerve	Passes on the lateral surface of serratus anterior muscle in midaxillary line.

Apex (Cervicoaxillary Canal)

It is directed upwards and medially towards the root of the neck (Fig. 4.2). It is truncated (not pointed) and corresponds to a triangular, oblique passage called the ***cervicoaxillary canal***. This canal is bounded:

- *Anteriorly*, by the posterior surface of clavicle.
- *Posteriorly*, by the superior border of the scapula and medial aspect of coracoid process.
- *Medially*, by the outer border of the first rib.

This canal gives passage to the axillary artery, axillary vein and brachial plexus in between the axilla and the neck.

Base or Floor

It is directed downwards. It is formed by skin, superficial and axillary fascia. Base of axilla extends from anterior to posterior axillary folds. Medially, it is continuous with the chest wall and laterally with the medial side of the arm. It is convex upwards.

Note: Axillary folds are folds of skin within which a margin of muscles is enclosed. *Anterior axillary fold* covers the lateral edge of pectoralis major muscle, and the *posterior axillary fold* covers the latissimus dorsi and teres major muscle.

Anterior Wall

It is formed by the following structures:

1. Pectoralis major in front (Fig. 4.4)
2. Clavipectoral fascia
3. Pectoralis minor.

Posterior Wall

It is formed by the following structures:

1. Subscapularis above (Plate 4.2)
2. Teres major
3. Latissimus dorsi below.

Plate 4.2: Muscles forming posterior wall of right axilla

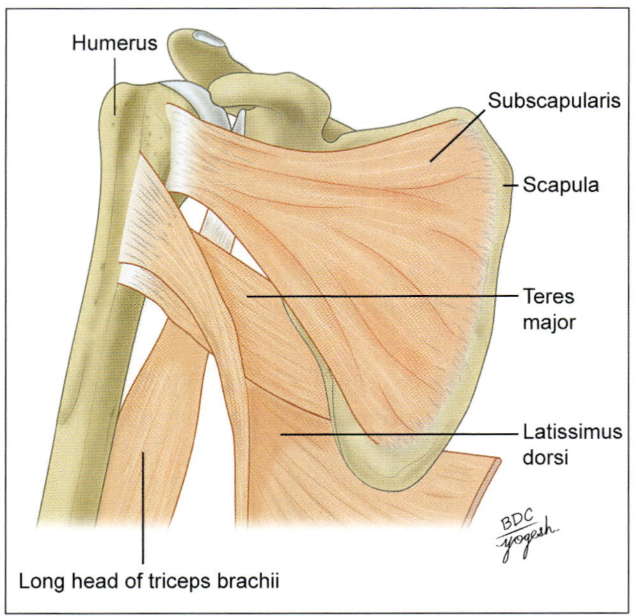

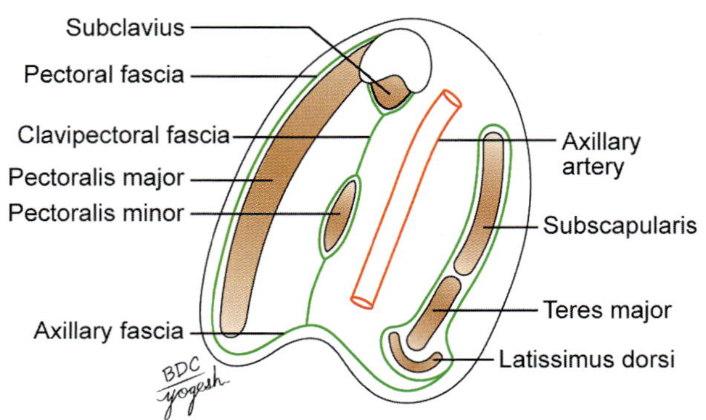

Fig. 4.4: Anterior and posterior walls and the base of the axilla with the axillary artery

Medial Wall

It is convex laterally and formed by the following structures:

1. Upper four ribs with their intercostal muscles.
2. Upper part of the serratus anterior muscle (Plates 4.1 and 4.3, Fig. 4.5).

Lateral Wall

It is very narrow because the anterior and posterior walls converge on it. It is formed by the following structures:

1. Upper part of the shaft of the humerus in the region of the bicipital groove.
2. Coracobrachialis and short head of the biceps brachii (Fig. 4.5).

CONTENTS OF AXILLA

1. Axillary artery and its branches (Plate 4.3, Figs 4.5 to 4.8)
2. Axillary vein and its tributaries
3. Infraclavicular part of the brachial plexus
4. Axillary lymph nodes
5. Long thoracic and intercostobrachial nerves

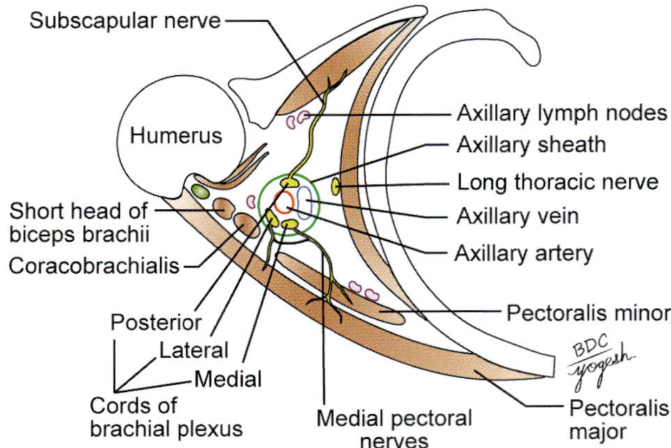

Fig. 4.5: Content of axilla (right)

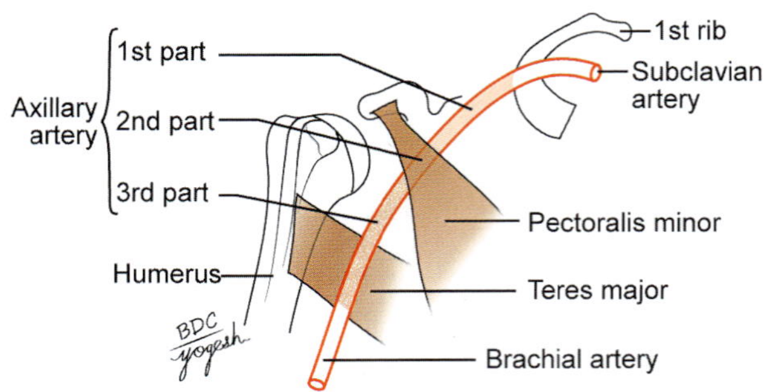

Fig. 4.6: The extent and parts of the axillary artery

6. Axillary tail of mammary gland
7. Axillary fat and areolar tissue in which the other contents are embedded.

CLINICAL ANATOMY

The axilla has abundant axillary hair. Infection of the hair follicles and sebaceous glands gives rise to boils, which are common in this area.

Competency:

AN10.2 Identify, describe and demonstrate the origin, extent, course, parts, relations and branches of axillary artery and tributaries of vein.

AXILLARY ARTERY

Axillary artery is the continuation of the subclavian artery. It extends from the outer border of the 1st rib to the lower border of the teres major muscle, where it continues as the brachial artery. Its direction varies with the position of the arm.

Parts

Axillary artery is crossed anteriorly by pectoralis minor muscle. The crossing of pectoralis minor muscle divides the axillary artery into the following three parts (Fig. 4.6, Flowchart 4.2):

1. **First part**, superior or proximal to the muscle.
2. **Second part**, posterior or deep to the muscle.
3. **Third part**, inferior or distal to the muscle.

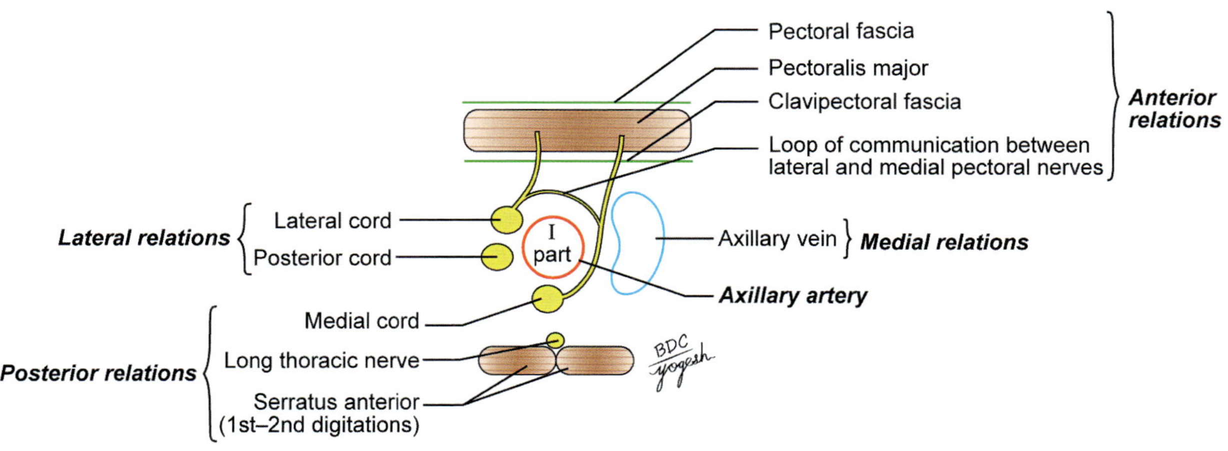

Fig. 4.7a: Diagrammatic relations of first part of axillary artery

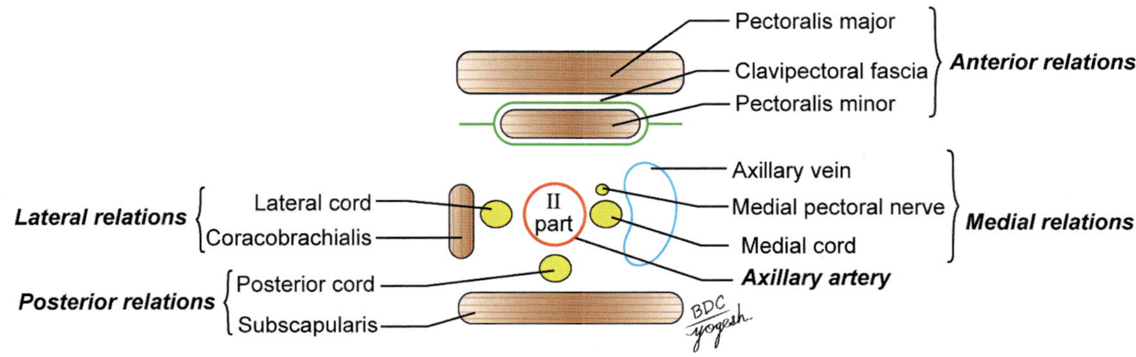

Fig. 4.7b: Diagrammatic relations of second part of axillary artery

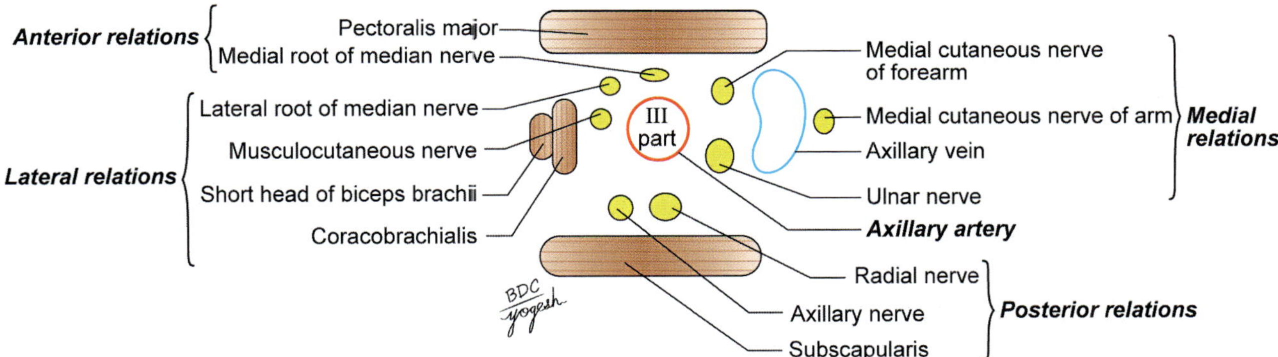

Fig. 4.7c: Diagrammatic relations of third part of axillary artery (proximal part)

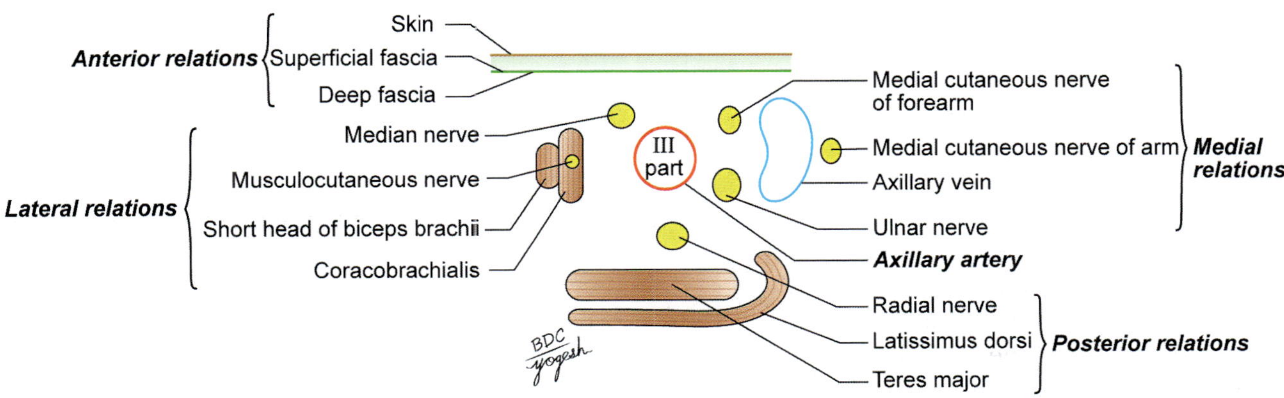

Fig. 4.7d: Diagrammatic relations of third part of axillary artery (distal part)

Plate 4.3: Content of right axilla

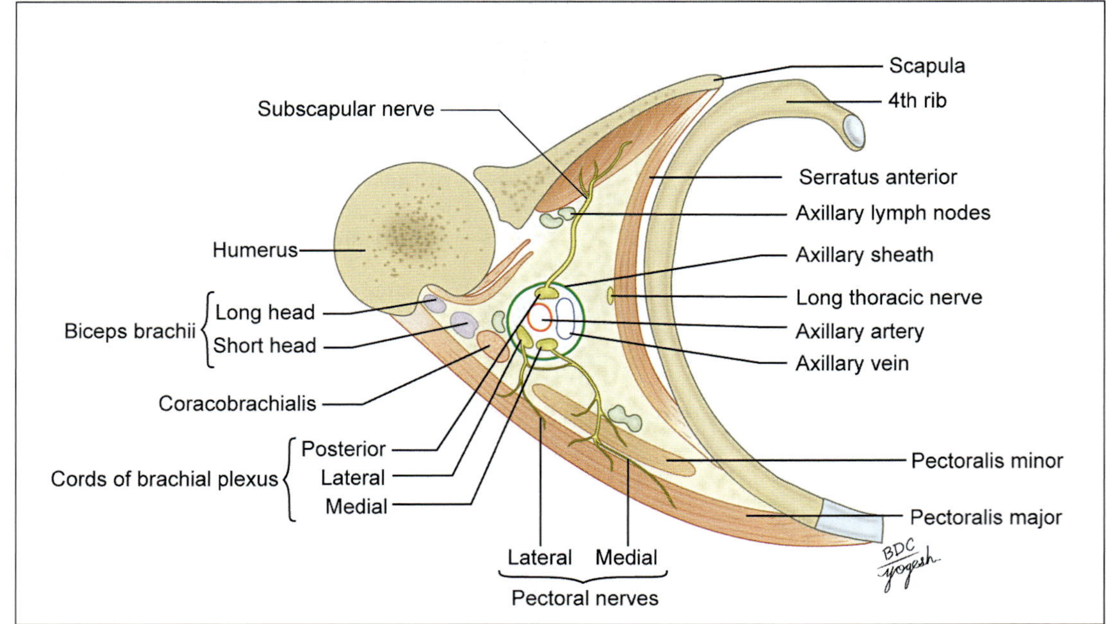

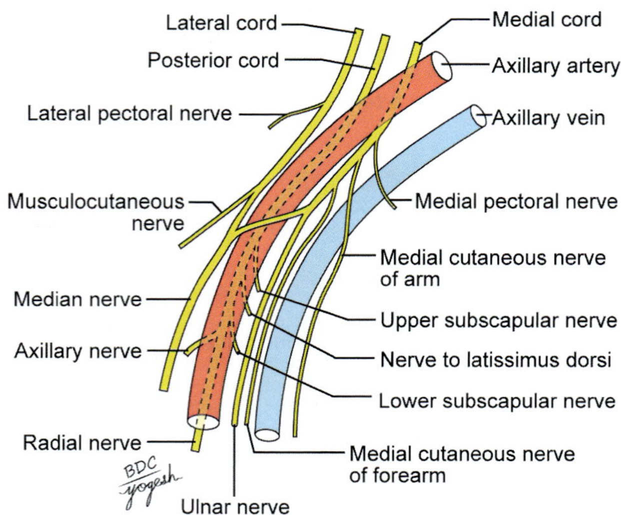

Fig. 4.8: Relation of the brachial plexus to the axillary artery

Flowchart 4.2: Axillary artery

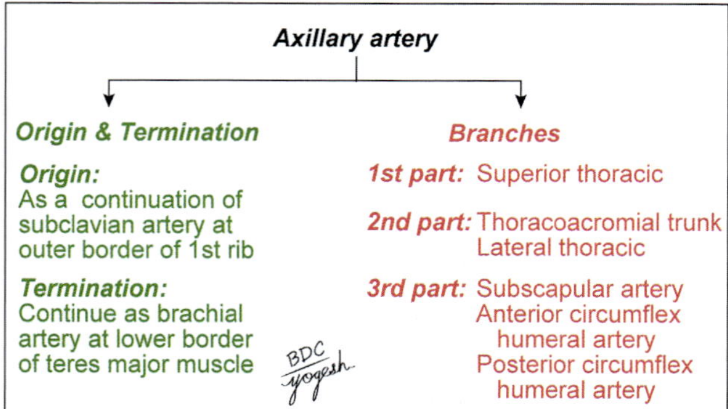

RELATIONS OF AXILLARY ARTERY

The axillary artery is related to the corresponding walls of axilla and accompanied by the axillary vein on the medial side (Plate 4.4). The first part of the axillary artery is enclosed (together with the brachial plexus) in the axillary sheath, derived from the prevertebral layer of deep cervical fascia. The other specific relations of axillary artery are described as relation of 1st, 2nd and 3rd parts are given below.

Relations of 1st Part

Anterior

1. Skin
2. Superficial fascia, platysma and supraclavicular nerves
3. Deep fascia
4. Clavicular part of the pectoralis major (Fig. 4.7a)
5. Clavipectoral fascia
6. Loop of communication between the lateral and medial pectoral nerves.

Posterior

1. Medial cord of brachial plexus
2. Nerve to serratus anterior
3. 1st and 2nd digitations of the serratus anterior
4. 1st intercostal space.

Lateral

1. Lateral and posterior cords of the brachial plexus.

Medial

1. Axillary vein.

Relations of 2nd Part

Anterior

1. Skin
2. Superficial fascia
3. Deep fascia
4. Pectoralis major
5. Pectoralis minor (Fig. 4.7b).

Plate 4.4: Relations of contents of axilla

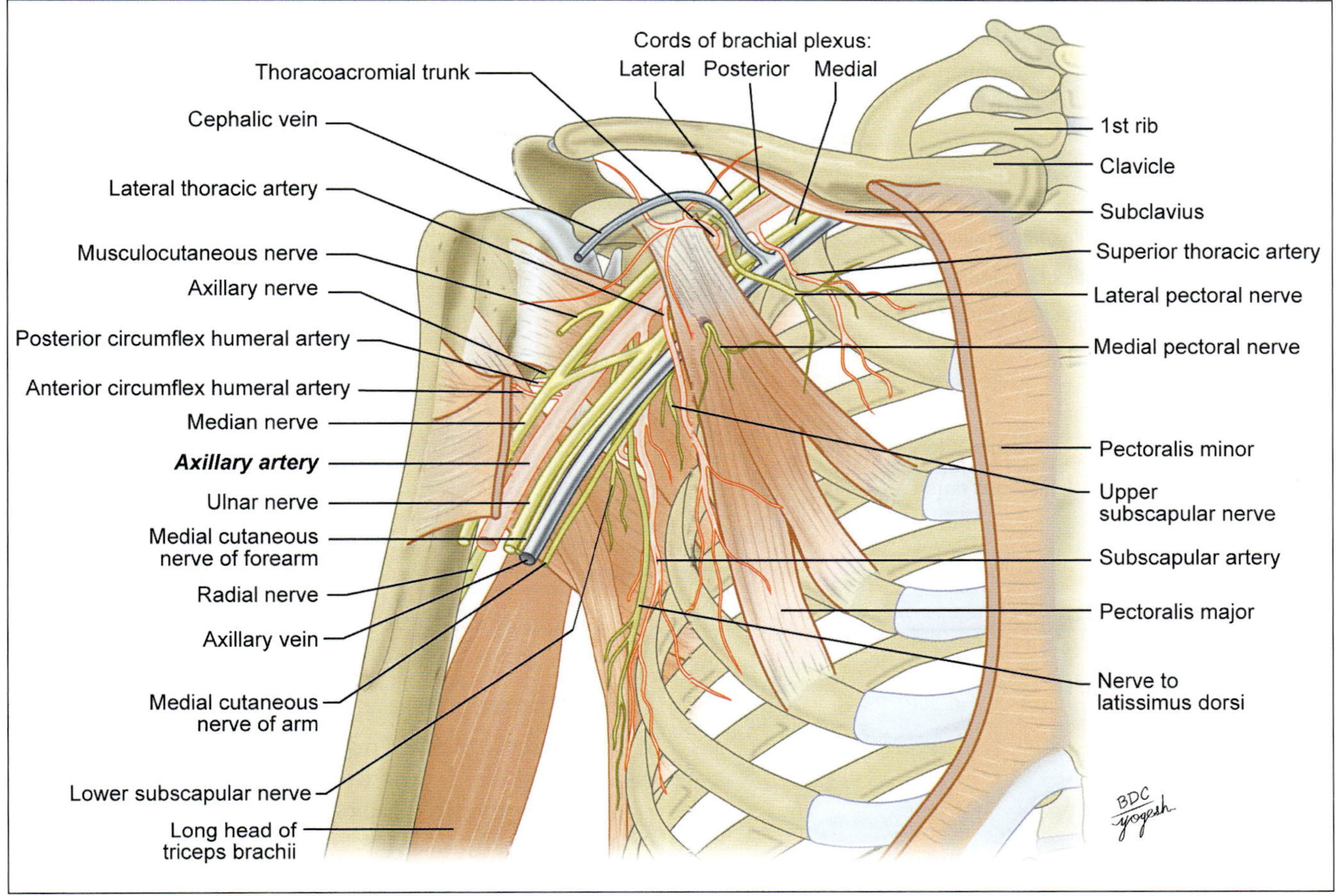

Posterior

1. Posterior cord of brachial plexus
2. Subscapularis.

Lateral

1. Lateral cord of brachial plexus (Fig. 4.8)
2. Coracobrachialis.

Medial

1. Medial cord of brachial plexus
2. Medial pectoral nerve
3. Axillary vein.

Relations of 3rd Part

Anterior

1. Skin
2. Superficial fascia
3. Deep fascia
4. Medial root of the median nerve
5. Pectoralis major (in the upper part only).

Posterior

1. Radial nerve (Plate 4.4)
2. Axillary nerve in the upper part
3. Subscapularis in the upper part
4. Tendons of the latissimus dorsi and the teres major in the lower part (Fig. 4.7d).

Lateral

1. Musculocutaneous nerve in the upper part (Fig. 4.8)
2. Lateral root of median nerve in the upper part
3. Trunk of median nerve in the lower part
4. Coracobrachialis.

Medial

1. Medial cutaneous nerve of the forearm
2. Ulnar nerve
3. Axillary vein
4. Medial cutaneous nerve of arm.

Branches

The axillary artery gives six branches, one from the 1st part, two from the 2nd part and three branches from the 3rd part (Plate 4.5, Fig. 4.9).

1st part:	Superior thoracic artery
2nd part:	Thoracoacromial trunk,
	Lateral thoracic artery
3rd part:	Subscapular artery
	Anterior circumflex humeral artery
	Posterior circumflex humeral artery.

Superior Thoracic Artery

It is a very small branch that arises from the 1st part of the axillary artery (near the subclavius). It runs along the superior border of pectoralis minor muscle. It supplies

Plate 4.5: Branches of axillary artery

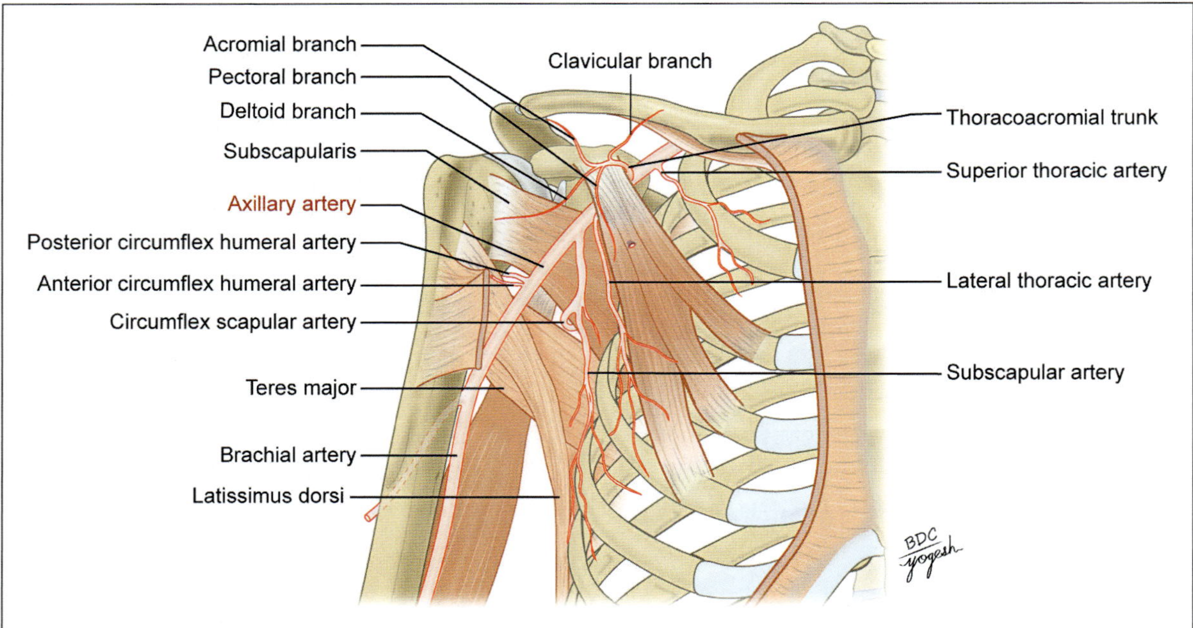

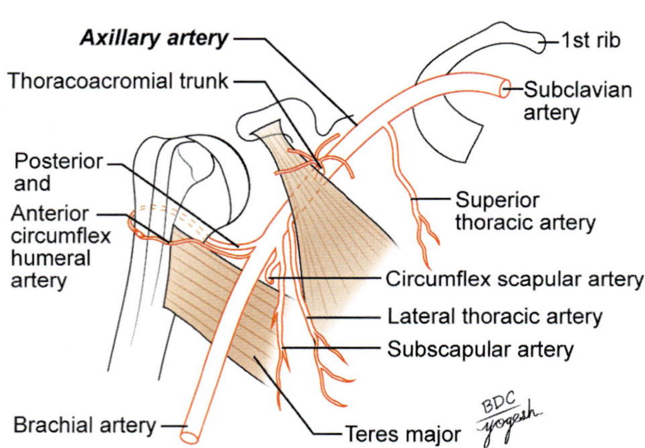

Fig. 4.9: The branches of the axillary artery

pectoralis major and minor muscles and the thoracic wall (Fig. 4.9).

Thoracoacromial (Acromiothoracic) Artery

It is a branch from the 2nd part of the axillary artery. It emerges at the upper border of the pectoralis minor, pierces the clavipectoral fascia and soon divides into the following four terminal radiating branches:

1. The *pectoral branch* passes between the pectoral muscles and supplies pectoral muscles and the breast.
2. The *deltoid branch* runs in the deltopectoral groove, along with the cephalic vein.
3. The *acromial branch* joins the anastomoses over the acromion process.
4. The *clavicular branch* runs superomedially deep to the pectoralis major and supplies the acromioclavicular joint and subclavius.

[*Mnemonic*: "ABCD": **A**cromial, **B**reast (pectoral), **C**lavicular, **D**eltoid).

Lateral Thoracic Artery

It is a branch of the 2nd part of the axillary artery. It emerges at, and runs along, the lower border of the pectoralis minor in close relation with the anterior group of axillary lymph nodes.

In females, the artery is large and gives off the lateral mammary branches to the breast.

Subscapular Artery

It is the largest branch of the axillary artery, arising from its 3rd part. It runs along the lower border of the subscapularis to terminate near the inferior angle of the scapula. It supplies the latissimus dorsi and the serratus anterior.

It gives off a large branch, the ***circumflex scapular artery***, which passes through the upper triangular intermuscular space and winds around the lateral border of the scapula between two slips of the teres minor to enter the infraspinous fossa. The subscapular artery and its branches give numerous branches that anastomoses around the scapula. It also gives ***thoracodorsal artery*** which runs inferiorly with the thoracodorsal nerve and supplies the latissimus dorsi.

Anterior Circumflex Humeral Artery

It is a small branch arising from the 3rd part of the axillary artery at the lower border of the subscapularis.

It passes laterally and anastomoses with the posterior circumflex humeral artery to form an arterial circle round the surgical neck of the humerus.

It gives off an *ascending branch*, which runs in the intertubercular sulcus, and supplies the head of the humerus and shoulder joint (Fig. 4.9).

Posterior Circumflex Humeral Artery

It is much larger than the anterior artery. It arises from the 3rd part of the axillary artery at the lower border of the subscapularis. It runs backwards, accompanied by the axillary nerve, passes through the *quadrangular intermuscular* space and ends by anastomosing with the anterior circumflex humeral artery around the surgical neck of the humerus.

It supplies the shoulder joint, the deltoid and the muscles bounding the quadrangular space.

It gives off a *descending branch,* which anastomoses with the ascending branch of the *profunda brachii artery*.

CLINICAL ANATOMY

Axillary arterial pulsations can be felt against the lower part of the lateral wall of the axilla. In order to check bleeding from the distal part of the limb (in injuries, operations and amputations), the artery can be effectively compressed against the humerus in the lower part of the lateral wall of the axilla.

AXILLARY VEIN

The axillary vein is the continuation of the basilic vein at the lower border of the teres major muscle. It runs upward on the medial side of the axillary artery (Fig. 4.10). At the outer border of the first rib, it becomes the subclavian vein.

Tributaries

1. Brachial veins (formed by venae comitantes along radial and ulnar arteries).

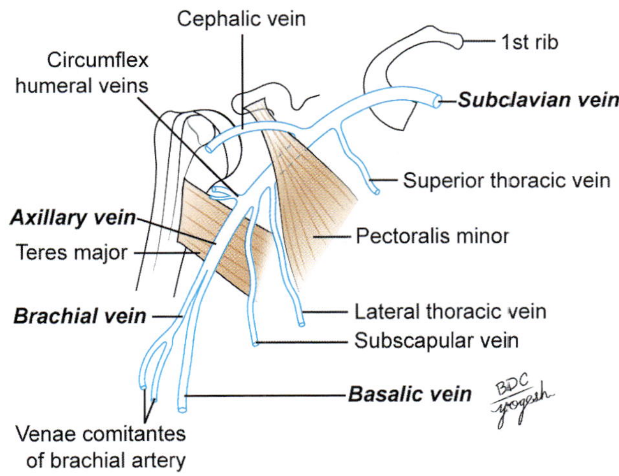

Fig. 4.10: Axillary vein: Formation and tributaries

2. Tributaries corresponding to the branches of axillary artery (except that of thoracoacromial trunk)
3. Cephalic vein.

Note: The axillary vein lies outside the axillary sheath, which permits the required expansion of the axillary vein during venous return. Veins accompanying branches of thoracoacromial artery drain directly into the cephalic vein. Lateral thoracic vein of upper limb is joined to superficial epigastric vein of lower limb by thoracoepigastric vein enabling blood to return to heart in blockage of inferior vena cava.

Old concept: The axillary vein is formed by union of basilic vein and brachial vein.

Competencies:

AN10.4 Describe the anatomical groups of axillary lymph nodes and specify their areas of drainage.

AN10.7 Describe axillary lymph nodes, areas of drainage and anatomical basis of their enlargement.

AXILLARY LYMPH NODES

The axillary lymph nodes are scattered in the fibrofatty tissue of the axilla. They are divided into the following five groups:

1. ***Anterior (pectoral) group*** lies along the lateral thoracic vessels, i.e. along the lower border of the pectoralis minor. They receive lymph from the upper half of the anterior wall of the trunk, and from the major part of the breast (Flowchart 4.3, Fig. 4.11).
2. ***Posterior (scapular) group*** lies along the subscapular vessels on the posterior axillary fold. They receive lymph from the posterior wall of the upper half of the trunk and from the axillary tail of the breast.
3. ***Lateral group*** lies along the upper part of the humerus, medial to the axillary vein. They receive lymph from the upper limb.
4. ***Central group*** lies in the fat of the upper axilla. They receive lymph from the preceding groups and drain into the apical group. They receive some direct vessels from the floor of the axilla.
5. ***Apical or infraclavicular group*** lies deep to the clavipectoral fascia, along the axillary vessels. They receive lymph from the central group, from the upper part of the breast and from the thumb and its web. The lymphatics from the thumb accompany the cephalic vein. Anterior and central groups of nodes are often involved in carcinoma breast.

Flowchart 4.3: Axillary lymph nodes

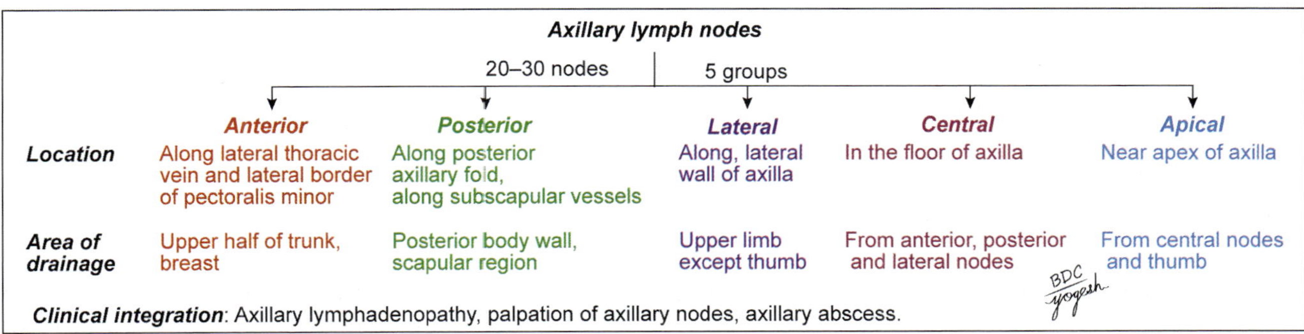

Axillary lymph nodes

20–30 nodes | 5 groups

	Anterior	*Posterior*	*Lateral*	*Central*	*Apical*
Location	Along lateral thoracic vein and lateral border of pectoralis minor	Along posterior axillary fold, along subscapular vessels	Along, lateral wall of axilla	In the floor of axilla	Near apex of axilla
Area of drainage	Upper half of trunk, breast	Posterior body wall, scapular region	Upper limb except thumb	From anterior, posterior and lateral nodes	From central nodes and thumb

Clinical integration: Axillary lymphadenopathy, palpation of axillary nodes, axillary abscess.

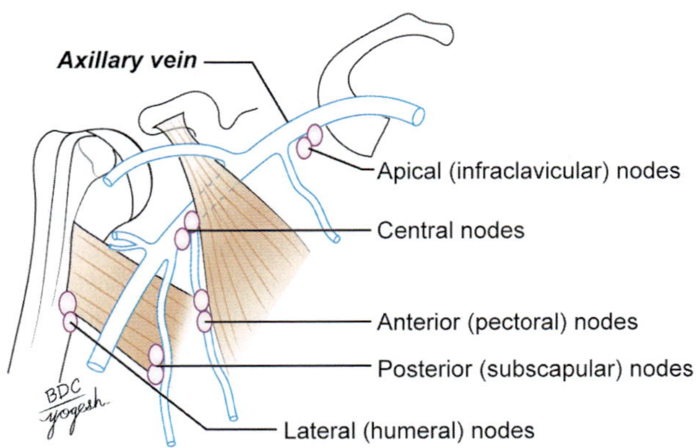

Fig. 4.11: The axillary lymph nodes

CLINICAL ANATOMY

- ***Axillary lymphadenopathy***: The axillary lymph nodes drain lymph not only from the upper limb but also from the breast and the anterior and posterior body walls above the level of the umbilicus. Therefore, infections or malignant growths in any part of their territory of drainage give rise to *axillary lymphadenopathy* (enlargement of the lymph nodes) (Fig. 4.12).
- **Bimanual examination** of axillary lymph nodes is important in clinical practice. Left axillary nodes have to be palpated by right hand. Right axillary nodes have to be palpated by left hand. An axillary abscess should be incised through the floor of the axilla, midway between the anterior and posterior axillary folds and nearer to the medial wall in order to avoid injury to the main vessels running along the anterior, posterior and lateral walls.
- The axillary tail of Spence of the breast comes in contact with anterior group of axillary nodes. Therefore, cancer involving axillary tail of the breast may be misdiagnosed as an enlarged lymph node.
- The central group of nodes is in close relationship with intercostobrachial nerve. Hence, enlarged nodes may compress this nerve and cause pain along the inner border of arm.
- ***Axillary abscess*** may occur due to pus formation in the enlarged and infected axillary nodes. It can be drained by giving incision in the floor of axilla midway between anterior and posterior axillary walls, near the medial wall (to avoid injury to major vessels and nerves).

SPINAL NERVE

There are 31 pairs of spinal nerves. Each spinal nerve is formed by union of dorsal root and ventral root. *Dorsal root* is sensory and is characterised by the presence of *spinal* or *dorsal root ganglion* and enters the dorsal horn and posterior funiculus of spinal cord. *Ventral root* is motor and arises from anterior horn cells of spinal cord (Fig. 4.13). The motor and sensory fibres get united in the spinal nerve, which divides into short dorsal ramus and long ventral ramus. Dorsal ramus supplies muscles and skin of back, whereas the ventral ramus supplies anterolateral part of trunk and limb.

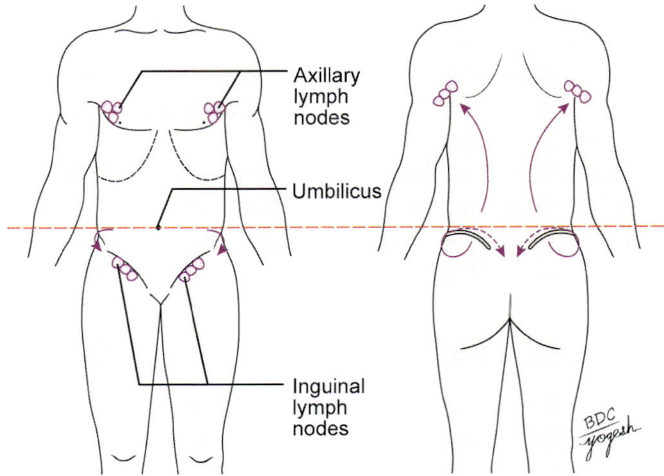

Fig. 4.12: Lymph above umbilicus drains into axillary lymph nodes while below umbilicus drains into inguinal group

Only the ventral primary rami form nerve plexuses. Brachial plexus is formed by ventral primary rami of C5–C8 and T1 segments of spinal cord.

Sympathetic fibres arising from lateral horn cells enter the ventral root and then the chain of sympathetic ganglion via grey rami communicantes. Postganglionic sympathetic fibres join spinal nerve through white rami communicantes.

Competencies:

AN10.3 Describe, identify and demonstrate formation, branches, relations, area of supply of branches, course and relations of terminal branches of brachial plexus.

AN10.5 Explain variations in formation of brachial plexus.

BRACHIAL PLEXUS

The brachial plexus is the nerve plexus that is derived from ventral (or anterior) primary rami of lower four cervical spinal nerves (C5–C8) and 1st thoracic spinal nerve (T1).

Components of Brachial Plexus

- Brachial plexus consists of the following components (Plate 4.4, Fig. 4.14, Flowchart 4.4):
  1. Roots: Ventral primary rami of C5–C8 and T1 nerves.
  2. Trunks: Three trunks derived from roots (upper, middle and lower).
  3. Divisions: Each trunk divides into anterior and posterior divisions.
  4. Cords: Divisions join to form three cords (medial, lateral and posterior).
  5. Branches: Various nerves arise from each cord.

[*Mnemonic*: "Ramu Tailor Drinks Cold Beer": **R**oots, **T**runks, **D**ivisions, **C**ords, **B**ranches]

- Relations of brachial plexus with clavicle: *Supraclavicular part* of brachial plexus includes roots and trunks, *retroclavicular part* includes divisions of trunks and *infraclavicular part* includes cords and their branches.

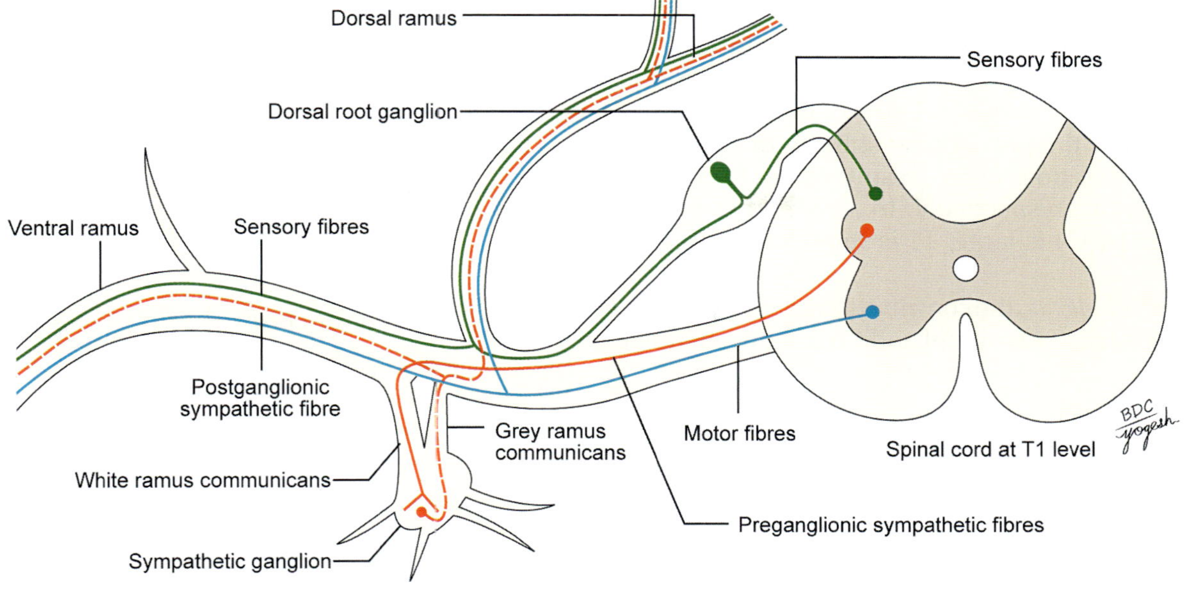

Fig. 4.13: Mixed fibres of a spinal nerve

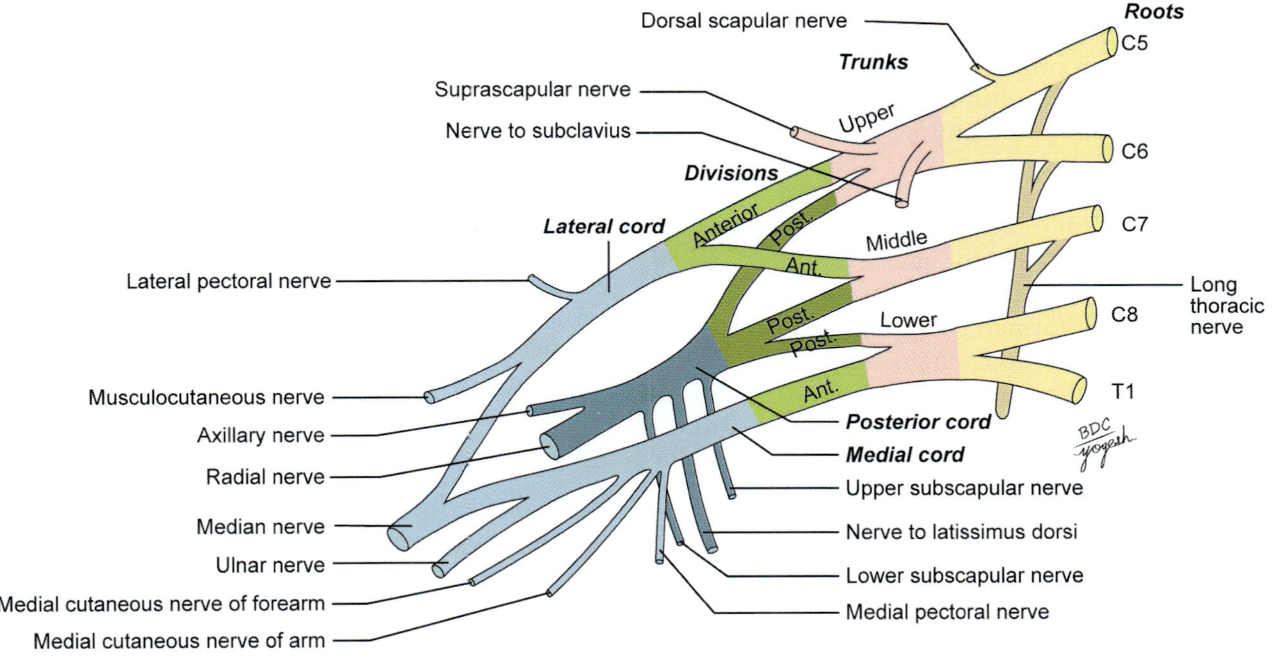

Fig. 4.14: The right brachial plexus

Flowchart 4.4: Brachial plexus

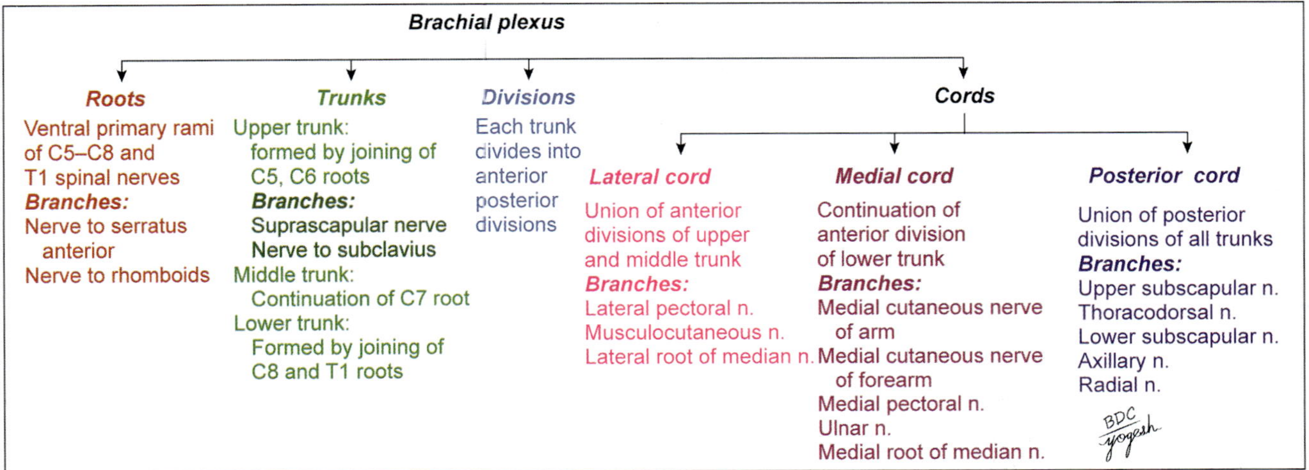

Roots

These are constituted by the ventral primary rami of spinal nerves C5–C8 and T1, with occasional contributions from the ventral primary rami of C4 and T2 (Fig. 4.14).

The origin of the plexus may shift by one segment, either upward or downward, resulting in a prefixed or postfixed plexus, respectively. In a *prefixed plexus*, the contribution by C4 is large, T1 is small and T2 is often absent.

In a *postfixed plexus*, the contribution by T1 is large, T2 is always present, C4 is absent and C5 is reduced in size.

Trunks

Roots of the brachial plexus join to form three trunks as follows:

1. *Upper trunk* formed by joining of C5 and C6 roots.
2. *Middle trunk* as a continuation of C7 root.
3. *Lower trunk* formed by joining C8 and T1 roots.

Trunks lie deep in the neck between scalenus anterior and scalenus medius muscles.

Divisions of the Trunks

Each trunk (three in number) divides into ventral and dorsal divisions (which ultimately supply the anterior and posterior aspects of the limb).

Cords and Branches

Divisions join to form three cords:

1. The *lateral cord* is formed by the union of ventral divisions of the upper and middle trunks (two divisions).
2. The *medial cord* is formed by the ventral division of the lower trunk (one division).
3. The *posterior cord* is formed by union of the dorsal divisions of all the three trunks (three divisions). These are named according to relation of cords to the 2nd part of axillary artery.

Branches

The root value of each branch is given in brackets.

Branches of the Roots

1. Nerve to serratus anterior (long thoracic nerve) (C5, C6, C7)
2. Nerve to rhomboids (dorsal scapular nerve) (C5)
3. Branches to longus colli and scaleni muscles (C5– C8) and branch to phrenic nerve (C4).

Branches of the Trunks

These arise only from the upper trunk:

1. Suprascapular nerve (C5, C6)
2. Nerve to subclavius (C5, C6).

Branches of the Cords

Branches of lateral cord

1. Lateral pectoral nerve (C5–C7)
2. Musculocutaneous nerve (C5–C7)
3. Lateral root of median nerve (C5–C7).

[*Mnemonic*: "**LML**"]

Branches of medial cord

1. Medial pectoral nerve (C8, T1)
2. Medial cutaneous nerve of arm (C8, T1)
3. Medial cutaneous nerve of forearm (C8, T1)
4. Ulnar nerve (C7, C8, T1)
5. Medial root of median nerve (C8, T1) (joins the lateral root to form the median nerve).

[*Mnemonic*: "**M4U**"]

Branches of posterior cord

1. Upper subscapular nerve (C5, C6)
2. Nerve to latissimus dorsi (C6–C8)
3. Lower subscapular nerve (C5, C6)
4. Axillary (circumflex) nerve (C5, C6)
5. Radial nerve (C5–C8, T1).

[*Mnemonic*: "**U**dit **N**ever **L**eave **A** **R**ainbow"]

In addition to the branches of the brachial plexus, the upper limb is also supplied near the trunk by the supraclavicular branches of the cervical plexus and by the intercostobrachial branch of the second intercostal nerve. Sympathetic nerves are distributed through the brachial plexus.

Kuntz's nerve is the communicating branch between T1 and T2 nerves, which carry sympathetic fibres from 3rd thoracic ganglion to the upper limb via T2 nerve.

Blood Supply of Brachial Plexus

Vertebral artery and thyrocervical trunk with its branches, the suprascapular and transverse cervical arteries, supply blood to the brachial plexus. These are the lifeline of this important plexus.

DISSECTION

After cleaning the branches of the axillary artery, proceed to clean the brachial plexus. It is formed by the ventral primary rami of the lower four cervicals (C5–C8) and the first thoracic (T1) nerves. The first and second parts of the axillary artery are related to the cords, and third part is related to the branches of the plexus.

Reflect upward carefully pectoralis major to visualise lateral pectoral nerve. Musculocutaneous nerve pierces coracobrachialis muscle. Lateral root of median nerve joins with medial root in front of 3rd part of axillary artery. Together, it forms a 'Y' shaped structure.

Reflect pectoralis major laterally to visualise medial pectoral nerve, which pierces the pectoralis minor muscle. The medial cutaneous nerve of arm is a very thin nerve that runs on medial side of axillary vein. The medial cutaneous nerve of forearm is a thin nerve and runs downward between axillary artery and vein, anterior to the thicker ulnar nerve.

Axillary nerve lies posterolateral to the axillary artery and leaves the axilla through the quadrangular muscular space. The radial nerve lies hidden behind the axillary artery. The upper and lower subscapular nerves and nerve to latissimus dorsi run downwards posterior to the axillary artery and vein, on the anterior surface of subscapularis muscle. Nerve to latissimus dorsi is larger and lies in between upper and lower subscapular nerves.

Long thoracic nerve passes on the lateral surface of serratus anterior muscle in midaxillary line.

Competency:

AN10.6 Explain the anatomical basis of clinical features of Erb's palsy and Klumpke's paralysis.

CLINICAL ANATOMY

Global total brachial plexus birth palsy is the most severe type of paralysis.

Erb's Paralysis

Erb's paralysis or palsy is the paralysis of arm caused by injury to upper trunk of brachial plexus [Wilhelm Heinrich Erb, German Neurologist, 1840–1921].

Site of injury: One region of the upper trunk of the brachial plexus is called Erb's point (Fig. 4.15). Six nerves meet here. Injury to the upper trunk causes Erb's paralysis.

Nerve roots involved: Mainly C5 and partly C6.

Causes of injury: Undue separation of the head from the shoulder, which is commonly encountered in the following:

1. Birth injury/difficult childbirth (Fig. 4.16)
2. Fall on the shoulder
3. During anaesthesia.

Muscles paralysed: Mainly biceps brachii, deltoid, brachialis and brachioradialis. Partly supraspinatus, infraspinatus and supinator.

Deformity and position of the limb:

- *Arm*: Hangs by the side; it is adducted and medially rotated.
- *Forearm*: Extended and pronated. The deformity is known as '***policeman's tip hand***' or '***waiter's tip hand***' or '***porter's tip hand***' (Fig. 4.17).

Disability: The following movements are lost.

- Abduction and lateral rotation of the arm at shoulder joint.
- Flexion and supination of the forearm.
- Biceps and supinator jerks are lost.
- Sensations are lost over a small area over the lower part of the deltoid.

Klumpke's Paralysis

Klumpke's paralysis or palsy is the injury of the lower trunk of brachial plexus, causing paralysis of hand muscles.

Site of injury: Lower trunk of the brachial plexus.

Cause of injury: Undue abduction of the arm, as in clutching something with the hands after a fall from a height, or sometimes in birth injury (Fig. 4.18, Flowchart 4.5).

Nerve roots involved: Mainly T1 and partly C8.

Muscles paralysed:

- Intrinsic muscles of the hand (T1).
- Ulnar flexors of the wrist and fingers (C8).

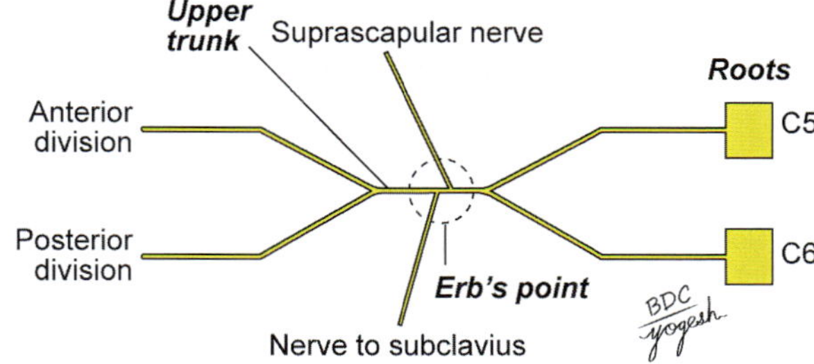

Fig. 4.15: Erb's point

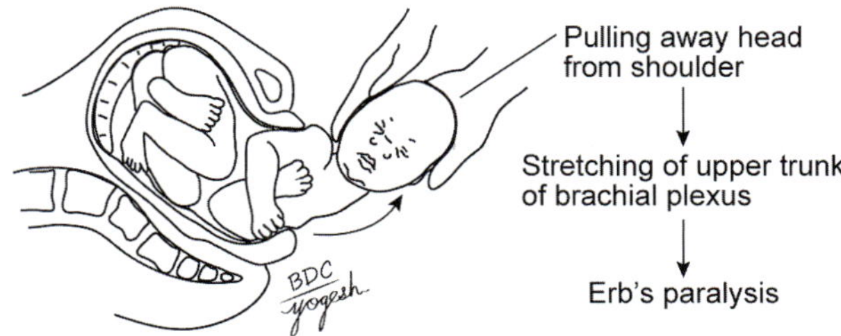

Fig. 4.16: Causes of injury in Erb's paralysis

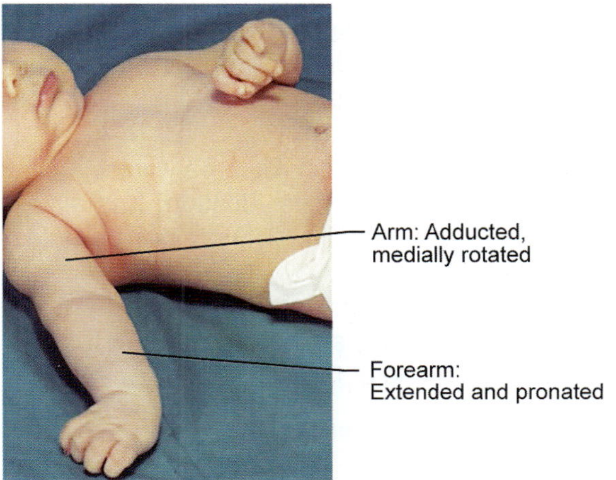

Fig. 4.17: Erb's paralysis of right arm

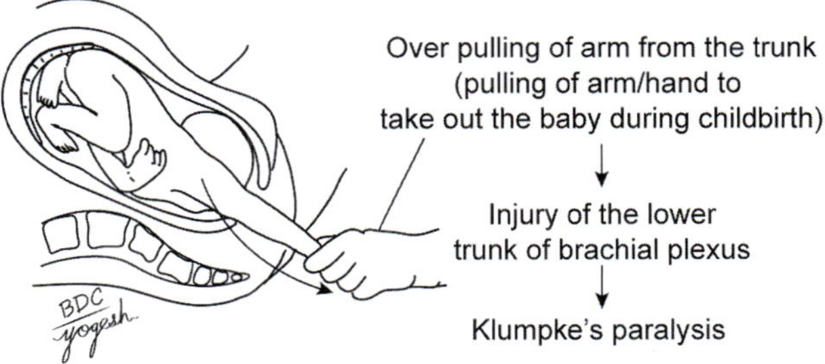

Fig. 4.18: Causes of injury in Klumpke's paralysis

Deformity and position of the hand: Claw hand due to the unopposed action of the long flexors and extensors of the fingers. In a claw hand, there is hyperextension at the metacarpophalangeal joints and flexion at the interphalangeal joints.

Disability:

- Complete claw hand (Fig. 4.19).
- Cutaneous anaesthesia and analgesia in a narrow zone along the ulnar border of the forearm and hand.
- *Horner's syndrome:* If T1 is injured proximal to white ramus communicantes to 1st thoracic sympathetic

Flowchart 4.5: Erb's and Klumpke's paralysis

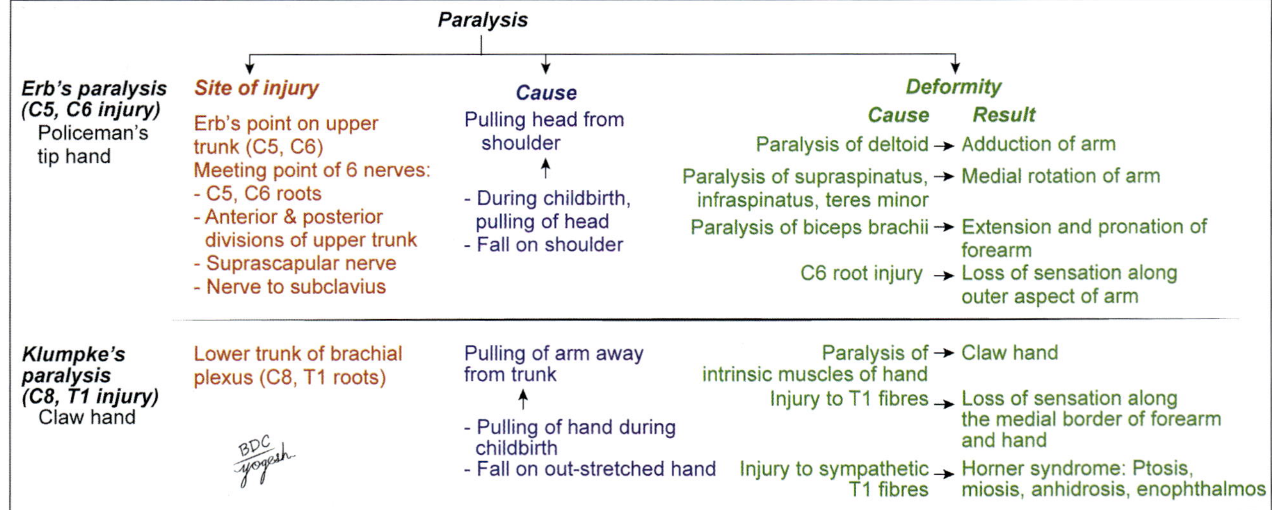

ganglion, there is ptosis, miosis, anhydrosis, enophthalmos and loss of ciliospinal reflex—may be associated. This is because of injury to sympathetic fibres to the head and neck that leave the spinal cord through nerve T1 (Fig. 4.20).

- *Vasomotor changes:* The skin area with sensory loss is warmer due to arteriolar dilation. It is also drier due to the absence of sweating as there is loss of sympathetic activity.
- *Trophic changes:* Long-standing case of paralysis leads to dry and scaly skin. The nails crack easily with atrophy of the pulp of fingers.

Injury to the Nerve to Serratus Anterior (Nerve of Bell)

Causes:

1. Sudden pressure on the shoulder from above.
2. Carrying heavy loads on the shoulder.

Deformity: Winging of the scapula, i.e. excessive prominence of the medial border of the scapula.

Normally, the pull of the muscle keeps the medial border against the thoracic wall.

Disability:

- Loss of pushing and punching actions. During attempts at pushing, there occurs winging of the scapula.
- Overhead abduction of shoulder girdle is partly affected due to intact trapezius muscle.

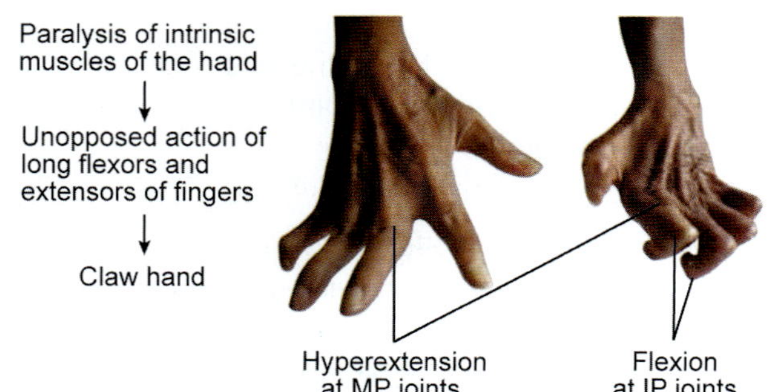

Fig. 4.19: Complete claw hand

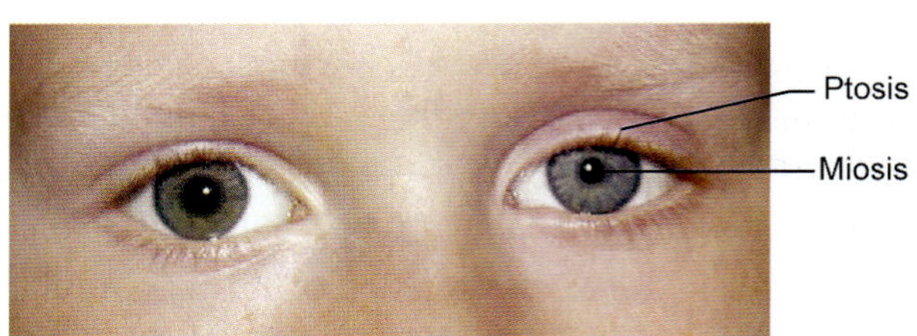

Fig. 4.20: Ptosis due to Horner's syndrome

Facts to Remember

- Apex of the axilla is known as *cervicoaxillary canal* and gives passage to axillary vessels and lower part of brachial plexus.
- Infraclavicular part of brachial plexus lies in the axilla.
- The fibre of sternoaponeurotic part of pectoralis major and latissimus dorsi twisted.
- Axillary sheath is derived from prevertebral fascia.
- Brachial plexus – ventral primary rami of C5–C8 and T1 – consists of roots, trunks, divisions, cords and branches.
- The radial nerve is the largest branch of the brachial plexus.
- *Horner's syndrome,* due to damaged sympathetic fibres from T1, shows ptosis, miosis, anhidrosis, enophthalmos and loss of ciliospinal reflex.
- Erb's paralysis – injury to the upper trunk – *'policeman's tip hand'* or *'waiter's tip hand'* or *'porter's tip hand'*
- Klumpke's paralysis – injury of the lower trunk – complete claw hand.

BDC's Anatomy *e*-book

1. Layout of axilla
2. Anastomoses and collateral circulation
3. Branches of brachial plexus
4. Sympathetic innervation of upper limb
5. Further reading
6. Viva voce questions

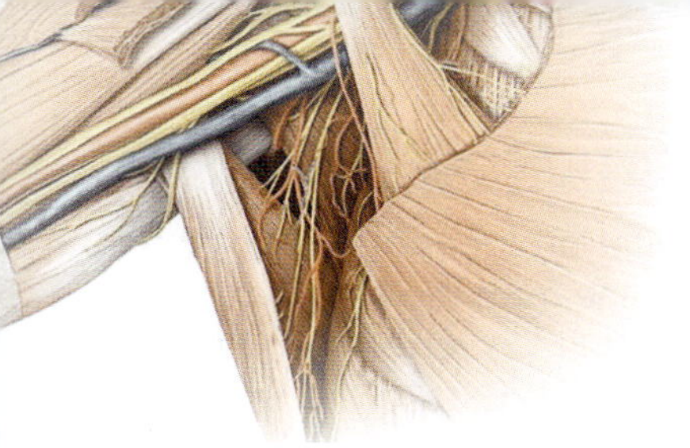

Chapter

5

Back

SURFACE LANDMARKS

1. ***Scapula (shoulder blade)*:** It is placed on the postero-lateral aspect of the upper part of the thorax. It extends from the 2nd to 7th ribs. Although it is thickly covered by muscles, most of its outline can be felt in the living subject.
   a. The ***acromion*** process lies at the top of the shoulder.
   b. The ***crest of the spine*** of the scapula runs from the acromion process medially and slightly downwards to the medial border of the scapula.
   c. The *medial border* and the *inferior angle* of the scapula can also be palpated (Fig. 5.1).
2. The ***8th rib*** is just below the inferior angle of the scapula. The lower ribs can be identified on the back by counting down from the 8th rib.
3. The ***iliac crest*** is a curved bony ridge lying below the waist. The anterior end of the crest is the *anterior superior iliac spine*. The *posterior superior iliac spine* is felt in a shallow dimple above the buttock, about 5 cm from the median plane.
4. The ***sacrum*** lies between the right and left dimples mentioned above. Usually, three *sacral spines* are palpable in the median plane.
5. The ***coccyx*** lies between the two buttocks in the median plane.
6. The spine of the 7th cervical vertebra or *vertebra prominens* is readily felt at the root of the neck. Higher up on the back of the neck, the *2nd cervical spine* can be felt about 5 cm below the *external occipital protuberance*. Other spines that can be recognised are T3 at the level of root of the spine of the scapula, L4 at the level of the highest point of the iliac crest and S2 at the level of the posterior superior iliac spine (Table 5.1).
7. The junction of the back of the head with that of the neck is indicated by the external occipital protuberance and the superior nuchal lines. The ***external occipital protuberance*** is a bony projection felt in the median plane on the back of the head at the upper end of the nuchal furrow (running vertically on the back of the neck).
8. The ***superior nuchal lines*** are indistinct curved ridges, which extend on either side from the protuberance to the mastoid process. The *nuchal furrow* extends to the external occipital protuberance above and to the spine of C7 below.

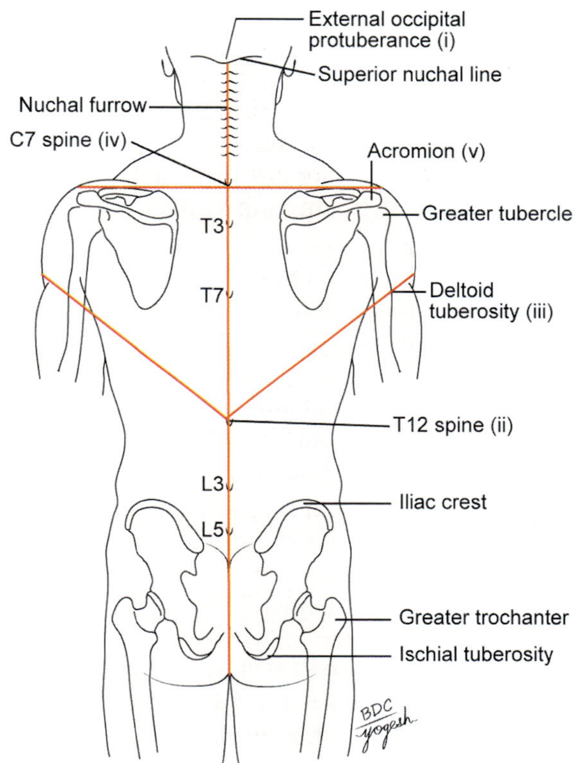

Fig. 5.1: Surface landmarks and lines of dissection

TABLE 5.1: Approximate levels of some spines on the back of the body

Vertebral spine	*Level*
C2	About 5 cm below the *external occipital protuberance*
C7	At the root of the neck
T2	Superior angle of the scapula
T3	Where crest of spine of the scapula meets its medial border
T7	Inferior angle of the scapula
L4	Highest point of iliac crests
S2	Posterior-superior iliac spine

SKIN AND FASCIAE OF THE BACK

Position

Humans mostly lie on their back. Therefore, the skin and fasciae of the back are adapted to sustain pressure of the body weight. Accordingly, the skin is thick and fixed to the underlying fasciae, the superficial fascia containing variable amount of fat is thick and strong and is connected to overlying skin by connective tissue, and the deep fascia is dense in texture. Hence, it is difficult to separate skin of back from underlying fascia.

Cutaneous Nerves

The cutaneous nerves of the back are derived from the *posterior primary rami* of the spinal nerves. Their distribution extends up to the posterior axillary lines.

1. The posterior primary rami of the spinal nerves C1, C7, C8, L4 and L5 do not give off any cutaneous branches. All twelve thoracic, L1–3 and five sacral nerves, however, give cutaneous branches.
2. Each posterior primary ramus divides into medial and lateral branches, both of which supply the erector spinae muscles, but only one of them, either medial or lateral, continues to become the cutaneous nerves.
3. In the upper half of the body (up to T6), the medial branches, and in the lower half of the body (below T6), the lateral branches of the posterior primary rami provide the cutaneous branches. Each cutaneous nerve divides into a smaller medial and a larger lateral branch before supplying the skin (Fig. 5.2).
4. The posterior primary rami supply the intrinsic muscles of the back and the skin covering them. The cutaneous distribution extends further laterally than the extensor muscles.
5. No posterior primary ramus *ever* supplies skin or muscles of a limb. The cutaneous branches of the posterior primary rami of nerves L1, 2, 3 and S1–3 are exceptions in this respect: They turn downwards unlike any other nerve and supply the skin of the gluteal region.

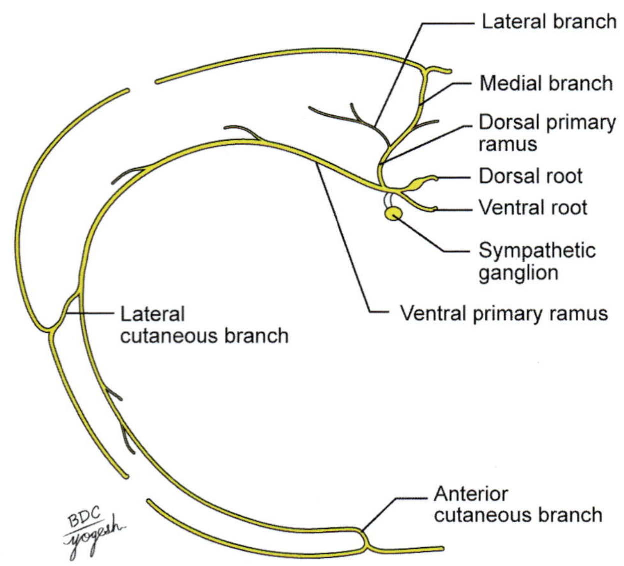

Fig. 5.2: Typical thoracic spinal nerve. The ventral or anterior primary ramus is the intercostal nerve

DISSECTION

Identify the external occipital protuberance (i) of the skull. Draw a line in the midline from the protuberance to the spine of the last thoracic (T12) vertebra (ii). Make incision along this line (Fig. 5.1). Extend the incision from its lower end to the deltoid tuberosity (iii) on the humerus which is present on lateral surface about the middle of the arm. Note that the arm is placed by the side of the trunk. Make another incision along a horizontal line from 7th cervical spine—vertebra prominens (iv) to the acromion process of scapula (v). Reflect the skin flap laterally.

Competency:

AN10.8 Describe, identify, and demonstrate the position, attachment, nerve supply, and actions of the trapezius and latissimus dorsi.

MUSCLES CONNECTING THE UPPER LIMB WITH THE VERTEBRAL COLUMN

Features

Muscles connecting the upper limb with the vertebral column are the posterior axio-appendicular muscles. These are grouped as follows (Figs 5.3a and b, Fig. 5.4, Flowchart 5.1, Plates 5.1 and 5.2):

1. Superficial layer
   - Trapezius
   - Latissimus dorsi
2. Deep layer
   - Levator scapulae
   - Rhomboid major
   - Rhomboid minor

The attachments of these muscles are given in Table 5.2, and their nerve supply and actions are shown in Table 5.3, Figs 5.3 to 5.6.

DISSECTION

Identify the attachments of trapezius muscle in the upper part of back; and that of latissimus dorsi in the lower part (Fig. 5.3b). Cut vertically through trapezius 5 cm lateral to the vertebral spines. Divide the muscle horizontally between the clavicle and spine of scapula; and reflect it laterally to identify the *accessory nerve* and its accompanying blood vessels, the *superficial branch of transverse cervical artery* and *vein*.

Look for the *suprascapular vessels* and *nerve*, deep to trapezius muscle, towards the scapular notch.

Cut through levator scapulae muscle midway between its two attachments and clean the dorsal scapular nerve (supplying the rhomboids) and accompanying blood vessels. Identify rhomboid minor from rhomboid major muscle.

Pull the medial or inner scapular border away from the chest wall for looking at the serratus anterior muscle.

Define attachments of latissimus dorsi muscle.

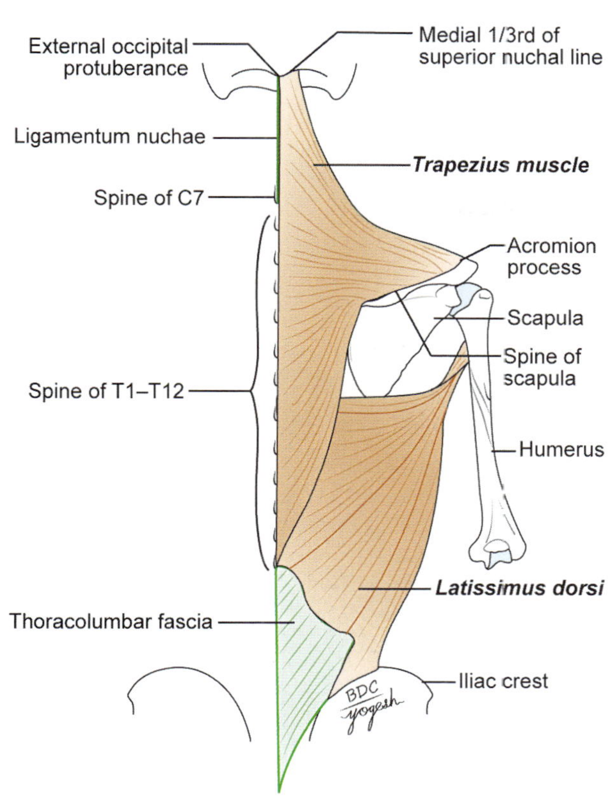

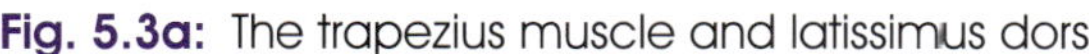

Fig. 5.3a: The trapezius muscle and latissimus dorsi

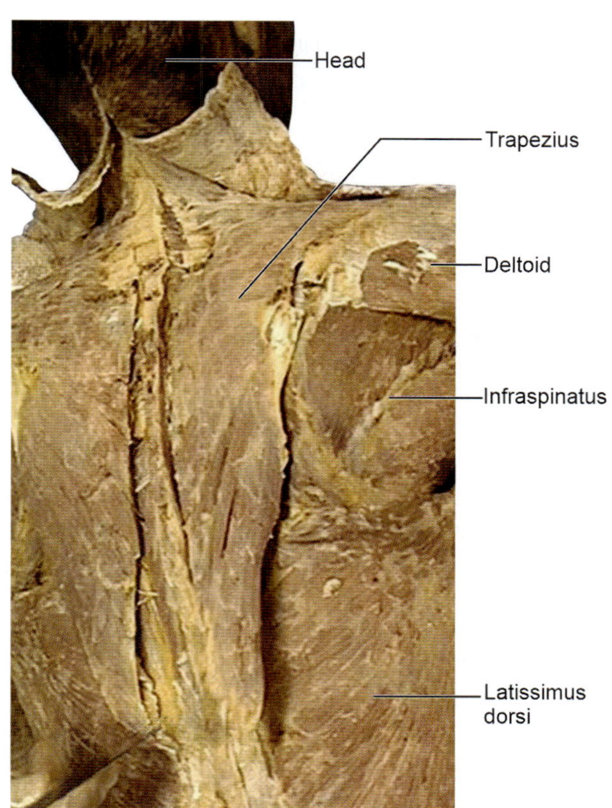

Fig. 5.3b: Dissection of the back showing superficial muscles

Flowchart 5.1: Muscles of back

Muscles of back

Muscle	Origin	Insertion	Innervation	Actions
Trapezius	External occipital protuberance Superior nuchal line Spines of C7–T12 vertebrae Ligamentum nuchae	Posterior border lateral third of clavicle Medial border of acromion Upper lip of crest of spine of scapula	Motor: Spinal part of XI cranial nerve Proprioceptive: C3, C4	Upper fibres: elevation of scapula Middle fibres: retraction of scapula Lower fibres: Overhead abduction of arm
Latissimus dorsi	Iliac crest Thoracolumbar fascia Spines of T7–T12 vertebrae Lower 3–4 ribs Inferior angle of scapula	Fibres twists upside down around lower border of teres major Inserts on floor bicipital groove	Thoracodorsal nerve (C6–C8)	Helps in swimming, rowing, climbing, pulling Adduction, extension, medial rotation of arm Violent expiration
Levator scapulae	Transverse processes of C1–C4 vertebrae	Medial border of scapula up to the root of spine	Dorsal scapular nerve (C5) C3, C4 fibres	Elevation of scapula
Rhomboid minor	Ligamentum nuchae and spine of C7 and T1	Root of spine	Dorsal scapular nerve (C5)	Retraction of scapula
Rhomboid major	Spines of T2–T5	Medial border of scapula below the root of spine	Dorsal scapular nerve (C5)	Retraction of scapula

ADDITIONAL FEATURES OF MUSCLES OF THE BACK

Trapezius

1. Developmentally, the trapezius is related to the sternocleidomastoid. Both of them develop from branchial arch mesoderm and are supplied by the spinal accessory nerve.
2. The principal action of the trapezius is to rotate the scapula during abduction of the arm beyond 90°.
3. The structures under cover of trapezius are shown in Plate 5.3 and Fig. 5.6 (for details, refer BDC's Anatomy eBook).
4. *Clinical testing*: Clinically, the muscle is tested by asking the patient to shrug their shoulder against resistance.

Latissimus Dorsi

1. This is the only muscle which connects the pelvic girdle and vertebral column to upper limb. It possesses extensive origin and narrow insertion.
2. The latissimus dorsi develops in the extensor compartment of the limb. Thereafter, it migrates to its wide attachment on the trunk, taking its nerve supply (thoracodorsal nerve) along with it (latus = wide). It is also called a ***swimmer's muscle***.

Plate 5.1: Latissimus dorsi and trapezius muscles.

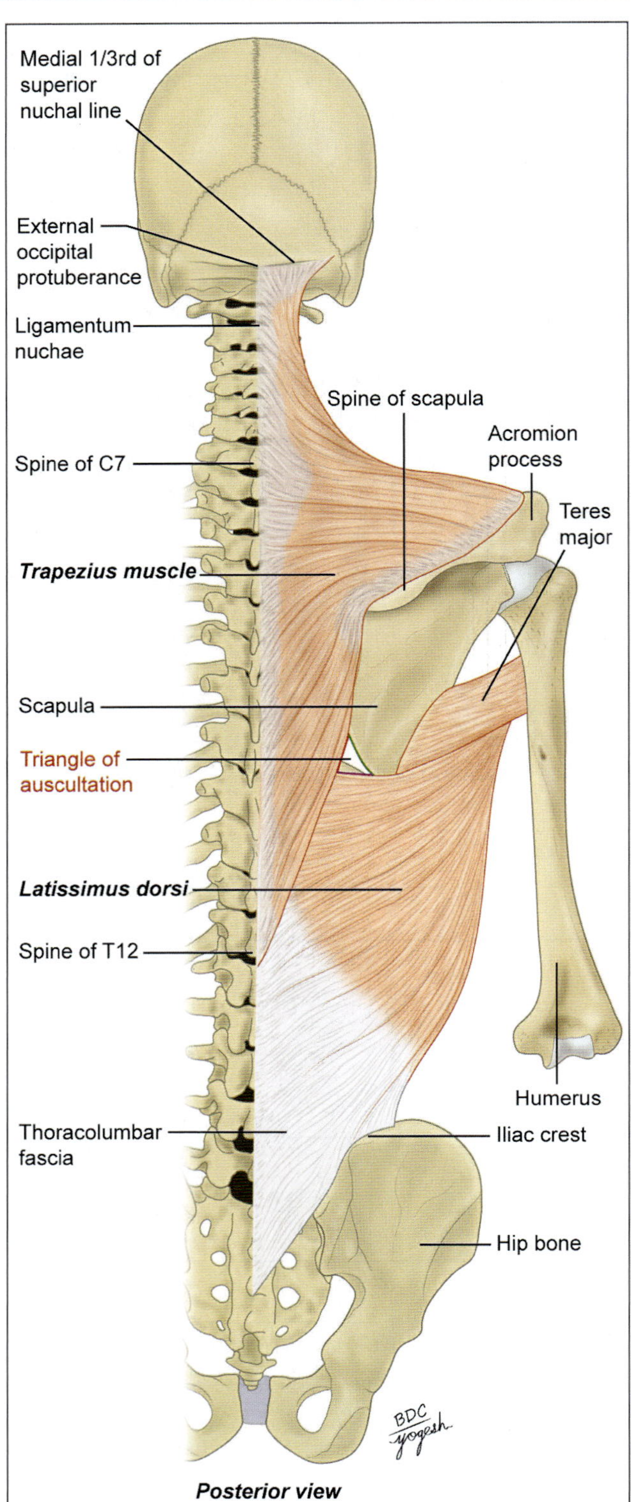

Plate 5.2: Levator scapulae, rhomboid major and rhomboid minor muscles.

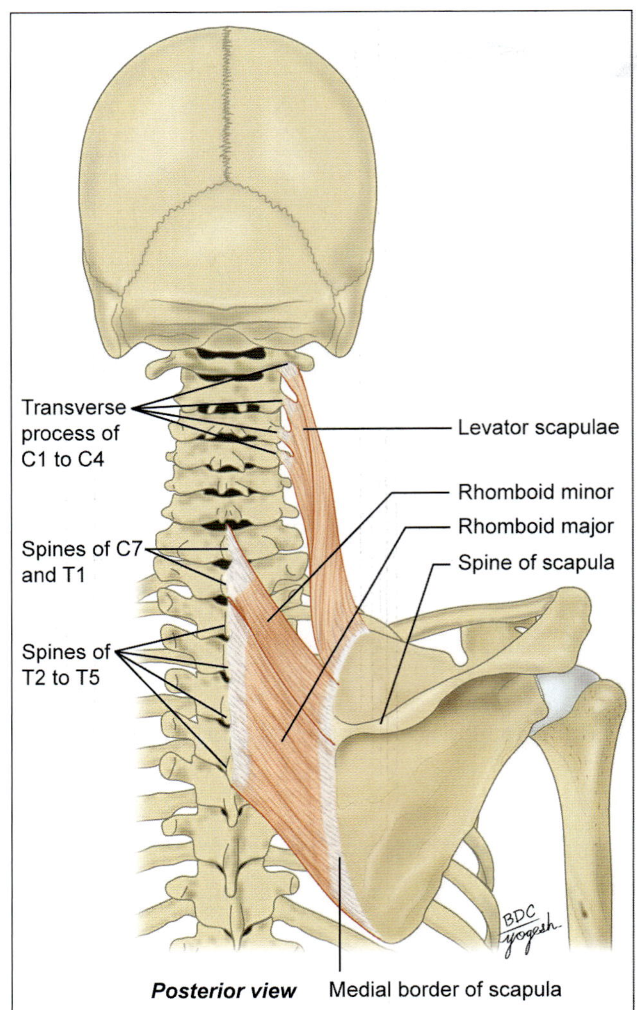

3. ***Clinical testing*:** The latissimus dorsi is tested clinically by feeling the contracting muscle in the posterior fold of the axilla after asking the patient to cough.

CLINICAL ANATOMY

- Musculocutaneous flap for breast reconstruction: In case of carcinoma of the breast, breast reconstruction surgery is required after mastectomy (removal of the breast). A musculocutaneous flap of latissimus dorsi with thoracodorsal nerve and thoracodorsal artery (branch of a subscapular artery) and venae comitantes may be used for breast reconstruction.
- *Cardiac support*: In patients with low cardiac output but not suitable for heart transplant, latissimus dorsi is wrapped around the heart, and this muscle is stimulated electrically using pacemaker along with heart. This procedure is called *cardiomyoplasty*.

Competency:

AN10.9 Describe the arterial anastomosis around the scapula and mention the boundaries of triangle of auscultation.

Triangle of Auscultation

Triangle of auscultation is a small triangular interval in the muscles of back (Fig. 5.7).

Boundaries

Medially — The lateral border of the trapezius
Laterally — The medial border of the scapula
Inferiorly — The upper border of the latissimus dorsi.
Floor of the triangle — It is formed by the 6th and 7th rib, and 6th intercostal space (ICS), and the rhomboid major.

Plate 5.3: Structures under cover of trapezius

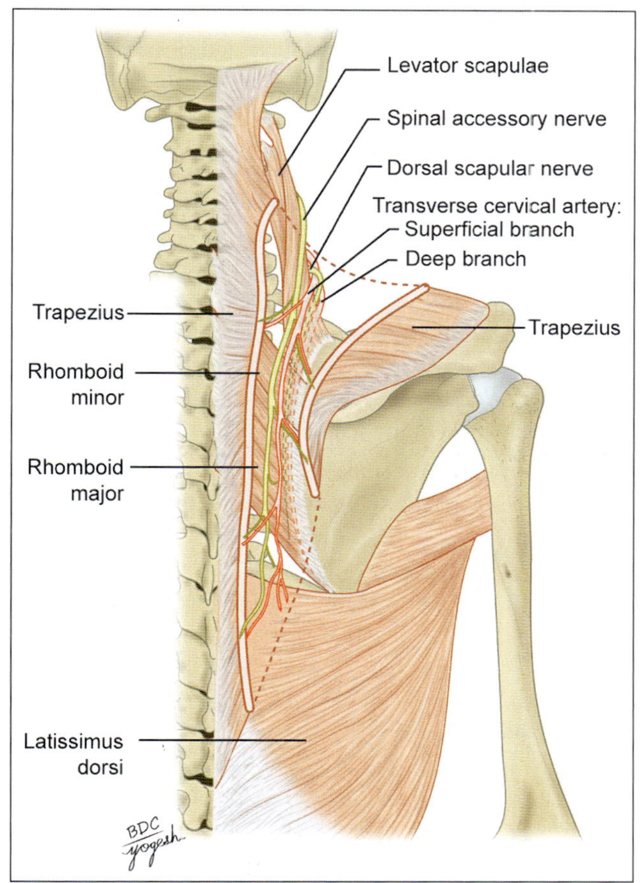

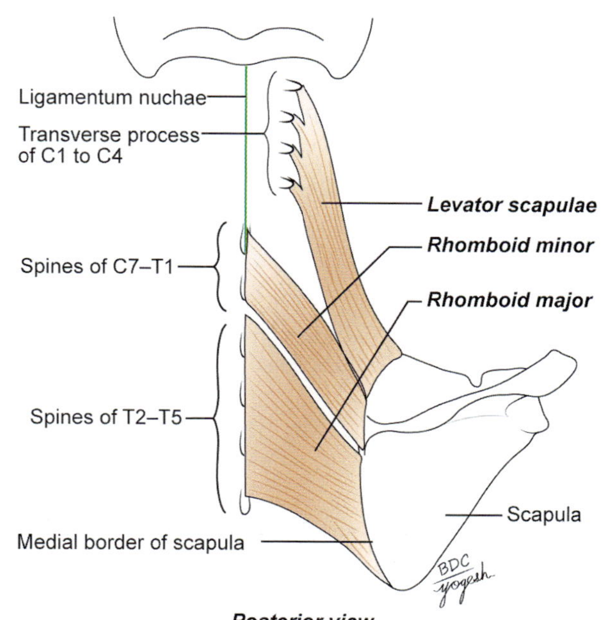

Fig. 5.4: The levator scapulae, the rhomboid minor and the rhomboid major muscles

This is the only part of the back which is not covered by big muscles. Respiratory sounds of apex of lower lobe heard through a stethoscope are better heard over this triangle on each side. On the left side, the cardiac orifice of the stomach lies deep to the triangle, and in days before X-rays were discovered, the sounds of swallowed liquids were auscultated over this triangle to confirm the oesophageal tumour (Fig. 5.3a).

Lumbar Triangle of Petit

Lumbar triangle of Petit is another small triangle surrounded by muscles (Fig. 5.7).

Boundaries

Medially — The lateral border of the latissimus dorsi

Laterally — The posterior border of the external oblique muscle of the abdomen.

TABLE 5.2: Attachments of muscles connecting the upper limb to the vertebral column (Figs 5.3 a–b, and 5.4)

Muscle	*Origin*	*Insertion*
Trapezius The right and left muscles together form a trapezium that covers the upper half of the back.	• Medial one-third of superior nuchal line • External occipital protuberance • Ligamentum nuchae • C7 spine • T1–T12 spines • Corresponding supraspinous ligaments	• *Upper fibres* into the posterior border of lateral one-third of clavicle • *Middle fibres* into the medial margin of the acromion process and upper lip of the crest of spine of the scapula • *Lower fibres* on the deltoid tubercle at the junction of medial and middle third of spine of scapula
Latissimus dorsi It covers a large area of the lower back, and is overlapped by the trapezius.	• Posterior one-third of the outer lip of iliac crest • Posterior layer of thoracolumbar fascia (thus attaching the muscle to the lumbar and sacral spines) • Spines of T7–T12, lower four ribs • Inferior angle of the scapula	The muscle winds a round the lower border of the teres major and forms the posterior fold of the axilla. The tendon is twisted upside down and is inserted into floor of the intertubercular sulcus
Levator scapulae	• Transverse processes of C1, C2 • Posterior tubercles of the transverse processes of C3, C4	Superior angle and upper part of medial border (up to the root of spine) of the scapula
Rhomboid minor	• Lower part of ligamentum nuchae • Spines C7 and T1	Base of the triangular area at the root of the spine of the scapula
Rhomboid major	• Spines of T2–T5 • Supraspinous ligaments	Medial border of scapula below the root of the spine

TABLE 5.3: Nerve supply and actions of muscles connecting the upper limb to the vertebral column

Muscle	*Nerve supply*	*Actions*
Trapezius	• Spinal part of accessory nerve (XI) • Branches from C3, C4 (proprioceptive)	• *Upper fibres* act with levator scapulae and elevate the scapula, as in shrugging. Upper fibres of both sides extend the neck • *Middle fibres* act with rhomboids and retract the scapula • *Upper and lower fibres* act with serratus anterior and rotate the scapula forwards around the chest wall, thus playing an important role in abduction of the arm beyond 90° (Fig. 5.5) • Steadies the scapula
Latissimus dorsi	Thoracodorsal nerve (C6–C8) (nerve to latissimus dorsi)	• Adduction, extension and medial rotation of the shoulder, as in swimming, rowing, climbing, pulling, folding the arm behind the back and scratching the opposite scapula • Helps in violent expiratory efforts like coughing, sneezing, etc. • Essentially a ***climbing*** muscle • Hold inferior angle of the scapula in place
Levator scapulae	• A branch from dorsal scapular nerve (C5) • Branches from C3, C4	• Helps in elevation of scapula • Steadies the scapula during movements of the arm
Rhomboid minor	Dorsal scapular nerve (C5)	• Retraction of scapula
Rhomboid major	Dorsal scapular nerve (C5)	

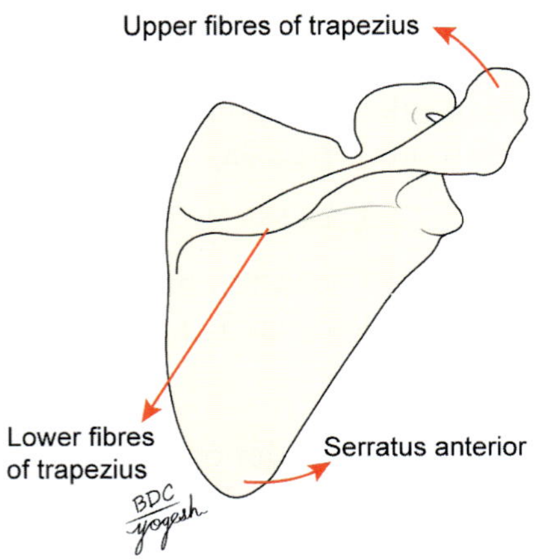

Fig. 5.5: Rotation of the scapula during abduction of the arm beyond 90°, brought about by the trapezius and the serratus anterior muscles

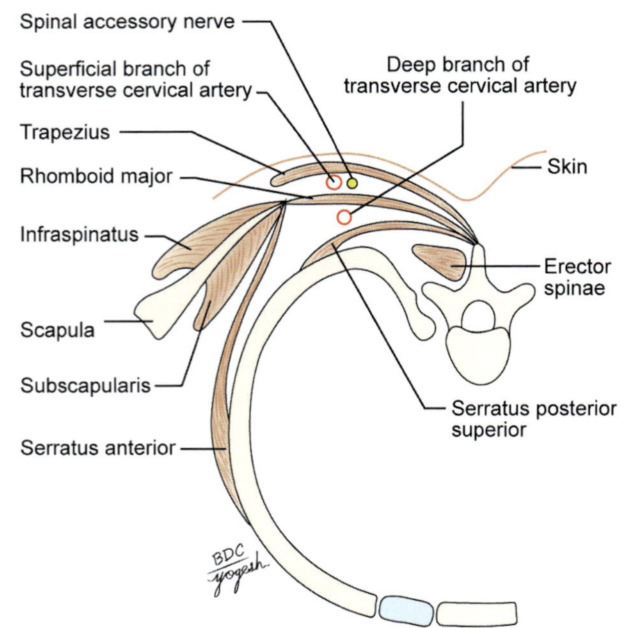

Fig. 5.6: Transverse section showing the arrangement of structures on the back

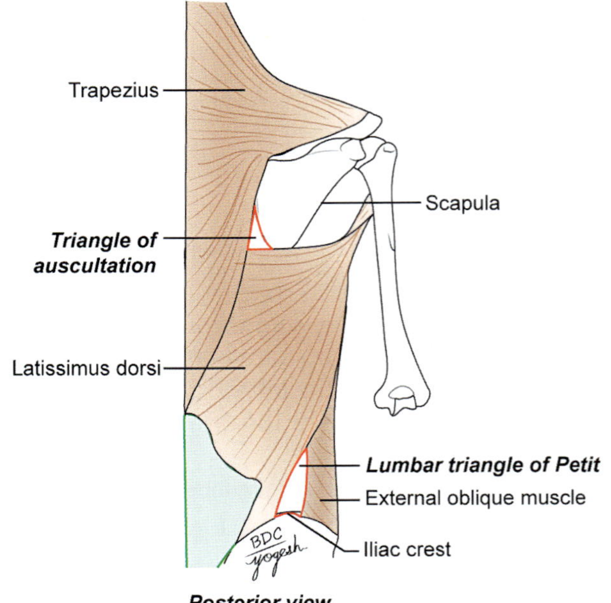

Fig. 5.7: The triangle of auscultation and lumbar triangle of Petit

Inferiorly — The iliac crest (which forms the base)

Floor of the triangle — It is formed by the internal oblique muscle of the anterior abdominal wall.

The occasional hernia at this site is called *lumbar hernia* (Fig. 5.4).

DISSECTION

After completing the dissection of the back, the limb with clavicle and scapula is detached from the trunk.

For detachment of the limb, muscles which need to be incised are trapezius, levator scapulae, rhomboid minor and major, serratus anterior, latissimus dorsi and sternocleidomastoid.

The sternoclavicular joint is opened to free clavicle from the sternum. Upper limb with clavicle and scapula is removed en bloc.

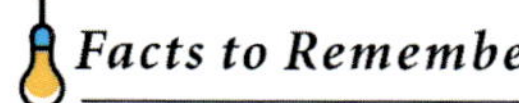

Facts to Remember

- The highest point of the iliac crests lies at the level of the L4 vertebral spine.
- The posterior-superior iliac spine lies at the level of the S2 vertebra.
- The posterior primary rami of the spinal nerves C1, C7, C8 and L4, L5 do not give off any cutaneous branches.
- Clinically, the trapezius is tested by asking the patient to shrug their shoulder against resistance.
- Trapezius is supplied by spinal root of XI nerve and C3–4 fibres.
- The latissimus dorsi and pectoralis major are *climbing muscles*.
- The dorsal scapular nerve supplies levator scapulae, rhomboid minor and rhomboid major.

BDC's Anatomy *e*-book

1. Structures under cover of the trapezius
2. Dorsal scapular nerve
3. Further reading
4. Viva voce questions

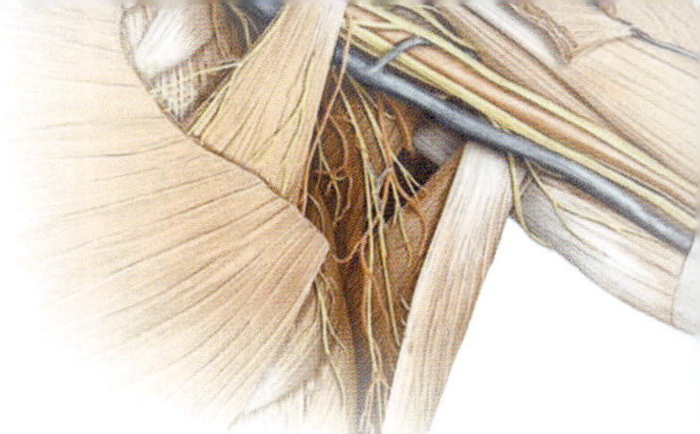

Chapter

6

Scapular Region

The shoulder or scapular region comprises structures closely related to and surrounding the shoulder joint. For a proper understanding of the region, revise some features of the scapula and the upper end of the humerus.

SURFACE LANDMARKS

1. a. The upper half of the humerus is covered on its anterior, lateral and posterior aspects by the *deltoid muscle*. This muscle is triangular and forms the rounded contour of the shoulder (Fig. 6.1).
   b. The *greater tubercle* of the humerus forms the most lateral bony point of the shoulder.
2. The *skin* covering the shoulder region is supplied by:
   a. The lateral supraclavicular nerve over the upper half of the deltoid.
   b. The upper lateral cutaneous nerve of the arm over the lower half of the deltoid.
   c. The dorsal rami of the upper thoracic nerves over the back, i.e. over the scapula.
3. The *superficial fascia* contains (in addition to some fat and cutaneous nerves) the inferolateral part of the platysma arising from the deltoid fascia.
4. The *deep fascia* covering the deltoid sends numerous septa between its fasciculi. The subscapularis, supraspinatus and infraspinatus fasciae provide origin to a part of the respective muscle.

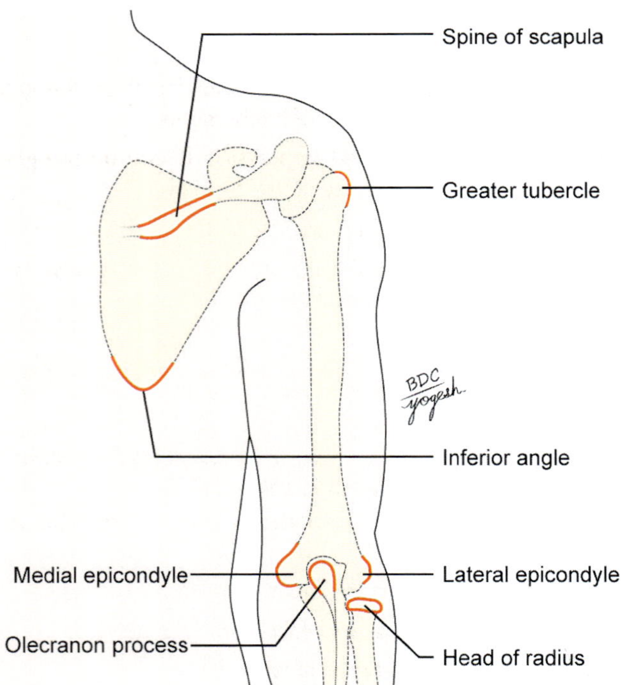

Fig. 6.1: Surface landmarks: Shoulder, arm and elbow regions

MUSCLES OF THE SCAPULAR REGION

Features

Muscles of scapular region are:

- Deltoid
- Supraspinatus
- Infraspinatus
- Teres minor
- Subscapularis
- Teres major

The deltoid is described below (Plate 6.1, Figs 6.2 to 6.4). The other muscles are described in Tables 6.1, 6.2, Plate 6.2, Figs 6.5 and 6.6.

Competency:
AN10.10 Describe and identify the deltoid and rotator cuff muscles along with their nerve supply and clinical anatomy.

DELTOID (DELTA-LIKE OR TRIANGULAR)

Origin

1. The anterior border and adjoining surface of the lateral 1/3rd of the *clavicle* (Plate 6.1, Fig. 6.2, Flowchart 6.1).
2. The lateral border of the *acromion process* where four septa of origin are attached (Fig. 6.2).
3. Lower lip of the crest of the *spine* of the scapula.

The acromial part of deltoid is an example of a *multipennate muscle*. Many fibres arise from four septa of origin that are attached above to the acromion process. The fibres converge onto three septa of insertion, which are attached to the deltoid tuberosity (Fig. 6.2).

Plate 6.1: Deltoid muscle

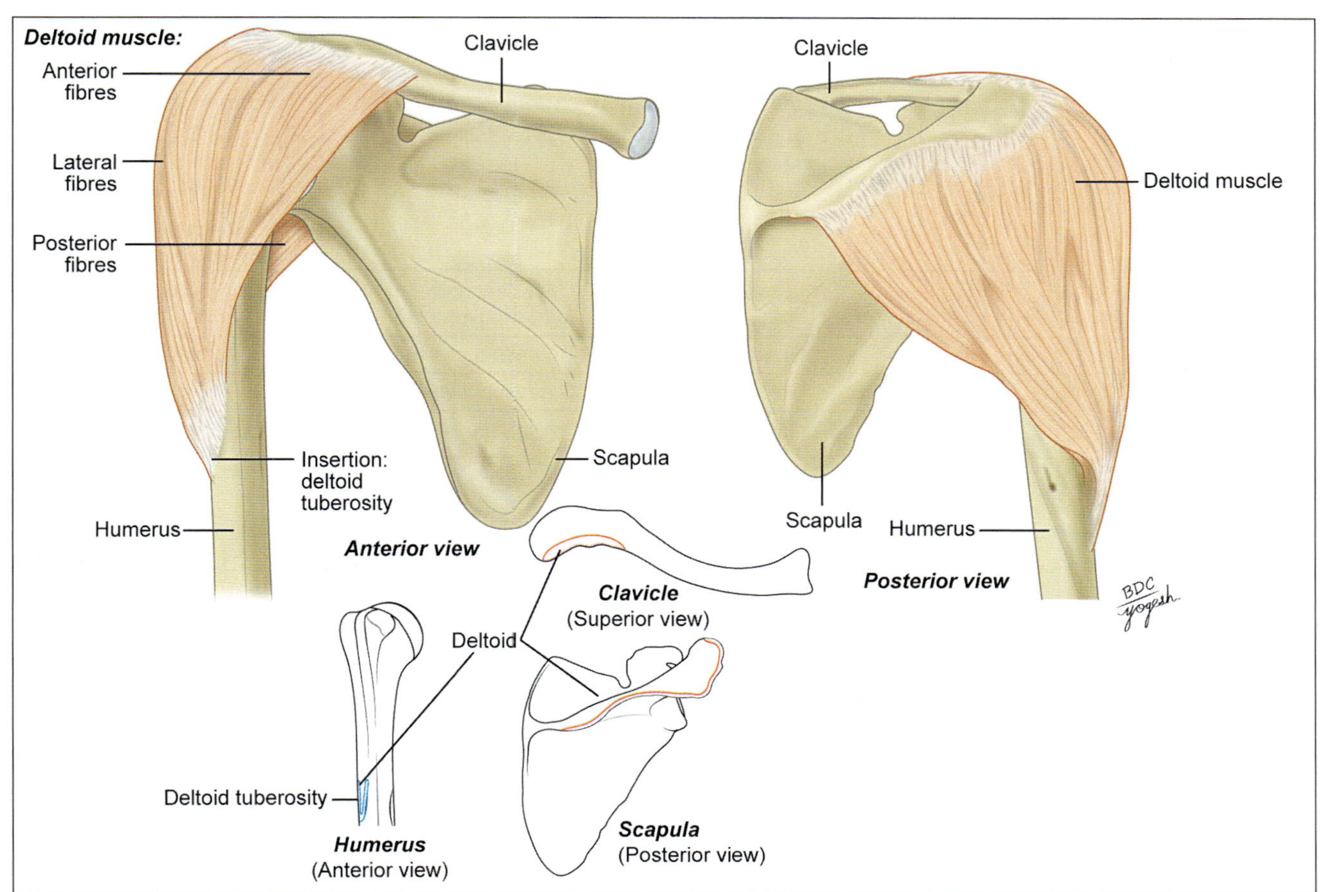

TABLE 6.1: Attachments of muscles of scapular region (except deltoid, Plate 6.2, Figs 6.5 and 6.6)

Muscle	*Origin*	*Insertion*
1. **Supraspinatus**	Medial 2/3rd of the supraspinous fossa of the scapula. The muscle passes as a tendon laterally beneath coracoacromial arch to blend with the capsule of shoulder joint. The tendon is separated from the arch by the subacromial bursa (Fig. 6.7).	Upper impression (facet) on the greater tubercle of the humerus
2. **Infraspinatus**	Medial 2/3rd of the infraspinous fossa of the scapula	Middle impression (facet) on the greater tubercle of the humerus
3. **Teres minor**	Upper 2/3rd of the dorsal surface of the lateral border of the scapula as 2 slips	Lowest impression (facet) on the greater tubercle of the humerus
4. **Subscapularis** (multipennate)	Medial 2/3rd of the subscapular fossa	Lesser tubercle of the humerus
5. **Teres major**	Lower 1/3rd of the dorsal surface of lateral border and inferior angle of the scapula	Medial lip of the bicipital groove of the humerus

TABLE 6.2: Nerve supply and actions of muscles of scapular region (except deltoid)

Muscle	*Nerve supply*	*Actions*
1. **Supraspinatus**	Suprascapular nerve (C5, C6)	Both supraspinatus and deltoid are involved in initiation of abduction and continuation of abduction (*Previous concept*: Supraspinatus acts as an abductor of the shoulder joint from 0°–15°)
2. **Infraspinatus**	Suprascapular nerve (C5, C6)	Lateral rotator of arm (*at shoulder joint*)
3. **Teres minor**	Axillary nerve (C5, C6)	Lateral rotator of arm (*at shoulder joint*)
4. **Subscapularis**	Upper and lower subscapular nerves (C5, C6)	Medial rotator and adductor of arm
5. **Teres major**	Lower subscapular nerve (C5, C6)	Medial rotator, adductor and extensor of arm

Flowchart 6.1: Muscles of scapular region

Muscles of scapular region

Muscle	Origin (scapula)	Insertion (humerus)	Innervation	Actions
Deltoid muscle	Anterior fibres: Anterior border of lateral 1/3 of clavicle Middle fibres: Acromion Posterior fibres: Lower lip of crest of spine of scapula	Deltoid tuberosity of humerus	Axillary nerve	Anterior fibres: Flexion and medial rotation of arm Middle fibres: Abduction (up to 90°) of arm Posterior fibres: Extension and lateral rotation of arm
Subscapularis	Medial 2/3 of subscapular fossa	Lesser tubercle	Upper and lower subscapular nerves	Medial rotations and adduction of arm
Supraspinatus	Supraspinous fossa	Greater tubercle	Suprascapular nerve	Initiation of abduction of arm
Infraspinatus	Infraspinous fossa	Greater tubercle	Suprascapular nerve	Lateral rotation of arm
Teres minor	Lateral border of scapula	Greater tubercle	Axillary nerve	Lateral rotation of arm

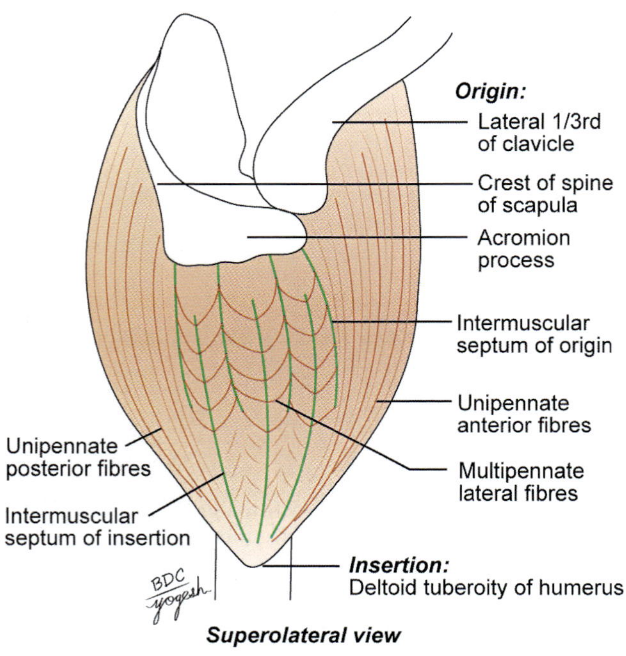

Fig. 6.2: The origin and insertion of the deltoid muscle

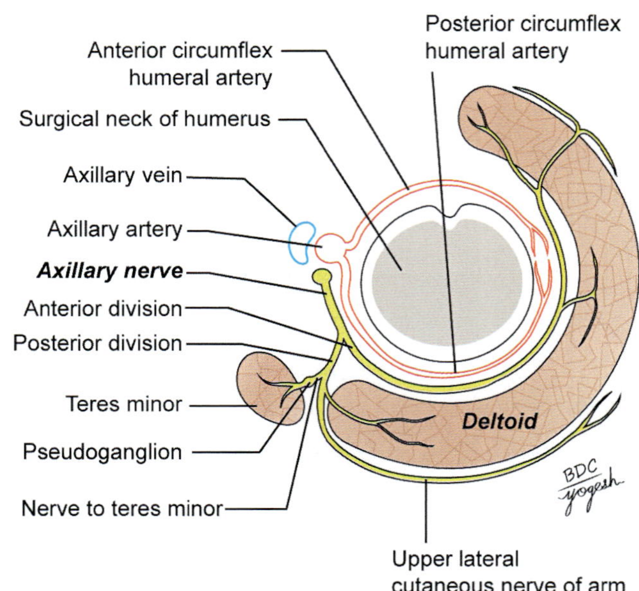

Fig. 6.3: Horizontal section of the deltoid region showing the axillary nerve and vessels around the surgical neck of humerus

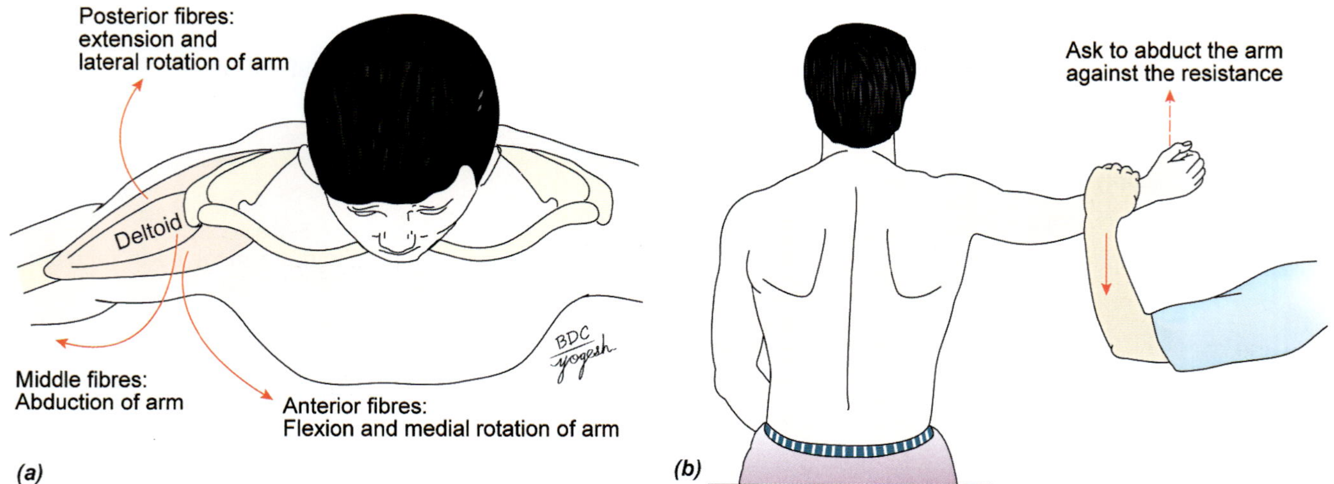

Figs 6.4a and b: (a) Actions of deltoid muscle and (b) clinical testing of deltoid muscle

Plate 6.2: Supraspinatus, infraspinatus, teres minor, teres major and subscapularis muscles

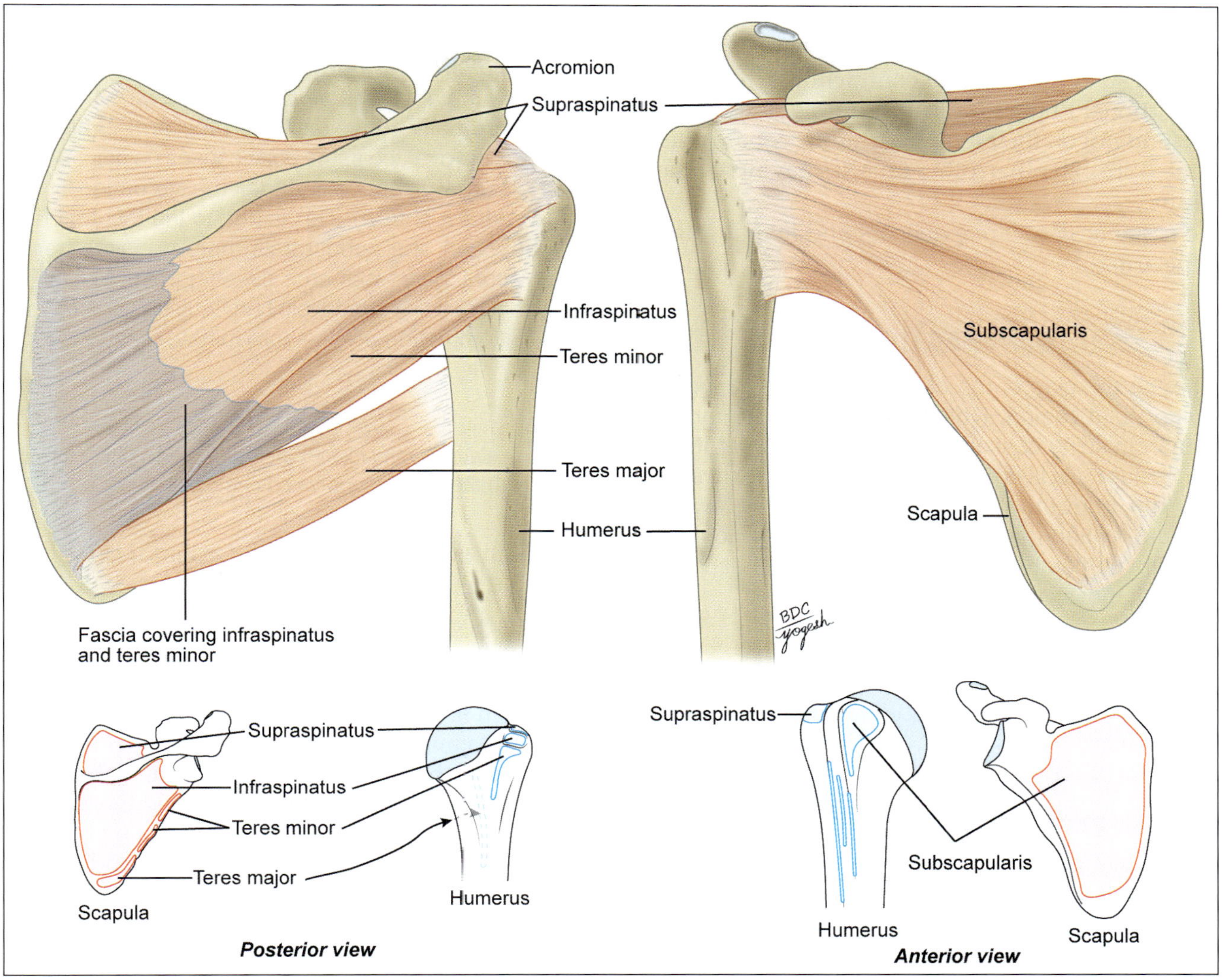

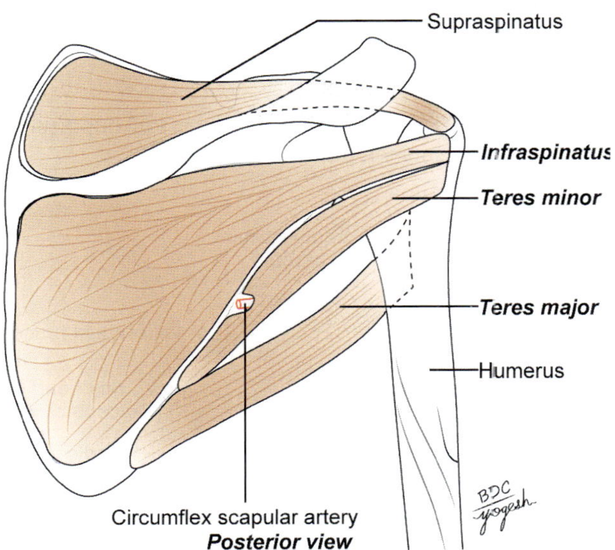

Fig. 6.5: The origins and insertions of the supraspinatus, infraspinatus and teres minor muscles of right side

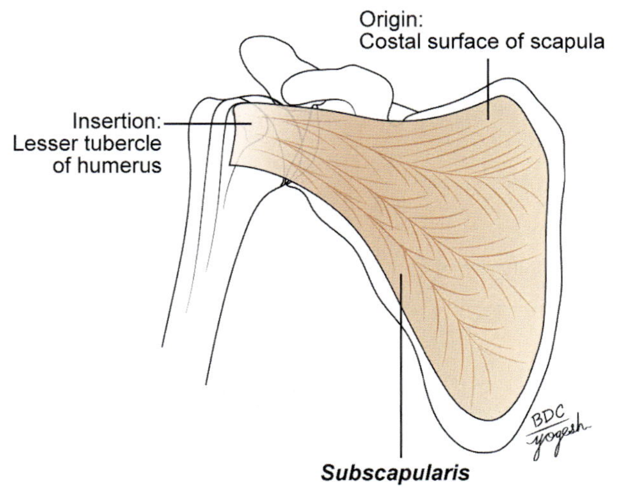

Fig. 6.6: The subscapularis muscle

Insertion

The V-shaped *deltoid tuberosity* of the humerus where three septa of insertion are attached.

Nerve Supply

Axillary nerve (C5, C6) (Fig. 6.3).

Actions

1. The *anterior fibres* are flexors and medial rotators of the arm (Fig. 6.4a).

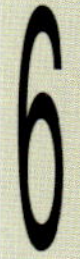

2. The *multipennate acromial fibres* are powerful abductors of the arm at the shoulder joint from beginning to 90°. A multipennate arrangement allows a large number of muscle fibres to be packed into a relatively small volume. As the strength of contraction of a muscle is proportional to the number of muscle fibres present in it (and not on their length), a multipennate muscle is much stronger than other muscles having the same volume.
3. The *posterior fibres* are extensors and lateral rotators of the arm.

DISSECTION

Define the margins of the deltoid muscle covering the shoulder joint region. Reflect the part of the muscle arising from spine of scapula downwards. Separate the infraspinatus muscle from teres major and minor muscles, which run from the lateral scapular border towards humerus. Axillary nerve accompanied with posterior circumflex humeral vessels lies on the deep aspect of the deltoid muscle.

Competency:

AN10.13 Explain anatomical basis of injury to axillary nerve during intramuscular injections.

CLINICAL ANATOMY

- Intramuscular injections (COVID-19 vaccination) are often given into the deltoid. They should be given in the middle of the muscle to avoid injury to the axillary nerve (Fig. 6.7). If injection is given in upper part of deltoid, axillary nerve may be damaged.
- The deltoid muscle is tested by asking the patient to abduct the arm against resistance applied with one hand, and feeling for the contracting muscle with the other hand (Fig. 6.4b).
- The tendon of the supraspinatus may undergo degeneration. This can give rise to calcification and even spontaneous rupture of the tendon.
- In ***subacromial bursitis***, pressure over the deltoid below the acromion process with the arm by the side causes pain. However, when the arm is abducted, pressure over the same point causes no pain, because the bursa disappears under the acromion process (***Dawbarn's sign***). This is due to the fact that during abduction, the subacromial bursa passes beneath the coracoacromial arch causing pain to disappear. Subacromial or subdeltoid bursitis is usually secondary to inflammation of the supraspinatus tendon.

Competency:

AN10.10 Describe and identify the deltoid and rotator cuff muscles along with their nerve supply and clinical anatomy.

Musculotendinous Cuff of the Shoulder or Rotator Cuff

The musculotendinous cuff of the shoulder is a fibrous sheath formed by the four flattened tendons, which blend with the capsule of the shoulder joint and strengthen it. The muscles which form the cuff arise from the scapula and are inserted into the lesser and greater tubercles of the humerus. They are the subscapularis, the supraspinatus, the infraspinatus and the teres minor (Plate 6.3, Fig. 6.8). Their tendons, while crossing the shoulder joint, become flattened and blend with each other on one hand, and with the capsule of the joint on the other hand, before reaching their points of insertion.

The cuff gives strength to the capsule of the shoulder joint all around except inferiorly. This explains why dislocations of the humerus occur commonly in an anteroinferior direction. Thus, rotator cuff rests on tuberosities, fused to the capsule, strengthens the capsule and steadies head of humerus.

[*Mnemonic:* The **SITS** muscles: Clockwise from top: **S**upraspinatus, **I**nfraspinatus, **T**eres minor, **S**ubscapularis]

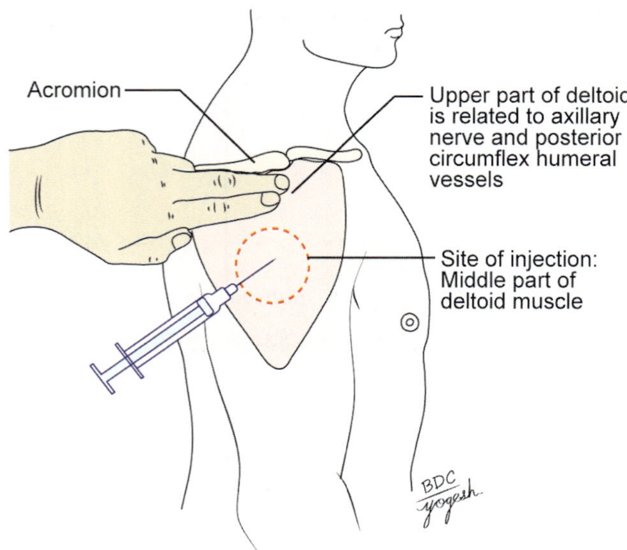

Fig. 6.7: Intramuscular injection in deltoid muscle

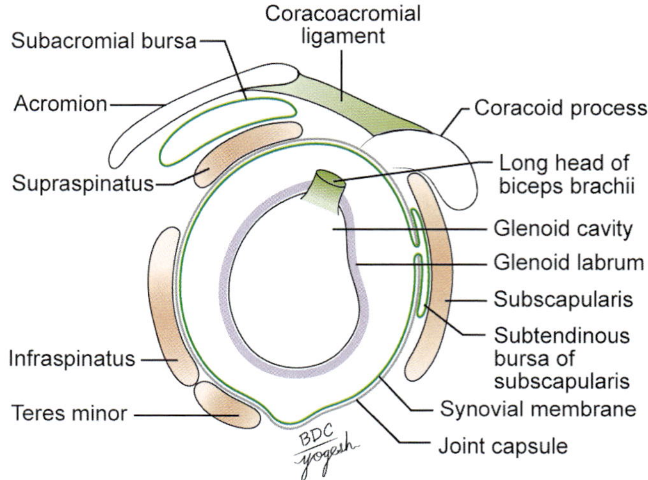

Fig. 6.8: Subacromial bursa with the musculotendinous cuff of the shoulder

Plate 6.3: Musculotendinous cuff of shoulder joint, subacromial bursa and insertion of muscles of rotator cuff muscles

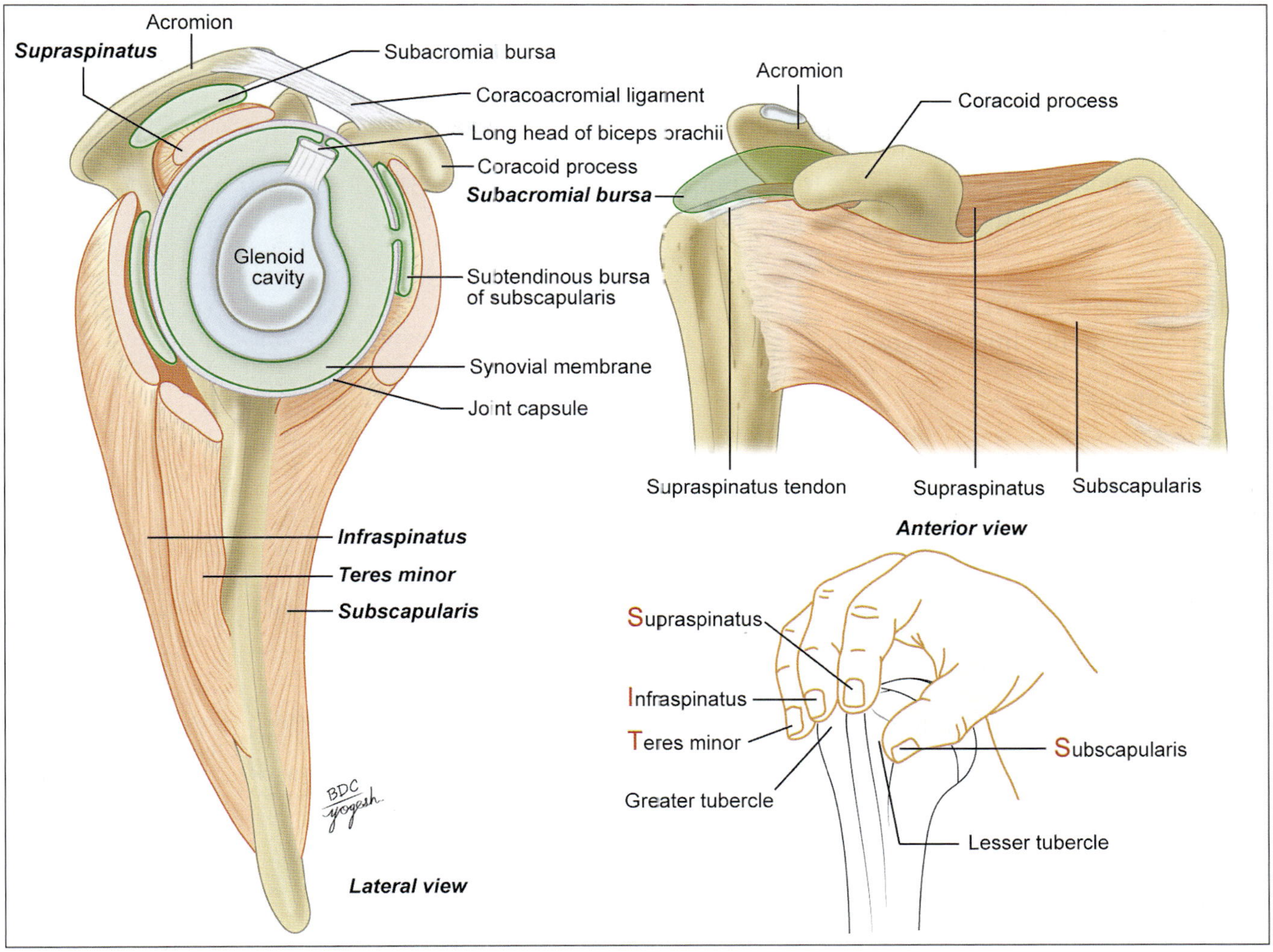

Subacromial Bursa

The subacromial bursa is the largest bursa of the body, situated below the coracoacromial arch and the deltoid muscle. Below the bursa, there are the tendon of the supraspinatus and the greater tubercle of the humerus (Fig. 6.8).

The subacromial bursa is of great value in the abduction of the arm at the shoulder joint.

a. It protects the supraspinatus tendon against friction with the acromion process.
b. During overhead abduction, the greater tubercle of the humerus passes under the acromion process; this is facilitated by the presence of this bursa.

Supraspinatus Tendinitis

Painful arc syndrome/rotator cuff syndrome: Pain starts at about 60° and lasts till 120° of abduction as supraspinatus muscle gets impinged between coracoacromial arch and greater tubercle of humerus. Further abduction of shoulder occurs after lateral rotation of humerus, which takes greater tubercle of humerus away from the coracoacromial arch. Then supraspinatus tendon is no longer impinged, and thus, no more pain occurs.

INTERMUSCULAR SPACES

The long head of triceps brachii spans the length of the arm arising from infraglenoid tubercle of scapula to the olecranon process of ulna. It lies medial to humerus. Teres minor crosses posterior aspect of the shoulder joint and origin of the long head as it passes from its origin from scapula to the humerus. The muscle is replaced by subscapularis on the anterior aspect of shoulder joint. Teres major also crosses the long head as it runs to bicipital groove for its insertion.

Thus potential spaces are formed between lateral border of scapula, medial aspect of humerus, long head of triceps brachii, teres minor or subscapularis and teres major muscles.

In the upper part, there is a quadrangular space laterally and upper triangular space medially. In the lower part is the lower triangular space (Plate 6.4, Fig. 6.9, Flowchart 6.2).

Quadrangular Space

Boundaries

Superior

1. Subscapularis in front.

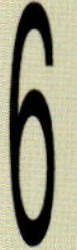

2. Capsule of the shoulder joint: This is the loose inferior part of the capsule of the shoulder joint. In anatomical position, the capsule lies in this space. The capsule gets taut as it is used up during abduction of the shoulder joint.
3. Inferior border of teres minor behind.

Inferior: Superior border of teres major.
Medial: Lateral border of long head of the triceps brachii.
Lateral: Surgical neck of the humerus.

Contents

1. Axillary nerve (Fig. 6.9)
2. Posterior circumflex humeral vessels.

Upper Triangular Space

Boundaries

Superior: Inferior border of teres minor.
Lateral: Medial border of long head of the triceps brachii.
Inferior: Superior border of teres major.

Contents

Circumflex scapular artery. It interrupts the origin of the teres minor and reaches the infraspinous fossa for anastomoses with the suprascapular artery and deep branch of transverse cervical artery.

Lower Triangular Space

It is diagonally opposite the upper triangular space.

Boundaries

Medial: Lateral border of long head of the triceps brachii.
Lateral: Medial border of humerus.
Superior: Lower border of teres major (Fig. 6.9).

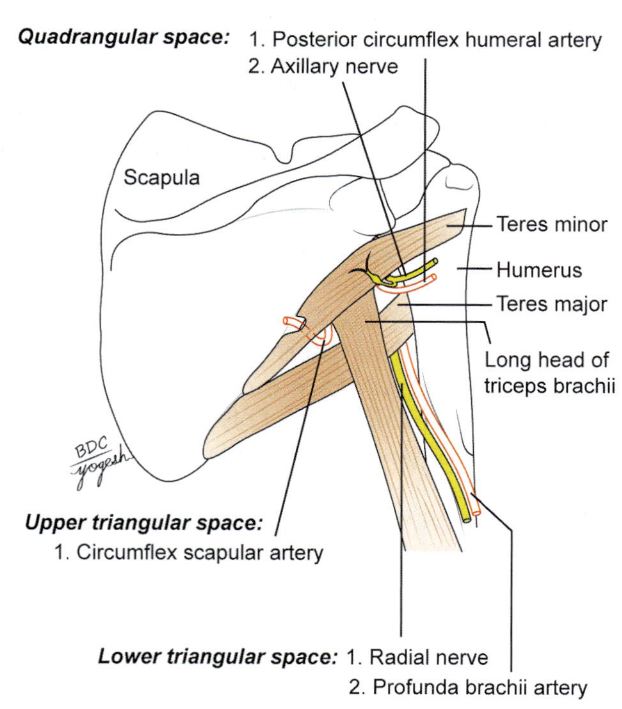

Fig. 6.9: The intermuscular spaces in the scapular region, including the quadrangular, upper triangular and lower triangular spaces

Plate 6.4: Intermuscular spaces in scapular region.

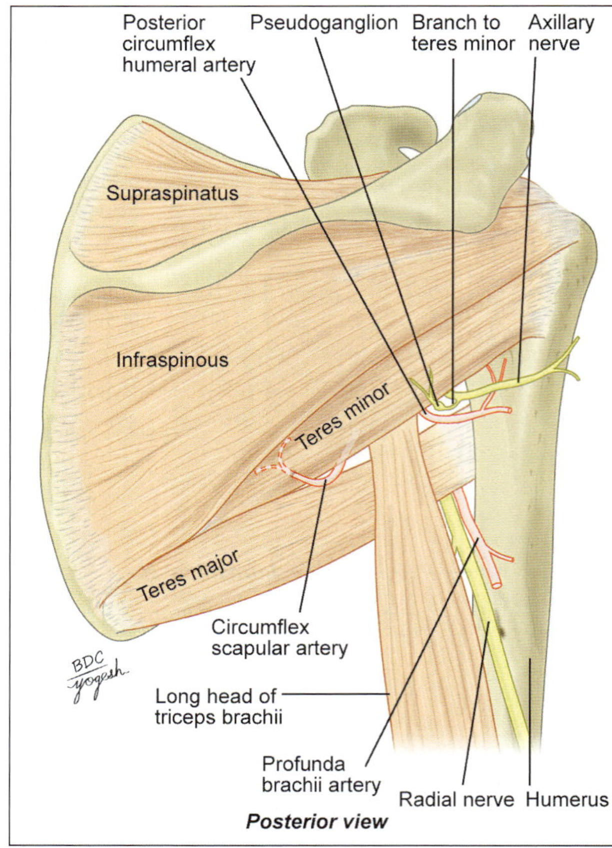

Contents

1. Radial nerve
2. Profunda brachii vessels.

DISSECTION

The quadrangular intermuscular space is a space in between the scapular muscles. The quadrangular space is bounded by teres minor above and teres major below; by the long head of triceps muscle medially and the surgical neck of humerus laterally. The axillary nerve accompanied with posterior circumflex humeral vessels lie in this space. Identify the nerve to the teres minor muscle (Fig. 6.9). Identify part of the capsule of the shoulder joint.

Another intermuscular space, the upper triangular space should be dissected. It is bounded by the teres minor muscle medially, long head of triceps laterally, and teres major muscle below.

Now the remaining 2/3rd of deltoid muscle can be reflected towards its insertion. Identify subscapularis muscle anteriorly.

Define the attachments of infraspinatus and cut muscle at the neck of scapula and reflect it on both sides.

Look for the structures covered with deltoid muscle.

Identify a lower triangular space, which is bounded above by the lower border of teres major muscle, medially by the long head of triceps brachii and laterally by the medial border of humerus. The radial nerve and profunda brachii vessels pass through the space.

Flowchart 6.2: Intermuscular spaces

	Quadrangular	Upper triangular	Lower triangular
Boundaries	Superior: Subscapularis, capsule of shoulder joint, teres minor Inferior: Teres major Medial: Triceps brachii Lateral: Humerus	Superior: Teres minor Inferior: Teres major Lateral: Triceps brachii	Superior: Teres major Medial: Triceps brachii Lateral: Humerus
Contents	1. Axillary nerve 2. Posterior circumflex humeral vessels	1. Circumflex scapular artery	1. Radial nerve 2. Profunda brachii vessels

Dissect and identify the arteries taking part in the anastomoses around scapula. These are suprascapular along upper border, deep branch of transverse cervical (dorsal scapular) along medial border and circumflex scapular along lateral border of scapula.

Competency:

AN10.13 Explain anatomical basis of injury to axillary nerve during intramuscular injections.

AXILLARY OR CIRCUMFLEX NERVE

Axillary or circumflex nerve is an important nerve because it supplies the deltoid muscle, which is the main abductor of the arm. Surgically, it is important because it is commonly involved in dislocations of the shoulder and in fractures of the surgical neck of the humerus.

The axillary nerve is a smaller terminal branch of the posterior cord of the brachial plexus (C5, C6).

Root value: Its root value is ventral rami of cervical 5, 6 segments of spinal cord.

Course

Axillary nerve courses through lower part of axilla into the quadrangular space, where it terminates by dividing into two branches (Fig. 6.3).

Relations and Branches

a. In the lower part of the axilla, the nerve runs downwards behind the third part of the axillary artery. Here, it lies on the subscapularis muscle. It is related medially to the radial nerve and laterally to the coracobrachialis. The nerve leaves the axilla by winding around the lower border of the subscapularis in close relation to the lowest part of the capsule of the shoulder joint, where it gives a branch to the capsule of the joint and enters the quadrangular space (Fig. 6.3).
b. The nerve then passes backwards through the quadrangular space. Here, it is accompanied by the posterior circumflex humeral vessels and has the following relations (Fig. 6.9).

   Superiorly:

   1. Subscapularis anteriorly or teres minor posteriorly.
   2. Lowest part of the capsule of the shoulder joint.

   Laterally: Surgical neck of humerus.

   Inferiorly: Teres major.

   Medially: Long head of the triceps brachii.

   In the quadrangular space, the nerve divides into anterior and posterior branches (Fig. 6.3).
c. The ***anterior branch*** is accompanied by the posterior circumflex humeral vessels. It winds around the surgical neck of the humerus, deep to the deltoid muscle supplying the deltoid and the skin over its anteroinferior part.
d. The ***posterior branch*** supplies the teres minor and the posterior part of the deltoid. The nerve to the teres minor bears a ***pseudoganglion***, i.e. fibrous tissue and fat without any neurons (Fig. 6.3). The posterior branch then pierces the deep fascia at the lower part of the posterior border of the deltoid and continues as the upper lateral cutaneous nerve of the arm.

CLINICAL ANATOMY

- The axillary nerve may be damaged by dislocation of the shoulder or by the fracture of the surgical neck of the humerus. The effects produced are:
  a. Rounded contour of shoulder is lost; greater tubercle of humerus becomes prominent (Fig. 6.10).
  b. Deltoid is paralysed, with loss of the power of abduction up to 90° at the shoulder.
  c. There is sensory loss over the lower half of the deltoid in a badge-like area called regimental badge (Fig. 6.10).

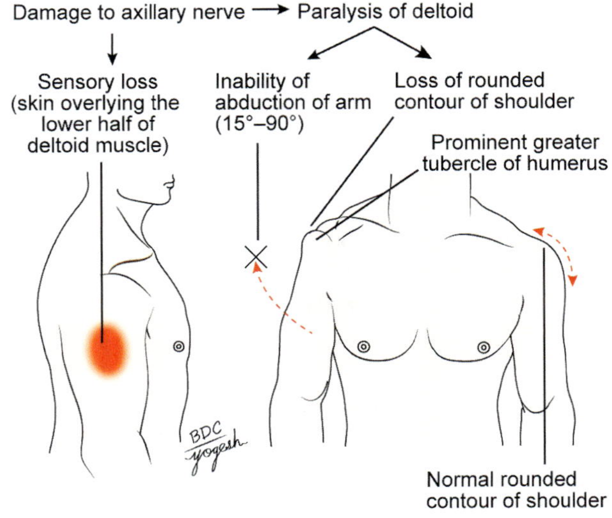

Fig. 6.10: Axillary nerve palsy

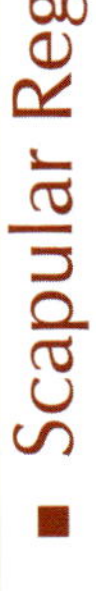

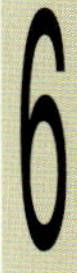

Competency:

AN10.9 Describe the arterial anastomosis around the scapula and mention the boundaries of triangle of auscultation.

ANASTOMOSES AROUND SCAPULA

Anastomoses Around the Body of the Scapula

It is formed by:

a. The *suprascapular artery*, a branch of the thyrocervical trunk (Fig. 6.11, Flowchart 6.3). It passes above suprascapular ligament and deep in to spinoglenoid ligament.
b. The *deep branch of the transverse cervical artery*, another branch of the thyrocervical trunk.
c. The *circumflex scapular artery*, a branch of the subscapular artery, which arises from the third part of the axillary artery.

Note that it is the anastomosis between branches of the 1st part of the subclavian artery and the branches of the 3rd part of the axillary artery. These arteries also anastomose with intercostal arteries.

Anastomoses Over the Acromion Process

It is formed by (Flowchart 6.3):

a. The acromial branch of the *thoracoacromial artery* (2nd part of axillary).
b. The acromial branch of the *suprascapular artery* (1st part of subclavian).
c. The acromial branch of the *posterior circumflex humeral artery* (3rd part of axillary).

Flowchart 6.3: Scapular anastomosis

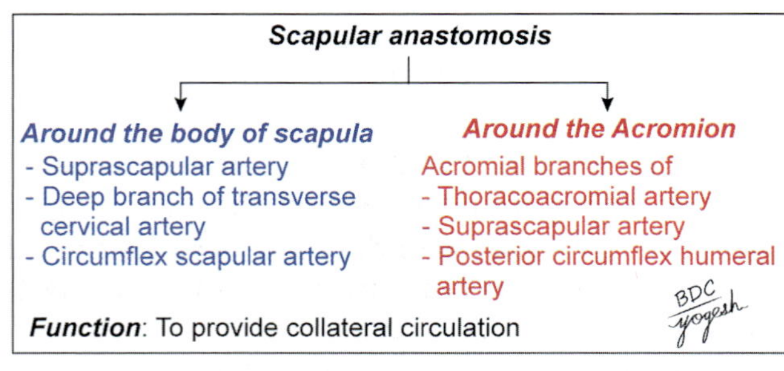

Note that this is the anastomosis between the first part of the subclavian artery and the branches of the second and third parts of the axillary artery (Fig. 6.11).

CLINICAL ANATOMY

The arterial anastomoses provide a collateral circulation through which blood can flow to the limb when the distal part of the subclavian artery, or the proximal part of the axillary artery is blocked (Fig. 6.11). Fracture of middle one-third of humerus causes injury to radial nerve as it lies in lower triangular space. This results in 'wrist drop'.

Facts to Remember

- Acromial fibres of the deltoid muscle are multipennate fibres.
- Muscles of rotator cuff (SITS): **S**upraspinatus, **I**nfraspinatus, **T**eres minor, **S**ubscapularis.
- Intramuscular injection should be given in the middle of the muscle as the upper part of the deltoid is related to the axillary nerve.
- Only circumflex scapular vessels pass through the upper triangular space.
- Branches of axillary nerve with accompanying blood vessels pass through the quadrangular intermuscular space.
- Radial nerve and profunda brachii vessels course through the lower triangular intermuscular space.
- Dawbarn's sign is seen in subacromial bursitis.

BDC's Anatomy *e*-book

1. Structures under cover of the deltoid
2. Forgotten muscle
3. Lift off test
4. Axillary nerve palsy
5. Further reading
6. Viva voce questions

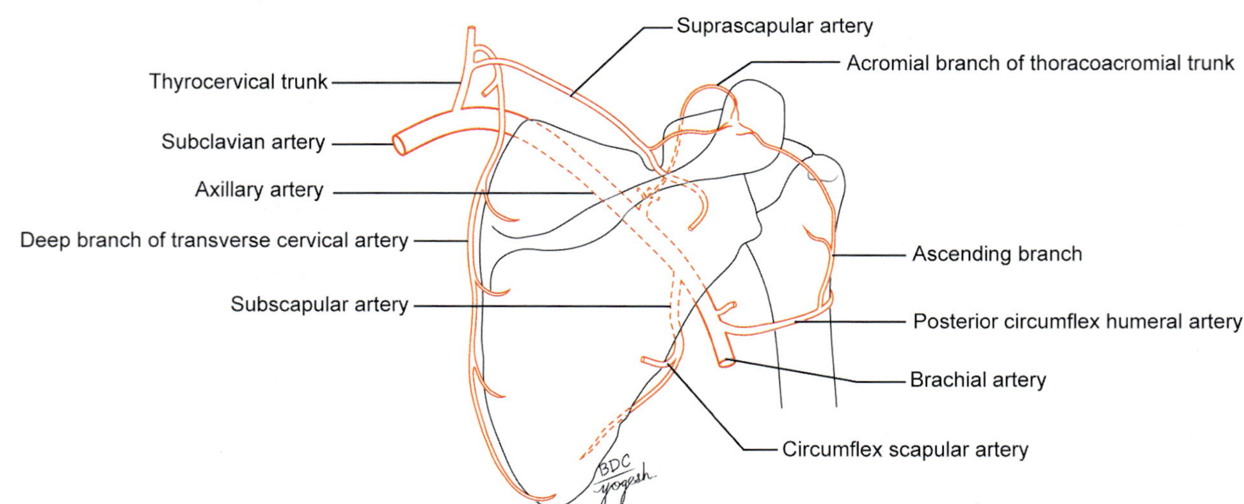

Fig. 6.11: Anastomoses around the scapula (dorsal aspect)

Chapter

7

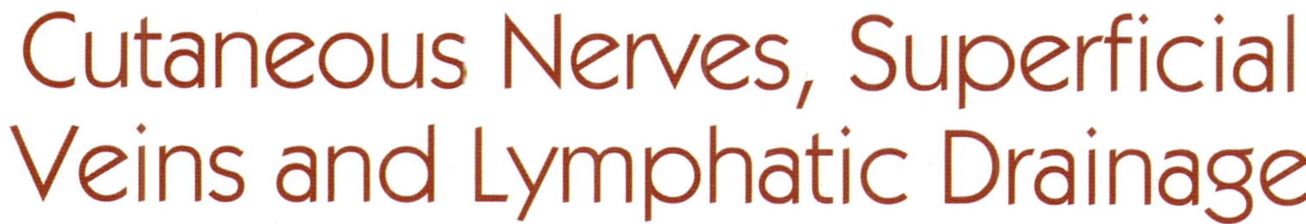

Cutaneous Nerves, Superficial Veins and Lymphatic Drainage

The superficial fascia seen after the reflection of skin contains cutaneous nerves, cutaneous or superficial veins and lymphatics. The cutaneous nerves are the continuation of the spinal nerves and carry sympathetic fibres for supplying the sweat glands, arterioles in the dermis and arrector pilorum muscles in relation to the hair follicle. Thus, the effects of sympathetic on the skin are sudomotor (increase sweat secretion), vasomotor (narrow the arterioles of skin) and pilomotor (contract arrector pilorum muscle to make the hair erect or straight), respectively.

The cutaneous nerves also carry sensation of pain, touch, temperature and pressure. Superficial veins are seen along with the cutaneous nerves. These are utilised for giving intravenous transfusions, cardiac catheterisation and taking blood samples. Lymphatic vessels, though important, are not easily seen in ordinary dissection.

CUTANEOUS NERVES

Position

The skin of the upper limb is supplied by 15 sets of cutaneous nerves (Table 7.1). Out of these, only one set (supraclavicular) is derived from the cervical plexus, and another nerve (intercostobrachial) is derived from the 2nd intercostal nerve. The remaining 13 sets are derived from the brachial plexus through the musculocutaneous, median, ulnar, axillary and radial nerves. Some branches arise directly from the medial cord of the plexus.

Peculiarities of Cutaneous Nerves of Upper Limb

1. The areas of distribution of peripheral cutaneous nerves do not necessarily correspond with those of individual spinal segments (areas of the skin supplied by individual spinal segments are called dermatomes). This is so because each cutaneous nerve contains fibres from more than one ventral ramus (of a spinal nerve), and each ramus gives fibres to more than one cutaneous nerve.
2. Adjacent areas of skin supplied by different cutaneous nerves overlap each other to a considerable extent. Therefore, the area of sensory loss after damage to a nerve is much less than the area of distribution of the nerve. The anaesthetic area is surrounded by an area in which the sensations are somewhat altered.
3. In both the upper and lower limbs, the nerves of the anterior or flexor surface have a wider area of distribution than those supplying the posterior or extensor surface.

Cutaneous Nerves of Upper Limb

The individual cutaneous nerves, from above downwards, are described below with their root values. Figures 7.1a and b show the cutaneous nerves of the upper limb.

1. ***Supraclavicular nerves*** (C3, C4): These are branches of the cervical plexus. They pierce the deep fascia in the neck, descend superficial to the clavicle and supply:
   a. The skin of the pectoral region up to the level of the second rib.
   b. Skin covering the upper half of the deltoid.
2. ***Upper lateral cutaneous nerve of the arm*** (C5, C6): It is the continuation of the posterior branch of the axillary nerve. It supplies the skin covering the lower half of the deltoid.
3. ***Lower lateral cutaneous nerve of the arm*** (C5, C6): It is a branch of the radial nerve given off in the radial groove. It supplies the skin of the lower half of the lateral side of the arm.
4. ***Intercostobrachial nerve*** (T2): It is the lateral cutaneous branch of the 2nd intercostal nerve. It crosses the axilla and supplies the skin of the upper half of the medial and posterior parts of the arm. It lies amongst the central group of axillary lymph nodes.
5. ***Medial cutaneous nerve of the arm*** (T1, T2): It is the smallest branch of the medial cord of the brachial plexus.
6. ***Posterior cutaneous nerve of the arm*** (C5): It is a branch of the radial nerve given off in the axilla. It supplies the skin of the back of the arm from the insertion of the deltoid to the olecranon process.
7. ***Lateral cutaneous nerve of the forearm*** (C5, C6): It is the continuation of the musculocutaneous nerve.

TABLE 7.1: The cutaneous nerves (Fig. 7.1)

Region supplied	*Nerve(s)*	*Root value*	*Derived from*
Upper part of pectoral region and skin over upper part of deltoid	Supraclavicular	C3, C4	Cervical plexus
ARM			
1. Upper medial part	Intercostobrachial (Figs 7.1a and b)	T2	2nd intercostal
2. Lower medial part	Medial cutaneous nerve of arm	T1, T2	Medial cord
3. Upper lateral part (including skin over lower part of deltoid)	Upper lateral cutaneous nerve of arm	C5, C6	Axillary nerve
4. Lower lateral part	Lower lateral cutaneous nerve of arm	C5, C6	Radial nerve
5. Posterior aspect	Posterior cutaneous nerve of arm	C5	Radial nerve
FOREARM			
1. Medial side	Medial cutaneous nerve of forearm	C8, T1	Medial cord
2. Lateral side	Lateral cutaneous nerve of forearm	C5, C6	Musculocutaneous
3. Posterior side	Posterior cutaneous nerve of forearm	C6–C8	Radial nerve
PALM			
1. Lateral two-thirds	Palmar cutaneous branch of median	C6, C7	Median
2. Medial one-third	Palmar cutaneous branch of ulnar	C8	Ulnar
DORSUM OF HAND			
1. Medial half, including proximal and middle phalanges of medial 1½ digits	Dorsal branch of ulnar	C8	Ulnar
2. Lateral half, including proximal and middle phalanges of lateral 3½ digits	Superficial terminal branch of radial	C6, C7	Radial
DIGITS			
Palmar aspect and dorsal aspect of distal phalanges			
1. Lateral 3½ digits	Palmar digital branch of median	C7	Median
2. Medial 1½ digits	Palmar digital branch of ulnar	C7, C8	Ulnar

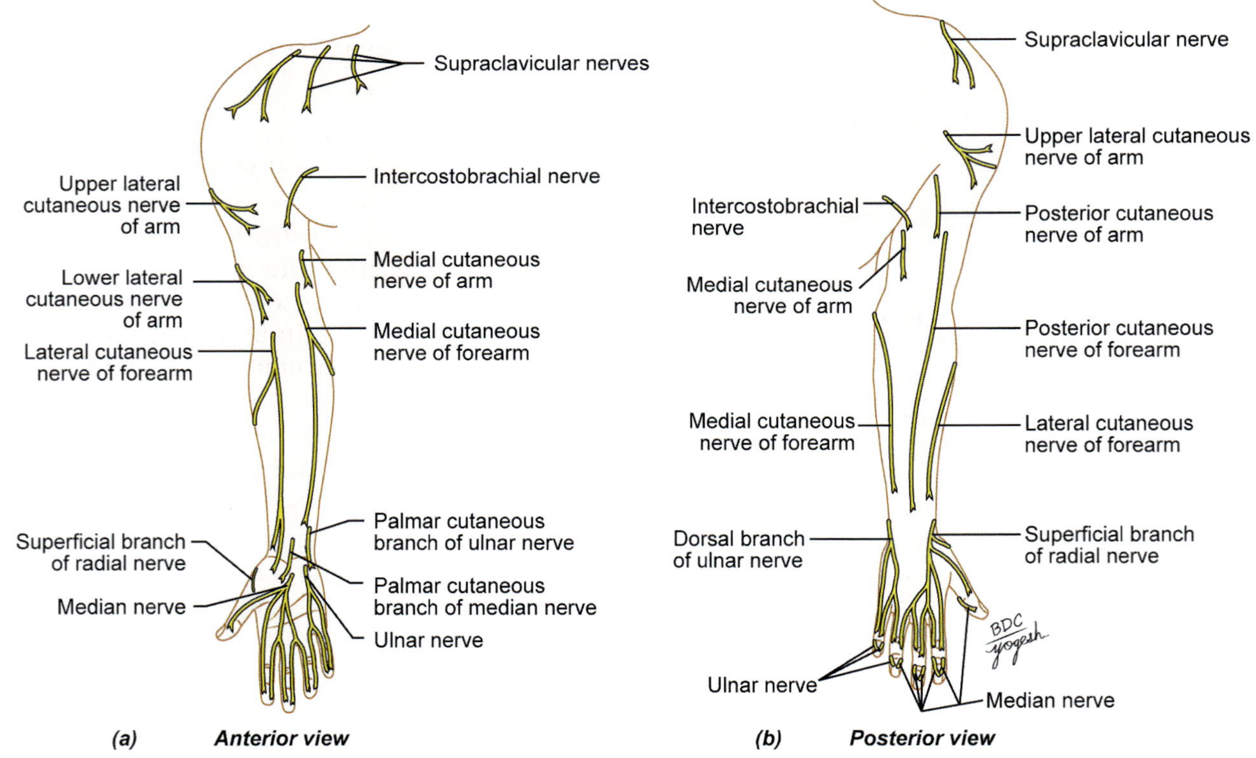

Fig. 7.1: The cutaneous nerves

It pierces the deep fascia just lateral to the tendon of the biceps 2–3 cm above the bend of the elbow and supplies the skin of the lateral side of the forearm, extending anteriorly to a small part of the ball of the thumb.

8. ***Medial cutaneous nerve of the forearm*** (C8, T1): It is a branch of the medial cord of the brachial plexus. It runs along the medial side of the axillary and brachial arteries and supplies the skin of the medial side of the forearm.

9. ***Posterior cutaneous nerve of the forearm*** (C6–C8): It arises from the radial nerve in the radial groove. It descends posterior to the lateral epicondyle and supplies the skin of the back of the forearm.
10. ***Median nerve*** gives off two sets of cutaneous branches in the hand.
    a. ***Palmar cutaneous branch*** (C6–C8): It arises a *short distance above the wrist*, lies *superficial to flexor retinaculum* and supplies skin over the lateral 2/3rd of the palm, including that over the thenar eminence (Fig. 7.1a).
    b. ***Palmar digital branches*** (C6–C8) are five in number and arise in the palm. The medial two branches are common palmar digital nerves; each divides near a digital cleft to form two *proper palmar digital nerves*. The lateral three branches are proper palmar digital nerves for the medial and lateral sides of the thumb and for the lateral side of the index finger. The various digital branches of the median nerve supply palmar skin of the lateral 3½ digits, the nail beds and skin on the dorsal aspect of the distal phalanges of the same digits (Fig. 7.1b).
11. ***Ulnar nerve*** gives off three sets of cutaneous nerves in hand.
    a. ***Palmar cutaneous branch*** (C7, C8): It arises in the middle of the forearm and descends, crossing *superficial to flexor retinaculum* and supplies skin of the medial 1/3rd of the palm.
    b. ***Palmar digital branches of the ulnar nerve*** (C7, C8) are two in number. They arise from the superficial terminal branch of the ulnar nerve just distal to the pisiform bone. The medial of the two branches is a proper palmar digital nerve for the medial side of the little finger. The lateral branch is a common palmar digital nerve which divides into two proper digital nerves for supply of adjacent sides of the ring and little fingers. Thus, it supplies skin of medial 1½ digits, their nail beds and skin on the dorsal aspects of distal phalanges of medial 1½ digits (Figs 7.1a and b).
    c. ***Dorsal branch of the ulnar nerve*** (C7, C8) arises about 6 cm above the wrist. It descends with the main trunk of the ulnar nerve almost to the pisiform bone. Here, it passes backwards to divide into three (sometimes two) dorsal digital nerves. Typically, the region of skin supplied by the dorsal branch covers the medial half of the back of the hand, and the skin on the dorsal aspect of the medial 1½ digits.
12. ***Superficial terminal branch of the radial nerve*** (C6–C8): It arises in front of the lateral epicondyle of the humerus. It descends through the upper 2/3rd of the forearm lateral to the radial artery, and then passes posteriorly about 7 cm above the wrist. While winding round the radius it pierces the deep fascia and divides into four or five small dorsal digital nerves. In all, the superficial terminal branch supplies the skin of the lateral half of the dorsum of the hand, and the dorsal surfaces of the lateral 3½ digits, including the thumb, except for the terminal portions supplied by the median nerve.

DISSECTION

Make one horizontal incision in the arm at its junction of upper 1/3rd and lower 2/3rd segments (*see* Fig. 3.3) and a vertical incision through the centre of arm and forearm till the wrist where another transverse incision is given.

Reflect the skin on either side on the front as well as on the back of the limb. Use this huge skin flap to cover the limb after the dissection.

Competency:

AN13.2 Describe dermatomes of upper limb.

DERMATOMES OF THE UPPER LIMB

Definition

- The area of skin supplied by one spinal segment is called a *dermatome.*
- A typical dermatome extends from the posterior median line to the anterior median line around the trunk. However, in the limbs, the dermatomes have migrated rather irregularly so that the original uniform pattern is disturbed.

Embryological Basis

- The early human embryo shows regular segmentation of the body. Each segment is supplied by the corresponding segmental nerve. In an adult, all structures, including the skin, developed from one segment, are supplied by their original segmental nerve.
- The limb may be regarded as an extension of the body wall, and the segments from which they are derived can be deduced from the spinal nerves supplying them. The limb buds arise in the area of the body wall supplied by the lateral branches of anterior primary rami. The nerves to the limbs represent these branches (Figs 7.2 to 7.4).

Peculiarities of Dermatomes of Upper Limb

1. The cutaneous innervation of the upper limb is derived:
    a. Mainly from segments C5–C8 and T1 of the spinal cord, and
    b. Partly from the overlapping segments from above, additional segments are found only at the proximal end of the limb (Fig. 7.5).
2. Since the limb bud appears on the ventrolateral aspect of the body wall, it is invariably supplied by the anterior primary rami of the spinal nerves. Posterior primary rami do not supply the limb.

    It is possible that the ventral and dorsal divisions of the trunks of the brachial plexus represent the anterior and posterior branches of the lateral cutaneous nerves.
3. There is a varying degree of ***segmental overlap*** of adjoining dermatomes so that the area of sensory loss

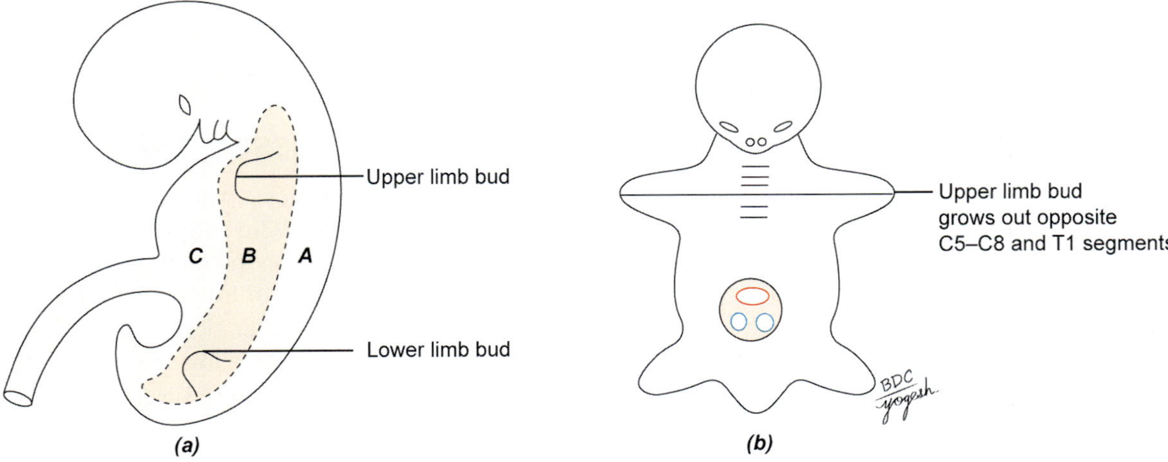

Figs 7.2a and b: (a) The body wall is supplied by (A) the posterior primary rami, (B) the lateral branches of the anterior primary rami and (C) the anterior branches of the anterior primary rami of the spinal nerves. The limb buds develop from the area supplied by the lateral branches of the anterior primary rami and (b) the upper limb bud grows out opposite C5 – C8 and T1 segments of the spinal cord.

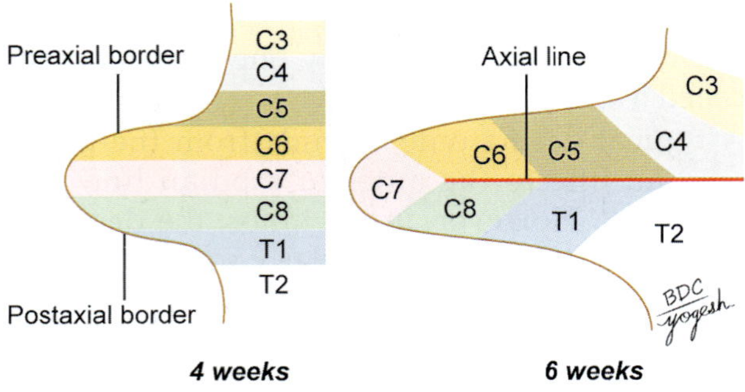

Fig. 7.3: Distribution of various segments in upper limb

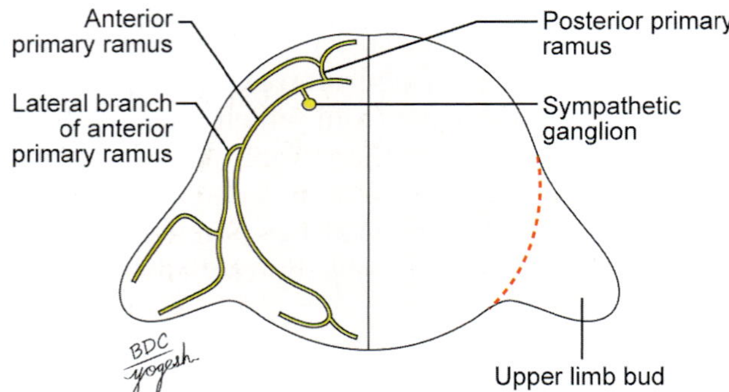

Fig. 7.4: The upper limb bud grows out from the part of the body wall supplied by the lateral cutaneous branches of the anterior primary rami of spinal nerves

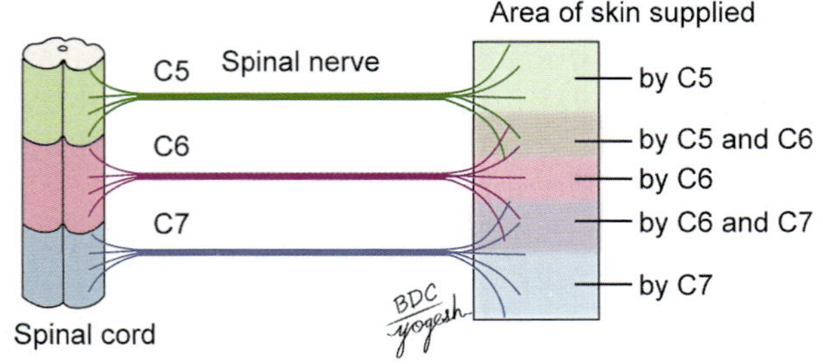

Fig. 7.5: Overlapping of the dermatomes

following damage to the cord or nerve roots is always less than the area of distribution of the dermatomes (Fig. 7.5).

4. Each limb bud has a cephalic and a caudal border, known as ***preaxial*** and ***postaxial borders***, respectively. In the upper limb, the thumb and radius lie along the preaxial border, and the little finger and ulna along the postaxial border.
5. The dermatomes of the upper limb are distributed in an orderly numerical sequence (Fig. 7.6).
   a. Along the preaxial border, by segments C3–C6 with overlapping of the dermatomes.
   b. The middle three digits (index, middle and ring fingers) and the adjoining area of the palm are supplied by segment C7.

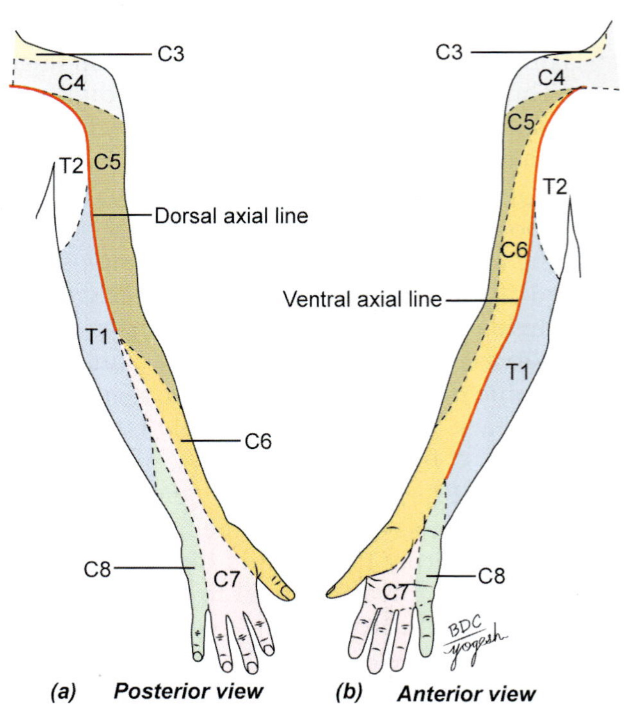

Fig. 7.6: Dermatomes of upper limb

c. The postaxial border is supplied (from below upwards) by segments C8, T1 and T2. There is overlapping of the dermatomes.

6. As the limb elongates, it rotates laterally and gets adducted and the central dermatome C7 gets pulled in such a way that these are represented only in the distal part of the limb and are buried proximally.

On the front of the limb, areas supplied by C5 and C6 segments adjoin the areas supplied by C8, T1 and T2 segments. There is a dividing line between them, known as the ***ventral axial line***, along which C7 is buried proximally. It reaches the skin just proximal to the wrist (Fig. 7.6).

On the back of the limb, C7 reaches the skin just proximal to the elbow. So the ***dorsal axial line*** ends more proximal to the ventral axial line. There is no overlapping across the ventral and dorsal axial lines (Fig. 7.6).

CLINICAL ANATOMY

- The area of sensory loss of the skin, following injuries of the spinal cord or of the nerve roots, conforms to the dermatomes. Therefore, the segmental level of the damage to the spinal cord can be determined by examining the dermatomes for touch, pain and temperature. Note that injury to a peripheral nerve produces sensory loss corresponding to the area of distribution of that nerve.
- The spinal segments do not lie opposite the corresponding vertebrae. In estimating the position of a spinal segment in relation to the surface of the body, it is important to remember that a vertebral spine is always *lower* than the corresponding spinal segment. As a rough guide, it may be stated that in the cervical region, there is a difference of one segment, e.g. the 5th cervical spine lies lower than the 5th cervical spinal segment. It overlies the 6th cervical spinal segment.

Spinal segments	*Spine of vertebra*
C1–C8	C1–C7
T1–T6	T1–T4
T7–T12	T5–T9
L1–L5	T10–T11
S1–S5 and Co1	T12–L1

Competency:

AN13.1 Describe and explain fascia of upper limb and compartments, veins of upper limb and its lymphatic drainage.

VEINS OF UPPER LIMB

The veins draining the upper limb are grouped as follows:

Superficial veins: These are located in the superficial fascia (Plate 7.1, Figs 7.8 and 7.9a–c). They include:

1. Dorsal venous arch
2. Cephalic vein
3. Basilic vein
4. Median cubital vein.

Deep veins: These are located deep in to the deep fascia. These include:

1. Venae comitantes that accompany the large arteries, such as radial, ulnar and brachial arteries.
2. Axillary vein.

SUPERFICIAL VEINS

Superficial veins of the upper limb assume importance in medical practice because these are most commonly used for intravenous injections and for withdrawing blood for testing.

General Features of Superficial Veins

1. Most of the superficial veins of the limb join together to form two large veins, cephalic (preaxial) and basilic (postaxial).
2. The superficial veins run away from pressure points. Therefore, they are absent in the palm (fist area), along the ulnar border of the forearm (supporting border) and in the back of the arm and trapezius region. This makes the course of the veins spiral from the dorsal to the ventral surface of the limb.
3. The preaxial vein is longer than the postaxial. In other words, the preaxial vein drains into the deep (axillary) vein more proximally (at the root of the limb) than the postaxial vein, which becomes deep in the middle of the arm.
4. The earlier a vein becomes deep the better, because the venous return is then assisted by muscular compression. The load of the preaxial (cephalic) vein is greatly relieved by the more efficient postaxial (basilic) vein through a short-circuiting channel (the median cubital vein situated in front of the elbow) and partly also by the deep veins through a perforator vein connecting the median cubital to the deep vein.
5. The superficial veins are accompanied by cutaneous nerves and superficial lymphatics and not by arteries. The superficial lymph nodes lie along the veins, and the deep lymph nodes along the arteries.
6. The superficial veins are best utilised for intravenous injections.

Dorsal Venous Arch

Dorsal venous arch lies on the dorsum of the hand (Fig. 7.7). Its afferents (tributaries) include:

1. Three dorsal metacarpal veins.
2. A dorsal digital vein from the medial side of the little finger.
3. A dorsal digital vein from the radial side of the index finger.
4. Two dorsal digital veins from the thumb.
5. Most of the blood from the palm courses through veins passing around the margins of the hand and also by perforating veins passing through the interosseous spaces.

Pressure on the palm during gripping fails to impede the venous return due to the mode of drainage of the palm into the dorsal venous arch.

Plate 7.1: Superficial veins of upper limb

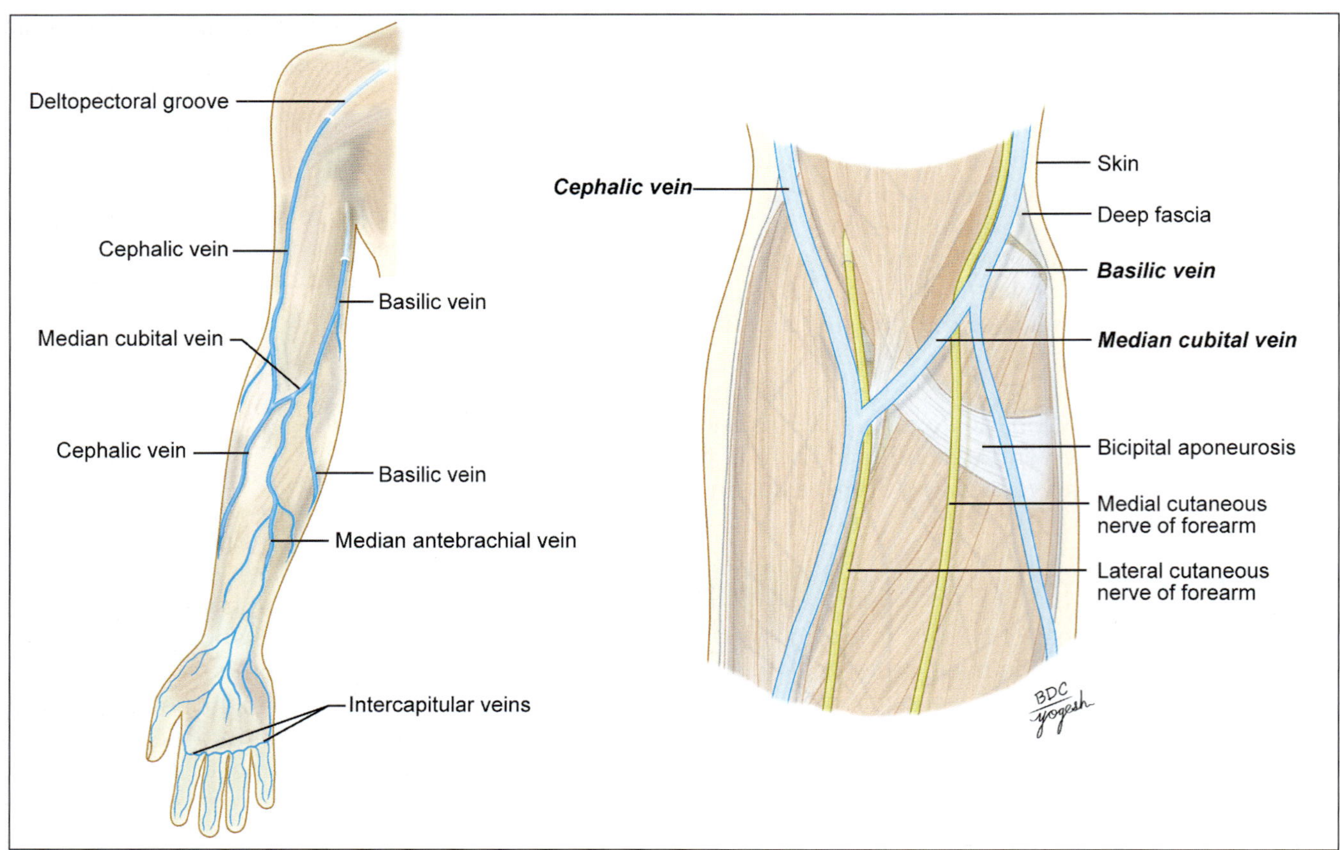

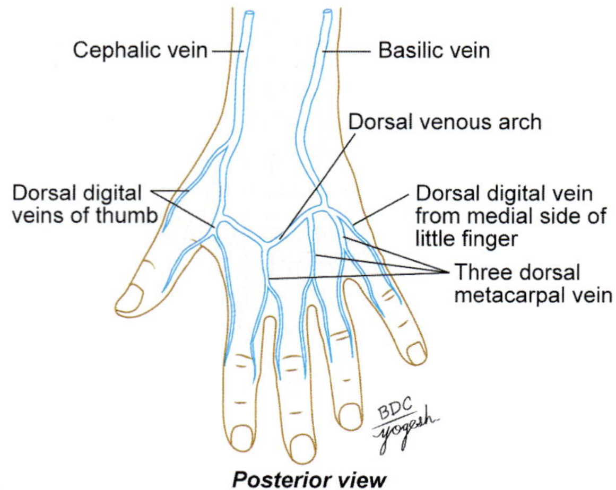

Fig. 7.7: Dorsal venous arch

The efferents of dorsal venous arch are the cephalic and basilic veins.

Cephalic Vein

Cephalic vein is the preaxial vein of the upper limb (cf. great saphenous vein of the lower limb). It begins from the lateral end of the dorsal venous arch.

It runs upwards:

1. Through the roof of the *anatomical snuffbox*.
2. Winds around the lateral border of the distal part of the forearm (Fig. 7.7).
3. Continues upwards in front of the elbow and along the lateral border of the biceps brachii.
4. Pierces the deep fascia at the lower border of the pectoralis major.
5. Runs in the deltopectoral groove up to the infraclavicular fossa.
6. It pierces the clavipectoral fascia and joins the axillary vein.

At the elbow, the greater part of its blood is drained into the basilic vein through the *median cubital vein* and partly also into the deep veins through the perforator vein.

It is accompanied by the lateral cutaneous nerve of the forearm and the terminal part of the radial nerve.

An *accessory cephalic vein* is sometimes present. It ends by joining the cephalic vein near the elbow.

Basilic Vein

Basilic vein is the postaxial vein of the upper limb (cf. short saphenous vein of the lower limb).

It begins from the medial end of the dorsal venous arch (Fig. 7.7).

It runs upwards:

1. Along the back of the medial border of the forearm,
2. Winds around this border near the elbow,
3. Continues upwards in front of the elbow (medial epicondyle) and along the medial margin of the biceps brachii up to the middle of the arm, where
   - It pierces the deep fascia, and
   - Runs along the medial side of the brachial artery up to the lower border of teres major where it becomes the axillary vein.

About 2.5 cm above the medial epicondyle of the humerus, it is joined by the median cubital vein.

It is accompanied by the posterior branch of the medial cutaneous nerve of the forearm and the terminal part of the dorsal branch of the ulnar nerve.

Median Cubital Vein

- Median cubital vein is a large communicating vein which shunts blood from the cephalic to the basilic vein (Fig. 7.8).
- It begins from the cephalic vein 2.5 cm below the bend of the elbow, runs obliquely upward and medially, and ends in the basilic vein 2.5 cm above the medial epicondyle. It is separated from the brachial artery by the bicipital aponeurosis.
- It may receive tributaries from the front of the forearm (median vein of the forearm) and is connected to the deep veins through a perforator vein, which pierces the bicipital aponeurosis. The perforator vein fixes the median cubital vein and thus makes it ideal for intravenous injections.

Median Vein of the Forearm

Median vein of the forearm begins from the palmar venous network and ends in any one of the veins in front of the elbow, mostly in median cubital vein.

DEEP VEINS

- Deep veins start as small venae comitantes running on each side of digital arteries. These continue proximally along superficial and deep palmar arches.
- Then, these course proximally to continue as venae comitantes of radial and ulnar arteries, which further join to form the brachial veins.
- Brachial veins lie on each side of brachial artery. These join the axillary vein at the lower border of teres major. Axillary vein is described in axilla (*see* Chapter 4).

Competency:

AN11.3 Describe the anatomical basis of venepuncture of cubital veins.

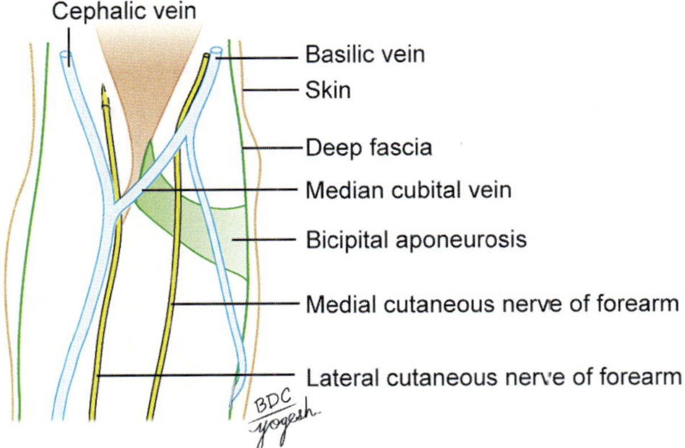

Fig. 7.8: Median cubital vein in the roof of cubital fossa

CLINICAL ANATOMY

- ***Venepuncture in the cubital fossa*:** The median cubital vein is the vein of choice for intravenous injections, for withdrawing blood from donors, and for cardiac catheterisation, because it is fixed by the perforator and does not slip away during piercing. When the median cubital vein is absent, the basilic vein is preferred over the cephalic vein because the former is a more efficient channel (Figs 7.10 and 7.11).
- The cephalic vein frequently communicates with the external jugular vein by means of a small vein, which crosses in front of the clavicle. In operations for removal of the breast (in carcinoma), the axillary lymph nodes are also removed, and it sometimes becomes necessary to remove a segment of the axillary vein also. In these cases, the communication between the cephalic vein and the external jugular vein enlarges considerably and helps in draining blood from the upper limb (Fig. 7.12).
- In case of fracture of the clavicle, the rupture of the communicating channel may lead to formation of a large haematoma, i.e. collection of blood.
- Basilic vein is preferred for right cardiac catheterisation as this vein has large diameter and easily accessible. In cardiac catheterisation, a long rubber tube (called catheter) is inserted in the heart to check the heart disease to know the functioning of the cardiac muscles and valve.

LYMPH NODES AND LYMPHATIC DRAINAGE

- When circulating blood reaches the capillaries, part of its fluid content passes through them into the surrounding tissue as *tissue fluid.* Most of this tissue fluid re-enters the capillaries at their venous ends. Some of it is, however, returned to circulation through a separate set of *lymphatic vessels.* These vessels begin as lymphatic capillaries, which drain into larger vessels.
- Along the course of these lymph vessels, there are groups of *lymph nodes.*
- Lymph vessels are difficult to see and special techniques are required for their visualisation.
- Lymph nodes are small bean-like structures that are usually present in groups. These are not normally palpable in the living subject.
- However, they often become enlarged in disease, particularly by infection or malignancy in the area from which they receive lymph. They then become palpable, and examination of these nodes provides valuable information regarding the presence and spread of disease.

Lymph Nodes

1. ***Axillary lymph nodes:*** The main lymph nodes of the upper limb are the *axillary lymph nodes*. These comprise anterior, posterior, lateral, central and apical groups. These have been described in Chapter 4 (*see* page 51).

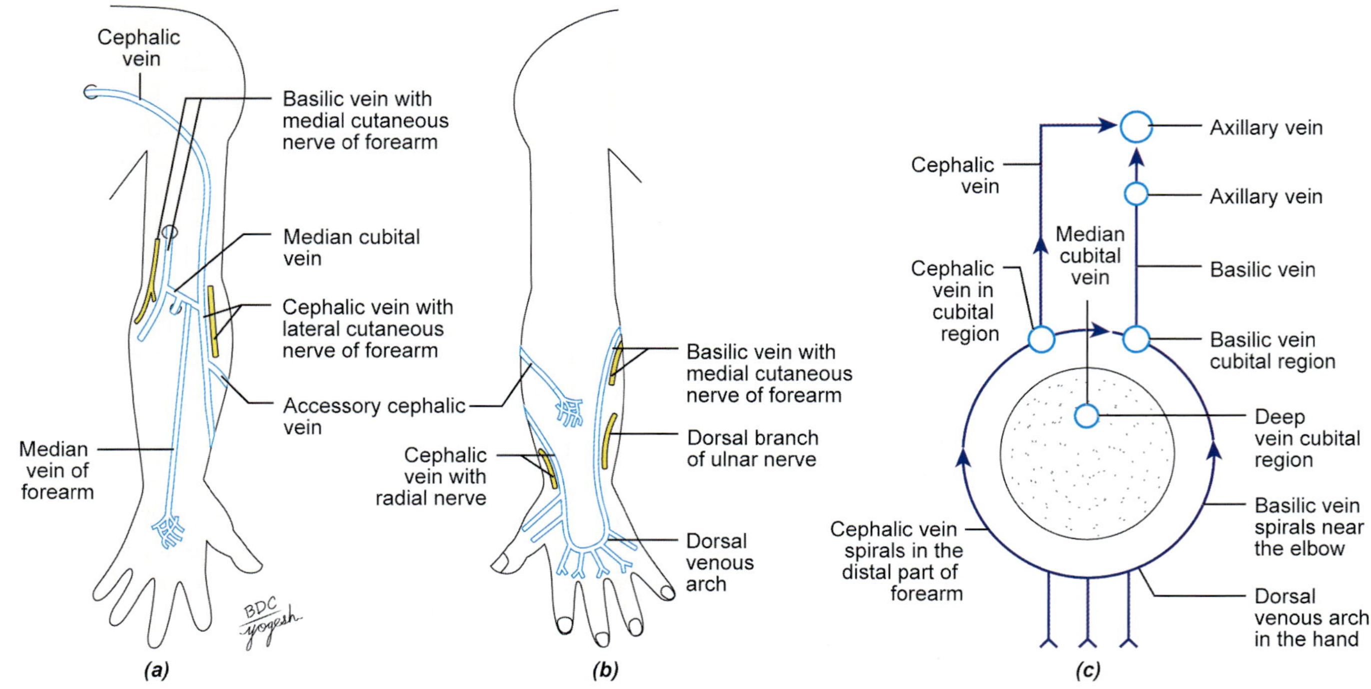

Figs 7.9a to c: The superficial veins of the upper limb: (a) On the front, (b) on the back of the limb, and (c) schematic representation

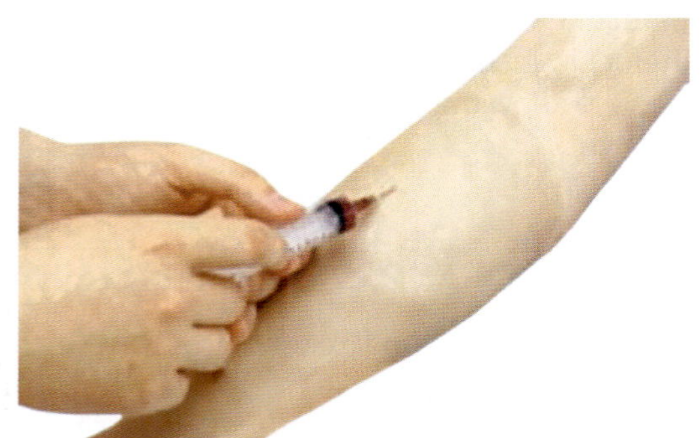

Fig. 7.10: Intravenous injection being given in the superficial vein of forearm

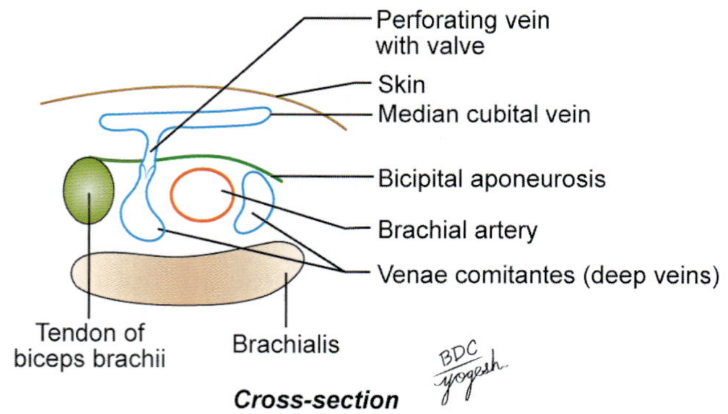

Fig. 7.11: Relations of median cubital vein

2. ***Infraclavicular nodes:*** They lie in or on the clavipectoral fascia along the cephalic vein. They drain the upper part of the breast and the thumb with its web.
3. ***Deltopectoral node:*** They lie in the deltopectoral groove along the cephalic vein. It is a displaced node of the infraclavicular set and drains similar structures.

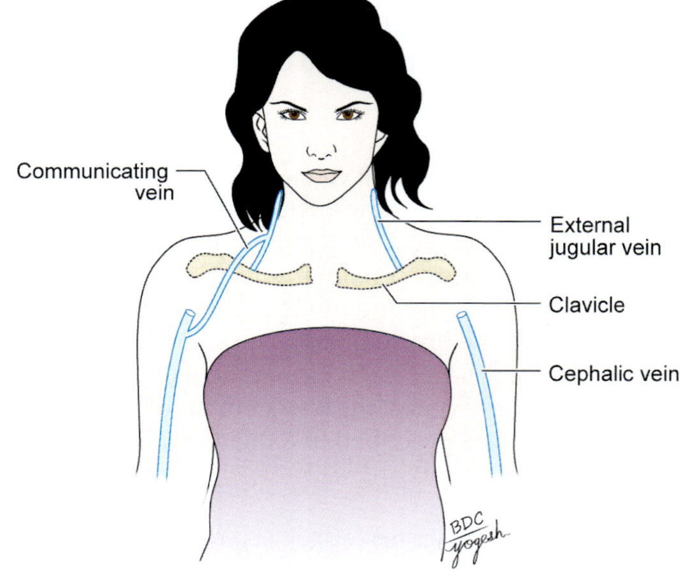

Fig. 7.12: A communicating vein helps in venous drainage from upper limb

4. ***Superficial cubital or supratrochlear nodes:*** They lie just above the medial epicondyle along the basilic vein. They drain the ulnar side of the hand and forearm. These are the most distal superficial lymph nodes in the upper limb.
5. A few other deep lymph nodes lie in the following regions:
   a. Along the medial side of the brachial artery.
   b. At the bifurcation of the brachial artery (deep cubital lymph node).
   c. Occasionally along the arteries of the forearm.

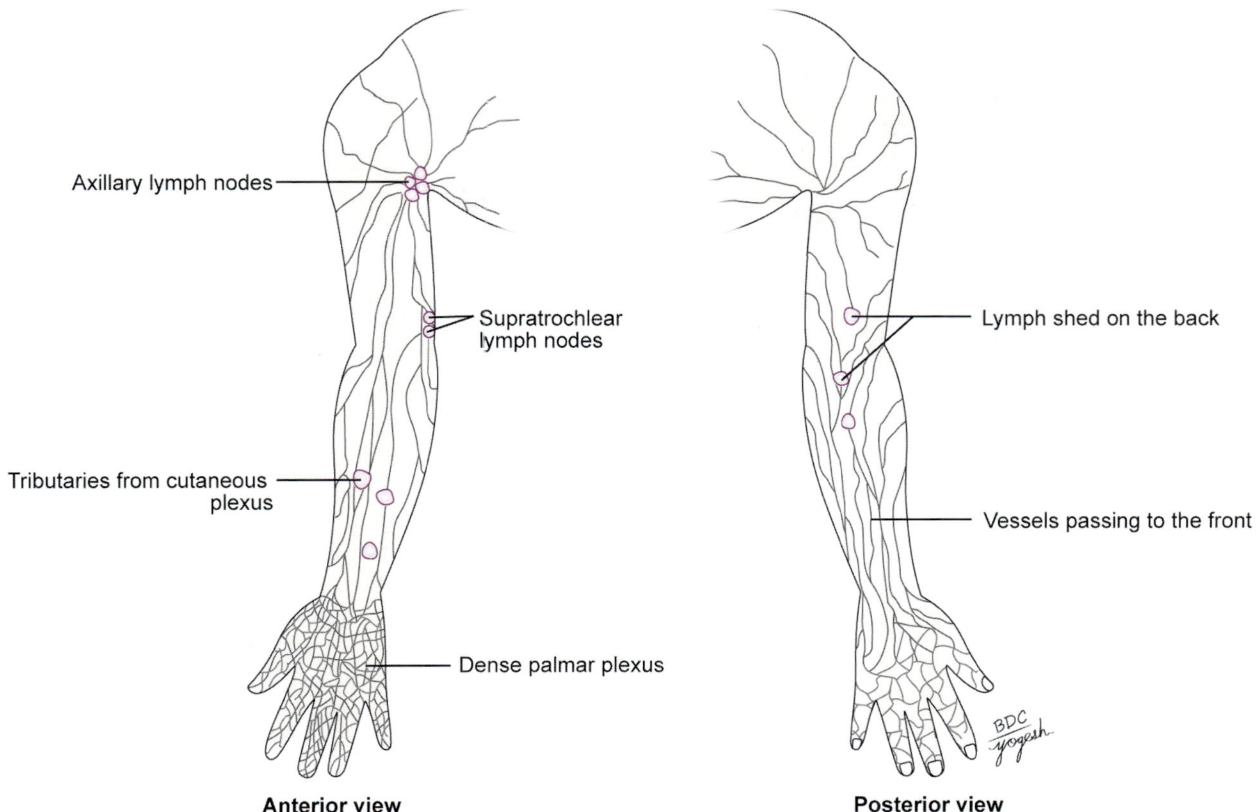

Fig. 7.13: The superficial lymphatics of the upper limb

Lymphatic Vessels

Superficial Lymphatics

Superficial lymphatics are much more numerous than the deep lymphatics. They collect lymph from the skin and subcutaneous tissues. Most of them ultimately drain into the axillary nodes, except for:

1. A few vessels from the medial side of the forearm, which drain into the superficial cubital nodes.
2. A few vessels from the lateral side of the forearm, which drain into the deltopectoral or infraclavicular nodes.

The dense *palmar plexus* drains mostly into the lymph vessels onto the dorsum of the hand, where these continue with the vessels of the forearm. Lymph vessels of the back of forearm and arm curve around their medial and lateral surfaces and ascend up to reach the floor of the axilla. Thus, there is a vertical area of *lymph shed* in the middle of back of forearm and arm (Fig. 7.13).

Deep Lymphatics

Deep lymphatics are much less numerous than the superficial lymphatics. They drain structures lying deep into the deep fascia. They run along the main blood vessels of the limb and end in the axillary nodes. Some of the lymph may pass through the deep lymph nodes present along the axillary vein, as mentioned above.

CLINICAL ANATOMY

- Inflammation of lymph vessels is known as ***lymphangitis***. In acute lymphangitis, the vessels may be seen through the skin as red, tender (painful to touch) streaks (Fig. 7.14).
- Inflammation of lymph nodes is called ***lymphadenitis***. It may be acute or chronic. The nodes enlarge and become palpable and painful (Fig. 7.15).
- Obstruction to lymph vessels can result in accumulation of tissue fluid in areas of drainage. This is called ***lymphoedema***. This may be caused by carcinoma because of surgical removal of lymph nodes (Fig. 7.16).
- Pain along the medial side of upper arm is due to pressure on the intercostobrachial nerve by enlarged central group of axillary lymph nodes.

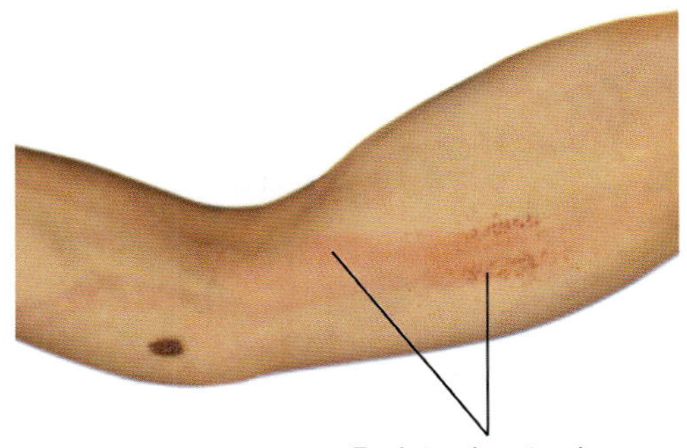

Fig. 7.14: Lymphangitis

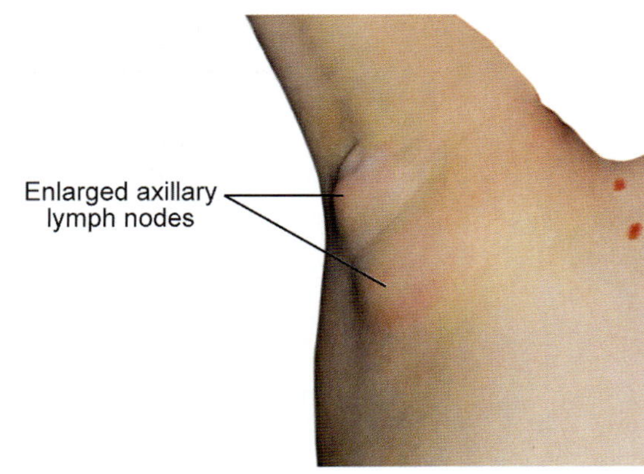

Fig. 7.15: Enlarged axillary lymph nodes

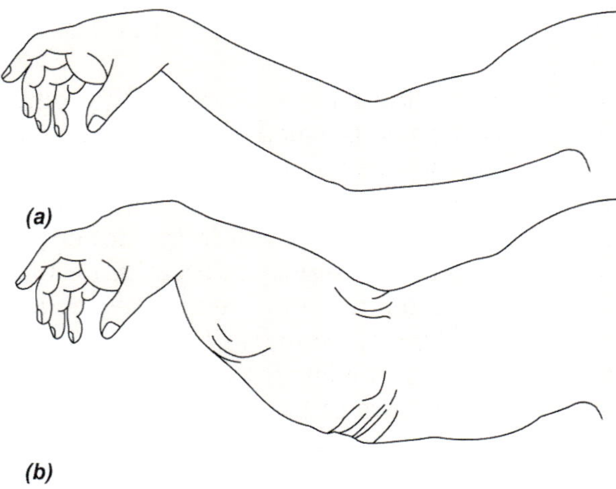

Figs 7.16a and b: (a) Normal upper limb and (b) lymphoedema due to removal of axillary lymph nodes in case of carcinoma of the breast

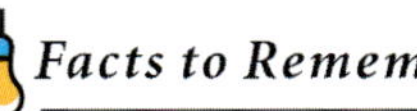

Facts to Remember

- Ventral axial line ends close to wrist joint, while dorsal axial line ends close to elbow joint.
- Dermatome is an area of skin supplied by single spinal segment through a pair of right and left spinal nerves through both its dorsal and ventral rami.
- There is no overlapping of the nerve supply across the axial lines.
- Intercostobrachial nerve (T2) is the lateral cutaneous branch of the 2nd intercostal nerve. It supplies the skin of the upper half of the medial and posterior parts of the arm.
- Cephalic vein begins in the 'anatomical snuffbox' and it is the longest superficial vein of the upper limb.
- The median cubital vein is the most commonly used vein for venipuncture. It is fixed due to perforators passing through the bicipital aponeurosis.
- The basilic vein is the most preferred vein for cardiac catheterisation.
- There is a vertical area of *lymph shed* in the middle of back of forearm and arm.

BDC's Anatomy *e*-book

1. Segment innervation of upper limb
2. Axial lines of upper limb
3. Common venous patterns in front of the elbow
4. Steps of venepuncture
5. Use of cephalic vein in haemodialysis
6. How is the lymph generated?
7. Further reading
8. Viva voce questions

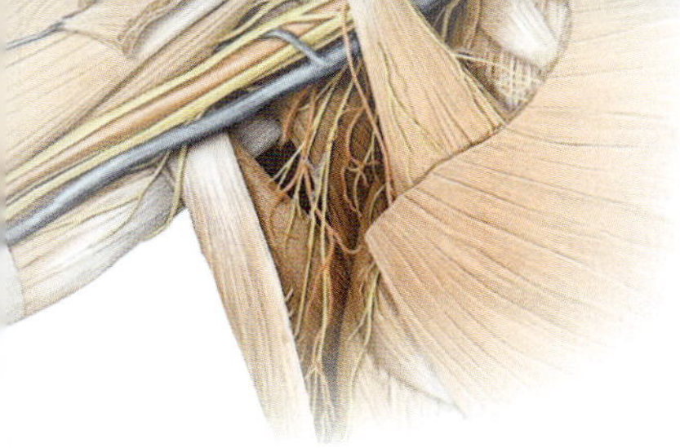

Chapter

8

Arm

The arm extends from the shoulder joint to the elbow joint. The skeleton of the arm is a 'solo' bone, the humerus. Medial and lateral intermuscular septa divide the arm into an anterior or flexor compartment and a posterior or extensor compartment to give each compartment its individuality and freedom of action. Since the structures in the front of arm continue across the elbow joint into the cubital fossa, the cubital fossa is also included in this chapter.

The arm is called *brachium*, so most of the structures in this chapter are named accordingly, like brachialis, coracobrachialis and brachial artery.

SURFACE LANDMARKS

The following landmarks can be felt in the living subject.

1. ***Greater tubercle of the humerus:*** It can be felt just below the acromion process, deep to the deltoid, when the arm is by the side of the trunk (Fig. 8.1).
2. ***Shaft of the humerus:*** It is felt only indistinctly because it is surrounded by muscles in its upper half. In the lower half, the humerus is covered anteriorly by the biceps brachii and brachialis and posteriorly by the triceps brachii.
3. ***Medial epicondyle of the humerus:*** It is a prominent bony projection on the medial side of the elbow. It is best seen and felt in a mid-flexed elbow.
4. ***Lateral epicondyle of the humerus:*** It is less prominent than the medial. It can be felt in the upper part of the depression on the posterolateral aspect of the elbow in the extended position of the forearm.
5. ***Medial and lateral supracondylar ridges:*** These are better defined in the lower portions of the medial and lateral borders of the humerus. They can be felt in the lower one-fourth of the arm as upward continuations of the epicondyles.
6. ***Deltoid muscle:*** It forms the rounded contour of the shoulder. The apex of the muscle is attached to the deltoid tuberosity located in the middle of the anterolateral surface of the humerus.
7. ***Coracobrachialis muscle:*** It forms an inconspicuous rounded ridge in the upper part of the medial side of the arm. Pulsations of the brachial artery can be felt in the depression behind it.
8. ***Biceps brachii muscle:*** It forms a conspicuous elevation on the front of the arm. Upon flexing the elbow, the contracting muscle becomes still more prominent. The tendon of the biceps can be felt in front of the elbow. The tendon is a guide to the brachial artery, which lies on its medial side.
9. ***Brachial artery:*** It can be felt in front of the elbow joint just medial to the tendon of the biceps brachii. Brachial pulsations are used for recording the blood pressure.
10. ***Ulnar nerve:*** It can be rolled by the palpating finger behind the medial epicondyle of the humerus. During leprosy, this nerve becomes thick and enlarged.
11. The superficial cubital veins can be made more prominent by applying tight pressure a round the arm and then contracting the forearm muscles by clenching and releasing the fist a few times. The ***cephalic vein*** runs upwards along the lateral border of the biceps. The ***basilic vein*** can be seen along the

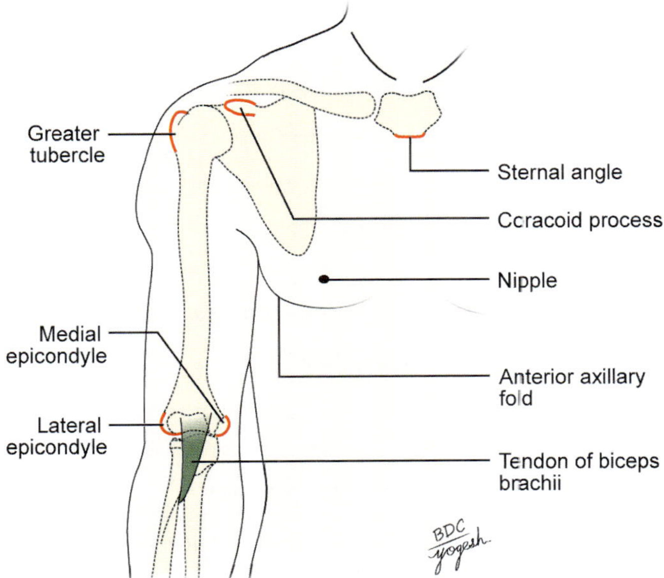

Fig. 8.1: Surface landmarks—front of upper arm

lower half of the medial border of the biceps. The cephalic and basilic veins are connected together in front of the elbow by the ***median cubital vein,*** which runs obliquely upwards and medially.

COMPARTMENTS OF THE ARM

The arm is divided into anterior and posterior compartments by extension of deep fascia, called the ***medial*** and ***lateral intermuscular septa*** (Fig. 8.2). These septa provide additional surface for the attachment of muscles. They also form planes along which nerves and blood vessels travel. The septa are well-defined only in the lower half of the arm and are attached to the medial and lateral borders and supracondylar ridges of the humerus.

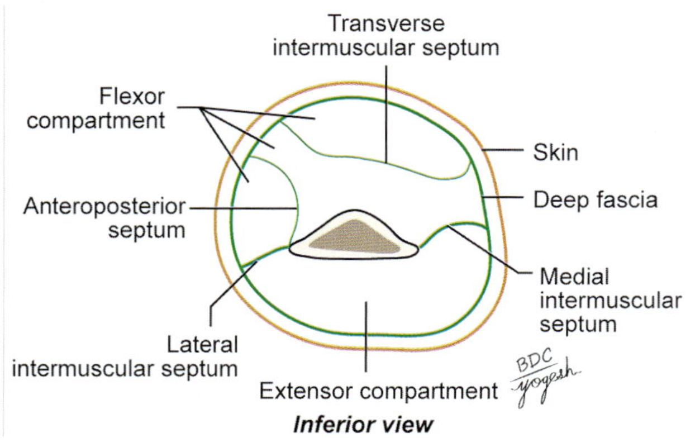

Fig. 8.2: Transverse section through the distal one-third of the arm, showing the intermuscular septa and the compartments

The medial septum is pierced by the ulnar nerve and the superior ulnar collateral artery; the lateral septum is pierced by the radial nerve and radial collateral artery or the anterior descending branch of the profunda brachii artery.

Two additional septa are present in the anterior compartment of the arm. The ***transverse septum*** separates the biceps from the brachialis and encloses the musculocutaneous nerve. The ***anteroposterior septum*** separates the brachialis from the muscles attached to the lateral supracondylar ridge; it encloses the radial nerve and the anterior descending branch of the profunda brachii artery.

Competency:

AN11.1 Describe and demonstrate muscle groups of upper arm with emphasis on biceps and triceps brachii.

ANTERIOR COMPARTMENT

The front or anterior compartment of the arm is homologous with flexor and medial compartments of the thigh. The flexor compartment of thigh lies posteriorly because the lower limb bud rotates medially.

MUSCLES

Muscles of the anterior compartment of the arm are the coracobrachialis, the biceps brachii and the brachialis (Fig. 8.3, Plates 8.1 and 8.2). They are described in Tables 8.1 and 8.2, Flowchart 8.1.

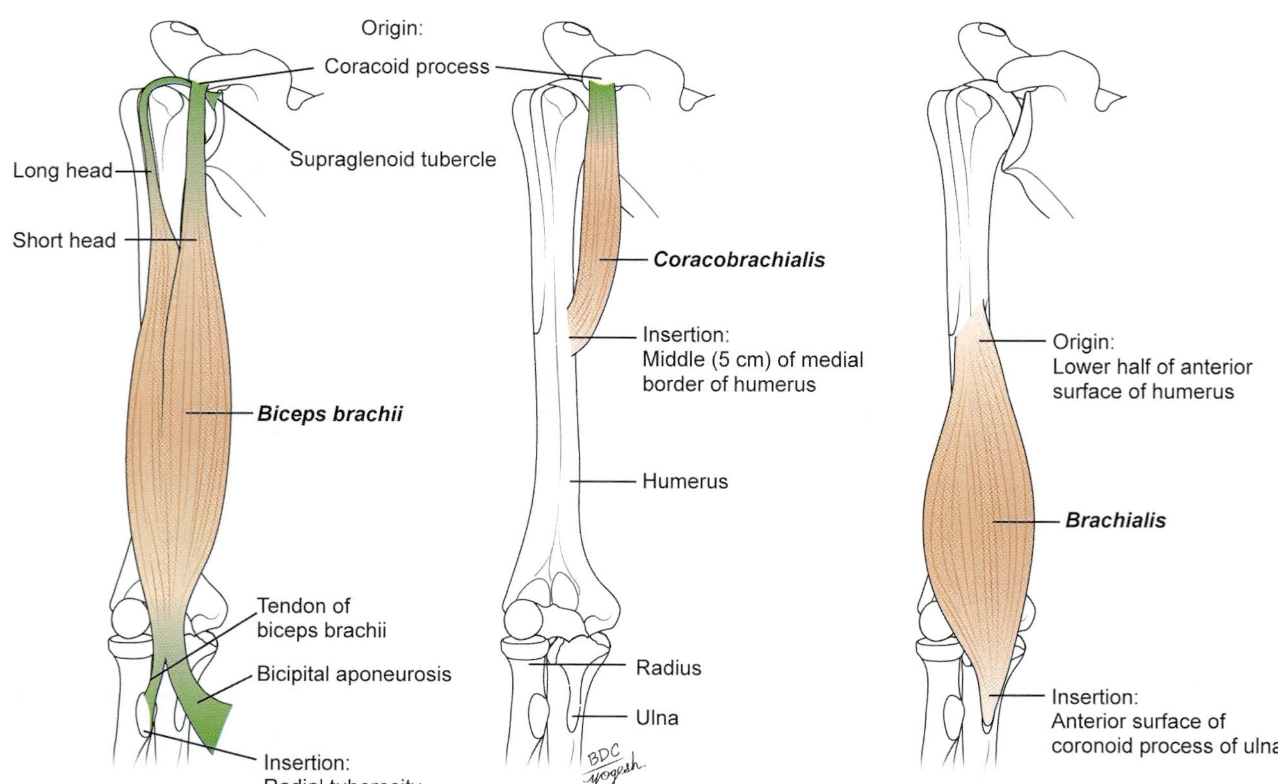

Fig. 8.3: Biceps brachii, coracobrachialis and brachialis muscles

Plate 8.1: Coracobrachialis, brachialis and biceps brachii muscles

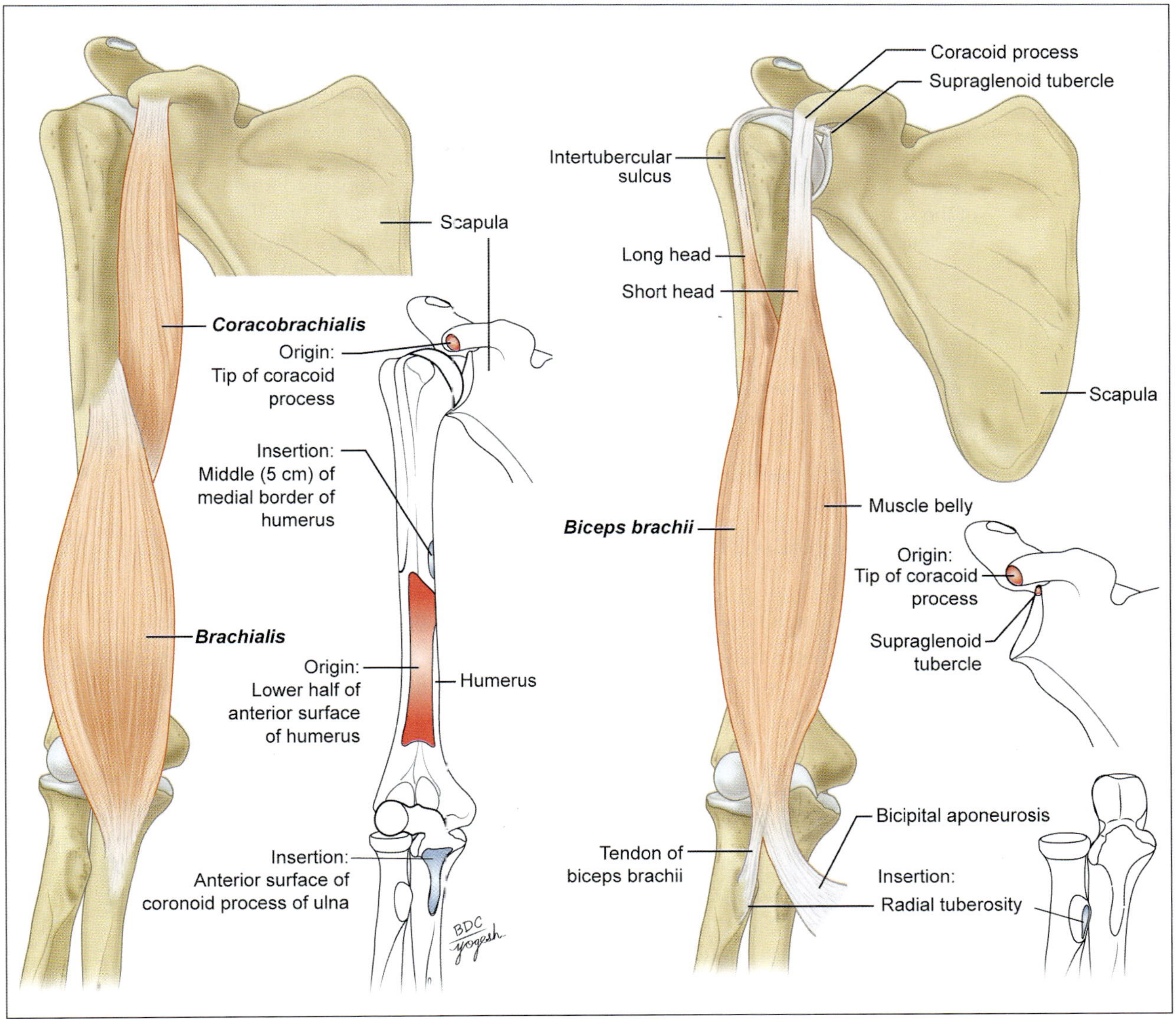

Scapula
Coracobrachialis
Origin: Tip of coracoid process
Insertion: Middle (5 cm) of medial border of humerus
Brachialis
Origin: Lower half of anterior surface of humerus
Humerus
Insertion: Anterior surface of coronoid process of ulna
Coracoid process
Supraglenoid tubercle
Intertubercular sulcus
Long head
Short head
Scapula
Muscle belly
Biceps brachii
Origin: Tip of coracoid process
Supraglenoid tubercle
Bicipital aponeurosis
Tendon of biceps brachii
Insertion: Radial tuberosity
BDC yogesh

Plate 8.2: Origin of long head and insertion of biceps brachii

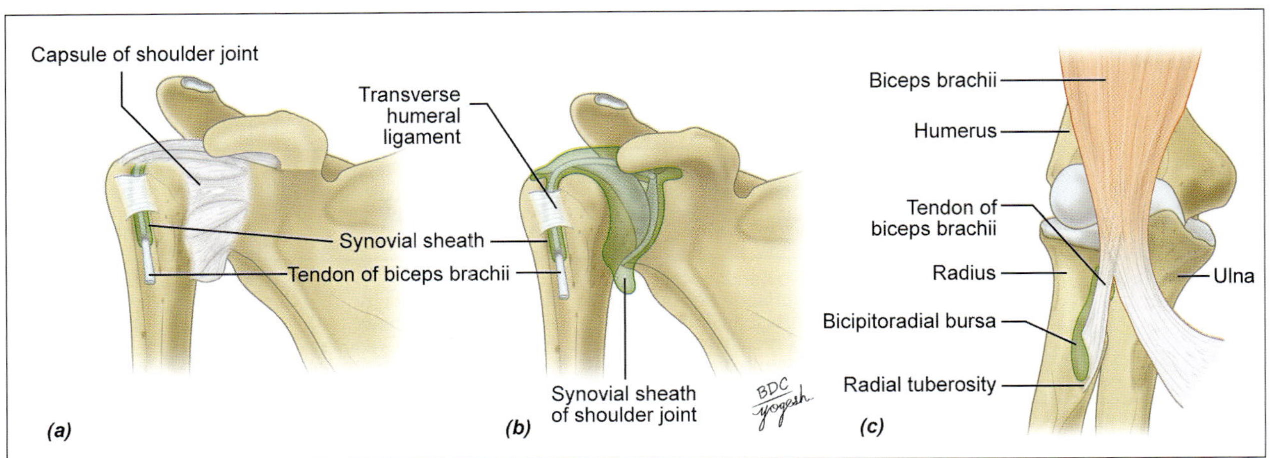

Morphological Importance of Coracobrachialis

Morphologically, the muscle is very important for the following reasons.

The coracobrachialis represents the *medial compartment*, which is so well developed in the thigh.

In some animals, it is a ***tricipital muscle***. In humans, the upper two heads have fused and musculocutaneous nerve passes between the two, and the lowest third head has disappeared. Persistence of the lower head in humans is associated with the

TABLE 8.1: Origin and insertion of muscles

Muscle	*Origin*	*Insertion*
1. **Coracobrachialis**	• The tip of the coracoid process with the short head of the biceps brachii	• The middle 5 cm of the medial border of the humerus
2. **Biceps brachii**	It has two heads of origin: 1. *Short head*: Arises with coracobrachialis from the tip of the coracoid process 2. *Long head:* Arises from the *supraglenoid tubercle* of the scapula and from the glenoidal labrum. The tendon is intracapsular (Plate 8.2a and b)	• Posterior rough part of the *radial tuberosity*. • The ***tendon*** is twisted; the anterior fibres become lateral and posterior fibres become medial. The tendon is separated from the anterior part of the tuberosity by a *bursa* (Plate 8.2c) • The tendon gives off an extension called the ***bicipital aponeurosis***, which extends to ulna and it separates median cubital vein from brachial artery
3. **Brachialis**	• Lower half of the front of the *humerus*, including both the anteromedial and anterolateral surfaces and the anterior border Superiorly, the origin embraces the insertion of the deltoid • Medial and lateral intermuscular septa	• Anterior surface of the *coronoid process* of the ulna and *ulnar tuberosity*

TABLE 8.2: Nerve supply and actions of muscles

Muscle	*Nerve supply*	*Actions*
1. **Coracobrachialis**	Musculocutaneous nerve	Flexes and adducts the arm at the shoulder joint
2. **Biceps brachii**	Musculocutaneous nerve	• It is strong supinator when the forearm is flexed • All screwing movements are done with it • It is a flexor of the elbow • The short head is a flexor of the arm • The long head prevents upwards displacement of the head of the humerus • It can be tested against resistance, as shown in Fig. 8.4
3. **Brachialis**	• Musculocutaneous nerve is motor • Radial nerve is proprioceptive	Flexes forearm at the elbow joint

Flowchart 8.1: Muscles of arm

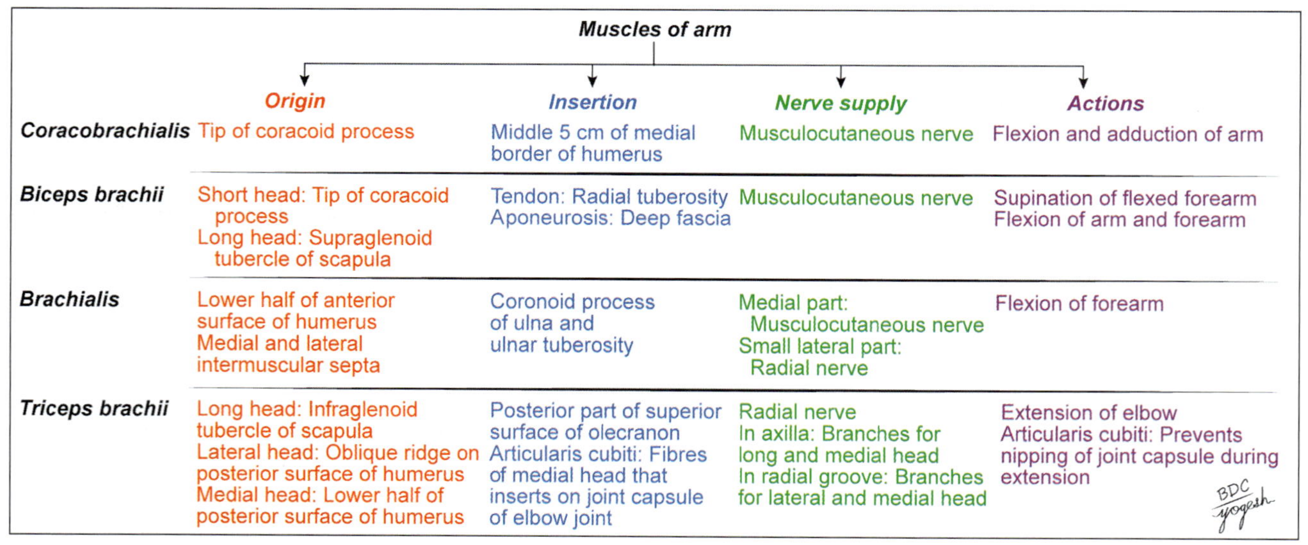

presence of *'ligament of Struthers'*, which is a fibrous band extending from the trochlear spine to the medial epicondyle of the humerus, to which the third head of the coracobrachialis is inserted, and from the lower part of which the pronator teres muscle takes origin. Beneath the ligament passes the median nerve or brachial artery or both.

CLINICAL ANATOMY

- ***Clinical testing of biceps brachii***: Physician holds the patient's wrist firmly, not letting it move. Patient is requested to flex the elbow against the resistance offered by physician's hand. One can see and palpate hardening biceps brachii muscle (Fig. 8.4).

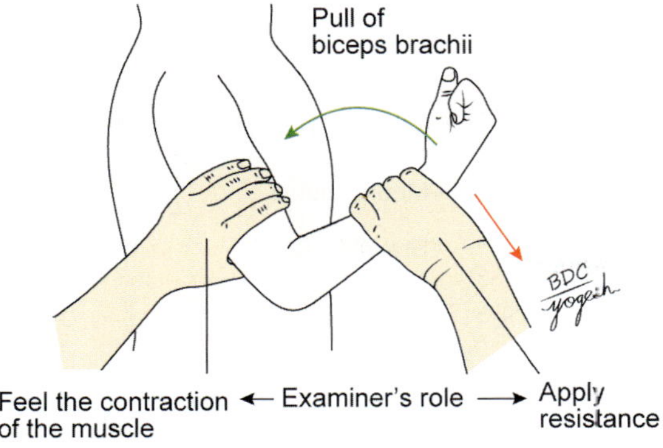

Fig. 8.4: Testing biceps brachii against resistance

Competency:

AN11.2 Identify and describe origin, course, relations, branches (or tributaries), termination of important nerves and vessels in arm.

NERVES

Musculocutaneous Nerve

The musculocutaneous nerve is the main nerve of the front of the arm and continues below the elbow as the lateral cutaneous nerve of the forearm (Flowchart 8.2, Plate 8.3).

It is a branch of the lateral cord of the brachial plexus, arising at the lower border of the pectoralis minor in the axilla.

Root Value

The root value of musculocutaneous nerve is ventral rami of C5–C7 segments of spinal cord.

Origin, Course and Termination

Musculocutaneous nerve arises from the lateral cord of brachial plexus in the lower part of the axilla. It accompanies the third part of the axillary artery. It then enters the front of arm, where it pierces coracobrachialis muscle.

Musculocutaneous nerve runs downwards and laterally between biceps brachii and brachialis muscles to reach the lateral side of the tendon of biceps brachii. It terminates by continuing as the lateral cutaneous nerve of forearm 2 cm above the bend of the elbow (Plate 8.3).

Flowchart 8.2: Musculocutaneous nerve

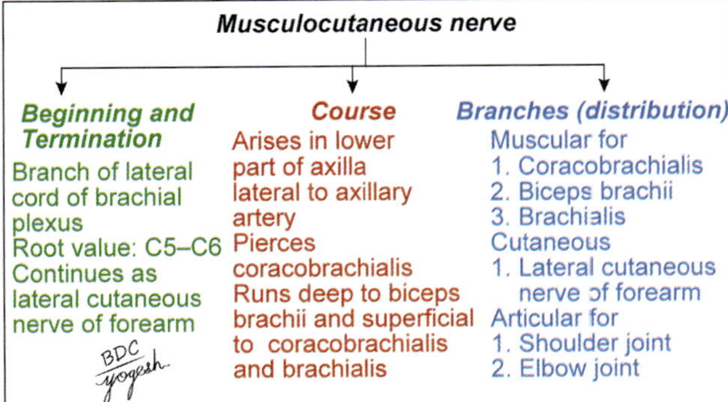

Plate 8.3: Musculocutaneous nerve

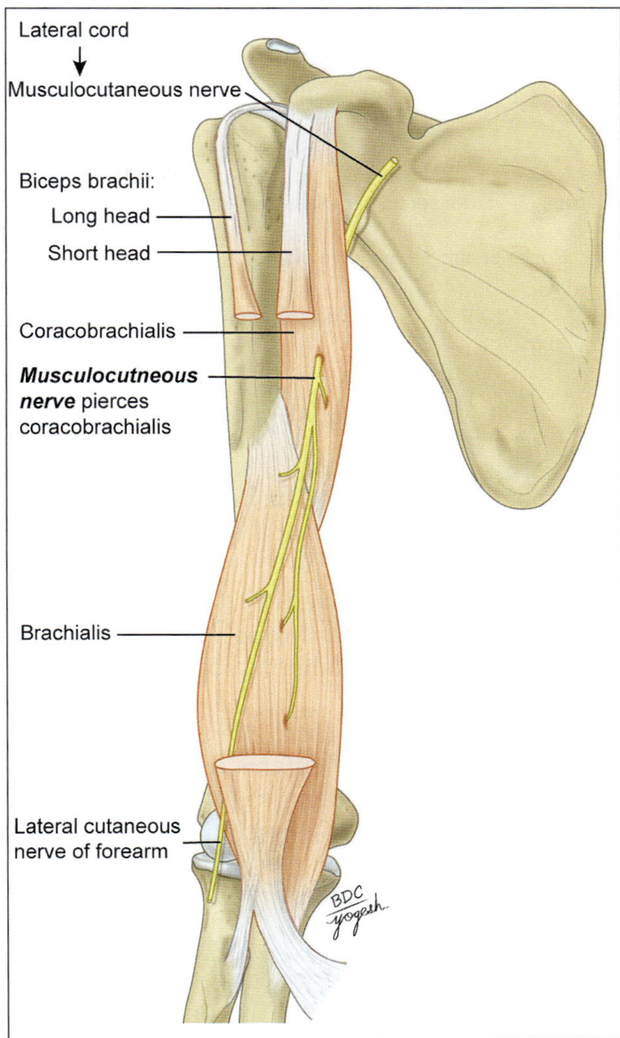

Relations

In the lower part of the axilla: It accompanies the third part of the axillary artery and has the following relations:

Anteriorly: Pectoralis major

Posteriorly: Subscapularis

Medially: Axillary artery and lateral root of the median nerve

Laterally: Coracobrachialis.

Musculocutaneous nerve leaves the axilla and enters the front of the arm by piercing the coracobrachialis.

In the arm: It runs downward and laterally between the biceps brachii and brachialis to reach the lateral side of the tendon of the biceps. It ends by piercing the fascia 2 cm above the bend of the forearm.

Branches and Distribution

A. ***Muscular branches:*** It supplies the following muscles of the front of the arm.
   1. Coracobrachialis
   2. Biceps brachii, long and short heads
   3. Brachialis (Plate 8.3, Fig. 8.5).

B. ***Cutaneous branches:*** Through the ***lateral cutaneous nerve of the forearm***, it supplies the skin of the

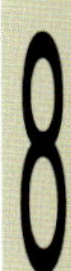

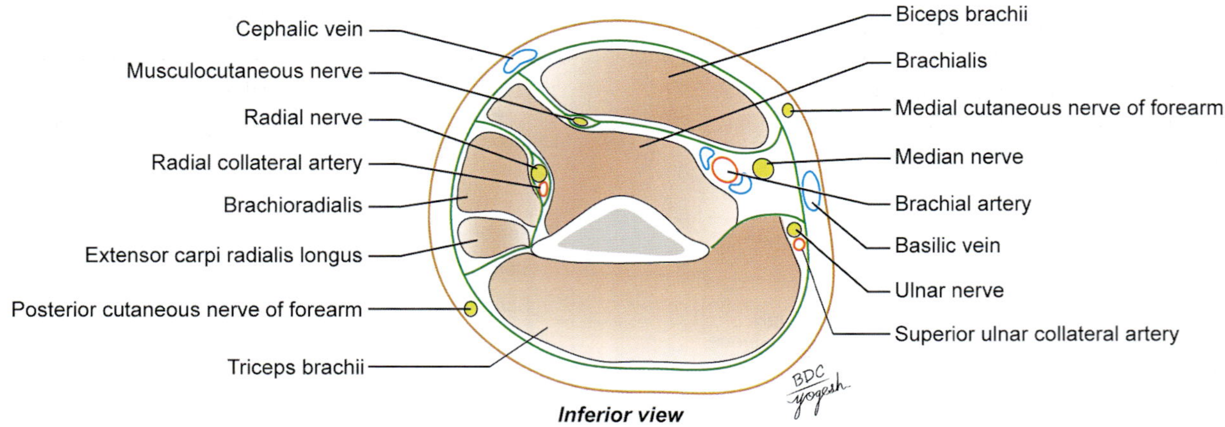

Fig. 8.5: Transverse section passing through the lower one-third of the arm

lateral side of the forearm from the elbow to the wrist, including the ball of the thumb.

C. *Articular branches*
   1. The elbow joint through its branch to the brachialis.
   2. The shoulder joint through a separate branch which enters the humerus along with its nutrient artery.

D. ***Communicating branches*:** The musculocutaneous nerve, through lateral cutaneous nerve of forearm communicates with the neighbouring nerves, namely the superficial branch of the radial nerve, the posterior cutaneous nerve of the forearm and the palmar cutaneous branch of the median nerve.

CLINICAL ANATOMY

***Biceps reflex*:** Musculocutaneous nerve is tested by biceps reflex. Tap the tendon of biceps with forearm pronated and partially extended at the elbow. Normal reflex is jerk-like flexion of elbow joint (Fig. 8.6).

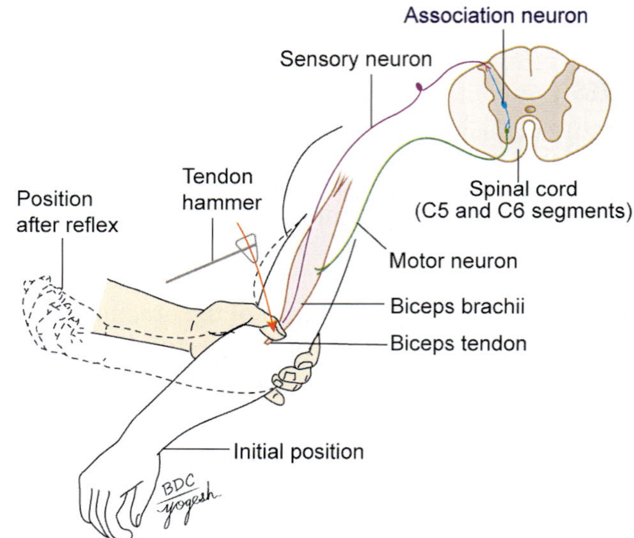

Fig. 8.6: Biceps tendon reflex

Median Nerve

Median nerve is closely related to the brachial artery throughout its course in the arm.

In the upper part, it is lateral to the artery; in the middle of the arm, it crosses the artery from lateral to the medial side and remains on the medial side of the artery right up to the elbow.

In the arm, the median nerve gives off a branch to the pronator teres just above the elbow and vascular branches to the brachial artery.

An articular branch to the elbow joint arises at the elbow.

Ulnar Nerve

Ulnar nerve runs on the medial side of the brachial artery up to the level of insertion of the coracobrachialis, where it pierces the medial intermuscular septum and enters the posterior compartment of the arm. It is accompanied by the superior ulnar collateral vessels.

At the elbow, it passes behind the medial epicondyle, where it can be palpated with a finger.

Radial Nerve

At the beginning of the brachial artery, the radial nerve lies posterior to the artery. Soon, the nerve leaves the artery by entering the radial (spiral) groove on the back of the arm, where it is accompanied by the profunda brachii artery.

In the lower part of the arm, the nerve appears again on the front of the arm, where it lies between the brachialis (medially) and the brachioradialis and extensor carpi radialis longus (laterally). Its branches will be discussed with the back of the arm.

DISSECTION

Make an incision in the middle of deep fascia of the upper arm right down up to the elbow joint. Reflect the flaps sideways.

The most prominent muscle seen is the biceps brachii. Deep to this, another muscle called brachialis is seen easily. In the fascial septum between the two muscles lies the musculocutaneous nerve (a branch of the lateral cord of brachial plexus). Trace the tendinous long head of biceps arising from the supraglenoid tubercle and the

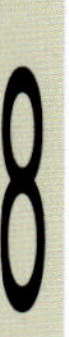

short head arising from the tip of the coracoid process of scapula. Identify coracobrachialis muscle on the medial side of biceps brachii. This muscle is easily identified as it is pierced by musculocutaneous nerve. Clean the branches of the nerve supplying all the three muscles dissected.

BRACHIAL ARTERY

Features

Brachial artery is the continuation of the axillary artery (Plate 8.4, Flowchart 8.3). It extends from the lower border of the teres major muscle to a point in front of the elbow, at the level of the neck of the radius, just medial to the tendon of the biceps brachii.

Beginning, Course and Termination

Brachial artery begins at the lower border of teres major muscle as a continuation of axillary artery (Fig. 8.7). It runs downwards and laterally in the front of arm and crosses the elbow joint. It ends at the level of the neck of radius in the cubital fossa by dividing into its two terminal branches, the radial and ulnar arteries.

Relations

1. It runs downwards and laterally from the medial side of the arm to the front of the elbow.
2. It is superficial throughout its extent and is accompanied by two venae comitantes.
3. Anteriorly, in the middle of the arm, it is crossed by the median nerve from the lateral to the medial side; and in front of the elbow, it is covered by the bicipital aponeurosis and the median cubital vein (Fig. 8.8).
4. Posteriorly, it is related to:
   a. The triceps brachii
   b. The radial nerve and the profunda brachii artery.

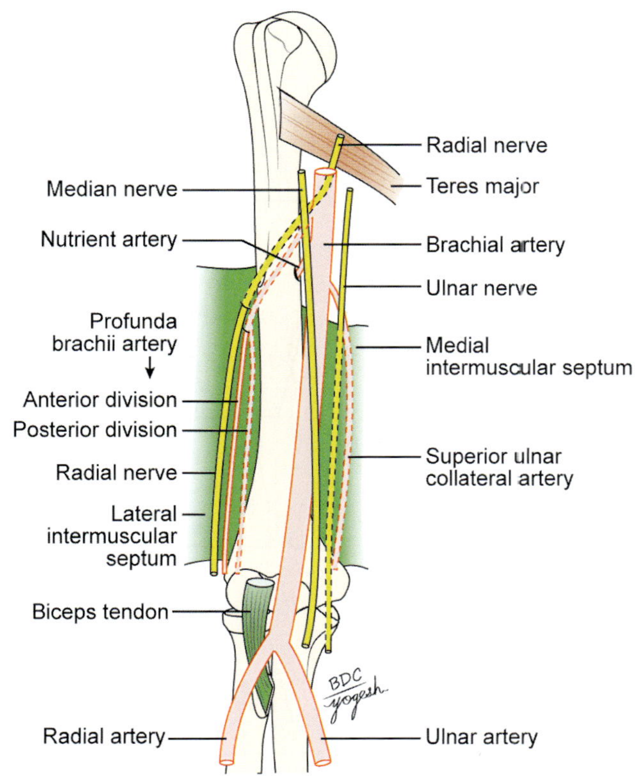

Fig. 8.7: The course and relations of the brachial artery

Plate 8.4: Relations of brachial artery

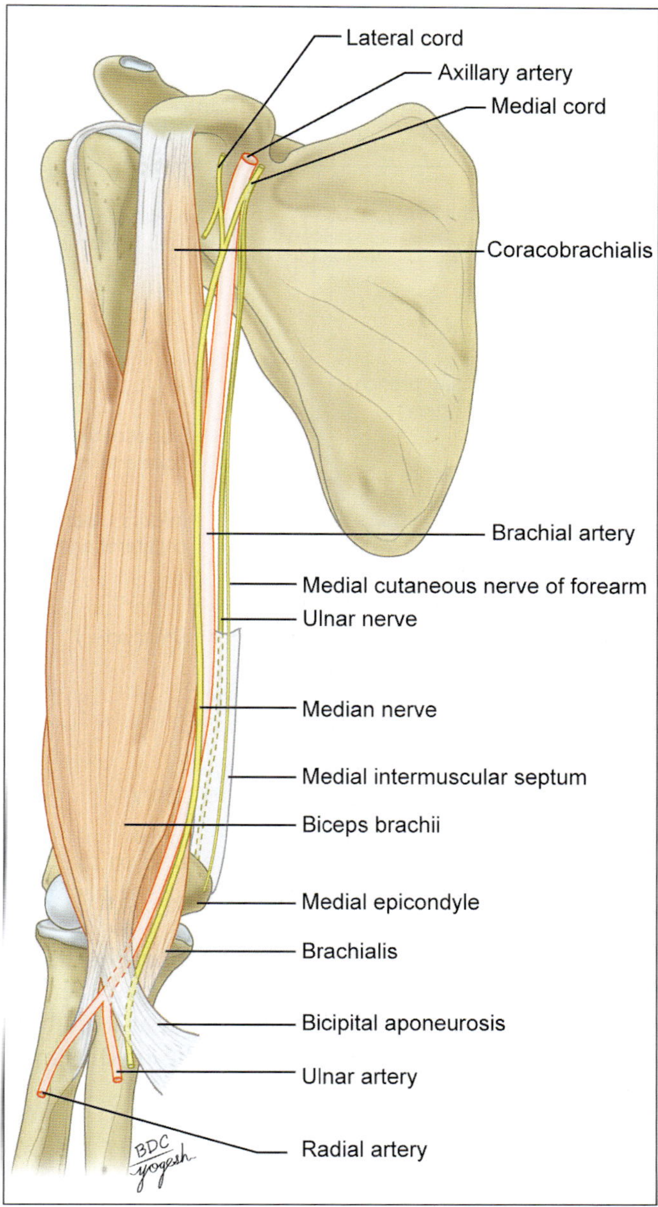

Flowchart 8.3: Brachial artery

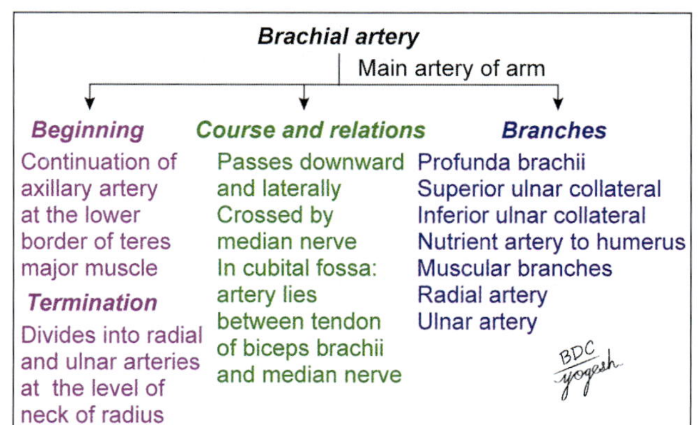

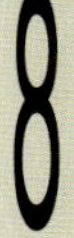

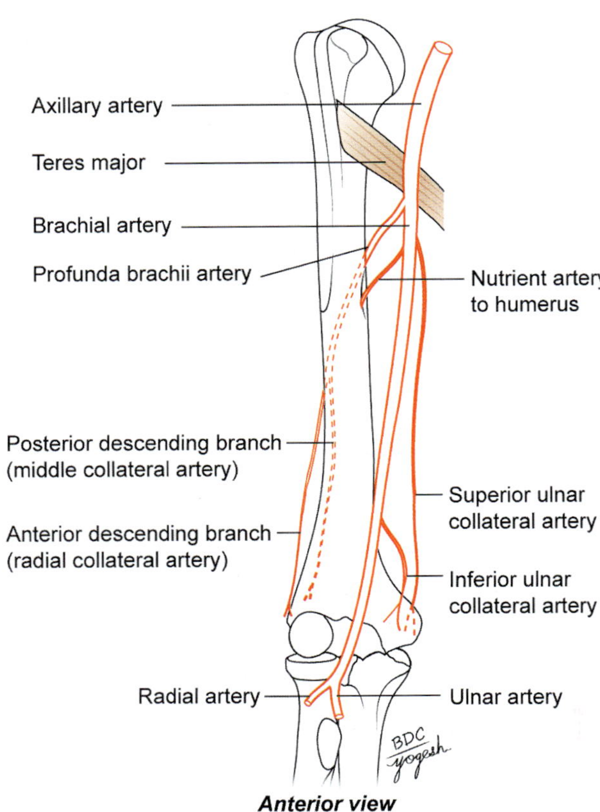

Fig. 8.8: Branches of brachial artery

5. Medially, in the upper part, it is related to the ulnar nerve and the basilic vein and in the lower part to the median nerve (Fig. 8.7).
6. Laterally, it is related to the coracobrachialis, the biceps brachii and the median nerve in its upper part, and to the tendon of the biceps brachii at the elbow.
7. At the elbow, the structures from the medial to the lateral side are:
   a. Median nerve
   b. Brachial artery
   c. Biceps brachii tendon
   d. Radial nerve on a deeper plane (*mnemonic*: MBBR).

Branches

1. Unnamed ***muscular branches***.
2. ***Profunda brachii artery:*** It arises just below the teres major and accompanies the radial nerve.
3. ***Superior ulnar collateral branch:*** It arises in the upper part of the arm and accompanies the ulnar nerve (Fig. 8.8).
4. A ***nutrient artery*** is given off to the humerus.
5. ***Inferior ulnar collateral*** (or supratrochlear) branch: It arises in the lower part and takes part in the anastomoses around the elbow joint.
6. The artery ends by dividing into two terminal branches, the ***radial*** and ***ulnar arteries***.

CLINICAL ANATOMY

- ***Brachial pulsations*** are felt or auscultated in front of the elbow just medial to the tendon of biceps for recording the blood pressure (Fig. 8.9). Figure 8.10 shows other palpable arteries.
- ***Compression of brachial artery:*** Although the brachial artery can be compressed anywhere along its course, it can be compressed most favourably in the middle of the arm, where it lies on the tendon of the coracobrachialis.
- Blood for blood gas analysis is collected from the brachial artery.

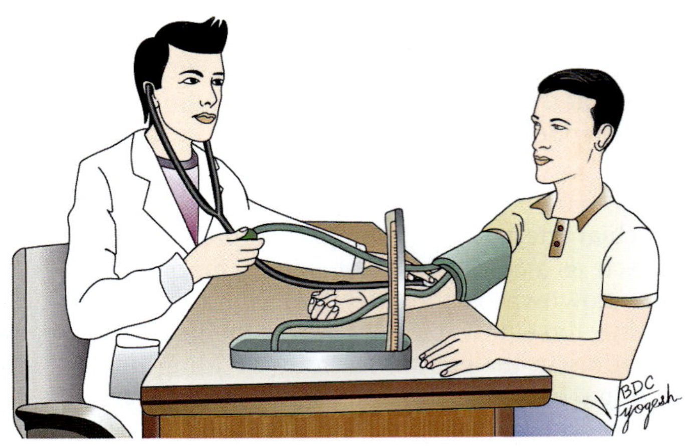

Fig. 8.9: Blood pressure being taken

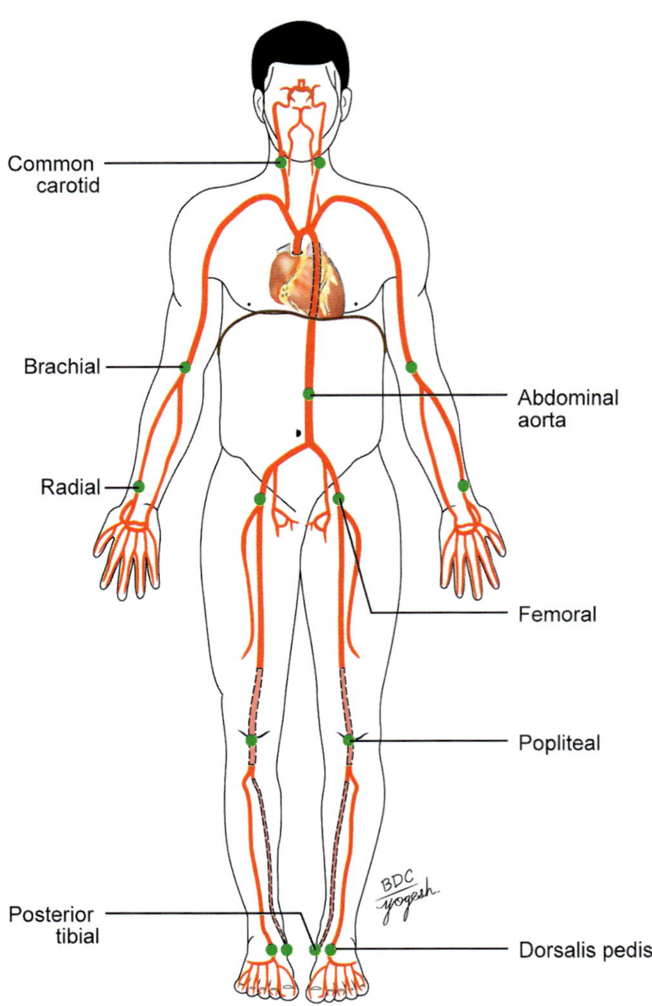

Fig. 8.10: Palpable arteries in the body

Competency:
AN11.6 Describe the anastomoses around the elbow joint.

ANASTOMOSES AROUND THE ELBOW JOINT

Anastomoses around the elbow joint link the brachial artery with the upper ends of the radial and ulnar arteries. They supply the ligaments and bones of the joint. The anastomoses can be subdivided into the following parts (Fig. 8.11):

A. *In front of the lateral epicondyle* of the humerus, the anterior descending (radial collateral) branch of the profunda brachii anastomoses with the radial recurrent branch of the radial artery (Figs 8.10a and b).
B. *Behind the lateral epicondyle* of the humerus, the posterior descending branch of the profunda brachii artery (middle collateral) anastomoses with the interosseous recurrent branch of the posterior interosseous artery.
C. *In front of the medial epicondyle* of the humerus, the inferior ulnar collateral branch of the brachial artery anastomoses with the anterior ulnar recurrent branch of the ulnar artery.
D. *Behind the medial epicondyle* of the humerus, the superior ulnar collateral branch of the brachial artery anastomoses with the posterior ulnar recurrent branch of the ulnar artery.

DISSECTION

Dissect the brachial artery as it lies on the medial side of the upper part of the arm medial to median nerve and lateral to ulnar nerve.

In the lower half of the upper arm, the brachial artery is seen lateral to the median nerve as the nerve crosses the brachial artery from lateral to medial side. Note that the median nerve and brachial artery are forming together a neurovascular bundle.

Ulnar nerve accompanied by the superior ulnar collateral branch of the brachial artery will be dissected later as it reaches the posterior (extensor) compartment of the upper arm after piercing the medial intermuscular septum.

Look for the radial nerve on the posterior aspect of artery before it enters the radial groove.

Clean the branches of brachial artery and identify other arteries which take part in the arterial anastomoses around the elbow joint.

Changes at the Level of Insertion of Coracobrachialis

1. *Bone*: The circular shaft of humerus becomes triangular below this level.
2. *Fascial septa*: The medial and lateral intermuscular septa become better defined from this level down (Fig. 8.7).
3. *Muscles*:
   a. Deltoid and coracobrachialis are inserted at this level (Fig. 8.3).

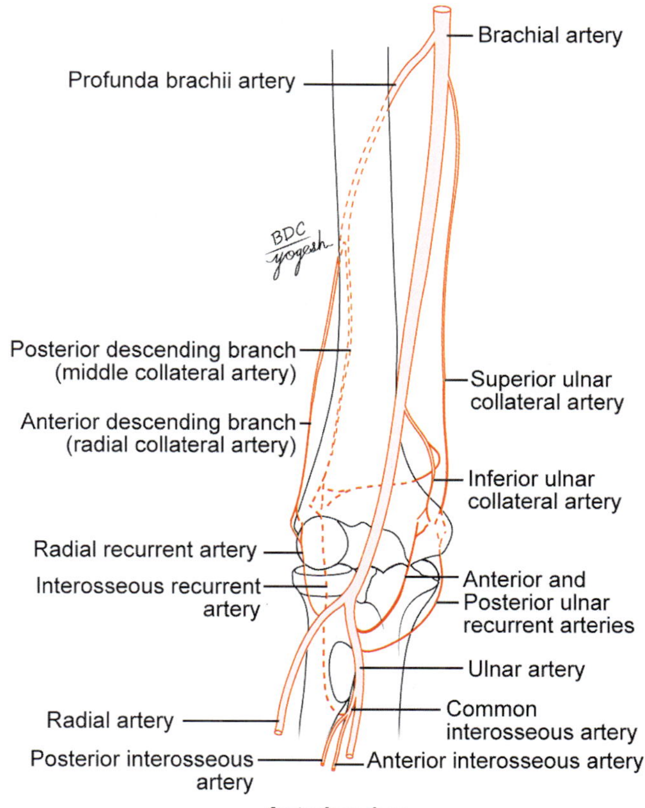

Fig. 8.11: Anastomosis around elbow

   b. Upper end of origin of brachialis.
   c. Upper end of origin of the medial head of triceps brachii.
4. *Arteries*:
   a. The brachial artery passes from the medial side of the arm to its anterior aspect.
   b. The profunda brachii artery runs in the spiral groove and divides into its anterior descending/ radial collateral artery and posterior descending/ middle collateral branches (Figs 8.7, 8.12a).
   c. The superior ulnar collateral artery originates from the brachial artery and pierces the medial intermuscular septum along with the ulnar nerve.
   d. The nutrient artery of the humerus enters the bone.
5. *Veins*:
   a. The basilic vein pierces the deep fascia (Fig. 8.12b).
   b. Two venae comitantes of the brachial artery may unite to form one brachial vein.
6. *Nerves*:
   a. The median nerve crosses the brachial artery from the lateral to the medial side (Fig. 8.7).
   b. The ulnar nerve pierces the medial intermuscular septum with the superior ulnar collateral artery and goes to the posterior compartment (Fig. 8.7).
   c. The radial nerve pierces the lateral intermuscular septum with the anterior descending (radial collateral) branch of the profunda brachii artery and passes from the posterior to the anterior compartment (Fig. 8.12a).

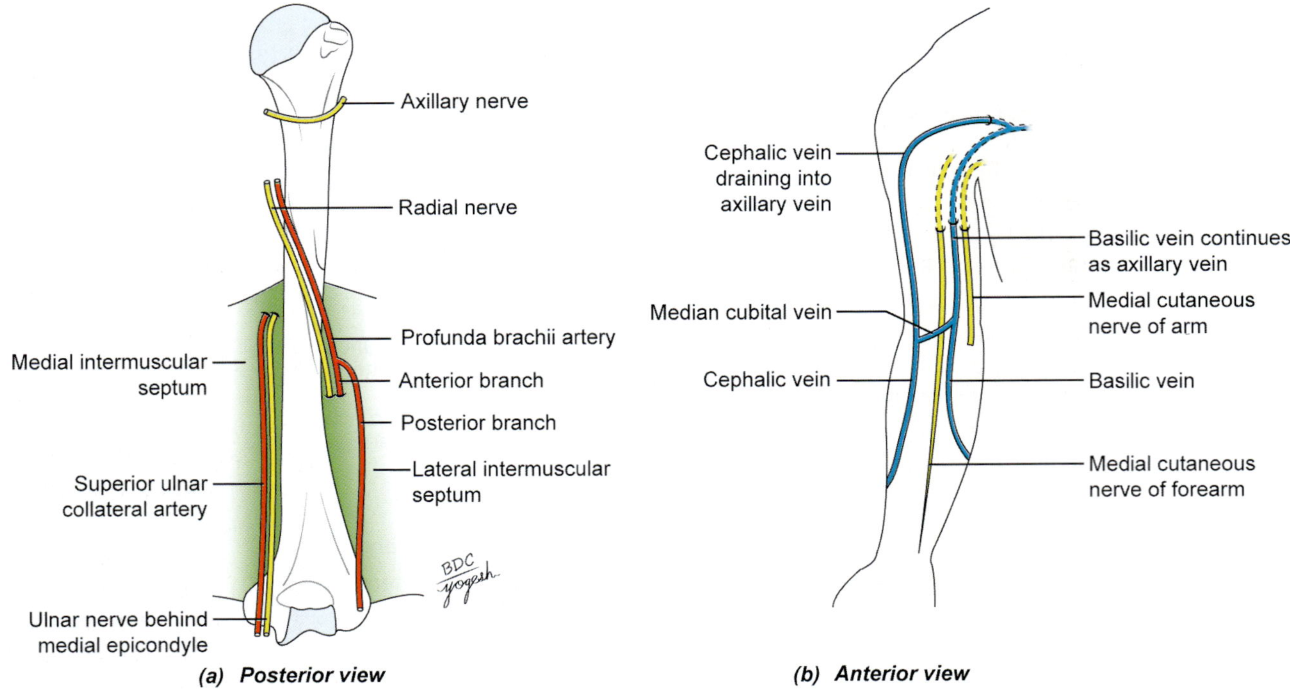

Figs 8.12a and b: Changes in positions of nerve, veins and arteries: (a) Back of arm and (b) front of arm and forearm

d. The medial cutaneous nerve of the arm pierces the deep fascia (Fig. 8.12b).

e. The medial cutaneous nerve of the forearm pierces the deep fascia (Fig. 8.12b).

Competency:

AN11.5 Identify and describe boundaries and contents of cubital fossa.

CUBITAL FOSSA

Features

Cubital (Latin *cubitus, elbow*) fossa is a triangular hollow situated on the front of the elbow. (It is homologous with the popliteal fossa of the lower limb situated on the back of the knee.) (Plate 8.5, Figs 8.13 to 8.17, Flowchart 8.4).

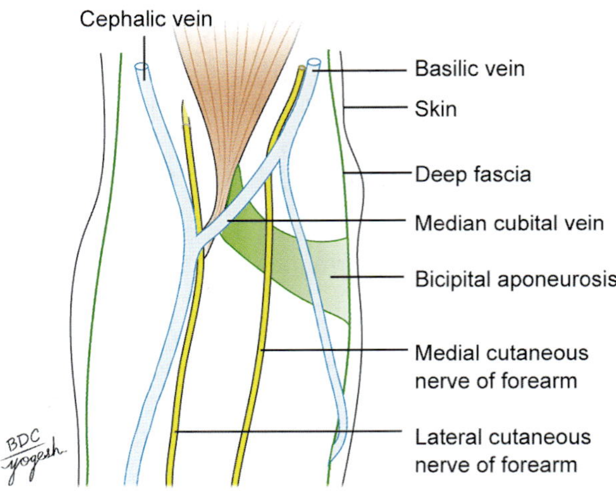

Fig. 8.14: Structures in the roof of the right cubital fossa

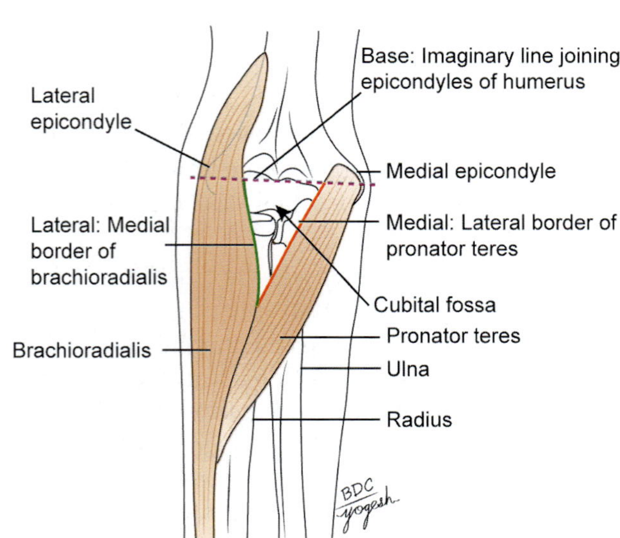

Fig. 8.13: Boundaries of the right cubital fossa

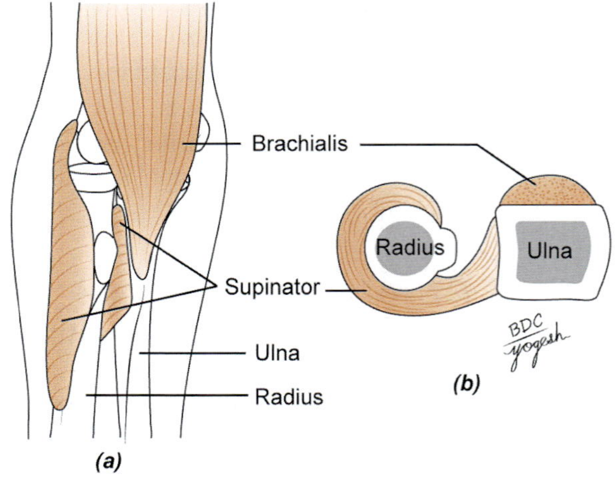

Figs 8.15a and b: The floor of the cubital fossa is formed by the brachialis and supinator muscles: (a) Surface view and (b) cross-sectional view

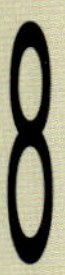

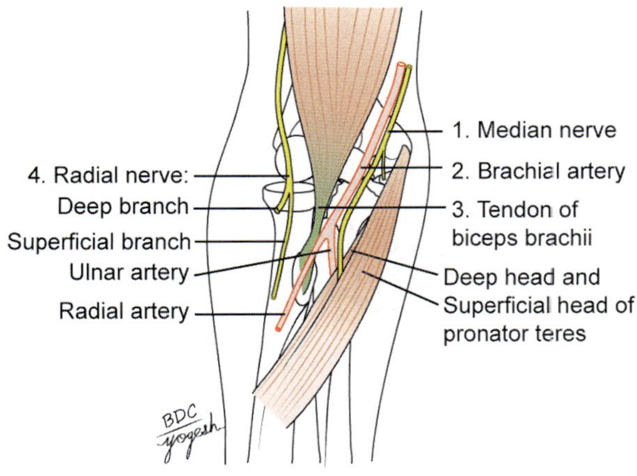

Fig. 8.16: Contents of right cubital fossa (schematic)

Flowchart 8.4: Cubital fossa

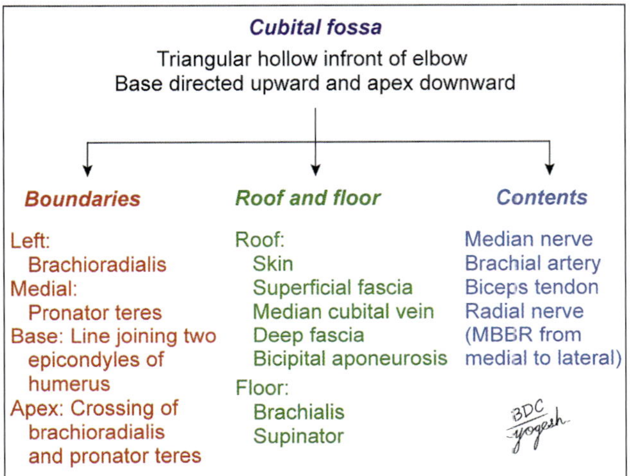

Boundaries

Laterally: Medial border of the brachioradialis (Plate 8.5, Fig. 8.13).

Medially: Lateral border of the pronator teres.

Base: It is directed upwards and is represented by an imaginary line joining the front of two epicondyles of the humerus.

Apex: It is directed downwards and is formed by the area where brachioradialis crosses the pronator teres muscle.

Roof

The roof of the cubital fossa (Plate 8.5, Fig. 8.14) is formed by:

a. Skin
b. Superficial fascia containing the median cubital vein joining the cephalic and basilic veins. The lateral cutaneous nerve of the forearm lies along with cephalic vein, and the medial cutaneous nerve of the forearm along with basilic vein.
c. Deep fascia
d. Bicipital aponeurosis.

Floor

It is formed by:

1. Brachialis (Plate 8.5, Figs 8.15a and b).
2. Supinator surrounding the upper part of radius.

Contents

The fossa is actually very narrow. The contents described are seen after retracting the boundaries. From medial to the lateral side, the contents are as follows:

1. ***Median nerve:*** It gives branches to flexor carpi radialis, palmaris longus and flexor digitorum superficialis and leaves the fossa by passing between the two heads of pronator teres (Fig. 8.17).
2. The termination of the ***brachial artery*** and the beginning of the ***radial*** and ***ulnar arteries*** lie in the fossa.

   The radial artery is smaller and more superficial than the ulnar artery. It gives off the *radial recurrent branch*. The *ulnar artery* goes deep to both heads of pronator teres and runs downwards and medially, being separated from the median nerve by the deep head of the pronator teres (Fig. 8.18).

   Ulnar artery gives off the *anterior ulnar recurrent*, the *posterior ulnar recurrent* and the *common interosseous* branches (Fig. 8.11).

   The common interosseous branch divides into the *anterior* and *posterior interosseous arteries*, and latter gives off the interosseous recurrent branch.
3. The tendon of the ***biceps brachii*** (Plate 8.5, Fig. 8.16).
4. ***Radial nerve:*** It descends down medial to lateral epicondyle to enter cubital fossa. In the fossa, it gives

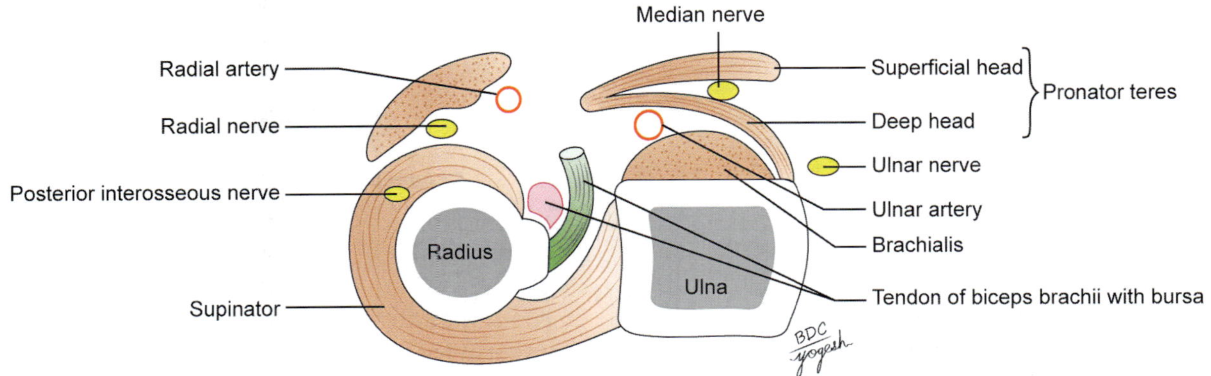

Fig. 8.17: Contents of the right cubital fossa seen in cross-section (anterior view)

Plate 8.5: Cubital fossa: Boundaries, floor, roof and contents

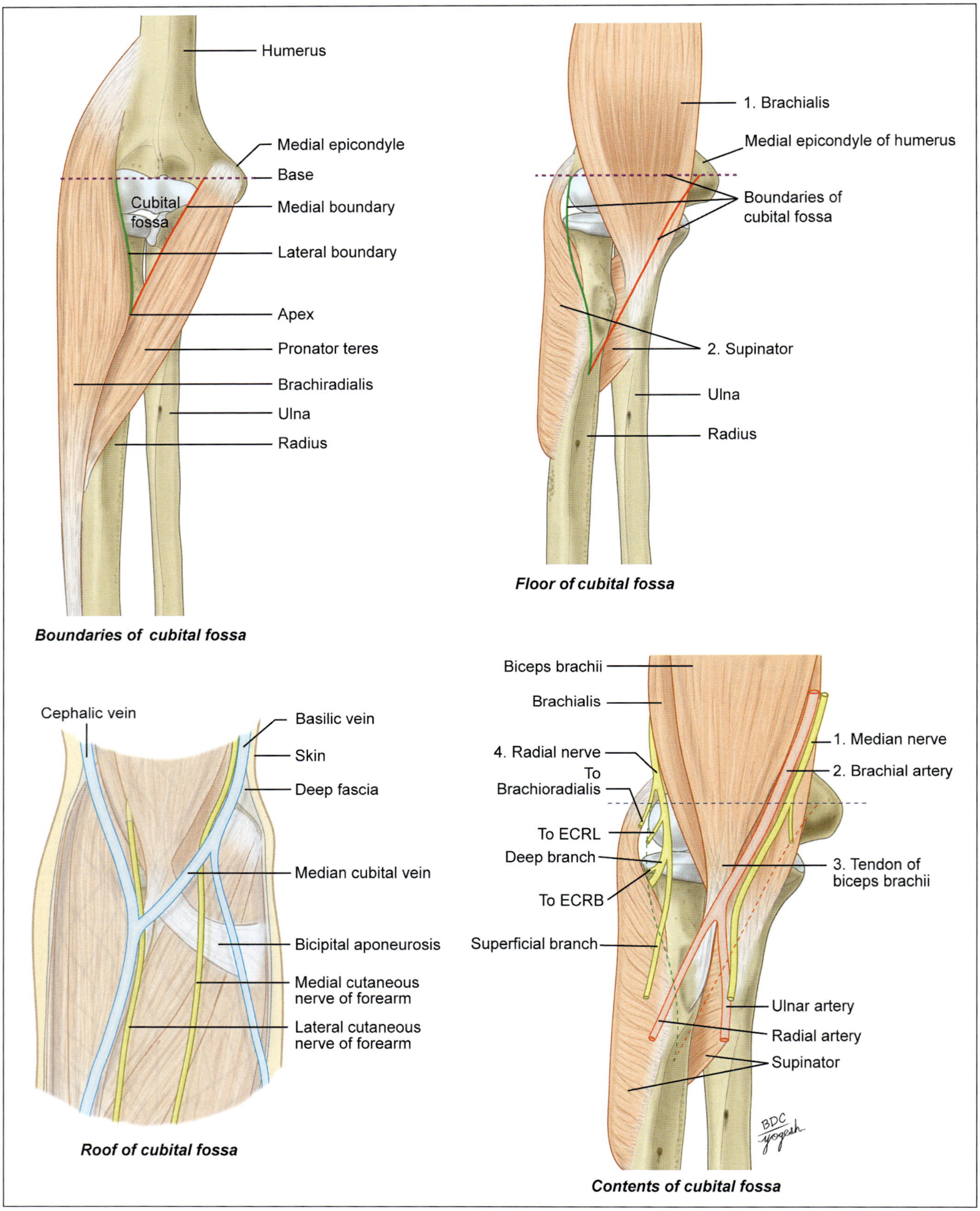

Humerus
Medial epicondyle
Base
Cubital fossa
Medial boundary
Lateral boundary
Apex
Pronator teres
Brachiradialis
Ulna
Radius

Boundaries of cubital fossa

1. Brachialis
Medial epicondyle of humerus
Boundaries of cubital fossa
2. Supinator
Ulna
Radius

Floor of cubital fossa

Cephalic vein
Basilic vein
Skin
Deep fascia
Median cubital vein
Bicipital aponeurosis
Medial cutaneous nerve of forearm
Lateral cutaneous nerve of forearm

Roof of cubital fossa

Biceps brachii
Brachialis
4. Radial nerve
To Brachioradialis
To ECRL
Deep branch
To ECRB
Superficial branch
1. Median nerve
2. Brachial artery
3. Tendon of biceps brachii
Ulnar artery
Radial artery
Supinator
BDC yogesh

Contents of cubital fossa

off the *posterior interosseous nerve* or deep branch of the radial nerve, which gives branches to extensor carpi radialis brevis and supinator. Then, it leaves the fossa by piercing the supinator muscle (Fig. 8.17).

The remaining *superficial branch* runs in the front of forearm for some distance.

[*Mnemonic*: **MBBR**: **M**edian nerve, **B**rachial artery, **B**iceps brachii tendon, **R**adial nerve]

CLINICAL ANATOMY

- The cubital region is important for the following reasons:
  a. ***Intravenous injections***: The *median cubital vein* is often the vein of choice for intravenous injections. It is used for introducing cardiac catheters to get sample of blood from various chambers of heart.
  b. ***Blood pressure measurement:*** The blood pressure is universally recorded by auscultating the brachial artery in front of the elbow (Fig. 8.9).
- The anatomy of the cubital fossa is useful while dealing with fracture around the elbow, like the supracondylar fracture of the humerus.

DISSECTION

Identify the structures (*see* text) present in the roof of a shallow cubital fossa located on the front of the elbow. Separate the lateral and medial boundaries formed respectively by the brachioradialis and pronator teres muscles (Plate 8.5). Clean the contents:

1. Median nerve on the medial side of brachial artery.
2. Terminal part of brachial artery bifurcating into radial and ulnar arteries.
3. The tendon of biceps brachii muscle between the brachial artery and radial nerve.
4. The radial nerve on a deeper plane on the lateral side of biceps tendon.

Identify brachialis and supinator muscles, forming the floor of cubital fossa.

POSTERIOR COMPARTMENT

Features

The region contains the triceps muscle, the radial nerve and the profunda brachii artery. The nerve and artery run through the muscle. The ulnar nerve runs through the lower part of this compartment.

Competency:
AN11.1 Describe and demonstrate muscle groups of upper arm with emphasis on biceps and triceps brachii.
Biceps has been described in Tables 8.1 and 8.2.

TRICEPS BRACHII MUSCLE

Origin

Triceps brachii muscle arises by the following three heads (Plate 8.6, Fig. 8.18):

1. ***Long head***: It arises from the infraglenoid tubercle of the scapula; it is the longest of the three heads (Fig. 8.19).
2. ***Lateral head***: It arises from an oblique ridge on the upper part of the posterior surface of the humerus, corresponding to the lateral lip of the radial (spiral) groove (Fig. 8.18).

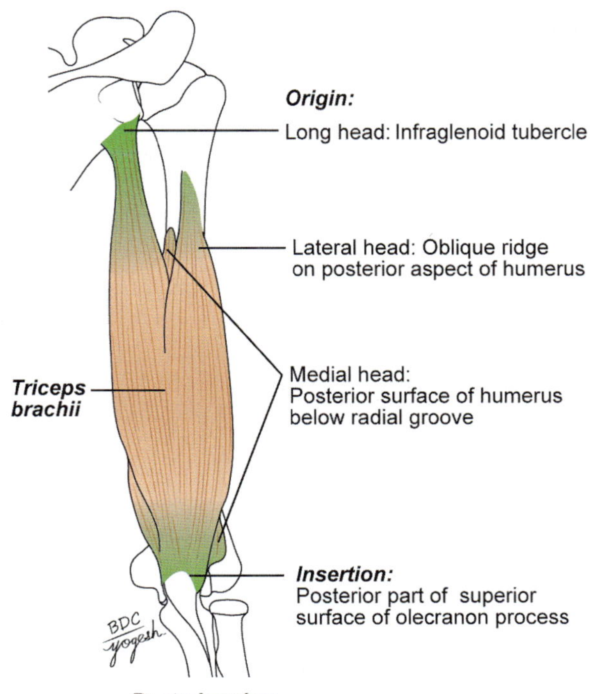

Fig. 8.18: The triceps brachii muscle

3. ***Medial head***: It arises from a large triangular area on the posterior surface of the humerus below the radial groove, as well as from the medial and lateral intermuscular septa. At the level of the radial groove, the medial head is medial to the lateral head.

Insertion

The long and lateral heads converge and fuse to form a superficial flattened tendon, which covers the medial head and is inserted into the posterior part of the superior surface of the ***olecranon process*** (Plate 8.6, Fig. 8.18).

The medial head is inserted partly into the superficial tendon and partly into the olecranon process. Although the medial head is separated from the capsule of the elbow joint by a small bursa, a few of its fibres are inserted into this part of the capsule. This prevents nipping of the capsule during extension of the arm. These fibres are referred to as the ***articularis cubiti*** or as the ***subanconeus***.

Nerve Supply

Each head receives a separate branch from the ***radial nerve*** (C7, C8). The branches arise in the axilla and in the radial groove.

Actions

The triceps is a powerful active ***extensor of the elbow***. The long head causes extension and adduction of arm at shoulder joint. It supports the head of the humerus in the abducted position of the arm. Gravity extends the elbow passively.

Electromyography has shown that the medial head of the triceps is active in all forms of extension, and the actions of the long and lateral heads are minimal, except when acting against resistance.

Plate 8.6: Triceps brachii muscle and radial nerve in the radial groove

Long head: Infraglenoid tubercle

Lateral head: Oblique ridge on the posterior aspect of humerus

Medial head: Posterior surface of humerus below radial groove

Insertion: Posterior part of superior surface of olecranon process

Triceps brachii

Radial nerve

Posterior cutaneous nerve of arm

Lateral head of triceps brachii and its nerve

Long head of triceps brachii and its nerve

Lower lateral cutaneous nerve of arm

Medial head of triceps brachii and its nerves

Radial nerve in spiral groove

Posterior cutaneous nerve of forearm

Lateral intermuscular septum

Branch to anconeus

Posterior view

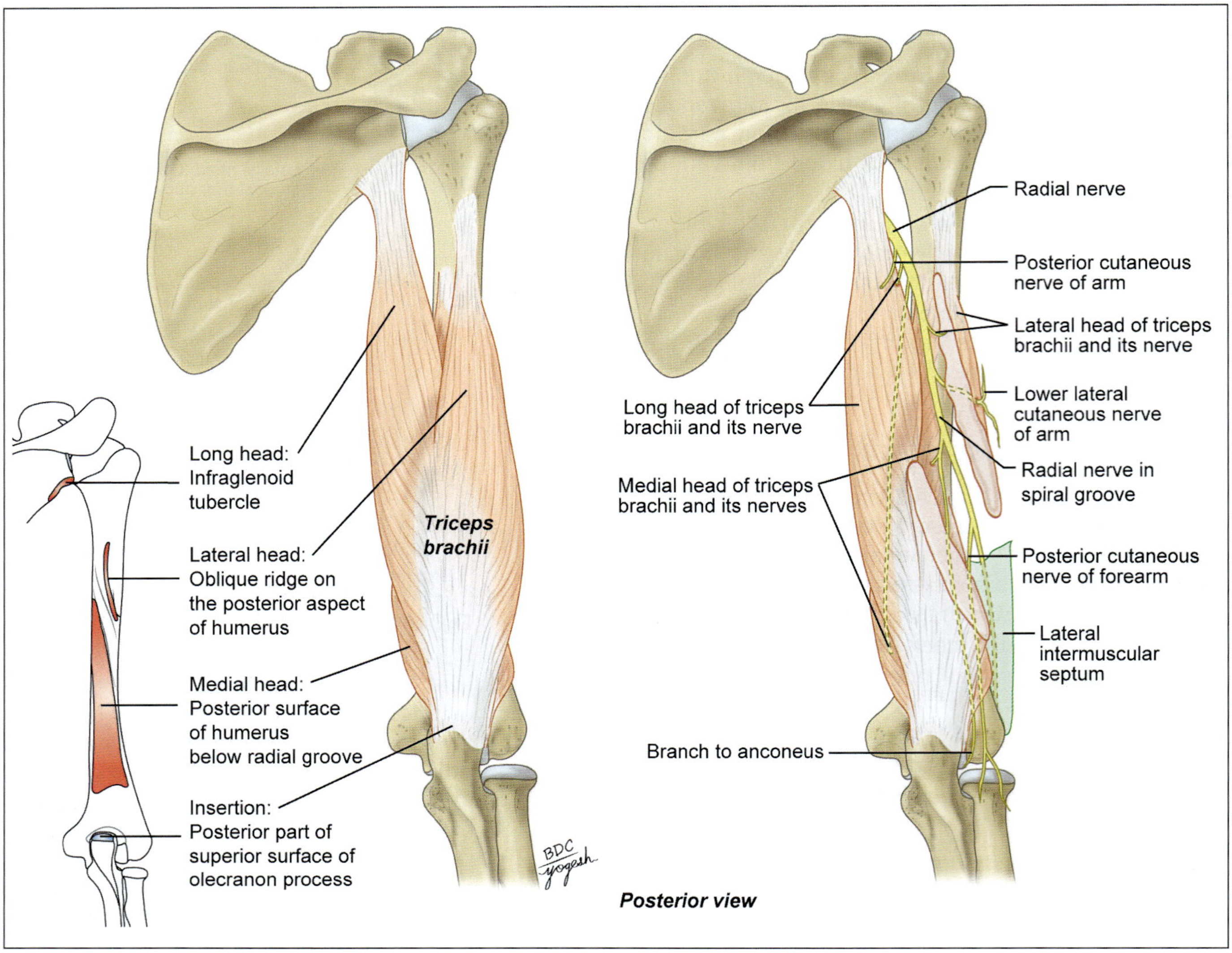

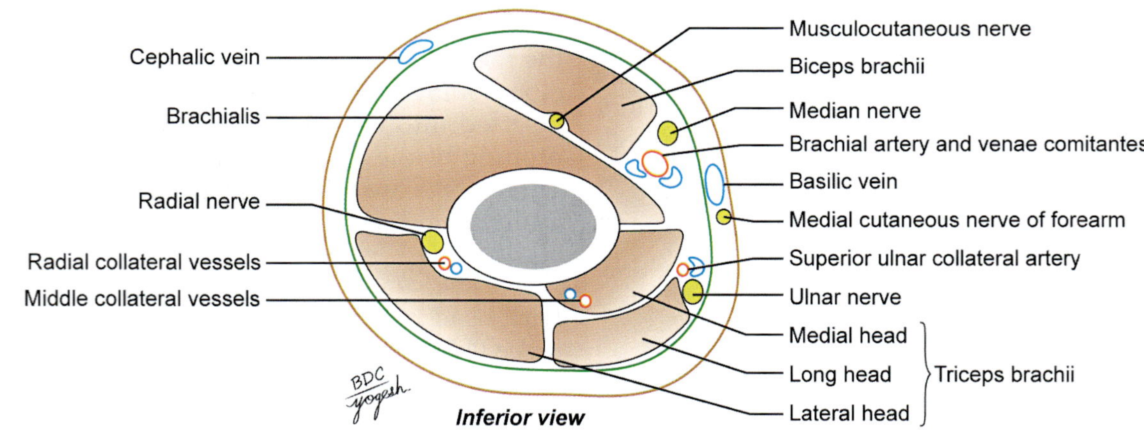

Fig. 8.19: Transverse section through the right arm a little below the insertion of the coracobrachialis and deltoid showing arrangement of three heads of the triceps and the radial nerve in the radial groove

CLINICAL ANATOMY

- In radial nerve injuries in the arm, the triceps brachii usually escapes complete paralysis because the two nerves supplying it, arising in the axilla.
- ***Clinical testing of triceps brachii***: Physician holds the flexed forearm firmly. Patient is requested to extend his elbow against the resistance of the physician's hand. The contracting triceps brachii is felt (Fig. 8.20).

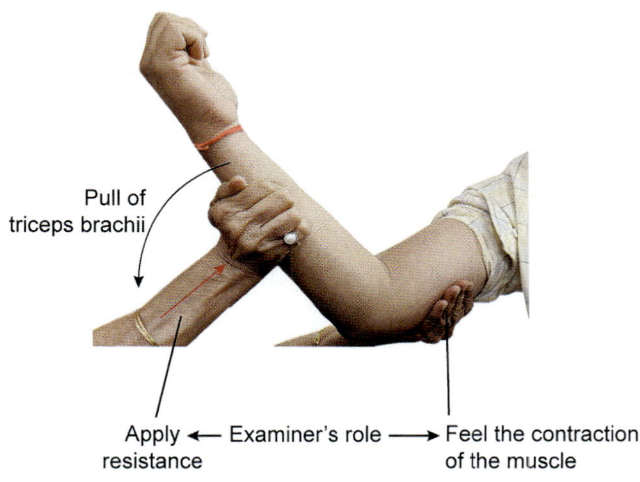

Fig. 8.20: Testing triceps brachii against resistance

DISSECTION

Reflect the skin of back of arm to view the triceps brachii muscle. Define its attachments and separate the long head of the muscle from its lateral head.

Radial nerve will be seen passing between the long head of triceps and medial border of the humerus. Note the continuity of radial nerve up to axilla. Carefully cut through the lateral head of triceps to expose radial nerve along with profunda brachii vessels. Note that the radial nerve lies in the radial groove, on the back of humerus, passing between the lateral head of triceps above and its medial head below. In the lower part of arm, the radial nerve lies on the front of elbow just lateral to the brachialis, dividing into two terminal branches in the cubital fossa.

The ulnar nerve (which was seen in the anterior compartment of arm till its middle) pierces the medial intermuscular septum with its accompanying vessels, reaches the back of elbow and may easily be palpated on the back of medial epicondyle of humerus.

RADIAL NERVE OR MUSCULOSPIRAL NERVE

Radial nerve is the largest branch of the posterior cord of the brachial plexus with a root value of C5–C8 and T1 (Flowchart 8.5).

Origin, Course and Termination

1. Radial nerve is given off from the posterior cord in the lower part of axilla.
2. It runs behind third part of axillary artery.
3. In the arm, it lies behind the brachial artery (Fig. 8.7).
4. It enters the lower triangular space to reach the oblique radial sulcus on the back of humerus (Fig. 8.12a).
5. The nerve reaches the lateral side of arm 5 cm below deltoid tuberosity and pierces lateral intermuscular septum to enter the anterior compartment of arm on its lateral aspect (Fig. 8.12a).
6. It descends down the medial to the lateral epicondyle into cubital fossa.

Flowchart 8.5: Radial nerve

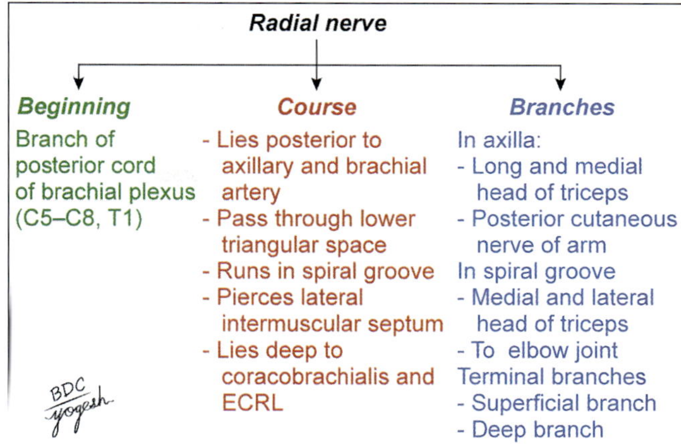

7. Radial nerve terminates by dividing into a *superficial* and a *deep branch* (*posterior interosseous nerve*) just below the level of lateral epicondyle.

Relations

a. **In the lower part of the axilla:** Here, the radial nerve passes downwards and has the following relations:
   - *Anteriorly:* 3rd part of the axillary artery
   - *Posteriorly:* Subscapularis, latissimus dorsi and teres major
   - *Laterally:* Axillary nerve and coracobrachialis
   - *Medially:* Axillary vein.

b. **In the upper part of the arm:** The radial nerve continues behind the brachial artery and passes posterolaterally (with the profunda brachii vessels) through the lower triangular space, below the teres major and between the long head of the triceps brachii and the humerus. It then enters the radial groove with the profunda vessels.

c. **In the radial groove:** The nerve runs downwards and laterally between the lateral and medial heads of the triceps brachii, in contact with the humerus. At the lower end of the groove, 5 cm below the deltoid tuberosity, the nerve pierces the lateral intermuscular septum (Fig. 8.12a) and passes into the anterior compartment of the arm to reach the cubital fossa, where it ends by dividing into superficial and deep branches (Fig. 8.17).

Branches and Distribution

Various branches of radial nerve are shown in Fig. 8.21.

Muscular Branches

1. Before entering the spiral groove, radial nerve supplies the long and medial heads of the triceps brachii.
2. In the spiral groove, it supplies the lateral and medial heads of the triceps brachii and the anconeus.
3. Below the radial groove, on the front of the arm, it supplies the brachialis with proprioceptive fibres. The brachioradialis and extensor carpi radialis longus are supplied with motor fibres (Fig. 8.21).

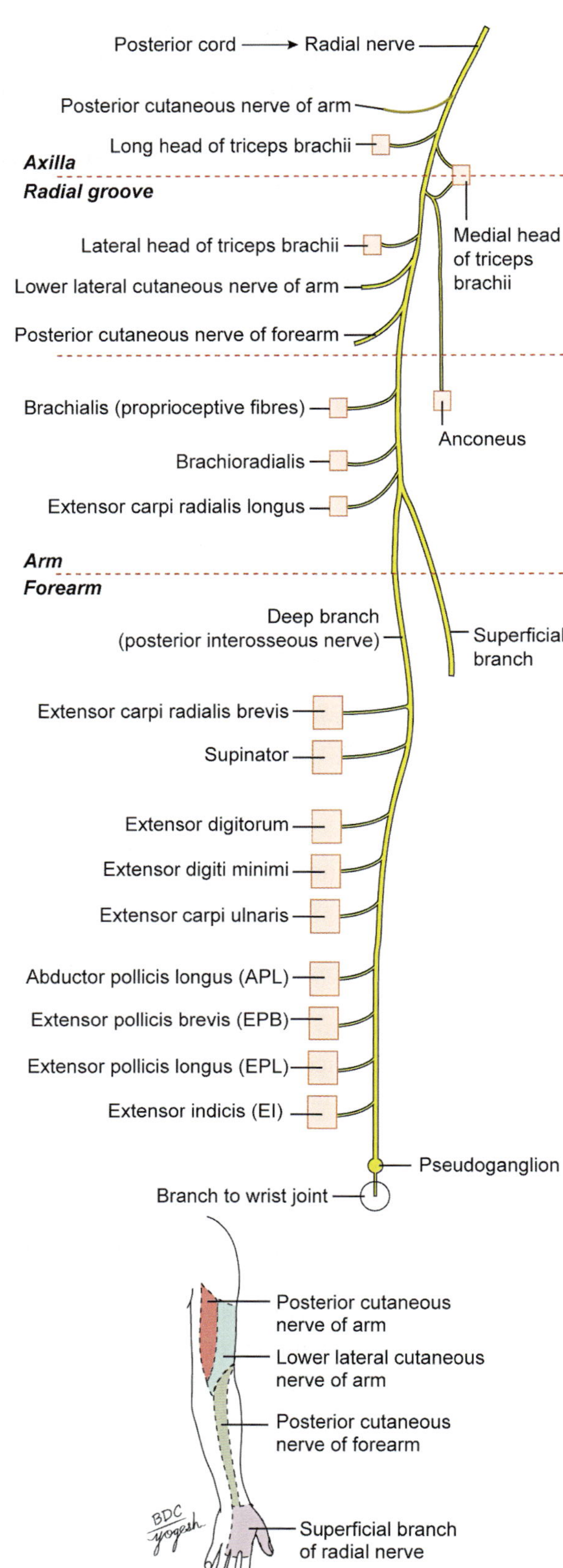

Fig. 8.21: Distribution of right radial nerve

Cutaneous Branches

1. In the axilla, radial nerve gives off the posterior cutaneous nerve of the arm, which supplies the skin on the back of the arm.
2. In the radial groove, the radial nerve gives off the lower lateral cutaneous nerves of the arm and the posterior cutaneous nerve of the forearm.

Articular Branches

The articular branches near the elbow supply the elbow joint.

Competencies:
AN11.4 Describe the anatomical basis of Saturday night paralysis.
AN12.13 Describe the anatomical basis of wrist drop.

CLINICAL ANATOMY

- ***Radial nerve injury:*** The radial nerve is very commonly damaged in the region of the radial (spiral) groove. The common causes of injury are as follows:
  a. Sleeping in an armchair with the limb hanging by the side of the chair (***Saturday night palsy***), or even the pressure of the crutch (***crutch paralysis***) (Figs 8.22a and b).
  b. Fractures of the shaft of the humerus. This results in the weakness and loss of power of extension at the wrist (wrist drop) (Fig. 8.23) and sensory loss over a narrow strip on the back of forearm, and on the lateral side of the dorsum of the hand (Fig. 8.24).
- *Wrist drop* is quite disabling because the patient cannot grip any object firmly in the hand without the synergistic action of the extensors.

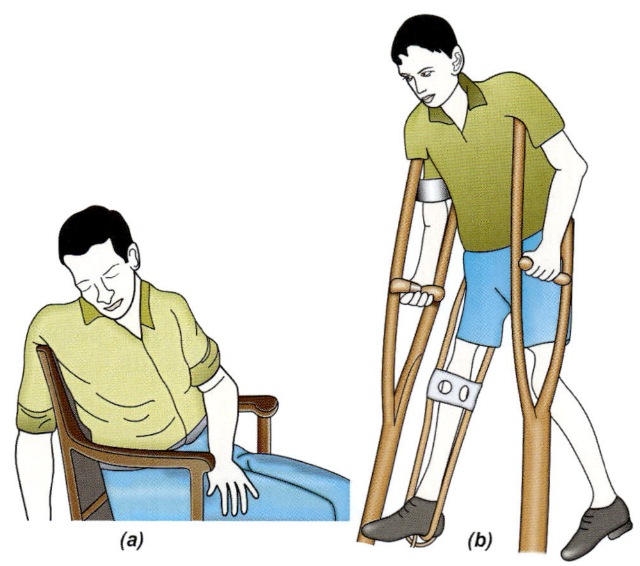

Figs 8.22a and b: Injury to radial nerve: (a) Saturday night palsy and (b) crutch paralysis

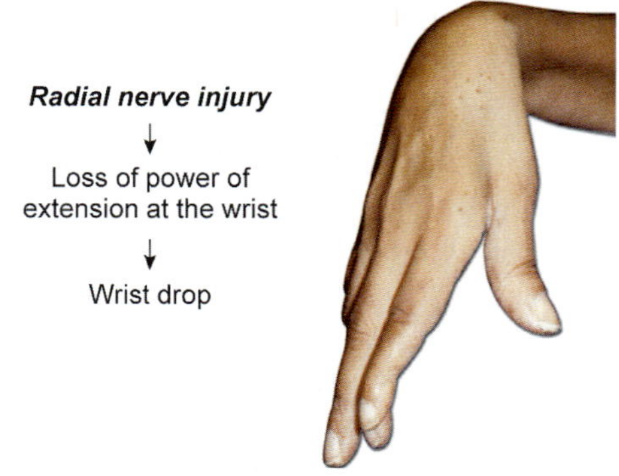

Fig. 8.23: Wrist drop

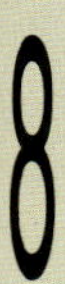

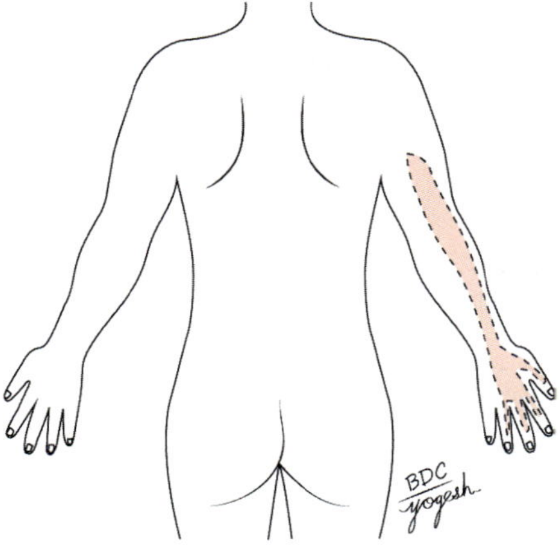

Fig. 8.24: Sensory loss over back of forearm and dorsum of hand

PROFUNDA BRACHII ARTERY

Profunda brachii artery is a large branch, arising just below the teres major. It accompanies the radial nerve through the radial groove, and before piercing the lateral intermuscular septum, it divides into the anterior and posterior descending branches, which take part in the anastomoses around the elbow joint (Fig. 8.8).

Branches

1. The ***anterior descending (radial collateral)*** artery is one of the terminal branches and represents the continuation of the profunda artery. It accompanies the radial nerve and ends by anastomosing with the radial recurrent artery in front of the lateral epicondyle of the humerus (Fig. 8.25).
2. The ***posterior descending (middle collateral)*** artery is the largest terminal branch, which descends in the substance of the medial head of the triceps. It ends by anastomosing with the interosseous recurrent artery behind the lateral epicondyle of the humerus (Fig. 8.25). It usually gives a branch which accompanies the nerve to the anconeus.

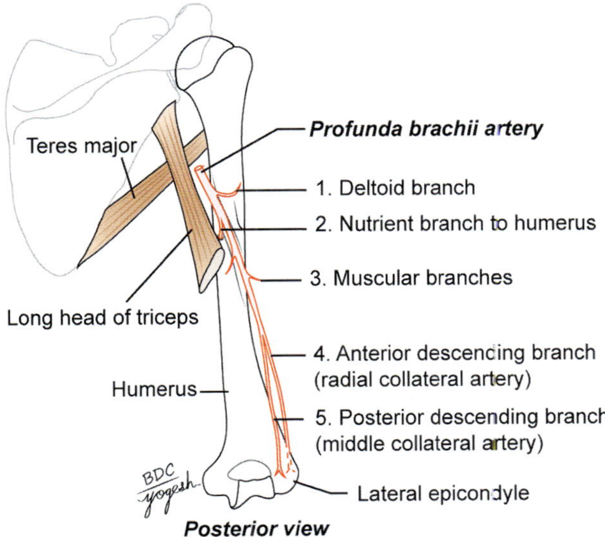

Fig. 8.25: Profunda brachii artery

3. The ***deltoid (ascending)*** branch ascends between the long and lateral heads of the triceps, and anastomoses with the descending branch of the posterior circumflex humeral artery.
4. The ***nutrient artery to the humerus*** is often present. It enters the bone in the radial groove just behind the deltoid tuberosity. However, it may be remembered that the main artery to the humerus is a branch of the brachial artery (Fig. 8.25).

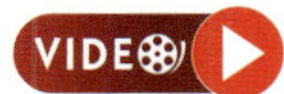

Video 1.8 Arm Muscles of the arm, Brachial artery, Cubital fossa—boundaries and contents, Back of arm—triceps brachii, radial nerve.

Facts to Remember

- The greater tubercle of humerus is the most lateral bony point of the shoulder.
- The coracobrachialis muscle is pierced by musculocutaneous nerve.
- Long head of biceps brachii muscle is intracapsular and extrasynovial at its origin.
- Biceps brachii is a strong supinator of the flexed elbow, besides being its flexor.
- The brachialis is the workhorse of the forearm flexion, whereas the medial head of the triceps is the workhorse of the forearm extension.
- Brachial pulse is commonly used for recording blood pressure.
- The median cubital vein is the most preferred vein for venepuncture.
- The ligament of Struthers is the fibrous band extending from the supracondylar spur to the medial epicondyle of the humerus.
- Medial root of median nerve crosses the axillary artery in front to join lateral root to form the median nerve.
- The order of structures from medial to lateral side in the cubital fossa (MBBR): median nerve, brachial artery, tendon of biceps brachii and radial nerve.
- Triceps brachii is the only active extensor of elbow joint. Gravity extends the joint passively.
- Radial groove gives passage to radial nerve and profunda brachii vessels.

BDC's Anatomy *e*-book

1. Bicipital aponeurosis
2. Biceps reflex
3. Recording of blood pressure
4. Musculocutaneous nerve palsy
5. Escape of triceps in radial nerve injuries
6. Further reading
7. Viva voce questions

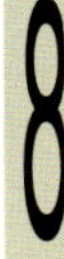

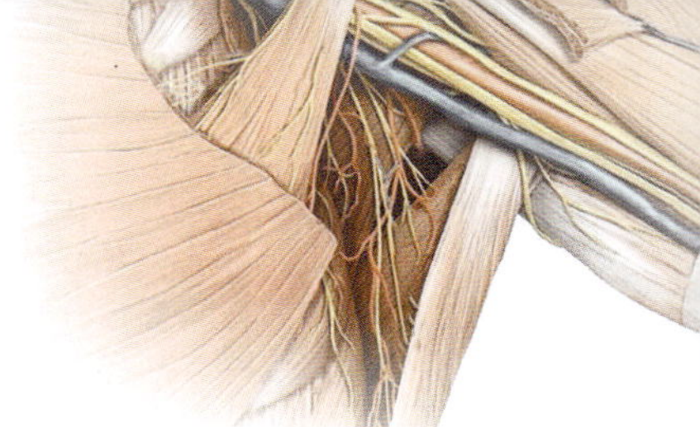

Chapter

9

Forearm and Hand

The forearm extends between the elbow and the wrist joints. Radius and ulna form its skeleton. These two bones articulate at both ends to form superior and inferior radioulnar joints. Their shafts are kept at optimal distance by the interosseous membrane. Muscles accompanied by nerves and blood vessels are present both on the front and the back of the forearm.

Hand is the most distal part of the upper limb, meant for carrying out diverse activities. Numerous muscles, tendons, bursae, blood vessels and nerves are artistically placed and protected in this region.

SURFACE LANDMARKS OF FRONT OF FOREARM

1. ***Epicondyles of the humerus:*** The medial epicondyle is more prominent than the lateral (Fig. 9.1). The posterior surface of the medial epicondyle is crossed by the *ulnar nerve,* which can be rolled under the palpating finger. Pressure on the nerve produces tingling sensations on the medial side of the hand (*see* Fig. 8.12a).
2. ***Tendon of the biceps brachii:*** It can be felt in front of the elbow. It can be made prominent by flexing the elbow joint against resistance. Pulsations of the brachial artery can be felt just medial to the tendon (*see* Fig. 8.16).
3. ***Head of the radius:*** It can be palpated in a depression on the posterolateral aspect of the extended elbow, distal to the lateral epicondyle. Its rotation can be felt during pronation and supination of the forearm.
4. ***Styloid process of the radius:*** It projects 1 cm lower than the styloid process of the ulna (Fig. 9.1). It can be felt in the upper part of the anatomical snuffbox.
5. ***Head of the ulna:*** It forms a surface elevation on the medial part of the posterior surface of the wrist when the hand is pronated.
6. ***Styloid process of the ulna:*** It projects downwards from the posteromedial aspect of the lower end of the ulna. Its tip can be felt on the posteromedial aspect of the wrist, where it lies about 1 cm above the tip of the styloid process of the radius (Fig. 9.1).

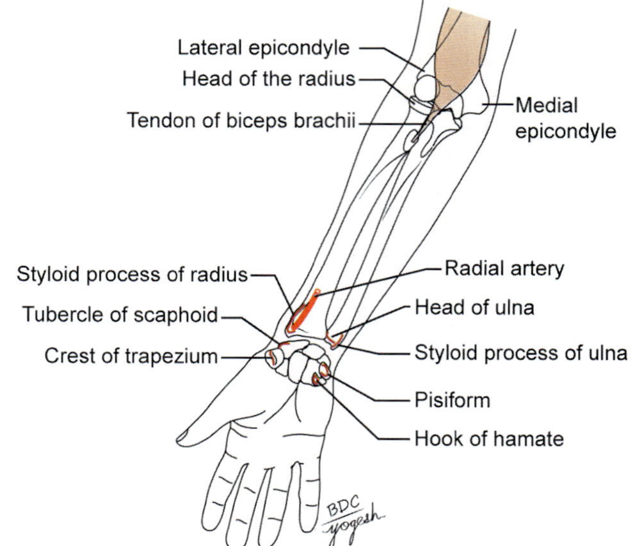

Fig. 9.1: Surface landmarks—front of forearm

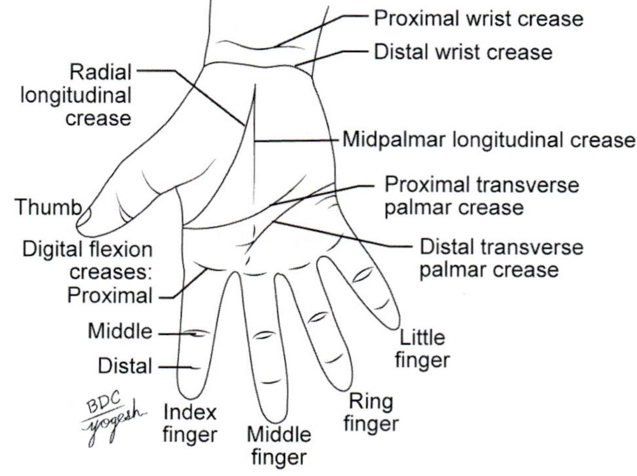

Fig. 9.2: Surface landmarks: Wrist and palm

7. ***Pisiform bone:*** It can be felt at the base of the hypothenar eminence (medially) where the tendon of the *flexor carpi ulnaris* terminates. It becomes visible and easily palpable at the medial end of the distal transverse crease (junction of forearm and hand) when the wrist is fully extended (Fig. 9.2).

8. ***Hook of the hamate:*** It lies one finger breadth below the pisiform bone, in line with the ulnar border of the ring finger. It can be felt only on deep palpation through the hypothenar muscles.
9. ***Tubercle of the scaphoid:*** It lies beneath the lateral part of the distal transverse crease in an extended wrist. It can be felt at the base of the thenar eminence in a depression just lateral to the tendon of the flexor carpi radialis (Fig. 9.1).
10. ***Tubercle (crest) of the trapezium:*** It may be felt on deep palpation inferolateral to the tubercle of the scaphoid.
11. The *brachioradialis* becomes prominent along the lateral border of the forearm when the elbow is flexed against resistance in the midprone position of the hand.
12. The *tendons of the flexor carpi radialis, palmaris longus* and *flexor carpi ulnaris* can be identified on the front of the wrist when the hand is flexed against resistance. The tendons lie in the order stated, from lateral to medial side (Fig. 9.3).
13. The pulsation of the *radial artery* can be felt in front of the lower end of the radius, just lateral to the tendon of the flexor carpi radialis.
14. The pulsations of the *ulnar artery* can be felt by careful palpation just lateral to the tendon of the flexor carpi ulnaris. Here, the ulnar nerve lies medial to the artery.
15. The *transverse creases* in front of the wrist are important landmarks. The proximal transverse crease lies at the level of the wrist joint, and distal crease corresponds to the proximal border of the flexor retinaculum.
16. The *median nerve* is very superficial in position at and above the wrist. It lies along the lateral edge of the tendon of the palmaris longus at the middle of the wrist.

Competency:
AN12.1 Describe and demonstrate important muscle groups of ventral forearm with attachments, nerve supply and actions.

MUSCLES OF FRONT OF FOREARM

The muscles of the front of the forearm may be divided into superficial and deep groups.

Components

The front of the forearm presents the following components for study.

1. Eight muscles: Five superficial and three deep.
2. Two arteries: Radial and ulnar.
3. Three nerves: Median, ulnar and radial.

These structures can be better understood by reviewing the long bones of the upper limb and having an articulated hand by the side.

SUPERFICIAL MUSCLES

There are five muscles in the superficial group (Plates 9.1 to 9.3, Figs 9.3 and 9.4):

1. Pronator teres
2. Flexor carpi radialis
3. Palmaris longus
4. Flexor carpi ulnaris
5. Flexor digitorum superficialis (Tables 9.1 and 9.2).

[*Mnemonic*: ***"Pretti Found Pamela for Fight":*** **P**ronator teres, **F**lexor carpi radialis, **P**almaris longus, **F**lexor carpi ulnaris, **F**lexor digitorum superficialis]

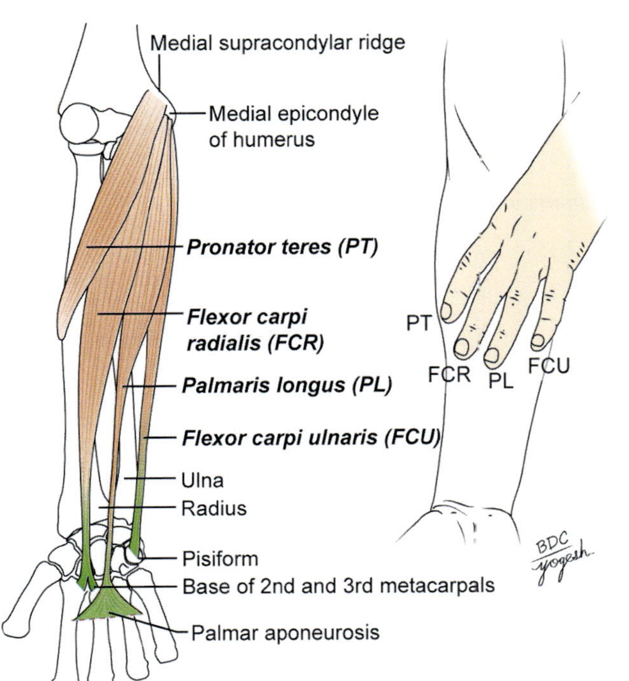

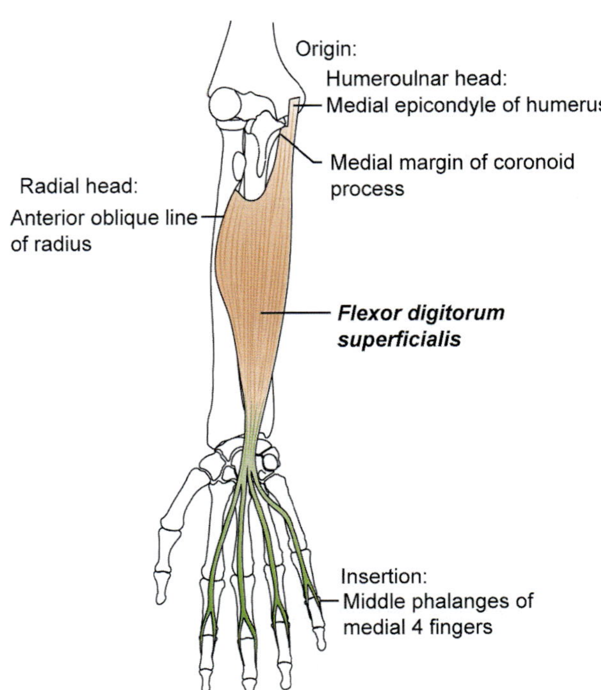

Fig. 9.3: The superficial muscles of the front of the right forearm

Plate 9.1: Pronator teres

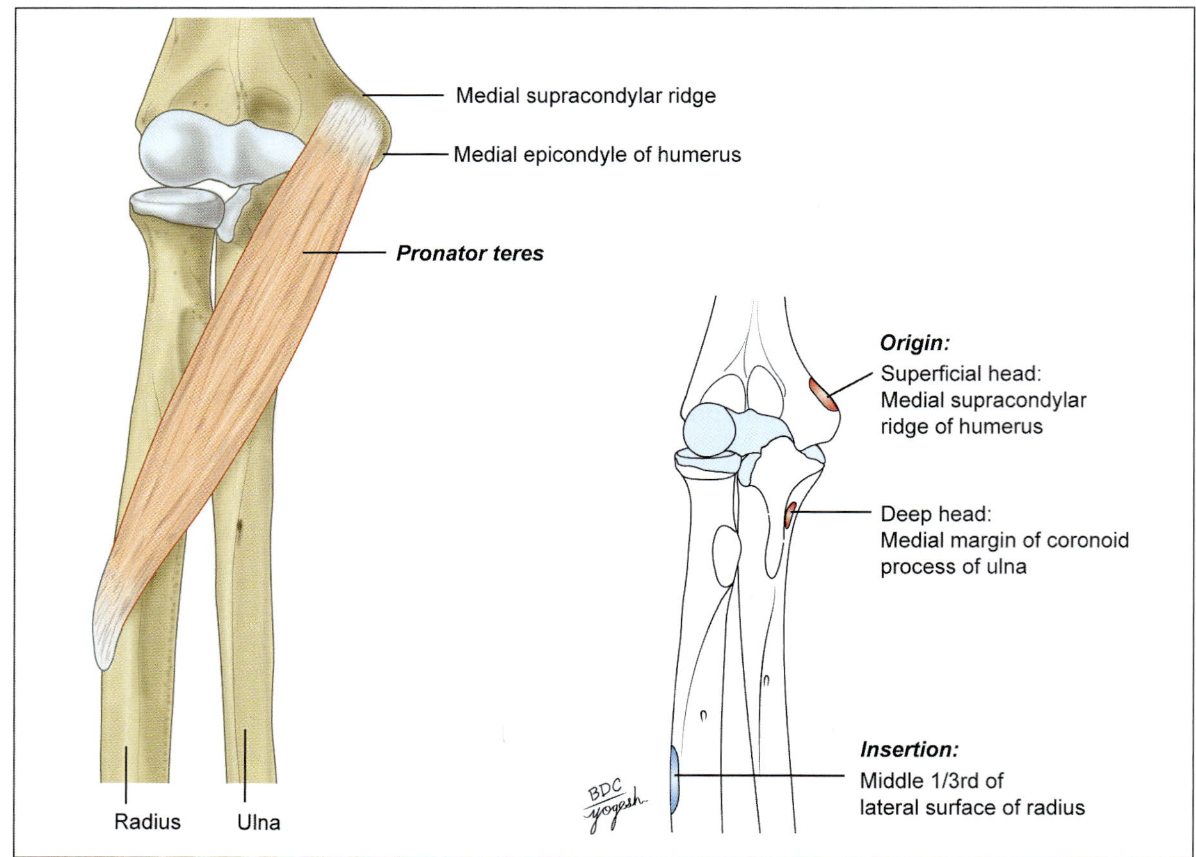

Plate 9.2: Flexor carpi radialis, palmaris longus and flexor carpi ulnaris

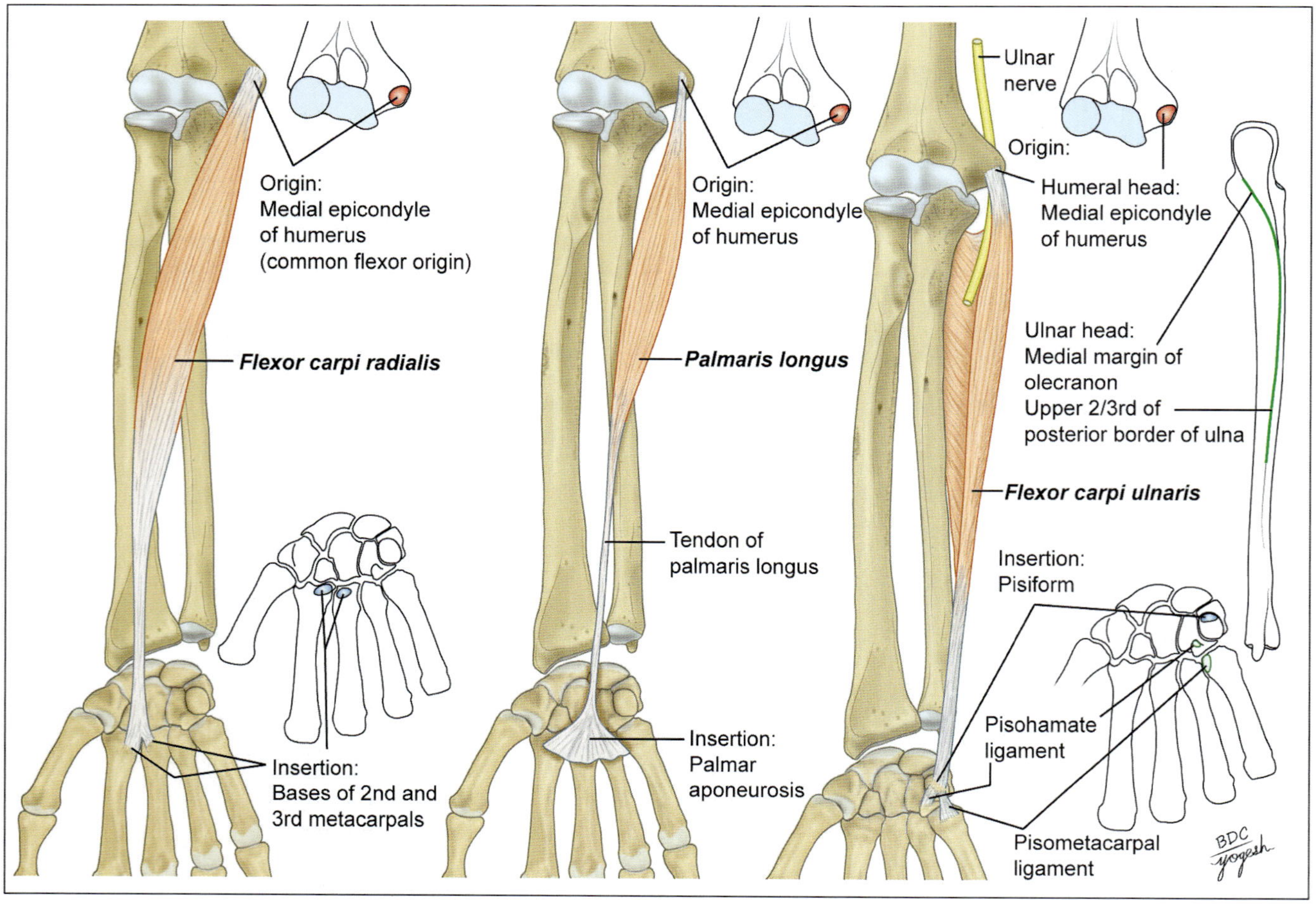

Origin:
Medial epicondyle of humerus (common flexor origin)
Flexor carpi radialis
Insertion:
Bases of 2nd and 3rd metacarpals

Origin:
Medial epicondyle of humerus
Palmaris longus
Tendon of palmaris longus
Insertion:
Palmar aponeurosis

Ulnar nerve
Origin:
Humeral head:
Medial epicondyle of humerus
Ulnar head:
Medial margin of olecranon
Upper 2/3rd of posterior border of ulna
Flexor carpi ulnaris
Insertion:
Pisiform
Pisohamate ligament
Pisometacarpal ligament
BDC yogesh

Plate 9.3: Flexor digitorum superficialis

Origin:
Humeroulnar head
Medial epicondyle of humerus
Medial margin of coronoid process
Radial head:
Anteior oblique line of radius

Median nerve
Ulnar artery

Flexor digitorum superficialis

Ulnar artery
Ulnar nerve
Median nerve

Insertion:
Middle phalanges of medial 4 fingers

BDC yogesh

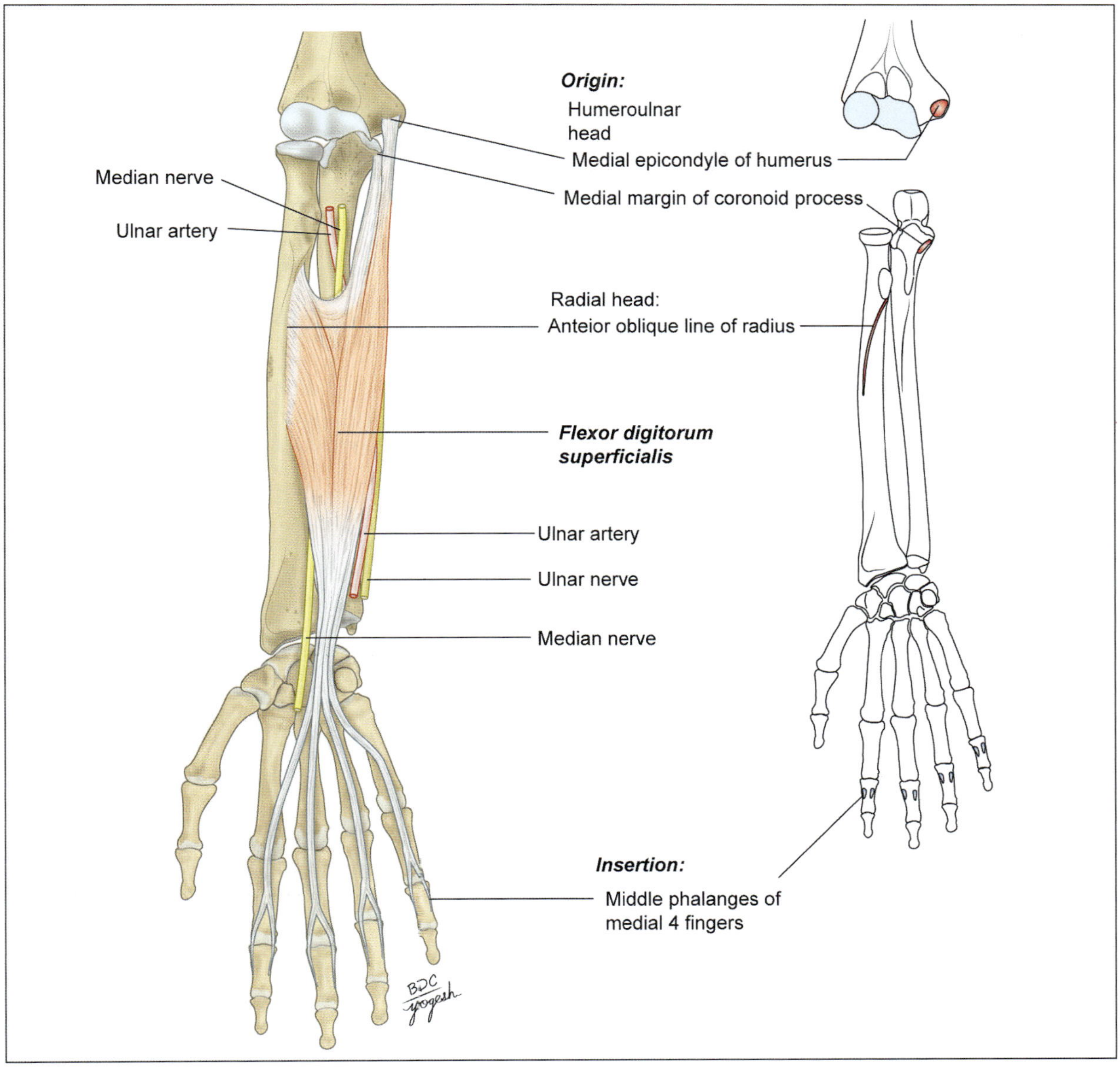

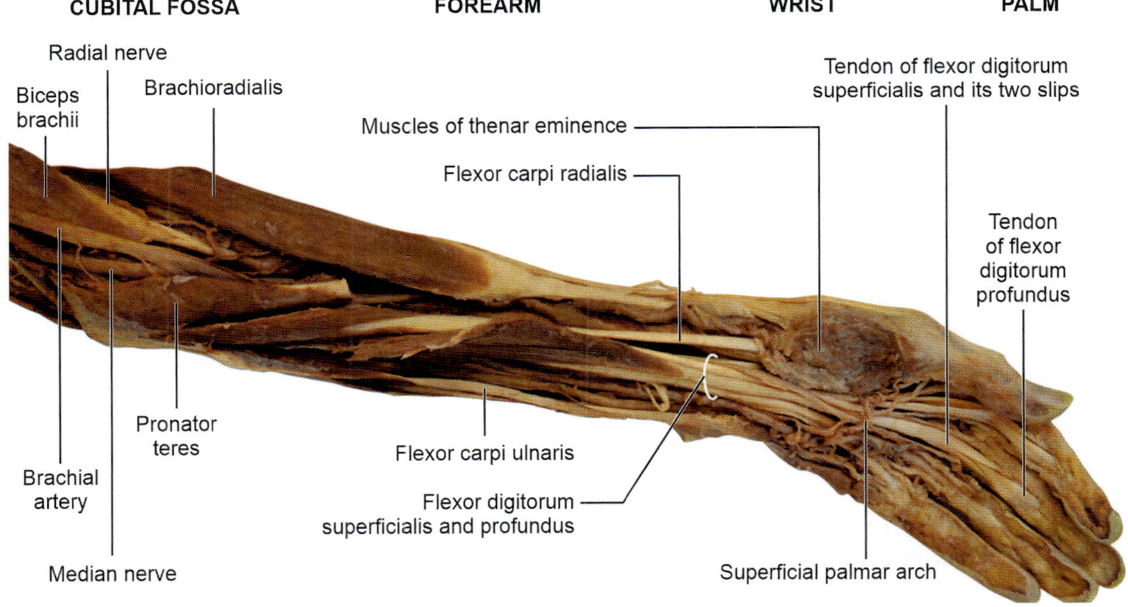

Fig. 9.4: Dissection of cubital fossa, front of the left forearm and palm

TABLE 9.1: Origin and insertion of the superficial muscles

Muscle	*Origin*	*Insertion*
1. **Pronator teres** (Fig.9.3)	Superficial head: Medial epicondyle of humerus Deep head: Medial margin of coronoid process of ulna	Middle of lateral aspect of shaft of radius
2. **Flexor carpi radialis**	Medial epicondyle of humerus	Bases of 2nd and 3rd metacarpal bones
3. **Palmaris longus**	Medial epicondyle of humerus	Flexor retinaculum and palmar aponeurosis
4. **Flexor digitorum superficialis** (Plate 9.3) • Humeroulnar head • Radial head	Medial epicondyle of humerus; medial border of coronoid process of ulna Anterior oblique line of shaft of radius	Muscle divides into 4 tendons. Each tendon divides into 2 slips, which are inserted on sides of **middle phalanx** of 2nd to 5th digits
5. **Flexor carpi ulnaris** • Humeral head • Ulnar head	Medial epicondyle of humerus Medial aspect of olecranon process and posterior border of ulna	**Pisiform** bone; insertion prolonged to hook of the hamate and base of 5th metacarpal bone (Plate 9.2)

TABLE 9.2: Nerve supply and actions of the superficial muscles

Muscle	*Nerve supply*	*Actions*
1. **Pronator teres**	Median nerve	Pronation of forearm
2. **Flexor carpi radialis**	Median nerve	Flexes and abducts hand at wrist joint
3. **Palmaris longus**	Median nerve	Flexes wrist joint
4. **Flexor digitorum superficialis**	Median nerve	Flexes middle phalanx of fingers and assists in flexing proximal phalanx and wrist joint
5. **Flexor carpi ulnaris**	Ulnar nerve	Flexes and adducts the hand at the wrist joint

Common Flexor Origin

All the superficial flexors of the forearm have a common origin from the front of the *medial epicondyle* of the humerus. This is called the common flexor origin (Plate 9.2).

Additional Features of Superficial Muscles

1. *Pronator teres:* Pronator teres comprise a big humeral and a smaller ulnar head. Between the two heads, the median nerve leaves the cubital fossa. Deep to the two heads exits ulnar artery from cubital fossa into the front of forearm. It forms medial boundary of the cubital fossa (Figs 9.3 and 9.4).
2. *Flexor carpi radialis:* It passes through a separate deep compartment of the flexor retinaculum. It is easily seen and is a guide to radial pulse, which lies lateral to the tendon (Fig. 9.4).
3. *Palmaris longus:* Palmaris longus (vestigial muscle) continues as palmar aponeurosis into the palm to protect the nerves and vessels there. Its tendon lies superficial to flexor retinaculum. It is known as "Fresher's nerve" as it looks like a nerve and may be cut by the fresher students.
4. *Flexor carpi ulnaris:* It is inserted into pisiform bone. Pisiform is a sesamoid bone in this tendon.
5. *Flexor digitorum superficialis:* Flexor digitorum superficialis comprises the humeroulnar and radial heads. The two heads of the muscle are joined by a fibrous arch. Median nerve and ulnar artery pass downwards deep to the fibrous arch (Plate 9.3). The part of muscle for middle ring and little fingers receive nerve supply from the median nerve in cubital fossa. Only the part for index finger receives nerve supply in middle of forearm.

DEEP MUSCLES

Deep muscles of the front of the forearm are (Tables 9.3 and 9.4, Plate 9.4, Fig. 9.5):
1. Flexor digitorum profundus
2. Flexor pollicis longus
3. Pronator quadratus.

Additional Points about the Flexor Digitorum Profundus

1. It is the most powerful and most bulky muscle of the forearm. It forms the muscular elevation seen and felt on the posterior surface of the forearm medial to the subcutaneous posterior border of the ulna (Fig. 9.5).
2. The main gripping power of the hand is provided by the flexor digitorum profundus.
3. The muscle is supplied by two different nerves. So, it is a ***hybrid muscle***.

Additional Points about the Flexor Pollicis Longus

1. The anterior interosseous nerve and vessels descend on the anterior surface of the interosseous membrane between the flexor digitorum profundus and the flexor pollicis longus.

TABLE 9.3: Origin and insertion of the deep muscles (Plate 9.4, Fig. 9.5)

Muscle	*Origin*	*Insertion*
1. **Flexor digitorum profundus** (composite or hybrid muscle)	• Upper 3/4th of the anterior and medial surface of the shaft of ulna • Upper 3/4th of the posterior border of ulna • Medial surface of the olecranon and coronoid processes of ulna • Adjoining part of the anterior surface of the interosseous membrane	• The muscle forms 4 tendons for the medial 4 digits, which enter the palm by passing deep to the flexor retinaculum in ulnar bursa and digital synovial sheaths • Opposite the proximal phalanx of the corresponding digit, the tendon perforates the tendon of the flexor digitorum superficialis (Plate 9.5) • Each tendon is inserted on the palmar surface of the base of the **distal phalanx** (Fig. 9.5)
2. **Flexor pollicis longus**	• Upper 3/4th of the anterior surface of the shaft of radius (Fig. 9.5) • Adjoining part of the anterior surface of the interosseous membrane	• The tendon enters the palm by passing deep to the flexor retinaculum • It is inserted into the palmar surface of the **distal phalanx** of the thumb
3. **Pronator quadratus**	Oblique ridge on the lower 1/4th of anterior surface of the shaft of ulna, and the area medial to it (Fig. 9.5)	• Superficial fibres into the lower 1/4th of the anterior surface and the anterior border of the radius • Deep fibres into the triangular area above the ulnar notch (*see* Fig. 2.18) of radius

TABLE 9.4: Nerve supply and actions of the deep muscles

Muscle	*Nerve supply*	*Actions*
1. **Flexor digitorum profundus**	• Medial half by ulnar nerve • Lateral half by anterior interosseous nerve (branch of median nerve)	• Flexor of distal phalanges after the flexor digitorum superficialis has flexed the middle phalanges • Secondarily, it flexes the other joints of the fingers and the wrist • It is the chief **gripping muscle**. It acts best when the wrist is extended
2. **Flexor pollicis longus**	Anterior interosseous nerve	• Flexes the distal phalanx of the thumb. Continued action may also flex the proximal joints crossed by the tendon
3. **Pronator quadratus**	Anterior interosseous nerve	• Superficial fibres pronate the forearm • Deep fibres bind the lower ends of radius and ulna

2. The tendon passes deep to the flexor retinaculum between the opponens pollicis and the oblique head of the adductor pollicis to enter the fibrous flexor sheath of the thumb. It lies in radial bursa (Fig. 9.6).

Competency:
AN12.9 Identify and describe fibrous flexor sheaths, ulnar bursa, radial bursa and digital synovial sheaths.

Synovial Sheaths of Flexor Tendons

1. ***Ulnar bursa (Common flexor synovial sheath)*:** The long flexor tendons of the fingers (flexor digitorum superficialis and profundus) are enclosed in a common synovial sheath while passing deep to the flexor retinaculum (carpal tunnel). The sheath has a parietal layer lining the walls of the carpal tunnel and a visceral layer closely applied to the tendons (Plate 9.5, Fig. 9.6). From the arrangement of the sheath, it appears that the synovial sac has been invaginated by the tendons from its lateral side. The synovial sheath extends upwards for 5.0 or 7.5 cm into the forearm and downwards into the palm up to the middle of the shafts of the metacarpal bones. It is important to note that the lower medial end is continuous with the digital synovial sheath of the little finger.
2. ***Radial bursa (Synovial sheath of the tendon of flexor pollicis longus)*:** This sheath is separate. Superiorly, it is coextensive with the common sheath, and inferiorly it extends up to the distal phalanx of the thumb (Fig. 9.6).
3. ***Digital synovial sheaths*:** The sheaths enclose the flexor tendons in the fingers and line the fibrous flexor sheaths. The digital sheath of the little finger is continuous with the ulnar bursa and that of the thumb with the radial bursa. However, the digital sheaths of the index, middle and ring fingers are separate and independent (Fig. 9.7).

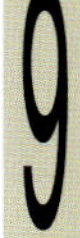

Plate 9.4: Deep muscles of front of forearm

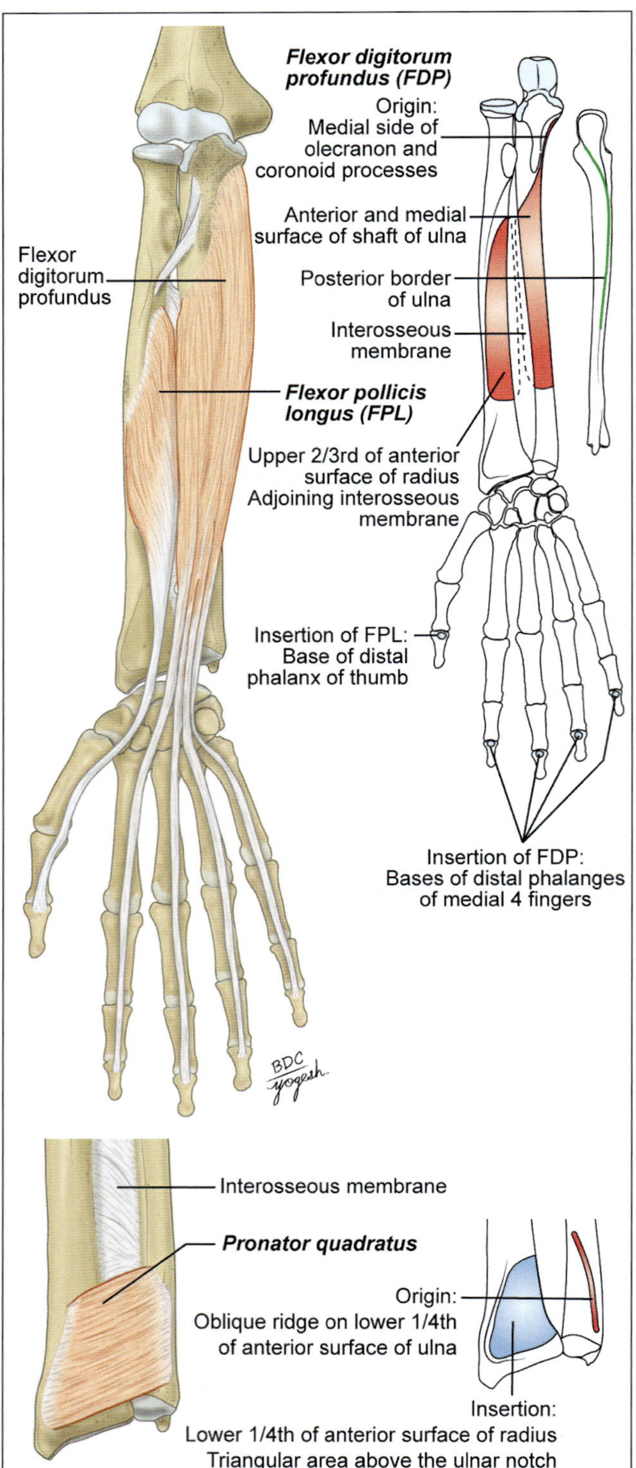

Plate 9.5: Synovial sheaths of the flexor tendons of hand

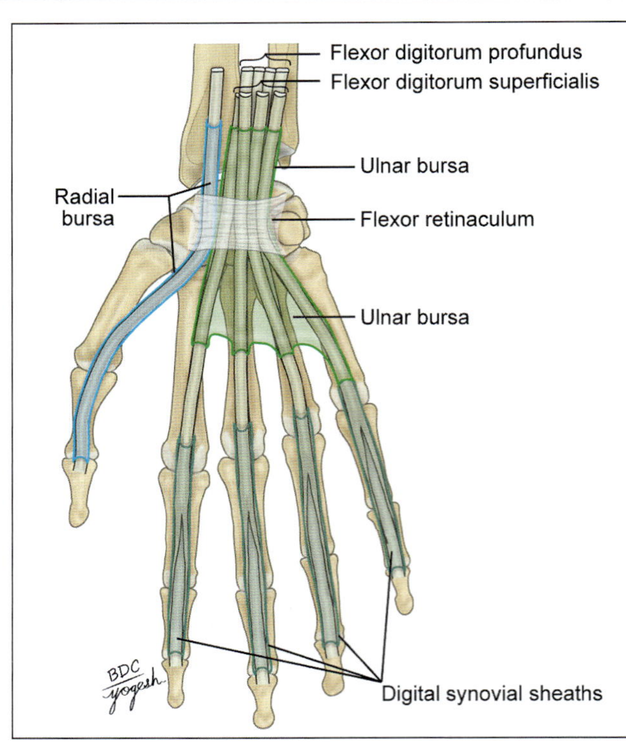

Plate 9.6: Vincula longa and brevia of the middle finger

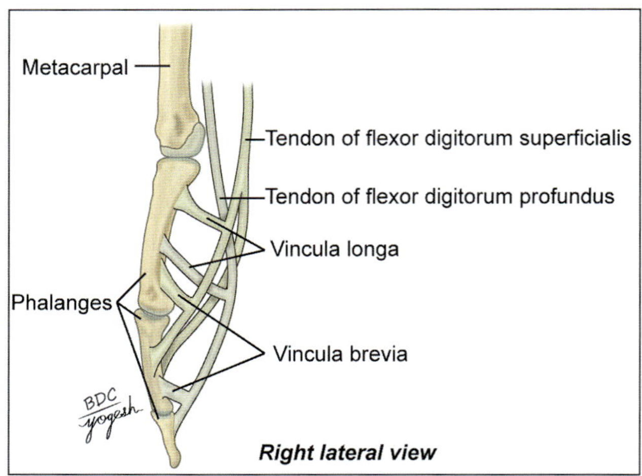

Vincula Longa and Brevia

The vincula longa and brevia are synovial folds, which connect the tendons to the phalanges. They transmit vessels to the tendons (Plate 9.6). These are the remnants of mesotendon.

DISSECTION

The skin of the forearm has already been reflected on each side. Cut through the superficial and deep fasciae to expose the superficial muscles of the forearm.

Superficial muscles

Identify these five superficial muscles. These are from lateral to medial side, pronator teres getting inserted into middle of radius, flexor carpi radialis reaching till the wrist, palmaris longus continuing with palmar aponeurosis, flexor digitorum superficialis passing through the palm and most medially the flexor carpi ulnaris getting inserted into the pisiform bone (Fig. 9.3).

Deep muscles

Cut through the origin of superficial muscles of forearm at the level of medial epicondyle of humerus and reflect them distally. This will expose the three deep muscles, e.g. flexor pollicis longus, flexor digitorum profundus and pronator quadratus.

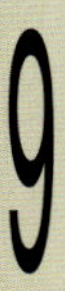

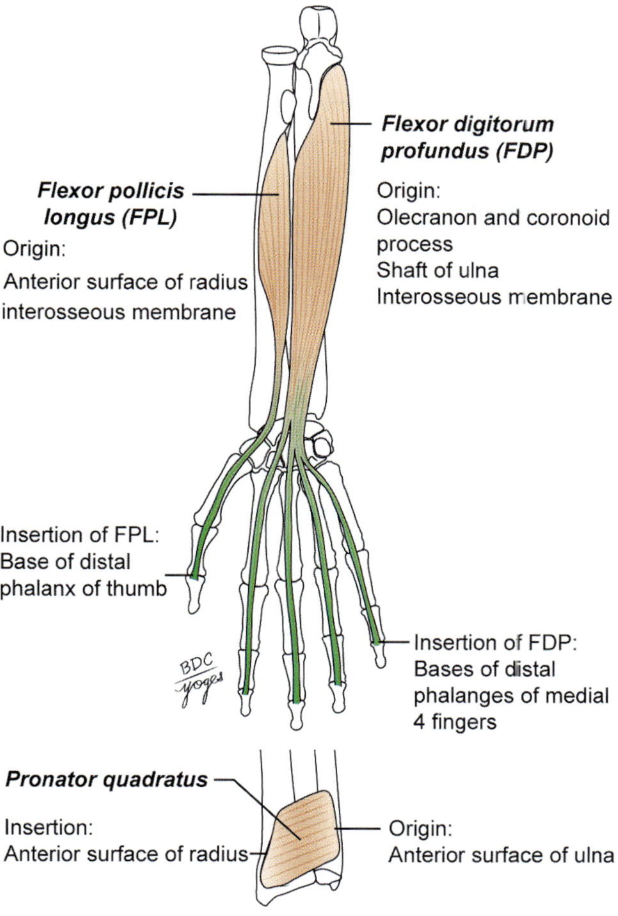

Fig. 9.5: Deep muscles of front of forearm

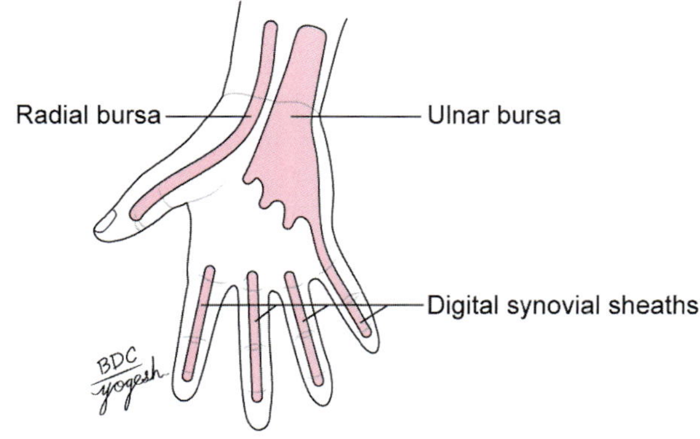

Fig. 9.6: The synovial sheaths of the flexor tendons, i.e. ulnar bursa, radial bursa and digital synovial sheaths

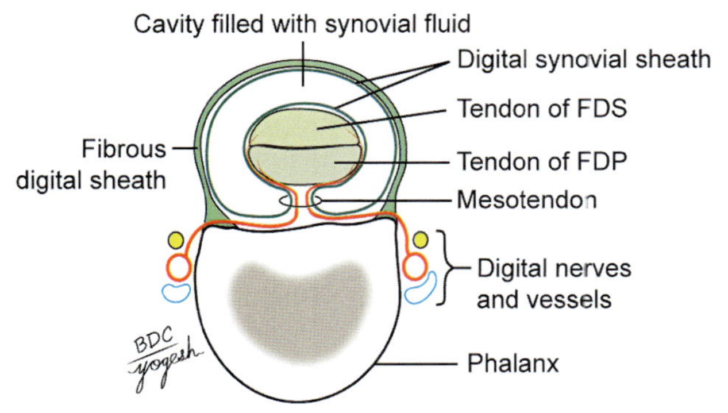

Fig. 9.7: Digital synovial sheath and mesotendon (cross-section of the digit)

Competency:

AN12.2 Identify and describe origin, course, relations, branches (or tributaries), termination of important nerves and vessels of forearm.

ARTERIES OF FRONT OF FOREARM

Features

The most conspicuous arteries of the forearm are the radial and ulnar arteries (Plate 9.7). However, they mainly supply the hand through the deep and superficial palmar arches. The arterial supply of the forearm is chiefly derived from the common interosseous branch of the ulnar artery, which divides into anterior and posterior interosseous arteries. The posterior interosseous artery is reinforced in the upper part and replaced in the lower part by the anterior interosseous artery.

RADIAL ARTERY

Beginning, Course and Termination

Radial artery (Fig. 9.8) is the smaller terminal branch of the brachial artery in the cubital fossa. It runs downwards to the wrist with a lateral convexity. It leaves the forearm by turning posteriorly and entering the anatomical snuffbox. As compared to the ulnar artery, it is quite superficial throughout its whole course. The radial artery continues as deep palmar arch in the palm. Its distribution in the hand is described later. It is the most commonly palpated artery (Fig. 9.9, Flowchart 9.1).

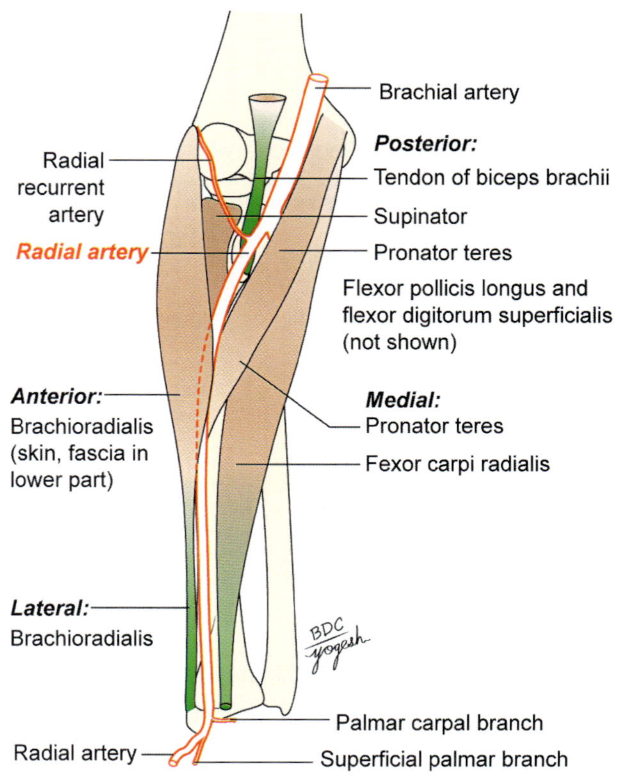

Fig. 9.8: Relations of radial artery

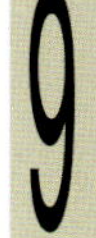

Plate 9.7: Blood vessels and nerves of front of the forearm

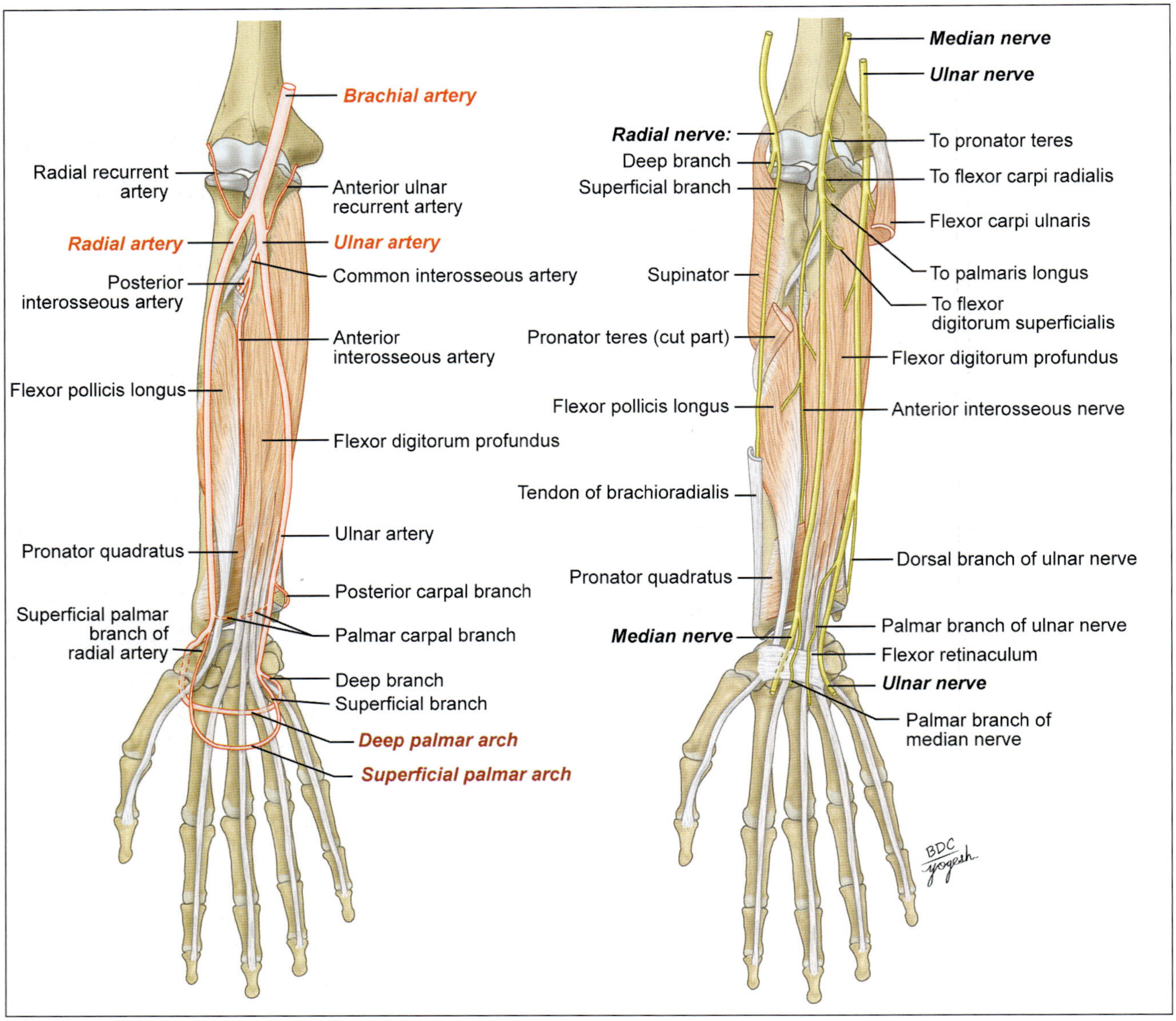

Brachial artery
Radial recurrent artery
Anterior ulnar recurrent artery
Radial artery
Ulnar artery
Posterior interosseous artery
Common interosseous artery
Anterior interosseous artery
Flexor pollicis longus
Flexor digitorum profundus
Pronator quadratus
Ulnar artery
Posterior carpal branch
Superficial palmar branch of radial artery
Palmar carpal branch
Deep branch
Superficial branch
Deep palmar arch
Superficial palmar arch

Median nerve
Ulnar nerve
Radial nerve:
Deep branch
Superficial branch
To pronator teres
To flexor carpi radialis
Flexor carpi ulnaris
Supinator
To palmaris longus
To flexor digitorum superficialis
Pronator teres (cut part)
Flexor digitorum profundus
Flexor pollicis longus
Anterior interosseous nerve
Tendon of brachioradialis
Pronator quadratus
Dorsal branch of ulnar nerve
Median nerve
Palmar branch of ulnar nerve
Flexor retinaculum
Ulnar nerve
Palmar branch of median nerve

Flowchart 9.1: Radial artery in forearm

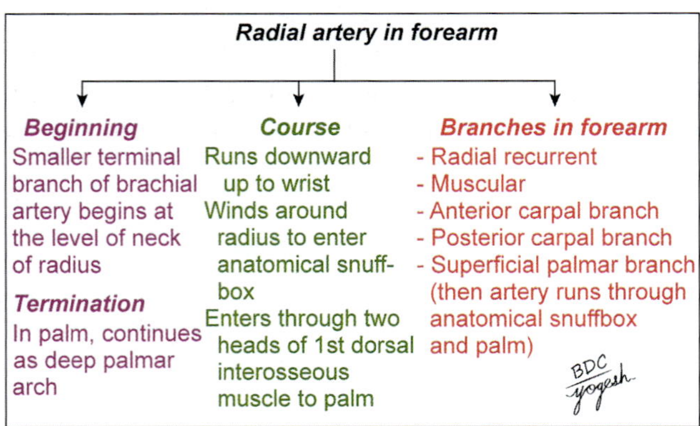

Relations

Anteriorly: It is overlapped by the brachioradialis in its upper part, but in the lower half, it is covered only by skin, superficial and deep fasciae.

Posteriorly: It is related to the tendon and muscles attached to anterior surface of radius, i.e. tendon of biceps brachii, supinator, flexor pollicis longus, radial head of flexor digitorum superficialis and pronator quadratus.

Medially: It is related to the pronator teres in the upper one-third and the tendon of the flexor carpi radialis in the lower two-thirds of its course (Figs 9.8 and 9.10).

Laterally: Brachioradialis in the whole extent and the radial nerve in the middle one-third.

The artery is accompanied by venae comitantes.

Branches in the Forearm

1. ***Radial recurrent artery:*** It arises just below the elbow, runs upwards deep to the brachioradialis and ends by anastomosing with the radial collateral artery (anterior branch of profunda brachii artery) in front of the lateral epicondyle of the humerus (*see* Fig. 8.11).
2. ***Muscular branches*** are given to the lateral muscles of the forearm.

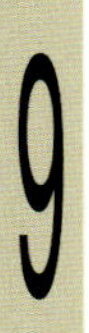

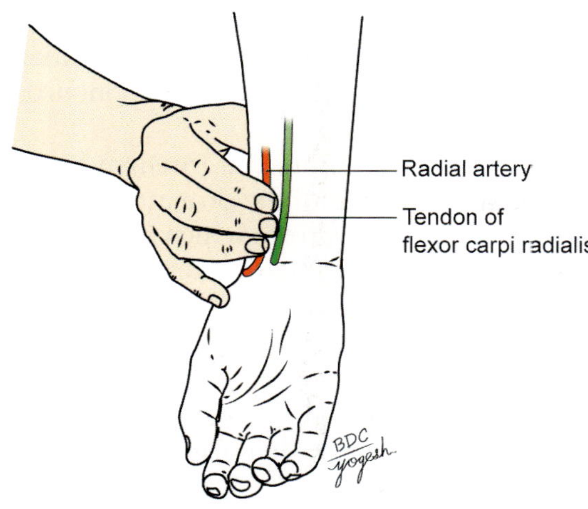

Fig. 9.9: Palpation of radial artery

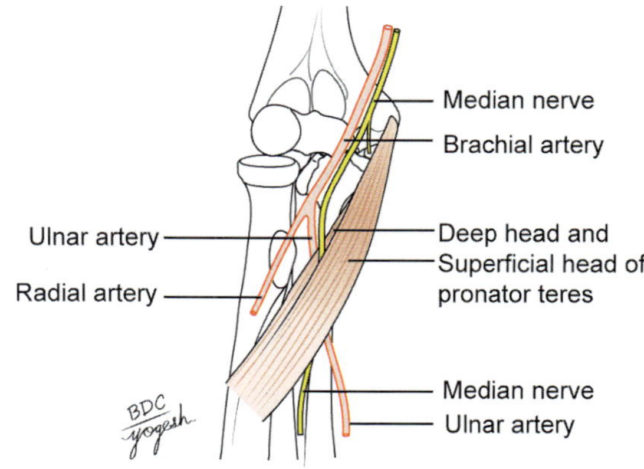

Fig. 9.10: Relations of the median nerve in right cubital fossa and its entry into the forearm

3. ***Palmar/anterior carpal branch:*** It arises near the lower border of the pronator quadratus, runs medially deep to the flexor tendons and ends by anastomosing with the palmar carpal branch of the ulnar artery in front of the middle of the recurrent branch of the deep palmar arch, to form a cruciform anastomosis. The palmar carpal arch supplies bones and joints at the wrist.
4. ***Dorsal/posterior carpal branch:*** It forms dorsal carpal arch with branch of ulnar artery.
5. ***Superficial palmar branch:*** It arises just before the radial artery leaves the forearm by winding backwards. The branch passes through the thenar muscles and ends by joining the terminal part of the ulnar artery to complete the superficial palmar arch (Fig. 9.29).

ULNAR ARTERY

Beginning, Course and Termination

Ulnar artery is the larger terminal branch of the brachial artery and begins in the cubital fossa (Fig. 9.10). The artery runs obliquely downwards and medially in the upper one-third of the forearm, but in the lower 2/3rd of the forearm, its course is vertical (Plate 9.7, Flowchart 9.2). It enters the palm by passing superficial to the flexor retinaculum. In palm, ulnar artery terminates by dividing into superficial and deep branches. Its distribution in the hand is described later.

Relations

Anteriorly: In its upper half, the artery is deep and is covered by muscles arising from common flexor origin and median nerve. The lower half of the artery is superficial and is covered only by skin and fascia (Fig. 9.4).

Posteriorly: It lies on brachialis and on the flexor digitorum profundus.

Medially: It is related to the ulnar nerve and to the flexor carpi ulnaris

Laterally: It is related to the flexor digitorum superficialis and median nerve.

The artery is accompanied by venae comitantes.

Flowchart 9.2: Ulnar artery

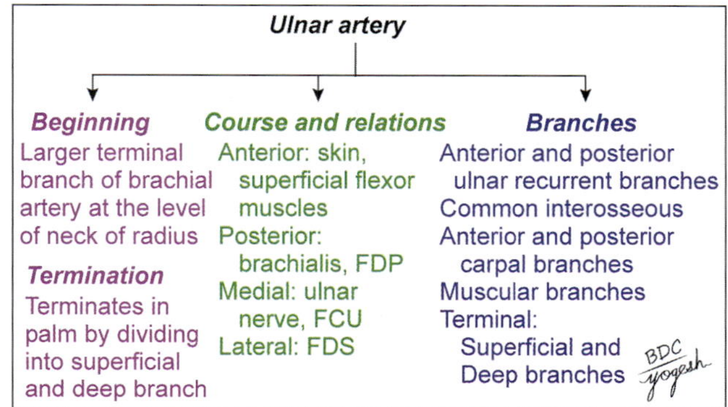

Branches

1. ***Anterior*** and ***posterior ulnar recurrent arteries:*** They anastomose around the elbow. The smaller anterior ulnar recurrent artery runs up and ends by anastomosing with the inferior ulnar collateral artery in front of the medial epicondyle. The larger posterior ulnar recurrent artery arises lower than the anterior and ends by anastomosing with the superior ulnar collateral artery behind the medial epicondyle (*see* Fig. 8.11).
2. ***Common interosseous artery*** (about 1 cm long): It arises just below the radial tuberosity. It passes backwards to reach the upper border of the interosseous membrane and end by dividing into the anterior and posterior interosseous arteries.

   The ***anterior interosseous artery*** is the deepest artery on the front of the forearm. It accompanies the anterior interosseous nerve. It descends on the surface of the interosseous membrane between the flexor digitorum profundus and the flexor pollicis longus (Plate 9.7). It pierces the interosseous membrane at the upper border of the pronator quadratus to enter the extensor compartment. The artery gives muscular branches to the deep muscles of the front of the forearm, nutrient branches to the radius and ulna and a *median artery*, which accompanies the median nerve.

   Near its origin, the ***posterior interosseous artery*** gives off the interosseous recurrent artery, which runs upwards, and ends by anastomosing with middle collateral artery (posterior branch of profunda brachii

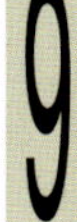

artery) behind the lateral epicondyle. The posterior interosseous artery passes through a gap above the interosseous membrane to the back of forearm (Fig. 8.10).

3. *Muscular branches* supply the medial muscles of the forearm.
4, 5. *Palmar* and *dorsal carpal branches:* They take part in the anastomoses around the wrist joint. The palmar carpal branch helps to form the palmar carpal arch.

The dorsal carpal branch arises just above the pisiform bone, winds backwards deep to the tendons and ends in the dorsal carpal arch. This arch is formed medially by the dorsal carpal branch of the ulnar artery and laterally by the dorsal carpal branch of the radial artery.

DISSECTION

Having dissected the superficial and deep group of muscles of the forearm, identify the terminal branches of the brachial artery, e.g. ulnar and radial arteries and their branches.

Radial artery follows the direction of the brachial artery (Plate 9.7).

Ulnar artery passes obliquely deep to heads of pronator teres and then runs vertically till the wrist. Carefully look for common interosseous branch of ulnar artery and its anterior and posterior branches.

NERVES OF FRONT OF FOREARM

Nerves of the front of the forearm are the median, ulnar and radial nerves. The radial and ulnar nerves run along the margins of the forearm and are never crossed by the corresponding vessels, which gradually approach them. The ulnar artery, while approaching the ulnar nerve, gets crossed by the median nerve (Plate 9.7).

MEDIAN NERVE

Median nerve is the main nerve of the front of the forearm. It also supplies the muscles of thenar eminence (Plate 9.7, Fig. 9.12, Flowchart 9.3).

The median nerve controls coarse movements of the hand, as it supplies most of the long muscles of the front of the forearm. It is, therefore, called the '*labourer's nerve*'.

Course

Median nerve lies medial to brachial artery and enters the cubital fossa. It is the most medial content of cubital fossa (Fig. 9.10). Then it enters the forearm to lie between flexor digitorum superficialis and flexor digitorum profundus. It lies adherent to the back of superficialis muscle. Then it reaches down the region of wrist where it lies deep and lateral to palmaris longus tendon. Lastly, it passes deep to flexor retinaculum through carpal tunnel to enter the palm (Plate 9.7).

Relations

1. In the cubital fossa, median nerve lies medial to the brachial artery, behind the bicipital aponeurosis and in front of the brachialis.
2. The median nerve enters the forearm by passing between the two heads of the pronator teres. Here, it crosses the ulnar artery from which it is separated by the deep head of the pronator teres (Fig. 9.10).
3. Along with the ulnar artery, the median nerve passes beneath the fibrous arch of the flexor digitorum superficialis, and runs deep to this muscle on the surface of the flexor digitorum profundus. It is accompanied by the median artery, a branch of the anterior interosseous artery. About 5 cm above the flexor retinaculum (wrist), it becomes superficial and lies between the tendons of the flexor carpi radialis (laterally) and the flexor digitorum superficialis (medially). It is overlapped by the tendon of the palmaris longus.
4. The median nerve enters the palm by passing deep to the flexor retinaculum through the carpal tunnel.

Branches

1. *Muscular branches* to pronator teres in lower part of arm and in cubital fossa to flexor carpi radialis, palmaris longus and flexor digitorum superficialis (Fig. 9.11)

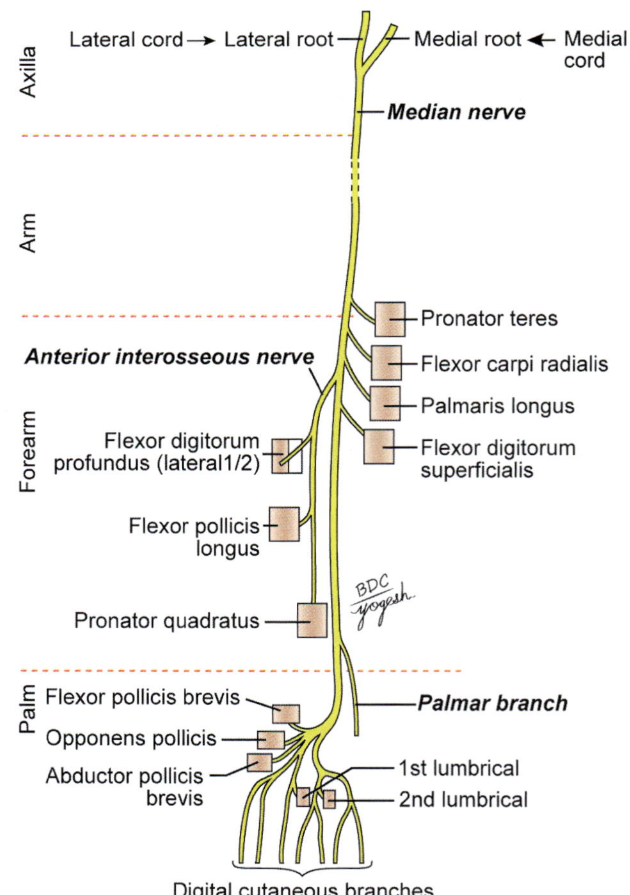

Fig. 9.11: Distribution of median nerve

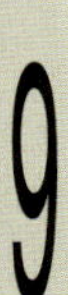

Flowchart 9.3: Median nerve

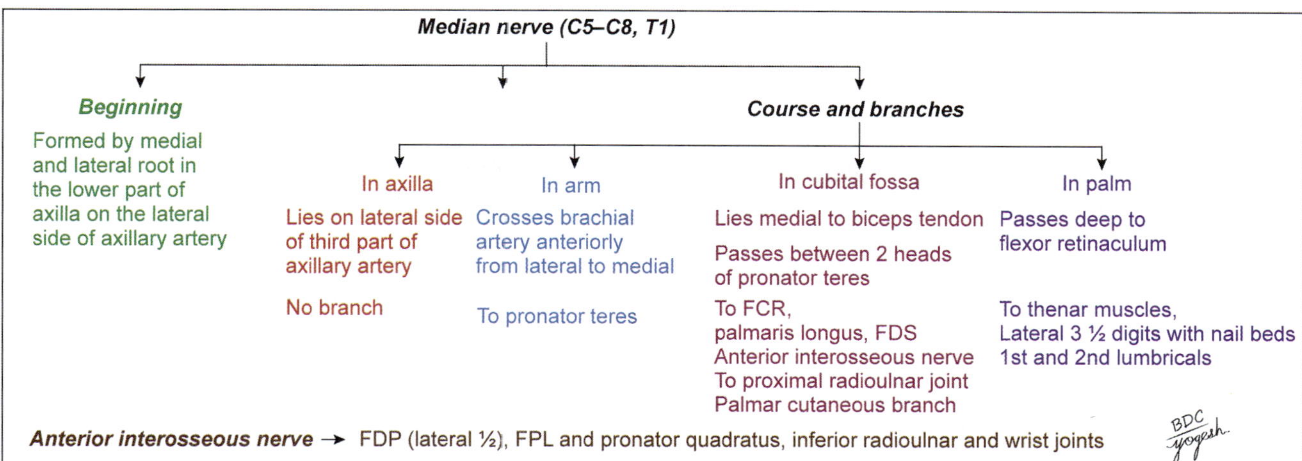

2. ***Anterior interosseous branch*** is given off in the upper part of the forearm. It supplies the flexor pollicis longus, the lateral half of the flexor digitorum profundus and the pronator quadratus. The nerve also supplies the distal radioulnar and wrist joints.
3. ***Palmar cutaneous branch*** arises a short distance above the flexor retinaculum, lies superficial to it and supplies the lateral 2/3rd part of skin of palm over the thenar eminence and the central part of the palm (*see* Fig. 7.1a).
4. ***Articular branches*** are given to the elbow joint and to the proximal radioulnar joint.
5. ***Vascular branches*** supply the radial and ulnar arteries.
6. ***Communicating branch*** is given to the ulnar nerve.

ULNAR NERVE

The ulnar nerve is also known as the ***'musician's nerve'*** because it controls fine movements of the fingers. Its course in the palm will be considered in the later part of this chapter.

Course

Ulnar nerve is palpable as it lies behind medial epicondyle of humerus and is ***not*** a content of cubital fossa (Plate 9.7, Flowchart 9.4).

It enters the forearm by passing between two heads of flexor carpi ulnaris, i.e. cubital tunnel, to lie along the lateral border of flexor carpi ulnaris in the forearm.

In the last phase, it courses *superficial* to the flexor retinaculum, covered by its superficial slip or volar carpal ligament to enter the region of palm.

Relations

1. At the elbow, the ulnar nerve lies behind the medial epicondyle of the humerus (Plate 9.7). It enters the forearm by passing between the two heads of the flexor carpi ulnaris.
2. In the forearm, the ulnar nerve runs on the medial part of the flexor digitorum profundus muscle.
3. At the wrist, the ulnar neurovascular bundle lies between the flexor carpi ulnaris and the flexor digitorum profundus. The bundle enters the palm by passing superficial to the flexor retinaculum, lateral to the pisiform bone (Plate 9.7).

Branches

1. ***Muscular***, to the flexor carpi ulnaris and the medial half of the flexor digitorum profundus.
2. ***Palmar cutaneous branch*** arises in the middle of the forearm and supplies the skin over the hypothenar eminence (*see* Fig. 7.1a) (medial 1/3rd of palm).

Flowchart 9.4: Ulnar nerve

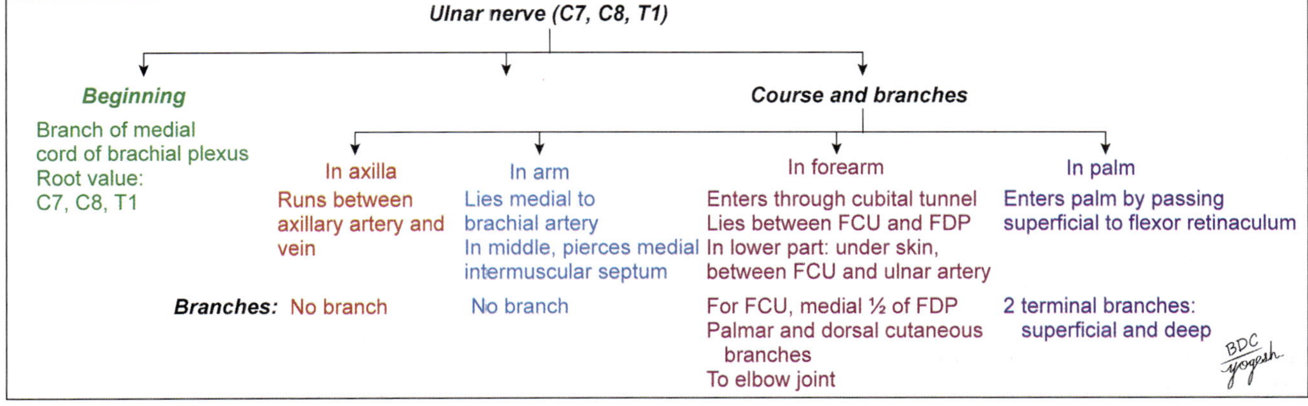

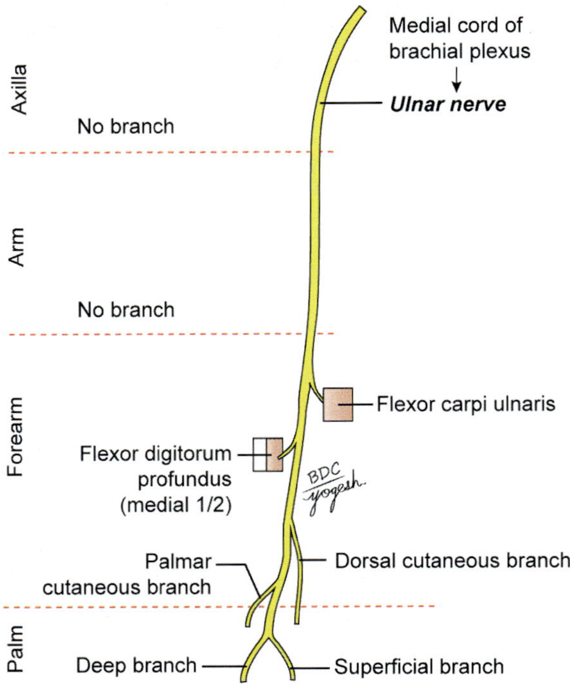

Fig. 9.12: Branches of ulnar nerve in forearm

3. ***Dorsal cutaneous branch*** arises 7.5 cm above the wrist, winds backwards and supplies the proximal parts of the medial 1½ digits and the adjoining area of the dorsum of the hand (*see* Fig. 7.1b).
4. ***Articular branches*** are given off to the elbow joint.

Its branches in the palm are shown in Fig. 9.33.

RADIAL NERVE

Course

The radial nerve divides into its two terminal branches in the cubital fossa just below the level of the lateral epicondyle of the humerus (Plate 9.7).

Branches

- The ***deep terminal branch*** (posterior interosseous nerve) soon enters the back of the forearm by passing through the supinator muscle. It will be studied further in back of forearm as posterior interosseous nerve.
- The ***superficial terminal branch*** (the main continuation of the nerve) runs down in front of the forearm. The superficial terminal branch of the radial nerve is closely related to the radial artery, only in the middle 1/3rd of the forearm. It is purely cutaneous.
- In the upper 1/3rd, it is widely separated from the artery, and in the lower 1/3rd it passes backwards under the tendon of the brachioradialis to reach the anatomical snuffbox from where it is distributed to the lateral half of the dorsum of the hand and to the proximal parts of the dorsal surfaces of the thumb, the index finger and lateral half of the middle finger (*see* Fig. 7.1b).
- Injury to this branch results in a small area of sensory loss over the root of the thumb.

DISSECTION

Median nerve is the chief nerve of the forearm. It enters the forearm by passing between two heads of pronator teres muscle. Its anterior interosseous branch is given off as it is leaving the cubital fossa. Identify median nerve *stuck* to the fascia on the deep surface of flexor digitorum superficialis muscle. Thus, the nerve lies deep to the flexor digitorum superficialis (Plate 9.3).

Dissect the anterior interosseous nerve as it lies on the interosseous membrane between flexor pollicis longus and flexor digitorum profundus muscles (Plate 9.7).

Identify the ulnar nerve situated behind the medial epicondyle. Trace it vertically down till the flexor retinaculum (Plate 9.7).

Trace the radial nerve and its two branches in the lateral part of the cubital fossa. Its deep branch is muscular and superficial branch is cutaneous (Plate 9.7).

PALMAR ASPECT OF WRIST AND HAND

Features

The human hand is designed:

1. For grasping,
2. For precise movements and
3. For serving as a tactile organ.

There is a big area in the motor cortex of brain for muscles of hand.

The skin of the palm is:

1. Thick for protection of underlying tissues.
2. Immobile because of its firm attachment to the underlying palmar aponeurosis.
3. Creased.

All of these characters increase the efficiency of the grip. The skin is supplied by spinal nerves C6–C8 (*see* Fig. 7.6a) through the median and ulnar nerves.

The superficial fascia of the palm is made up of dense fibrous bands, which bind the skin to the deep fascia (palmar aponeurosis) and divide the subcutaneous fat into small tight compartments, which serve as water-cushions during firm gripping. The fascia contains a subcutaneous muscle, the ***palmaris brevis***, which helps in improving the grip by steadying the skin on the ulnar side of the hand. The superficial metacarpal ligament, which stretches across the roots of the fingers over the digital vessels and nerves, is a part of this fascia.

The deep fascia is specialised to form:

1. The flexor retinaculum at the wrist.
2. The palmar aponeurosis in the palm.
3. The fibrous flexor sheaths in the fingers.

All three form a continuous structure, which holds the tendons in position and thus increases the efficiency of the grip.

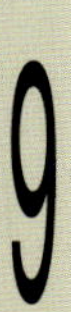

DISSECTION

1. A horizontal incision at the distal crease of front of the wrist has already been made.
2. Make a vertical incision from the centre of the above incision through the palm to the centre of the middle finger (Fig. 9.13).
3. Make one horizontal incision along the distal palmar crease.
4. Make an oblique incision starting 3 cm distal to incision no. 2 and extend it till the tip of the distal phalanx of the thumb.

Thus the skin of the palm gets divided into three areas. Reflect the skin of lateral and medial flaps on their respective sides. The skin of the intermediate flap is reflected distally towards the distal palmar crease. Further the skin of middle finger is to be reflected on either side.

Superficial fascia and deep fascia

Remove the superficial fascia to clean the underlying deep fascia.

Deep fascia is modified to form the flexor retinaculum at wrist, palmar aponeurosis in the palm and fibrous flexor sheaths in the digits. Identify the structures on its superficial surface. Divide the flexor retinaculum between the thenar and hypothenar eminences, carefully preserving the underlying median nerve and long flexor tendons.

Identify long flexor tendons enveloped in their synovial sheaths, including the digital synovial sheaths.

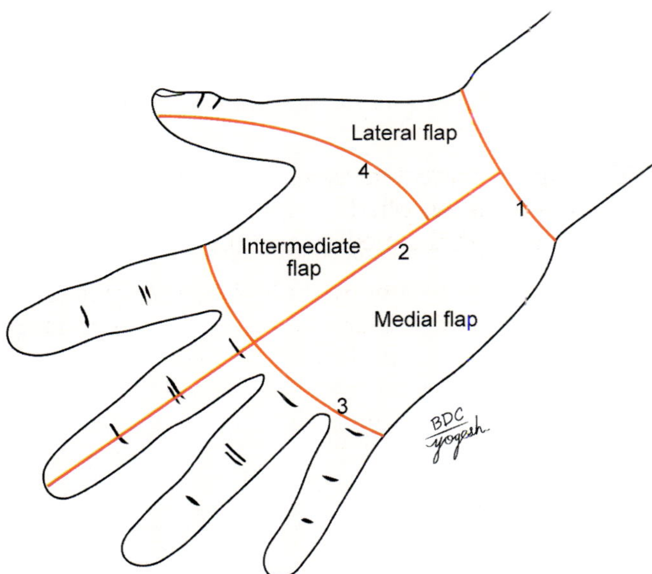

Fig. 9.13: Incisions of palm and digits (1–4)

Competency:
AN12.3 Identify and describe flexor retinaculum with its attachments.

Flexor Retinaculum

Flexor retinaculum (Latin *to hold back*) is a strong fibrous band, which bridges the anterior concavity of the carpus and converts it into a tunnel, the *carpal tunnel* (Plates 9.8 and 9.9, Figs 9.14 and 9.15). The thenar and hypothenar muscles arise from the retinaculum.

Attachments

Medially, to:
1. Pisiform bone
2. Hook of the hamate.

Laterally, to:
1. Tubercle of the scaphoid, and
2. Crest of the trapezium.

On either side, the retinaculum has a slip:
1. The lateral *deep slip* is attached to the medial lip of the groove on the trapezium, which is thus converted into a tunnel for the tendon of the flexor carpi radialis.
2. The medial *superficial slip* ***(volar carpal ligament)*** is also attached to the pisiform bone. The ulnar vessels and nerves pass deep to this slip (Plate 9.9).

Relations

Structures passing superficial to the flexor retinaculum

These are:
1. The palmar cutaneous branch of the median nerve (Fig. 9.14)
2. The tendon of the palmaris longus
3. The palmar cutaneous branch of the ulnar nerve
4. The ulnar vessels
5. The ulnar nerve.

Structures passing deep to the flexor retinaculum

These are:
1. The median nerve (Fig. 9.14)
2. Four tendons of the flexor digitorum superficialis
3. Four tendons of the flexor digitorum profundus
4. The tendon of the flexor pollicis longus
5. The ulnar bursa
6. The radial bursa
7. The tendon of the flexor carpi radialis lies between the retinaculum and its deep slip in the groove on the trapezium (Fig. 9.15).

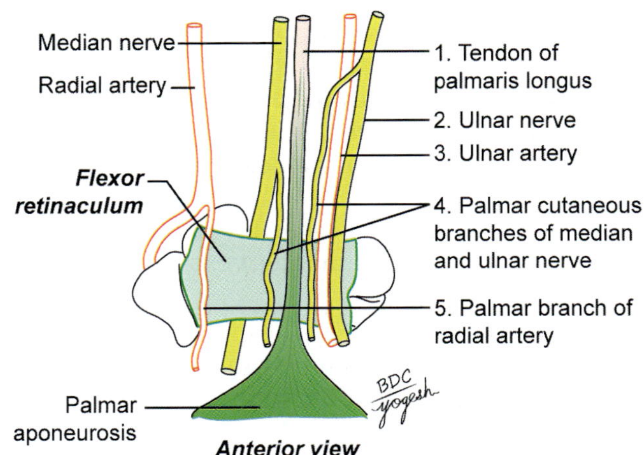

Fig. 9.14: Superficial relations of flexor retinaculum

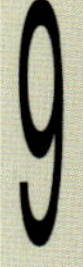

Plate 9.8: Flexor retinaculum and its superficial relations

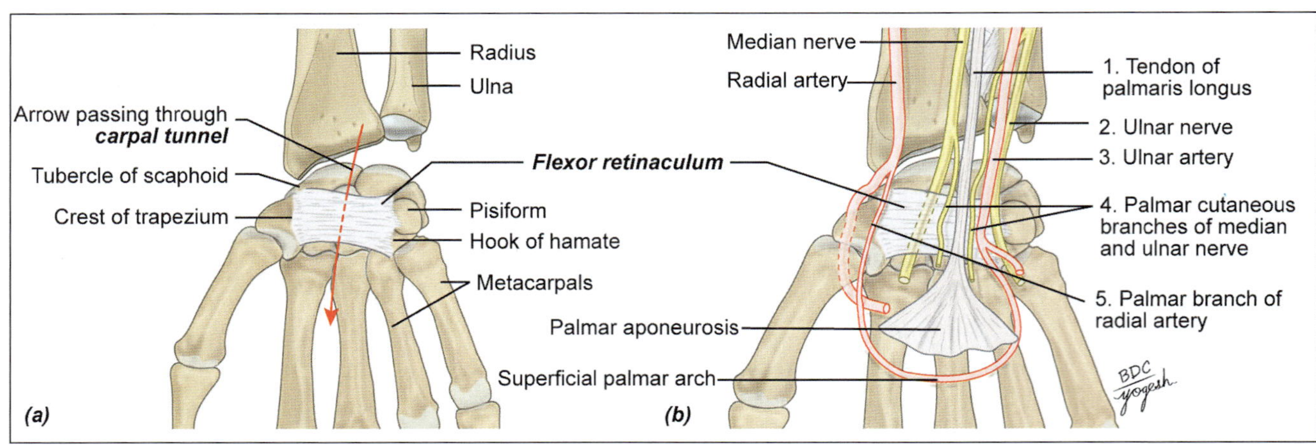

Plate 9.9: Carpal tunnel and structures passing through it

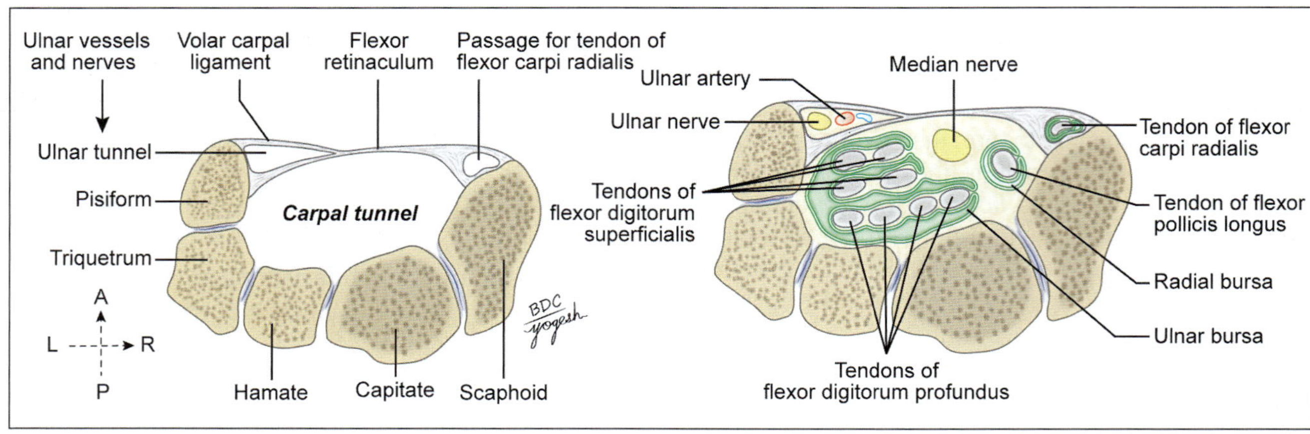

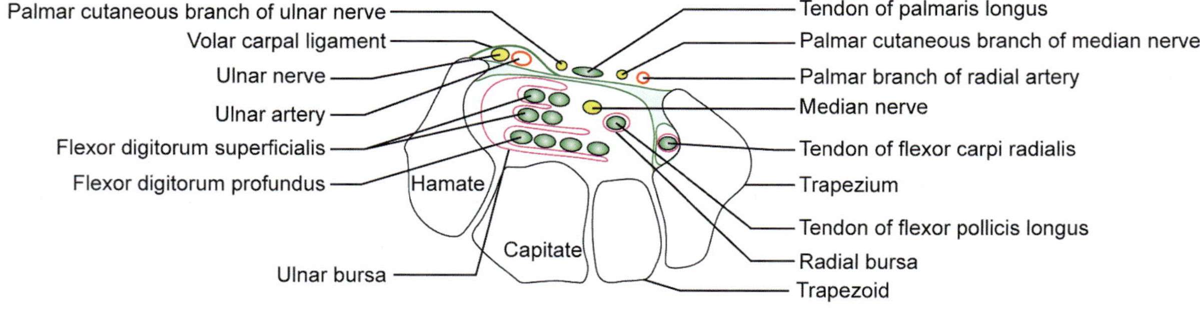

Fig. 9.15: Relations of flexor retinaculum (cross-section)

Palmar Aponeurosis

This term is often used for the entire deep fascia of the palm (Fig. 9.16). However, it is better to restrict this term to the central part of the deep fascia of the palm, which covers the superficial palmar arch, the long flexor tendons, the terminal part of the median nerve and the superficial branch of the ulnar nerve.

Features

Palmar aponeurosis is triangular in shape. It has apex, base and medial and lateral margins/borders.

1. The ***apex***, which is proximal, blends with the flexor retinaculum and is continuous with the tendon of the palmaris longus.
2. The ***base*** is directed distally. It divides into superficial and deep strata, superficial is attached to dermis. Deep strata divides into four slips opposite the heads of the metacarpals of the medial four digits. Each slip divides into two parts, which are continuous with the fibrous flexor sheaths. Extensions pass to the deep transverse metacarpal ligament, the capsule of the metacarpophalangeal joints and the sides of the base of the proximal phalanx. The digital vessels and nerves, and the tendons of the lumbricals emerge through the intervals between the slips.
3. From the ***lateral*** and ***medial margins*** of the palmar aponeurosis, the lateral and medial *palmar septa* pass backwards and divide the palm into compartments (Fig. 9.16).

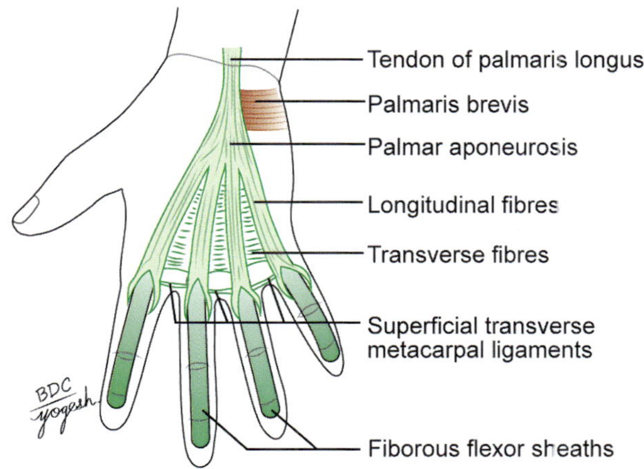

Fig. 9.16: The deep fascia of the hand forming the palmar aponeurosis and fibrous flexor sheaths

Functions

Palmar aponeurosis fixes the skin of the palm and thus improves the grip. It also protects the underlying tendons, vessels and nerves.

CLINICAL ANATOMY

Dupuytren's contracture: This condition is due to inflammation involving the ulnar side of the palmar aponeurosis. There is thickening and contraction of the aponeurosis. As a result, the proximal phalanx and later the middle phalanx become flexed and cannot be straightened. The terminal phalanx remains unaffected. The ring finger is most commonly involved (Fig. 9.17).

Fibrous Flexor Sheaths of the Fingers

The fibrous flexor sheaths are made up of the deep fascia of the fingers. The fascia is thick and arched.

It is attached to the sides of the phalanges and across the base of the distal phalanx. Proximally, it is continuous with a slip of the palmar aponeurosis. In this way, a blind osseofascial tunnel is formed, which contains the long flexor tendons enclosed in the digital synovial sheath (Plate 9.10).

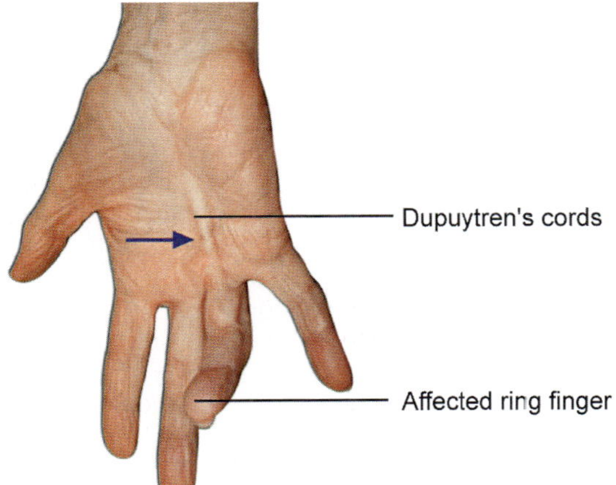

Fig. 9.17: Dupuytren's contracture

Plate 9.10: Fibrous flexor sheath of middle finger and its contents

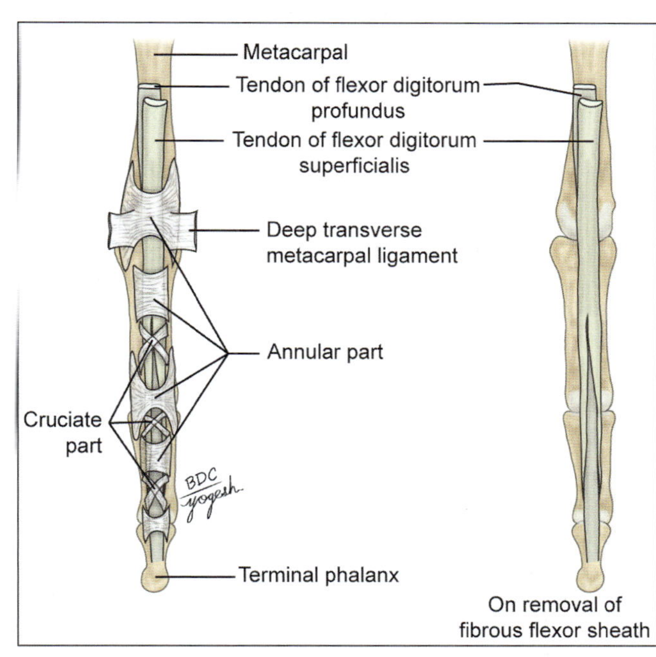

Functions

The fibrous sheath is thick opposite the phalanges and thin opposite the joints to permit flexion. The sheath holds the tendons in position during flexion of the digits.

Competency:
AN12.5 Identify and describe small muscles of hand. Also describe movements of thumb and muscles involved.

INTRINSIC MUSCLES OF HAND

Features

The intrinsic muscles of the hand serve the function of adjusting the hand during gripping and also for carrying out fine, skilled movements. Their attachments, nerve supply and actions are given in Tables 9.5 and 9.6.

There are 20 muscles in the hand. These are (Plates 9.11 to 9.14, Figs 9.18 to 9.20, Flowchart 9.5):

A. i. *Three muscles of thenar eminence* (Plate 9.11)
   1. Abductor pollicis brevis
   2. Flexor pollicis brevis
   3. Opponens pollicis

   ii. *One adductor of thumb:* Adductor pollicis (Plate 9.12).

B. Four hypothenar muscles (Plate 9.11, Fig. 9.16)
   1. Palmaris brevis (Fig. 9.16)
   2. Abductor digiti minimi
   3. Flexor digiti minimi
   4. Opponens digiti minimi

   Muscles (2) to (4) are muscles of hypothenar eminence.

C. Four lumbricals (Plate 9.13, Fig. 9.20)

D. Four palmar interossei (Plate 9.14)

E. Four dorsal interossei (Plate 9.14)

These muscles are described in Tables 9.5 and 9.6.

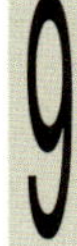

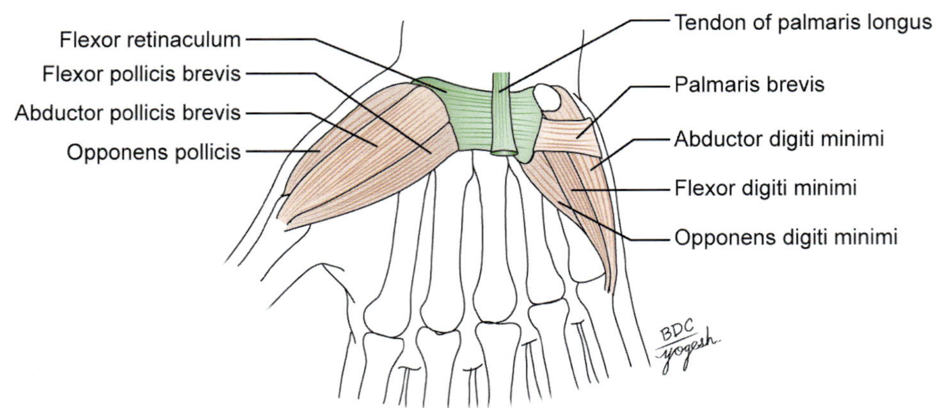

Fig. 9.18: Thenar and hypothenar muscles

TABLE 9.5: Origin and insertion of small muscles of the hand

Name	*Origin*	*Insertion*
Muscles of thenar eminence		
Abductor pollicis brevis	Tubercle of scaphoid Crest of trapezium Flexor retinaculum	Lateral side of base of proximal phalanx of thumb
Flexor pollicis brevis	Crest of trapezium Capitate bones Flexor retinaculum	Lateral side of base of proximal phalanx of thumb
Opponens pollicis	Crest of trapezium Flexor retinaculum	Lateral half of palmar surface of the shaft of metacarpal bone of thumb
Adductor of thumb		
Adductor pollicis	*Oblique head*: Capitate bone and bases of 2nd–3rd metacarpals *Transverse head*: Shaft of 3rd metacarpal	Medial side of base of proximal phalanx of thumb
Muscle of medial side of palm		
Palmaris brevis	Flexor retinaculum	Skin of palm on medial side
Muscles of hypothenar eminence		
Abductor digiti minimi	Pisiform bone	Medial side of base of proximal phalanx of little finger
Flexor digiti minimi	Hook of hamate Flexor retinaculum	Medial side of base of proximal phalanx of little finger
Opponens digiti minimi	Hook of hamate Flexor retinaculum	Medial border of 5th metacarpal bone
Lumbricals		
Lumbricals (4) Arise from 4 tendons of flexor digitorum profundus	1st: Lateral side of tendon of flexor digitorum profundus of index finger 2nd: Lateral side of same tendon of middle finger 3rd: Adjacent sides of same tendons of middle and ring fingers 4th: Adjacent sides of same tendons of ring and little fingers	Tendons cross the radial side of metacarpophalangeal joints and are inserted via *dorsal digital expansion* into dorsum of bases of distal phalanges of corresponding digits
Palmar interossei		
Palmar (4)	1st: Medial side of base of 1st metacarpal (MC) 2nd: Medial side of shaft of 2nd MC 3rd: Lateral side of shaft of 4th MC 4th: Lateral side of shaft of 5th MC	Medial side of base of proximal phalanx of thumb or 1st digit via *dorsal digital expansion* into dorsum of bases of distal phalanges of corresponding digits
Dorsal interossei		
Dorsal (4)	1st: Adjacent sides of shafts of 1st and 2nd MC 2nd: Adjacent sides of shafts of 2nd and 3rd MC 3rd: Adjacent sides of shafts of 3rd and 4th MC 4th: Adjacent sides of shafts of 4th and 5th MC	Via *dorsal digital expansion* into dorsum of bases of distal phalanges of corresponding digits

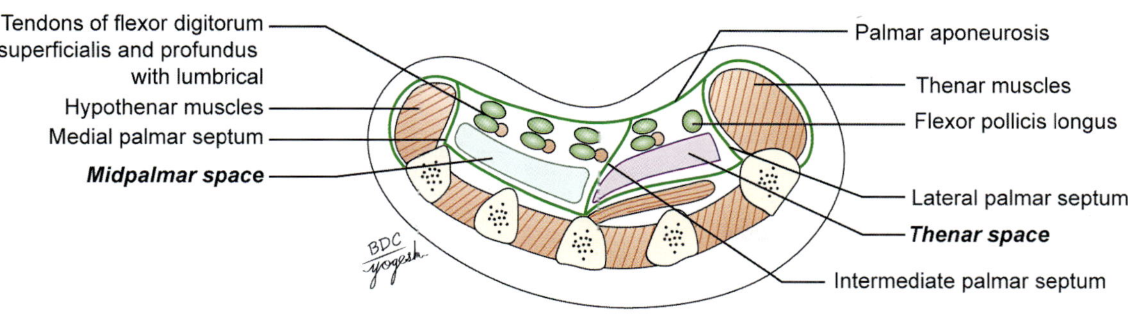

Fig. 9.19: Cross-section of hand (superior view)

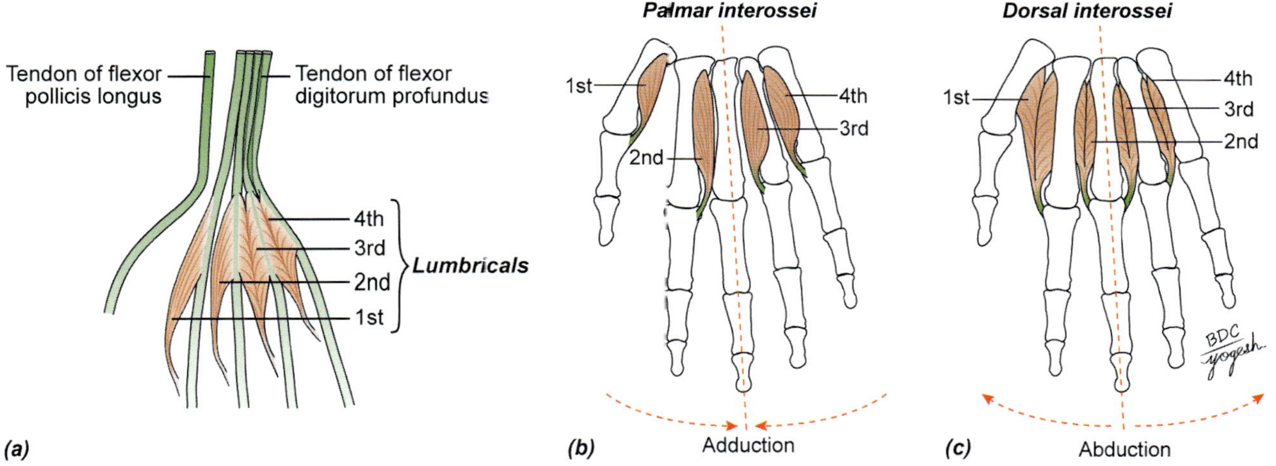

Figs 9.20a to c: Lumbricals and interossei muscles

TABLE 9.6: Nerve supply and actions of small muscles of the hand

Muscle	*Nerve supply*	*Actions*
Muscles of thenar eminence		
Abductor pollicis brevis	Median nerve	Abduction of thumb
Flexor pollicis brevis	Median nerve	Flexes metacarpophalangeal joint of thumb
Opponens pollicis	Median nerve	Opposes thumb towards the fingers (pulls thumb medially and forward across palm)
Adductor of thumb		
Adductor pollicis	Deep branch of ulnar nerve, which ends in this muscle	Adduction of thumb
Muscle of medial side of palm		
Palmaris brevis	Superficial branch of ulnar nerve	Wrinkles skin to improve grip of palm
Muscles of hypothenar eminence		
Abductor digiti minimi	Deep branch of ulnar nerve	Abducts little finger
Flexor digiti minimi	Deep branch of ulnar nerve	Flexes little finger
Opponens digiti minimi	Deep branch of ulnar nerve	Pulls fifth metacarpal forward as in cupping the palm
Lumbricals		
Lumbricals (4)	1st and 2nd: Median nerve 3rd and 4th: Deep branch of ulnar nerve	Flex metacarpophalangeal joints extend interphalangeal joints of 2nd–5th digits (Fig. 9.21)
Palmar interossei		
Palmar (4)	Deep branch of ulnar nerve	Palmar interossei adduct fingers towards centre of third digit or middle finger (Fig. 9.22)
Dorsal interossei		
Dorsal (4)	Deep branch of ulnar nerve	Dorsal interossei abduct fingers from centre of 3rd digit. Both palmar and dorsal interossei flex the metacarpophalangeal joints and extend the interphalangeal joints (Fig. 9.22)

Plate 9.11: Thenar muscles and hypothenar muscles

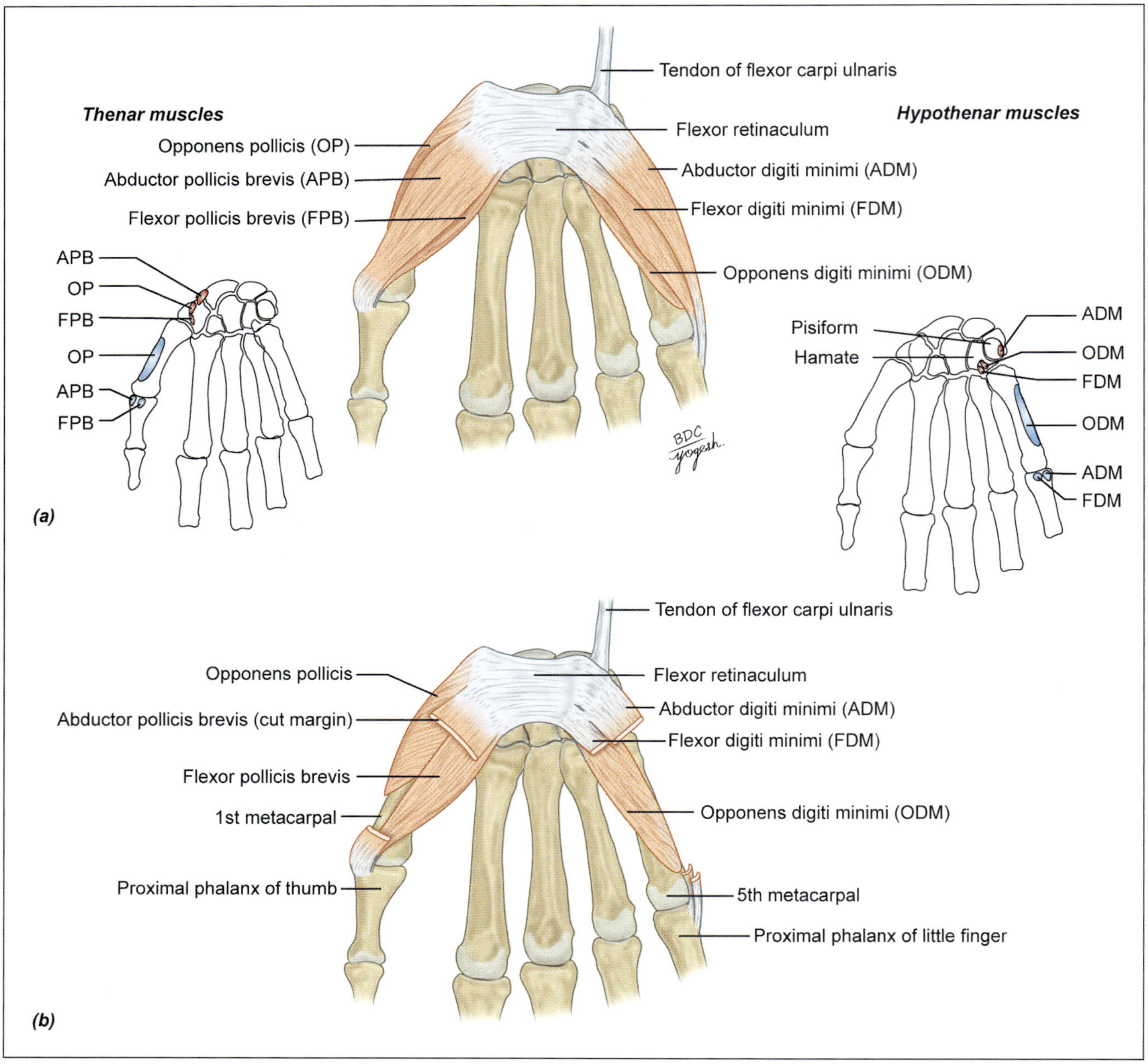

Plate 9.12: Adductor pollicis muscle

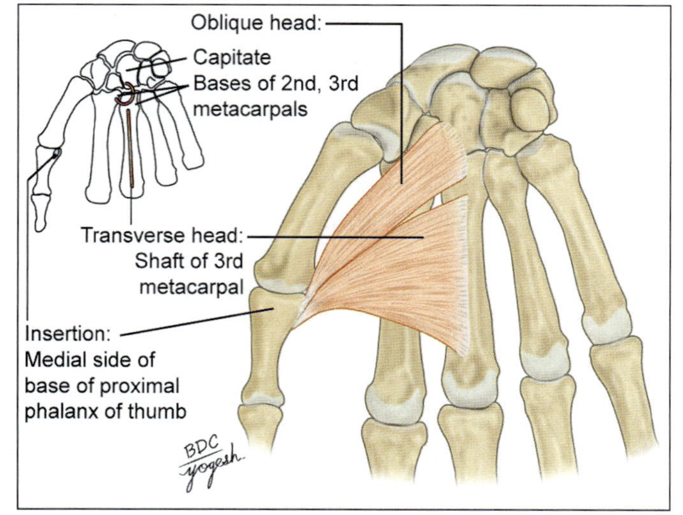

Actions of Thenar Muscles

In studying the actions of the thenar muscles, it must be remembered that the movements of the thumb take place in planes at right angles to those of the other digits because the thumb (1st metacarpal) is rotated medially through 90° (Fig. 9.23). Flexion and extension of the thumb take place in the plane of the palm, while abduction and adduction occur at right angles to the plane of palm.

Movement of the thumb across the palm to touch the other digits is known as 'opposition'. This movement is a combination of flexion and medial rotation.

Actions of Dorsal Interossei

All dorsal interossei cause abduction of the digits away from the line of the middle finger. This movement occurs in the plane of palm (Fig. 9.20) in contrast to the movement of thumb, where abduction occurs at

Plate 9.13: Lumbrical muscles and long flexor tendons of hand

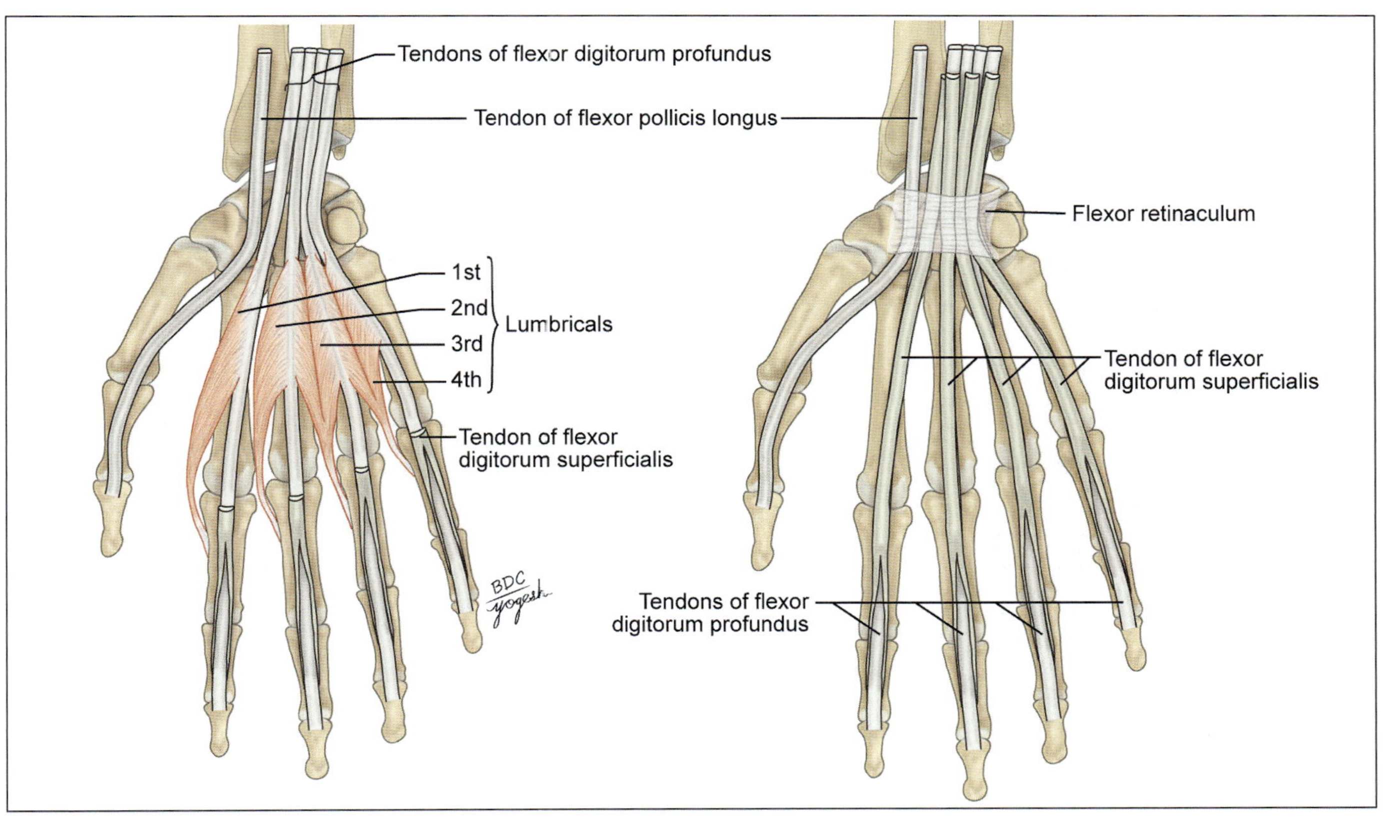

Plate 9.14: Palmar and dorsal interossei muscles of hand

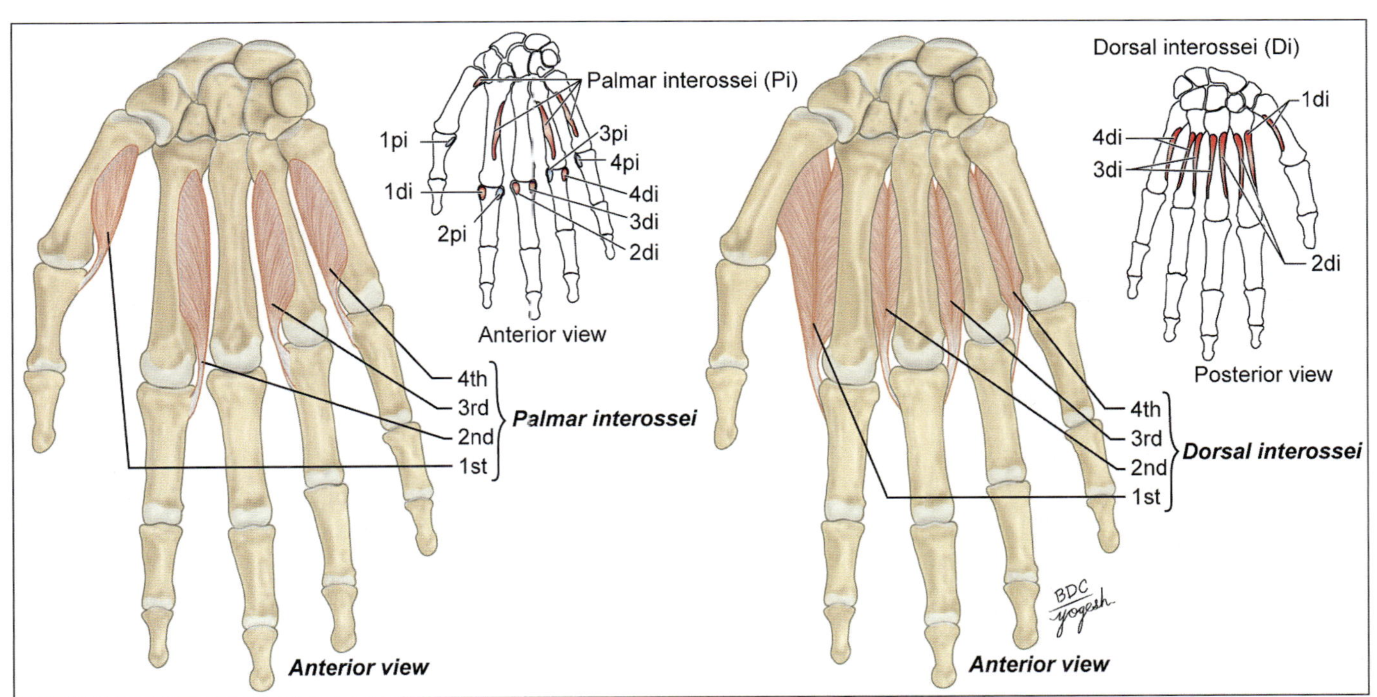

right angles to the plane of palm (Fig. 9.20). Note that movement of the middle finger to either the medial or lateral side constitutes abduction. Also note that the 1st and 5th digits do not require dorsal interossei as they have their own abductors.

Testing of Some Intrinsic Muscles

1. ***Pen/pencil test*** *for abductor pollicis brevis:* Lay the hand flat on a table with the palm directed upwards. Ask the patient to touch with his thumb a pen/pencil held in front of the palm (Fig. 9.24).

Flowchart 9.5: Muscles of hand

Muscle	Origin	Insertion	Actions
Abductor pollicis brevis	Flexor retinaculum, tubercle of scaphoid, crest of trapezium	Base of proximal phalanx of thumb	Abduction of thumb
Flexor pollicis brevis	Superficial head: Flexor retinaculum Deep head: Crest of trapezium, capitate bone	Base of proximal phalanx of thumb	Flexion of thumb
Opponens pollicis	Flexor retinaculum, crest of trapezium	Lateral side of palmar surface of shaft of 1st metacarpal	Opposition of thumb (pulls thumb medially and forward)
Abductor digiti minimi	Pisiform	Base of proximal phalanx of little finger	Abduction of little finger
Flexor digiti minimi	Flexor retinaculum Hook of hamate	Base of proximal phalanx of little finger	Flexion of little finger
Opponens digiti minimi	Flexor retinaculum Hook of hamate	Medial surface of shaft of 5th metacarpal bone	Opposition of tip of the little finger and thumb
Lumbricals 4 small, worm-like muscles	From tendons of FDP 1st and 2nd - Unipennate 3rd and 4th - Bipennate	Crosses lateral to MP joint to insert on dorsal digital expansion	Flexion at MP joint Extension at proximal and distal IP joints
Palmar interossei 1 to 4 from lateral to medial Unipennate	Sides of metacarpals (Unipennate) 1st & 2nd: Medial side 3rd & 4th: Lateral side	Dorsal digital expansion 1st & 2nd: Medial side 3rd & 4th: Lateral side	Adduction of fingers
Dorsal interossei 1 to 4 from lateral to medial	Adjacent sides of metacarpals (Bipennate)	Dorsal digital expansion 1st and 2nd: Lateral side 3rd and 4th: Medial side	Abduction of fingers

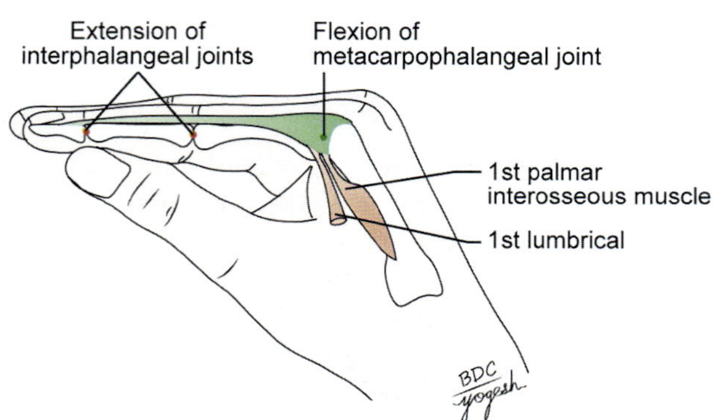

Fig. 9.21: Actions of lumbricals and interossei: lumbrical–interossei complex

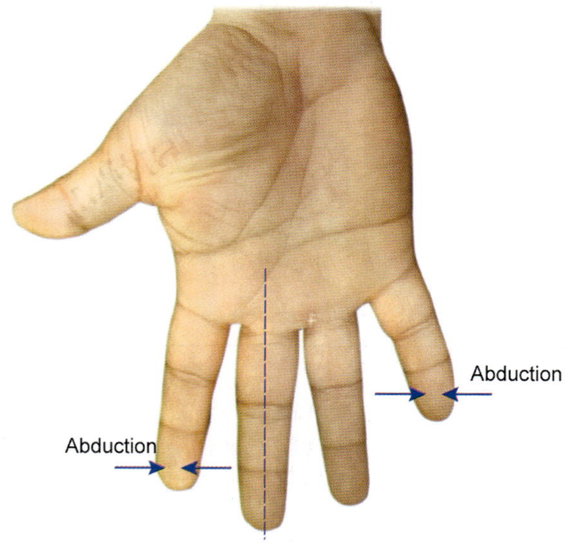

Fig. 9.22: The planes of movements of the fingers

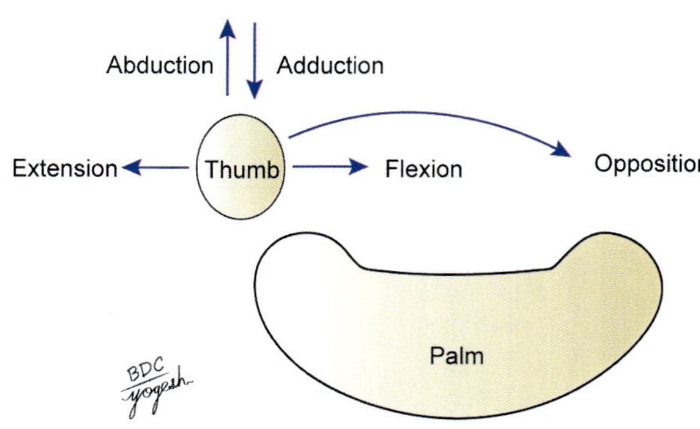

Fig. 9.23: The planes of movements of the thumb

2. *Test for opponens pollicis:* Ask the patient to touch the proximal phalanx of 2nd to 5th digits with the tip of thumb.
3. ***Interossei***
   a. ***Dorsal interossei*** are tested by asking the subject to spread out the fingers against resistance. As index finger is abducted, one feels 1st dorsal interosseous (Fig. 9.25).
   b. ***Palmar interossei*** and *adductor pollicis* are tested by placing a piece of paper between the fingers (Fig. 9.26), between thumb and index finger, and seeing how firmly it can be held (Fig. 9.27).

[*Mnemonic:* ***Interossei muscles: Actions of dorsal vs. palmar in hand "PAd and DAb":*** The **P**almar **Ad**duct and the **D**orsal **Ab**duct. Use your hand to dab with a pad.]

4. ***Froment's sign*** (**book test**) for the *adductor pollicis* muscle: When the patient is asked to grasp a book firmly between the thumb and other fingers of both hands, the terminal phalanx of the thumb on the

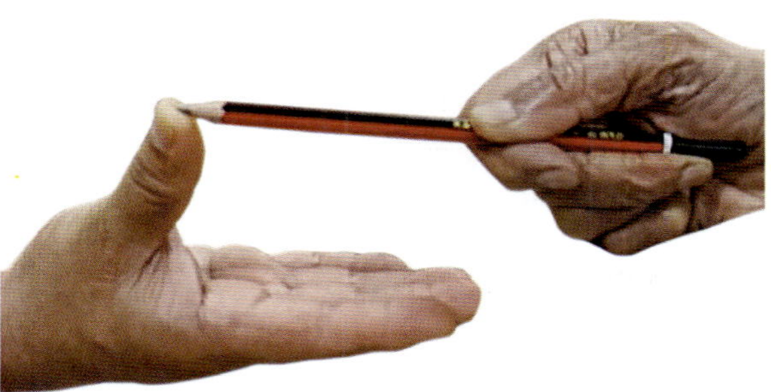

Fig. 9.24: Pen test for abductor pollicis brevis (median nerve)

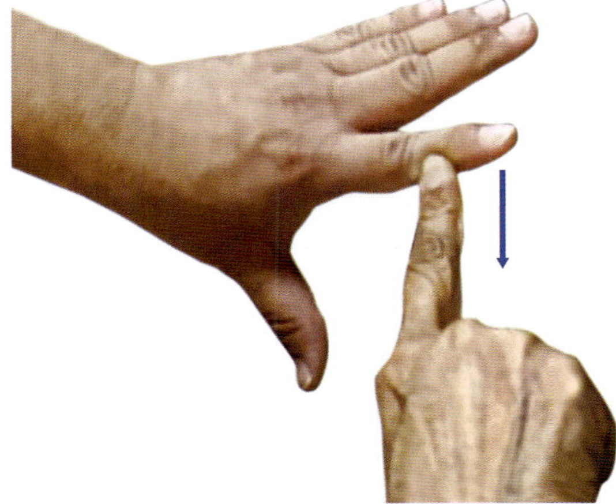

Fig. 9.25: Testing first dorsal interosseous muscle of hand (median nerve)

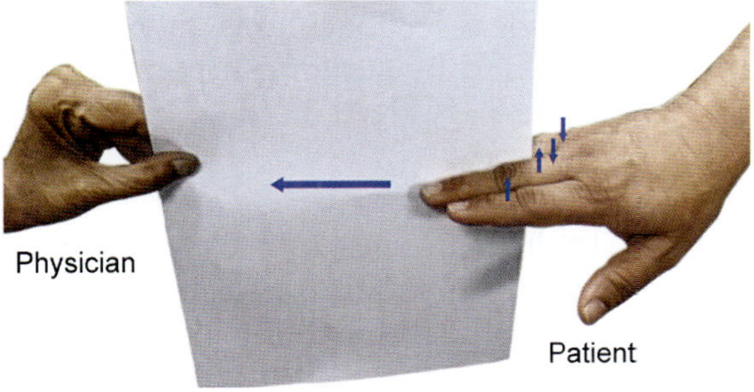

Fig. 9.26: Test for palmar interossei (ulnar nerve)

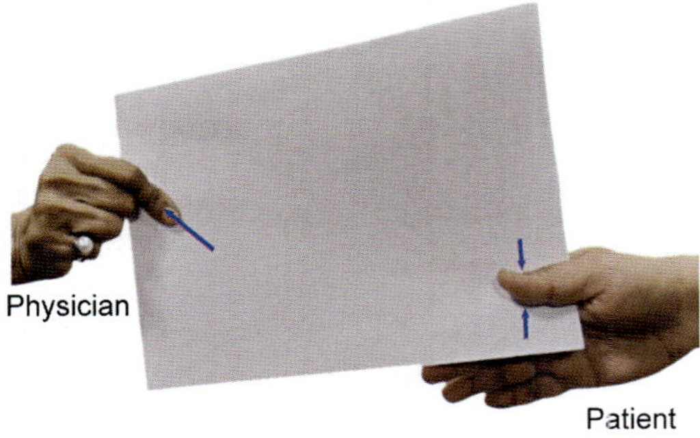

Fig. 9.27: Testing adductor pollicis (ulnar nerve)

paralysed side becomes flexed at the interphalangeal joint (by the flexor pollicis longus, which is supplied by the median nerve) (Fig. 9.28).

5. The *lumbricals* and *interossei* are tested by asking the subject to flex the fingers at the metacarpophalangeal joints against resistance.

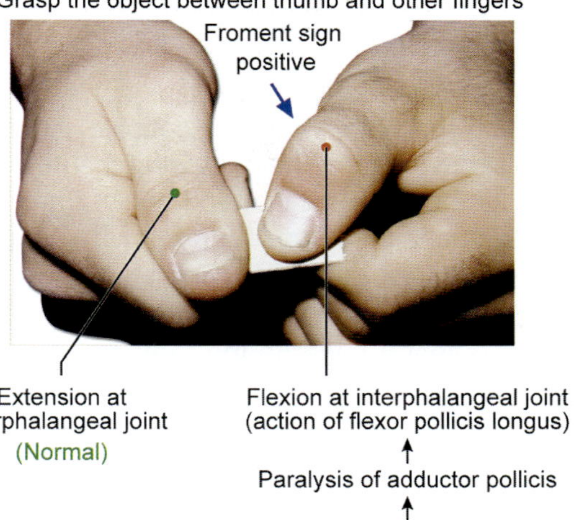

Fig. 9.28: Froment's test (ulnar nerve)

DISSECTION

Clean the thenar and hypothenar muscles. Carefully preserve the median nerve and superficial and deep branches of ulnar nerve, which supply these muscles.

Abductor pollicis brevis is the lateral muscle; flexor pollicis brevis is the medial one. Both these form the superficial lamina. The deeper lamina is constituted by opponens pollicis (Plate 9.11).

Cut through the abductor pollicis brevis and flexor pollicis brevis to expose the opponens pollicis. These three muscles constitute the muscles of thenar eminence.

Incise flexor pollicis brevis in its centre and reflect its two parts. This will reveal the tendon of flexor pollicis longus and adductor pollicis on a deeper plane. The three muscles of thenar eminence are supplied by thick recurrent branch of median nerve (Fig. 9.12).

On the medial side of hand, identify thin palmaris brevis muscle in the superficial fascia. It receives a twig from the superficial branch of ulnar nerve.

Hypothenar eminence is comprised by abductor digiti minimi medially, flexor digiti minimi just lateral to it. Deep to both these lies opponens digiti minimi. Identify these three muscles and trace their nerve supply from deep branch of ulnar nerve.

Between the two eminences of the palm, deep to palmar aponeurosis, identify the superficial palmar arch formed mainly by superficial branch of ulnar and superficial palmar branch of radial artery. Identify its common and proper digital branches.

Clean, dissect and preserve the branches of the median nerve and superficial division of ulnar nerve in the palm lying between the superficial palmar arch and long flexor tendons (Fig. 9.15).

Lying on a deeper plane are the tendons of flexor digitorum superficialis muscle. Dissect the peculiar mode of its insertion in relation to that of tendon of flexor digitorum profundus.

Cut through the tendons of flexor digitorum superficialis 5 cm above the wrist. Divide both ends of superficial

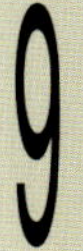

palmar arch. Reflect them distally towards the metacarpophalangeal joints.

Identify four tendons of flexor digitorum profundus diverging in the palm with four delicate muscles, the lumbricals, arising from them. Dissect the nerve supply to these lumbricals. The first and second are supplied from median and third and fourth from the deep branch of ulnar nerve (*see* Plate 9.15).

Divide the flexor digitorum profundus 5 cm above the wrist and reflect it towards the metacarpophalangeal joints. Trace one of its tendons to its insertion into the base of distal phalanx of one finger.

Competency:

AN12.7 Identify and describe course and branches of important blood vessels and nerves in hand.

ARTERIES OF HAND

Features

Arteries of the hand are the terminal parts of the ulnar and radial arteries. Branches of these arteries unite and form anastomotic channels called the superficial and deep palmar arches (Plate 9.15, Plate 9.6, Flowchart 9.6).

ULNAR ARTERY

It enters the palm by passing superficial to the flexor retinaculum but deep to the volar carpal ligament (Plate 9.15, Fig. 9.29). It ends by dividing into the *superficial palmar branch*, which is the main continuation of the artery, and the *deep palmar branch*. These branches take part in the formation of the superficial palmar arch and deep palmar arch, respectively.

The deep branch of the ulnar artery arises in front of the flexor retinaculum immediately beyond the pisiform bone. Soon, it passes between the flexor and abductor digiti minimi to join and complete the *deep palmar arch*.

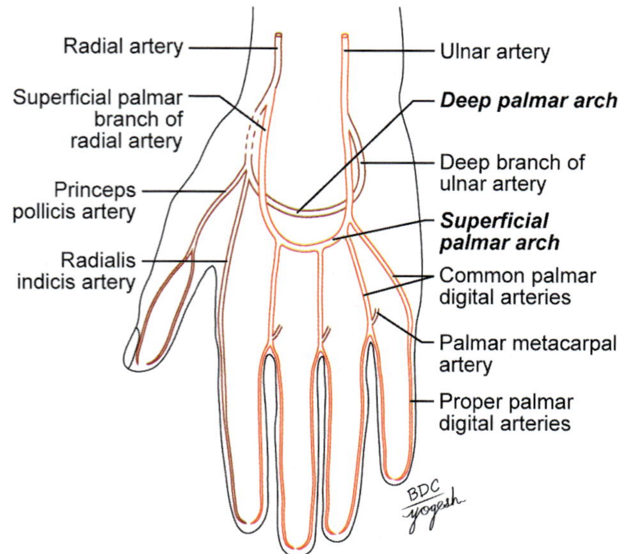

Fig. 9.29: The superficial and deep palmar arches

Flowchart 9.6: Palmar arterial arches

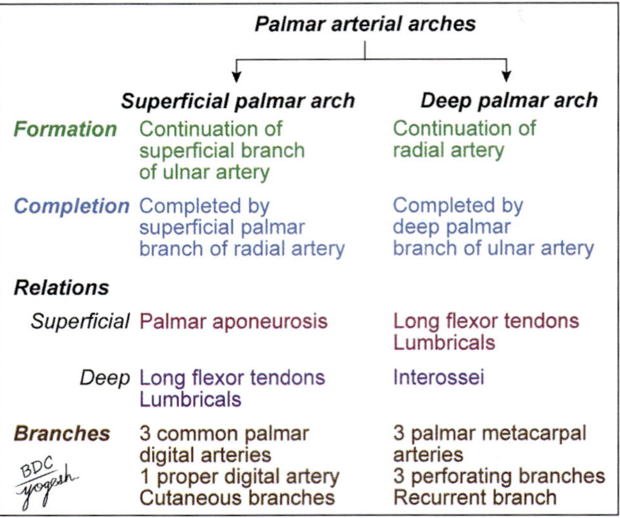

Palmar arterial arches

	Superficial palmar arch	***Deep palmar arch***
Formation	Continuation of superficial branch of ulnar artery	Continuation of radial artery
Completion	Completed by superficial palmar branch of radial artery	Completed by deep palmar branch of ulnar artery
Relations		
Superficial	Palmar aponeurosis	Long flexor tendons Lumbricals
Deep	Long flexor tendons Lumbricals	Interossei
Branches	3 common palmar digital arteries 1 proper digital artery Cutaneous branches	3 palmar metacarpal arteries 3 perforating branches Recurrent branch

SUPERFICIAL PALMAR ARCH

The arch represents an important anastomosis between the ulnar and radial arteries. The convexity of the arch is directed towards the fingers, and its most distal point is situated at the level of the distal border of the fully extended thumb.

Formation

The superficial palmar arch is formed as the direct continuation of the superficial palmar branch ulnar artery beyond the flexor retinaculum. On the lateral side, the arch is completed by superficial palmar branch of radial artery (Plate 9.15, Fig. 9.29).

Relations

The superficial palmar arch lies deep to the palmaris brevis and the palmar aponeurosis. It crosses the palm over the flexor digiti minimi, the flexor tendons of the fingers, the lumbricals and the digital branches of the median nerve.

Branches

Superficial palmar arch gives off ***three common digital branches*** and ***one proper digital branch***, which supply the medial 3½ digits. The lateral three common digital branches are joined by the corresponding palmar metacarpal arteries from the deep palmar arch. It also gives ***cutaneous branches*** to the skin of palm.

CLINICAL ANATOMY

The radial artery is used for feeling the (arterial) pulse at the wrist. The pulsations can be felt well in this situation because of the presence of the flat radius with pronator quadratus muscle behind the artery (Fig. 9.10).

RADIAL ARTERY

Course

Radial artery runs obliquely downwards and backwards from the site of 'radial pulse' to reach the anatomical

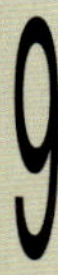

Plate 9.15: Superficial and deep palmar arch

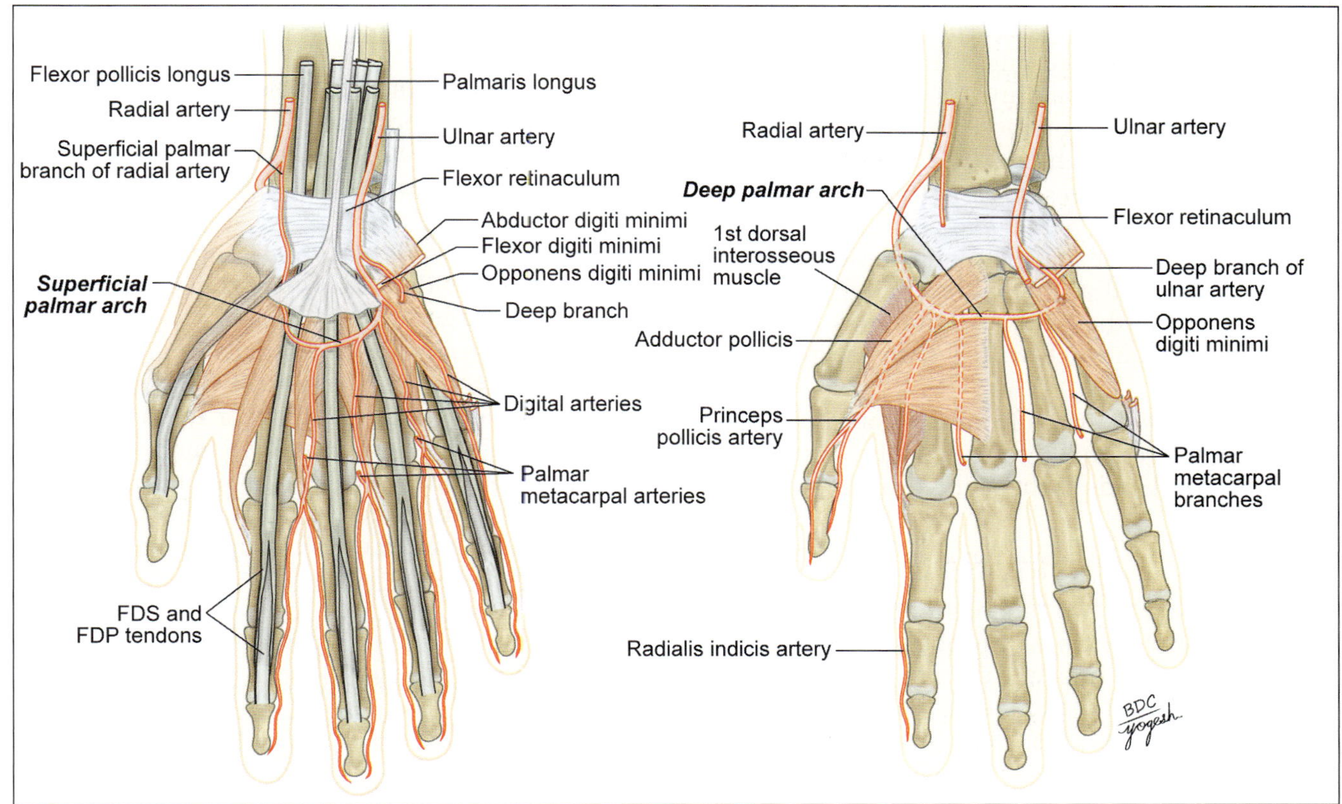

snuffbox. From there, it passes forwards to reach 1st interosseous space and then into the palm.

Relations

1. It leaves the forearm by winding backwards a around the wrist.
2. It passes through the "anatomical snuffbox" where it lies deep to the tendons of the abductor pollicis longus, the extensor pollicis brevis and the extensor pollicis longus and superficial to the lateral ligament of the wrist joint. It is also crossed by the digital branches of the radial nerve. The artery is superficial to the lateral ligament of the wrist joint, the scaphoid and the trapezium
3. It reaches the proximal end of the 1st interosseous space and passes between the two heads of the 1st dorsal interosseous muscle to reach the palm.
4. In the palm, the radial artery runs medially. At first, it lies deep to the oblique head of the adductor pollicis and then passes between the two heads of this muscle to form *deep palmar arch* (Fig. 9.29).

Branches

Dorsum of hand: On the dorsum of the hand, the radial artery gives off:

1. A branch to the lateral side of the dorsum of the thumb.
2. ***First dorsal metacarpal artery:*** This artery arises just before the radial artery passes into the interval between the two heads of the first dorsal interosseous muscle. It at once divides into two branches for the adjacent sides of the thumb and the index finger.

Palm: In the palm (deep to the oblique head of the adductor pollicis), the radial artery gives off:

1. The ***princeps pollicis artery***, which divides at the base of the proximal phalanx into two branches for the palmar surface of the thumb (Fig. 9.29).
2. The ***radialis indicis artery*** descends between the first dorsal interosseous muscle and the transverse head of the adductor pollicis to supply the lateral side of the index finger.

DEEP PALMAR ARCH

Deep palmar arch provides a channel connecting the radial and ulnar arteries in the palm (another channel is the superficial palmar arch). It is situated deep to the long flexor tendons.

Formation

The deep palmar arch is formed mainly by the terminal part of the radial artery and is completed medially at the base of the 5th metacarpal bone by the deep palmar branch of the ulnar artery (Fig. 9.29).

Relations

The arch lies on the proximal parts of the shafts of the metacarpals and on the interossei, under cover of the oblique head of the adductor pollicis, the flexor tendons of the fingers and the lumbricals. The deep branch of the ulnar nerve lies within the concavity of the arch.

Branches

1. From its convexity, i.e. from its distal side, the arch gives off ***three palmar metacarpal arteries***, which run distally in the 2nd, 3rd and 4th spaces, supply the medial four metacarpals and terminate at the finger clefts by joining the common digital branches of the superficial palmar arch (Fig. 9.29).
2. Dorsally, the arch gives off ***three*** (proximal) ***perforating digital arteries,*** which pass through the medial three interosseous spaces to anastomose with the dorsal metacarpal arteries. The digital perforating arteries connect the palmar digital branches of the superficial palmar arch with the dorsal metacarpal arteries.
3. ***Recurrent branch*** arises from the concavity of the arch, passes proximally to supply the carpal bones and joints, and ends in the palmar carpal arch.

DISSECTION

Deep to the lateral two tendons of flexor digitorum profundus muscle, note an obliquely placed muscle extending from two origins, i.e. from the shaft of the third metacarpal bone and the bases of 2nd and 3rd metacarpal bones and adjacent carpal bones to the base of proximal phalanx of the thumb. This is *adductor pollicis* (Plate 9.12). Reflect the adductor pollicis muscle from its origin towards its insertion. Identify the deeply placed interossei muscles.

Identify the radial artery entering the palm between two heads of first dorsal interosseous muscle and then between two heads of adductor pollicis muscle turning medially to join the deep branch of ulnar artery to complete the deep palmar arch (Fig. 9.29). Identify the deep branch of ulnar nerve lying in its concavity. Carefully preserve it, including its multiple branches. Deep branch of ulnar nerve ends by supplying the adductor pollicis muscle. It may supply deep head of flexor pollicis brevis also.

Lastly, define four small palmar interossei and four relatively bigger dorsal interossei muscles (Plates 9.13 and 9.14).

NERVES OF HAND

ULNAR NERVE

Ulnar nerve is the main nerve of the hand (like the lateral plantar nerve in the foot).

The ulnar nerve is also known as the '***musician's nerve***' because it controls fine movements of the fingers.

Course

The ulnar nerve lies superficial to the flexor retinaculum, covered only by the superficial slip of the retinaculum (volar carpal ligament). It terminates by dividing into a superficial and a deep branch.

Superficial branch is cutaneous. The deep branch passes through the muscles of the hypothenar eminence to lie in the concavity of the deep palmar arch to end in the adductor pollicis (Fig. 9.15).

Relations

1. The ulnar nerve enters the palm by passing superficial to the flexor retinaculum, where it lies between the pisiform bone and the ulnar vessels. Here, the nerve divides into its superficial and deep terminal branches (Plate 9.16).
2. The ***superficial terminal branch*** supplies the palmaris brevis and divides into two digital branches for the medial 1½ fingers (Plate 9.16).
3. The ***deep terminal branch*** accompanies the deep branch of the ulnar artery. It passes backwards between the abductor and flexor digiti minimi, and then between the opponens digiti minimi and the fifth metacarpal bone, lying on the hook of the hamate. Finally, it turns laterally within the concavity of the deep palmar arch. It ends by supplying the adductor pollicis muscle.

Branches

Superficial Terminal Branch

1. *Muscular branch*: To palmaris brevis.
2. *Cutaneous branches*: Two palmar digital nerves supply the medial 1½ fingers with their nail beds (Fig. 9.21).

The *medial branch* supplies the medial side of the little finger.

The *lateral branch* is a *common palmar digital nerve*. It divides into two proper palmar digital nerves for the adjoining sides of the ring and little fingers. The common palmar digital nerve communicates with the median nerve (Figs 9.30 and 9.31).

Deep Terminal Branch

1. *Muscular branches*:
   a. At its origin, the deep branch supplies three muscles of hypothenar eminence (Plate 9.16).
   b. As the nerve crosses the palm, it supplies the medial two lumbricals and eight interossei.
   c. The deep branch terminates by supplying the adductor pollicis and occasionally the deep head of the flexor pollicis brevis.
2. An *articular branch* supplies the wrist joint.

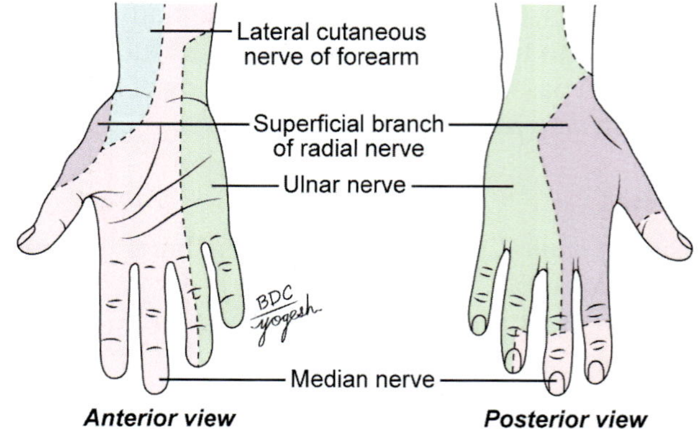

Fig. 9.30: Cutaneous innervation of palm and dorsum of hand

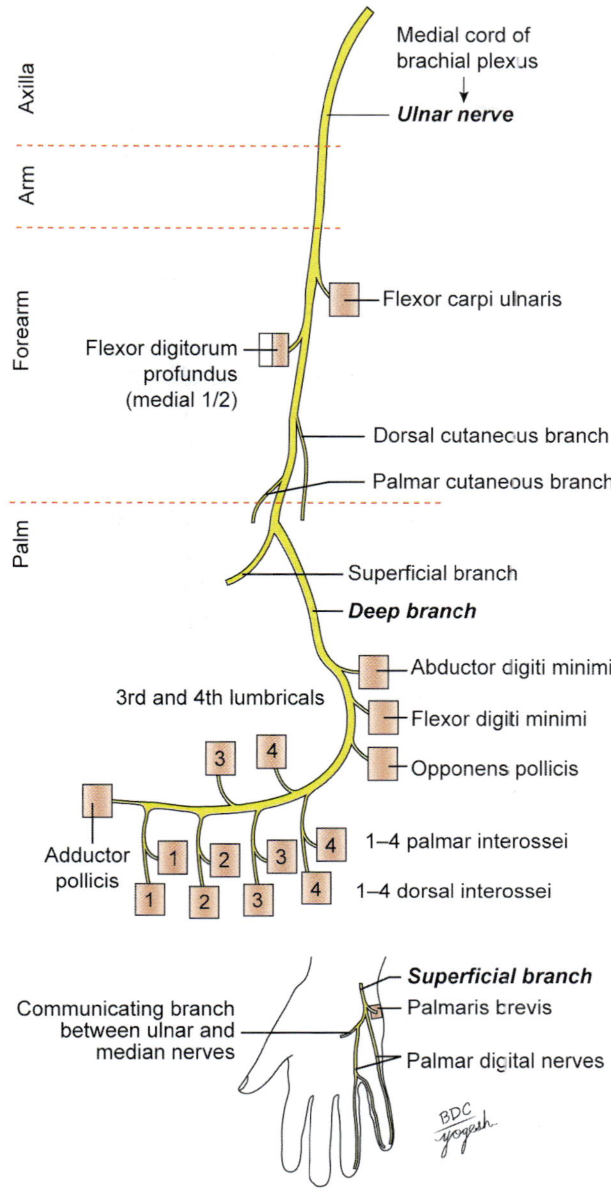

Fig. 9.31: Distribution of the branches of the ulnar nerve

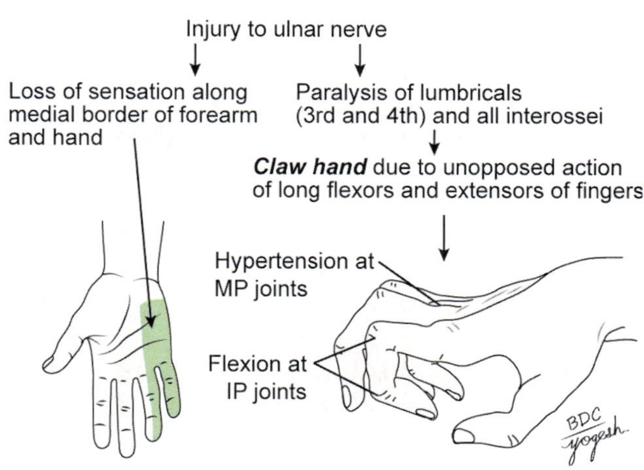

Fig. 9.32: Ulnar nerve injury (MP joint: Metacarpophalangeal joint, IP joint: Interphalangeal joint)

CLINICAL ANATOMY

Ulnar nerve injuries

- The ulnar nerve is commonly injured at the elbow, behind the medial epicondyle, or distal to elbow as it passes between two heads of flexor carpi ulnaris (cubital tunnel) or at the wrist in front of the flexor retinaculum.

Ulnar nerve injury at the elbow

- Flexor carpi ulnaris and the medial half of the flexor digitorum profundus get paralysed.
- Due to this paralysis, the medial border of the forearm becomes flattened. An attempt to produce flexion at the wrist results in abduction of the hand. The tendon of the flexor carpi ulnaris does not tighten on making a fist. Flexion of the terminal phalanges of the ring and little fingers is lost.
- The ulnar nerve controls fine movements of the fingers through its extensive motor distribution to the short muscles of the hand. There is ***ulnar claw hand*** as well (described below).

Ulnar nerve lesion at the wrist

- Produces '***ulnar claw hand' or 'Spinster claw deformity',*** which is characterised by the following signs:
  a. *Motor loss*: Hyperextension at the metacarpophalangeal joints and flexion at the interphalangeal joints, involving the ring and little fingers—more than the index and middle fingers (Fig. 9.32). The intermetacarpal spaces are hollowed out due to wasting of the interosseous muscles. Claw hand deformity is more obvious in wrist lesions as the profundus muscle is spared. This causes marked flexion of the terminal phalanges (***action of paradox***).
  b. *Sensory loss*: It is confined to the medial one-third of the palm and the palmar and dorsal surfaces of the medial 1½ fingers, including their nail beds (Figs 9.32).
  c. *Vasomotor changes:* The skin areas with sensory loss are warmer due to arteriolar dilatation; it is also dry due to the absence of sweating because of loss of sympathetic supply.
  d. *Trophic changes:* Long-standing cases of paralysis lead to dry and scaly skin. The nails crack easily with atrophy of the pulp of fingers.
  e. The patient is unable to spread out the fingers due to paralysis of the dorsal interossei. The power of adduction of the thumb and flexion of the ring and little fingers are lost. It should be noted that median nerve lesions are more disabling. In contrast, ulnar nerve lesions leave a relatively efficient hand.

MEDIAN NERVE

The median nerve is important because of its role in controlling the movements of the thumb, which are crucial in the mechanism of gripping by the hand (Plate 9.16).

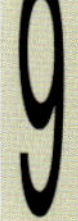

Plate 9.16: Median and ulnar nerves in palm

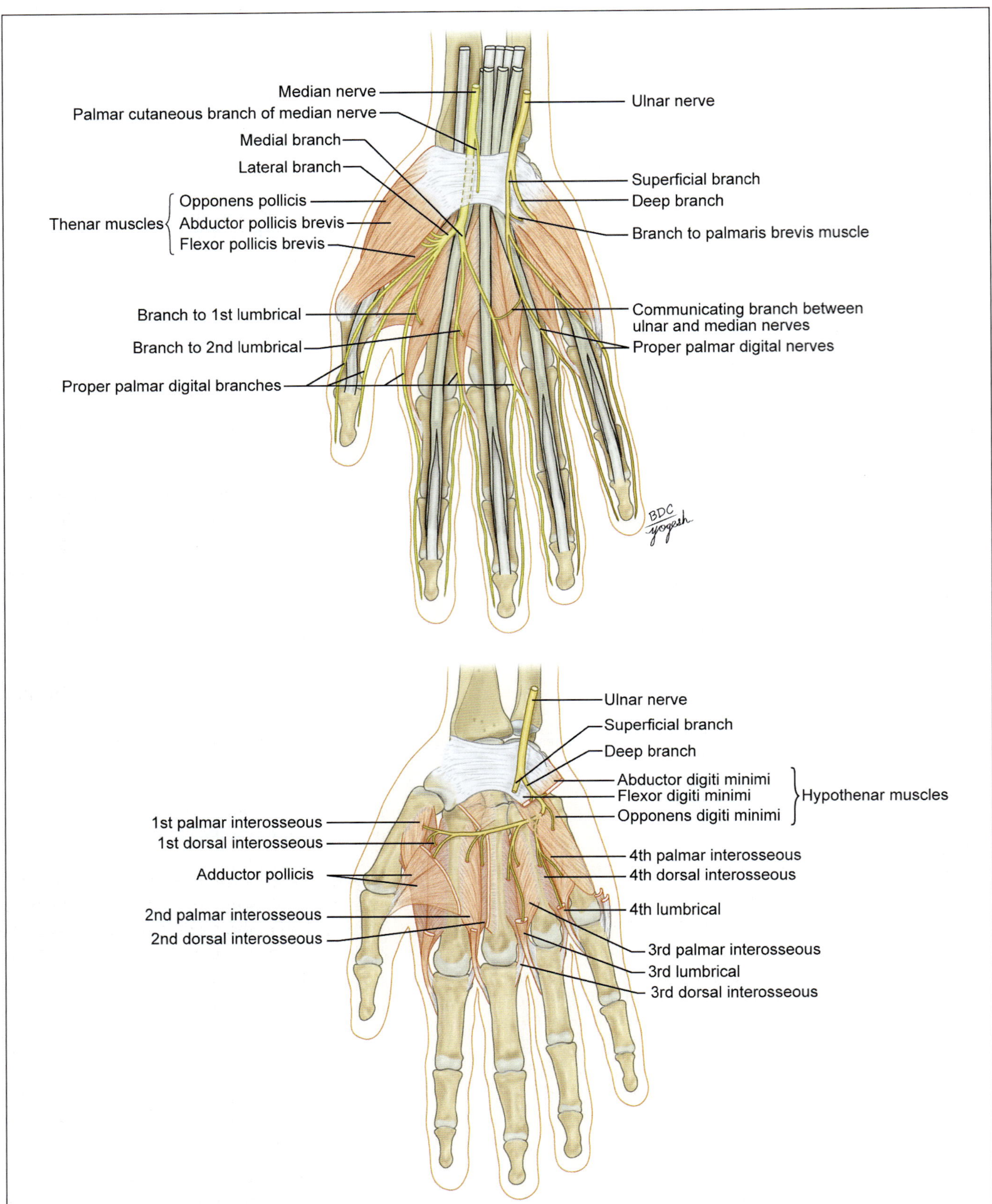

The median nerve controls coarse movements of the hand, as it supplies most of the long muscles of the front of the forearm. It is, therefore, called the ***labourer's nerve***. It is also called '***eye of the hand***' as it is sensory to most of the hand.

Course

Median nerve lies deep to flexor retinaculum in the carpal tunnel and enters the palm (Plate 9.16) and terminates by dividing into lateral and medial divisions.

Relations

1. The median nerve enters the palm by passing deep to the flexor retinaculum, where it lies in the narrow space of the carpal tunnel in front of the ulnar bursa, enclosing the flexor tendons. Immediately below the retinaculum, the nerve divides into lateral and medial divisions (Plate 9.16).
2. The ***lateral division*** gives off a muscular branch to the ***thenar muscles*** and three digital branches for the lateral 1½ digits, including the thumb. The muscular branch curls upwards around the distal border of the retinaculum and supplies the thenar muscles.

   Out of the three digital branches, two supply the thumb and one the lateral side of the index finger. The digital branch to the index finger also supplies the ***1st lumbrical*** (Fig. 9.33).
3. The medial division divides into two common digital branches for the second and third interdigital clefts, supplying the adjoining sides of the index, middle and ring fingers. The lateral common digital branch also supplies the ***2nd lumbrical***.

Branches

In the hand, the median nerve supplies:

a. Five muscles, namely the abductor pollicis brevis, the flexor pollicis brevis, the opponens pollicis and the 1st and 2nd lumbrical muscles.
b. Palmar skin over the lateral 3½ digits with their nail beds.

Competencies:
AN12.4 Explain anatomical basis of carpal tunnel syndrome.
AN12.8 Describe anatomical basis of claw hand.

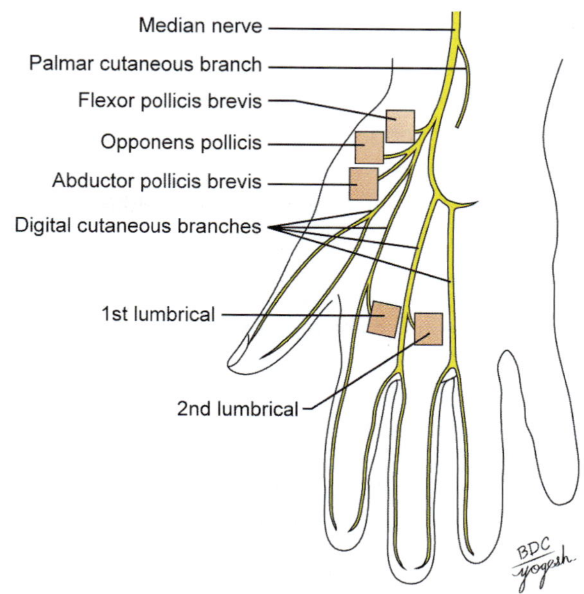

Fig. 9.33: Distribution of the median nerve in the hand

CLINICAL ANATOMY

Median nerve injuries above or at the level of the elbow

- When the median nerve is injured above the level of the elbow, as might happen in *supracondylar fracture of the humerus*, the following features are seen:
  1. The flexor pollicis longus and lateral half of flexor digitorum profundus are paralysed. The patient is unable to bend the terminal phalanx of the thumb and index finger when the proximal phalanx is held firmly by the clinician (to eliminate the action of the short flexors) (Fig. 9.34). Similarly, the terminal phalanx of the middle finger can be tested.
  2. The forearm is kept in a supine position due to paralysis of the pronators.
  3. The hand is adducted due to paralysis of the flexor carpi radialis, and flexion at the wrist is weak.
  4. Flexion at the interphalangeal joints of the index and middle fingers is lost so that the index and the middle (to a lesser extent) fingers tend to remain straight while making a fist. This is called ***pointing index finger***, occurs due to paralysis of long flexors of the digit (Fig. 9.35). When both index and middle fingers remain straight, the condition is called ***hand of benediction deformity***.
  5. ***Ape thumb*** or monkey-like thumb deformity is present due to paralysis of the thenar muscles (Fig. 9.36).
  6. The area of sensory loss corresponds to its distribution in the hand.
  7. Vasomotor and trophic changes: The skin on lateral 3½ digits is warm, dry and scaly. The nails get cracked easily (Fig. 9.37).
  8. ***Pen test*** done for abductor pollicis brevis (Fig. 9.24)

Carpal tunnel syndrome (CTS)

- Involvement of the median nerve in carpal tunnel at wrist has become a very common entity (Figs 9.15 and 9.38).
  1. This syndrome consists of motor, sensory, vasomotor and trophic symptoms in the hand caused by compression of the median nerve in the carpal tunnel. Examination reveals wasting of thenar eminence (ape-like hand), hypoaesthesia to light touch on the palmar aspect of lateral 3½ digits. However, the skin over the thenar eminence is *not affected* as the branch of median nerve supplying it arises in the forearm (Fig. 9.30).
  2. ***Froment's sign/book holding test***: The patient is unable to hold the book with thumbs and other fingers (Fig. 9.28).
  3. ***Paper holding test***: The patient is unable to hold paper between thumb and fingers. Both these tests are positive because of paralysis of thenar muscles.
  4. *Motor changes:* ***Ape thumb***/monkey-like thumb deformity (Fig. 9.39), loss of opposition of thumb. Index and middle fingers lag behind while making the fist due to paralysis of 1st and 2nd lumbrical muscles (Fig. 9.38).

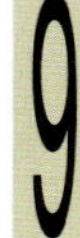

5. *Sensory changes:* Loss of sensations on lateral 3½ digits, including the nail beds and distal phalanges on dorsum of hand (Fig. 9.38).
6. *Vasomotor changes:* The skin areas with sensory loss are warmer due to arteriolar dilatation; it is also drier due to absence of sweating due to loss of sympathetic supply.
7. *Trophic changes:* Long-standing cases of paralysis lead to dry and scaly skin. The nails crack easily with atrophy of the pulp of fingers (Fig. 9.38).

- CTS occurs both in males and females between the age of 25 and 70. They complain of intermittent attacks of pain in the distribution of the median nerve on one or both sides. The attacks frequently occur at night. Pain may be referred proximally to the forearm and arm. It is more common because of excessive work on the computer. ***Phalen's test*** (Fig. 9.39) is attempted for CTS.

Complete claw hand

- If both median and ulnar nerves are paralysed, the result is complete claw hand (Fig. 9.40).

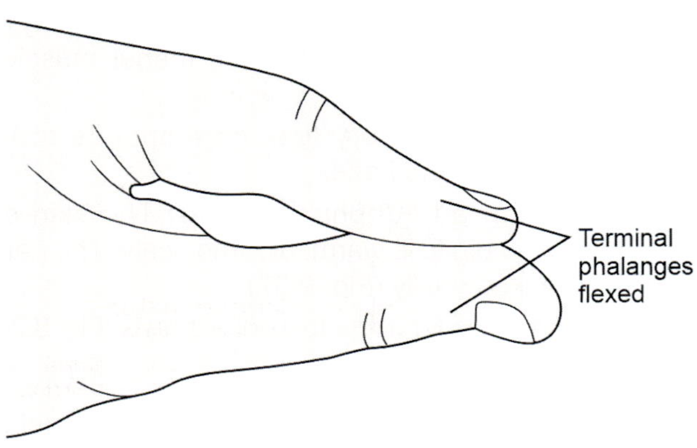

Fig. 9.34: Testing for anterior interosseous nerve

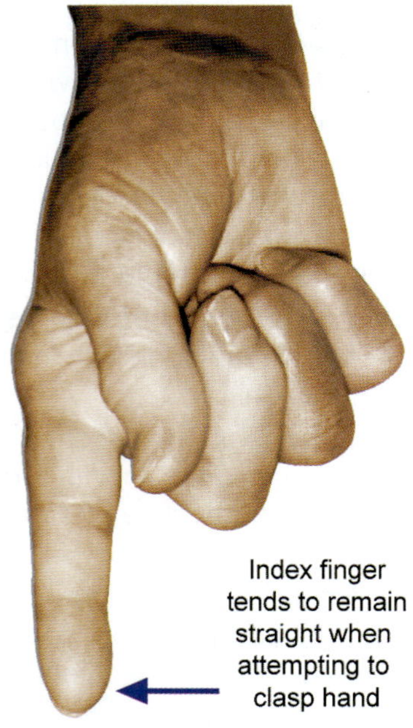

Fig. 9.35: Pointing index finger

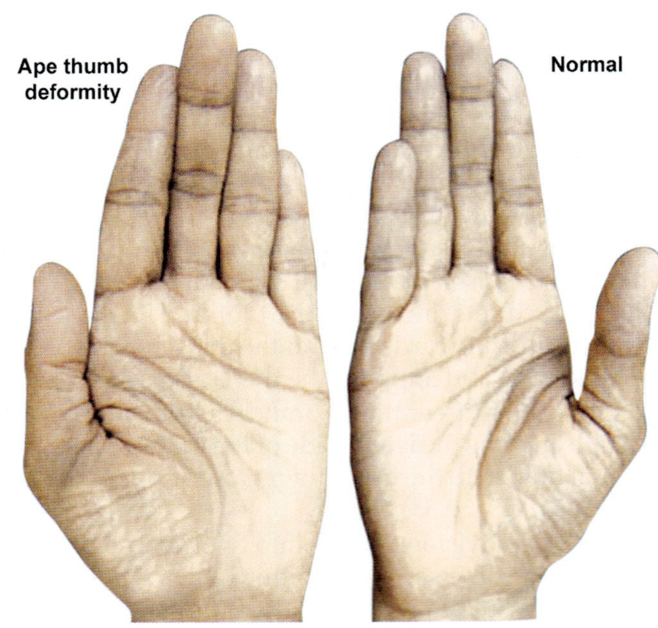

Fig. 9.36: Ape-like thumb deformity

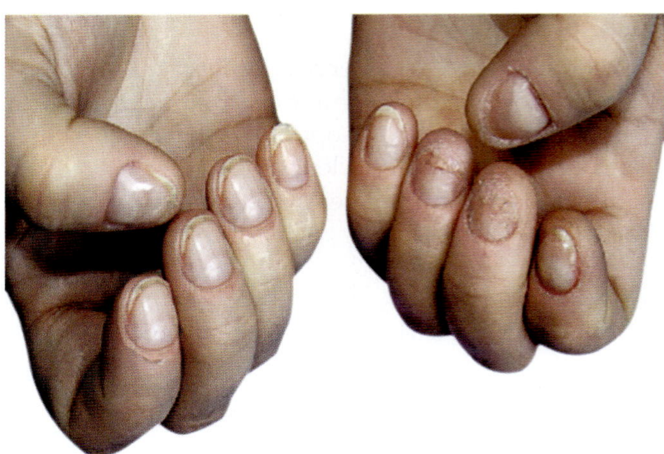

Fig. 9.37: Vasomotor and trophic changes in left hand

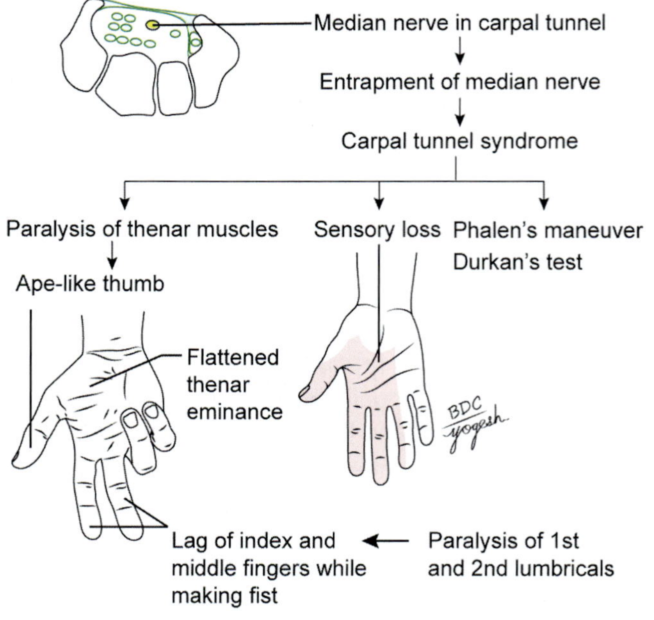

Fig. 9.38: Carpal tunnel syndrome or median nerve palsy

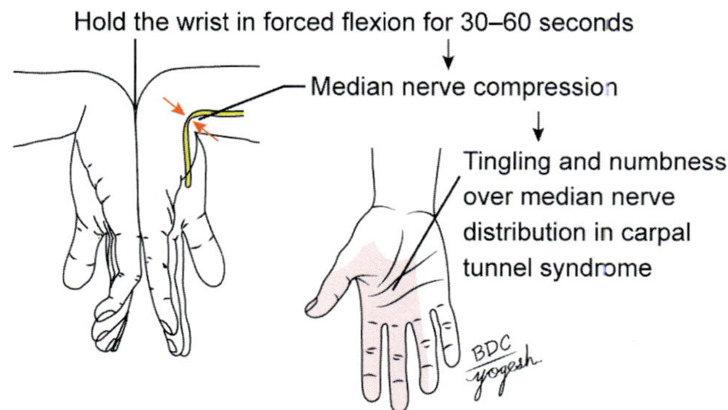

Fig. 9.39: Phalen's test: Acutely flexed wrist causes pain in carpal tunnel syndrome

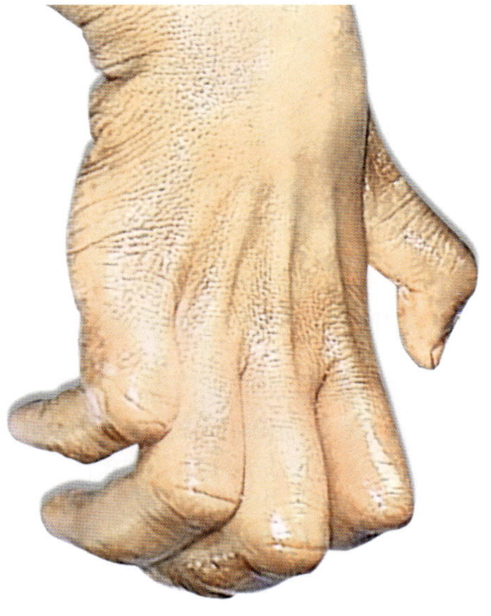

Fig. 9.40: Complete claw hand

RADIAL NERVE

The part of the radial nerve seen in the hand is a continuation of the superficial terminal branch. It reaches the dorsum of the hand (after winding a round the anatomical snuffbox on the lateral side of the radius) and divides into 4 dorsal digital branches, which supply the skin of the digits as follows (Fig. 9.41):

1st: Lateral side of thumb
2nd: Medial side of thumb
3rd: Lateral side of index finger
4th: Contiguous sides of index and middle fingers
5th: Contiguous sides of middle and ring fingers.

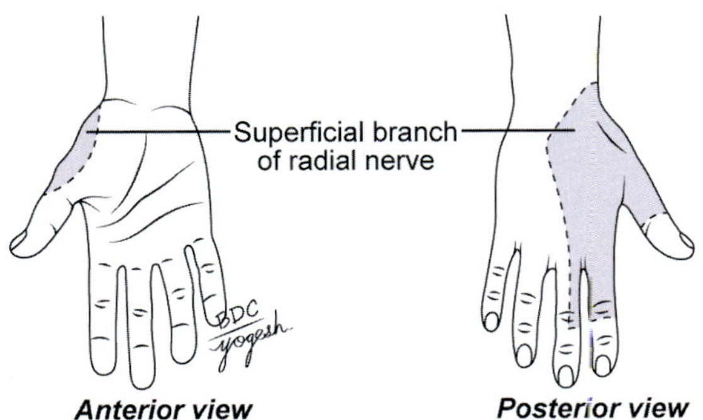

Fig. 9.41: Sensory loss in injury to superficial branch of radial nerve

Note that skin over the dorsum of the distal phalanges is supplied by the median nerve (not radial) (Fig. 9.41). Sensory loss is less because of the overlapping of nerves.

Competency:
AN12.10 Explain infection of fascial spaces of palm.

FASCIAL SPACES OF HAND

The spaces of the hand and their boundaries are clinically important. The arrangement of fasciae and the fascial septa in the hand is such that many spaces are formed. These spaces are of surgical importance because they may become infected and distended with pus. The important spaces are as follows (Plate 9.17, Fig. 9.42, Flowchart 9.7):

A. ***Palmar spaces***
   1. Pulp space of the fingers
   2. Midpalmar space
   3. Thenar space
B. ***Dorsal spaces***
   1. Dorsal subcutaneous space
   2. Dorsal subaponeurotic space
C. ***The forearm space of Parona.***

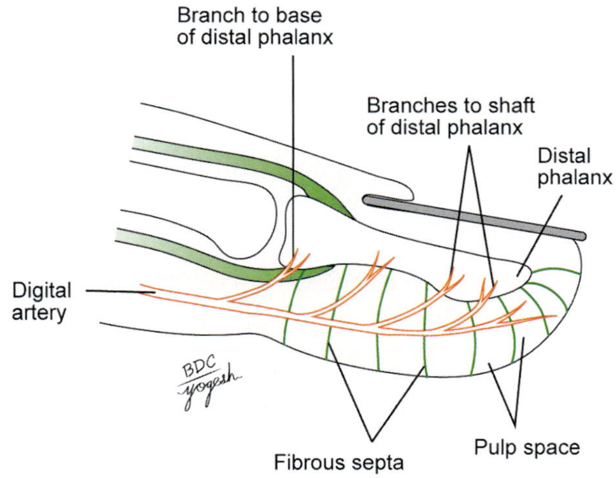

Fig. 9.42: The digital pulp space

Flowchart 9.7: Midpalmar and thenar space

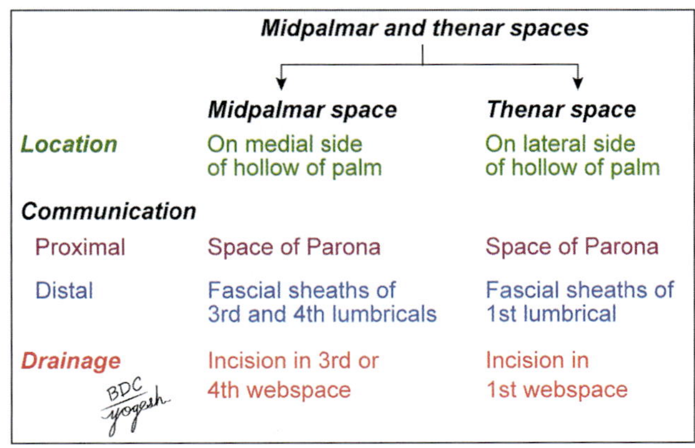

Midpalmar and thenar spaces	Midpalmar space	Thenar space
Location	On medial side of hollow of palm	On lateral side of hollow of palm
Communication		
Proximal	Space of Parona	Space of Parona
Distal	Fascial sheaths of 3rd and 4th lumbricals	Fascial sheaths of 1st lumbrical
Drainage	Incision in 3rd or 4th webspace	Incision in 1st webspace

Plate 9.17: Thenar, hypothenar and pulp spaces of hand

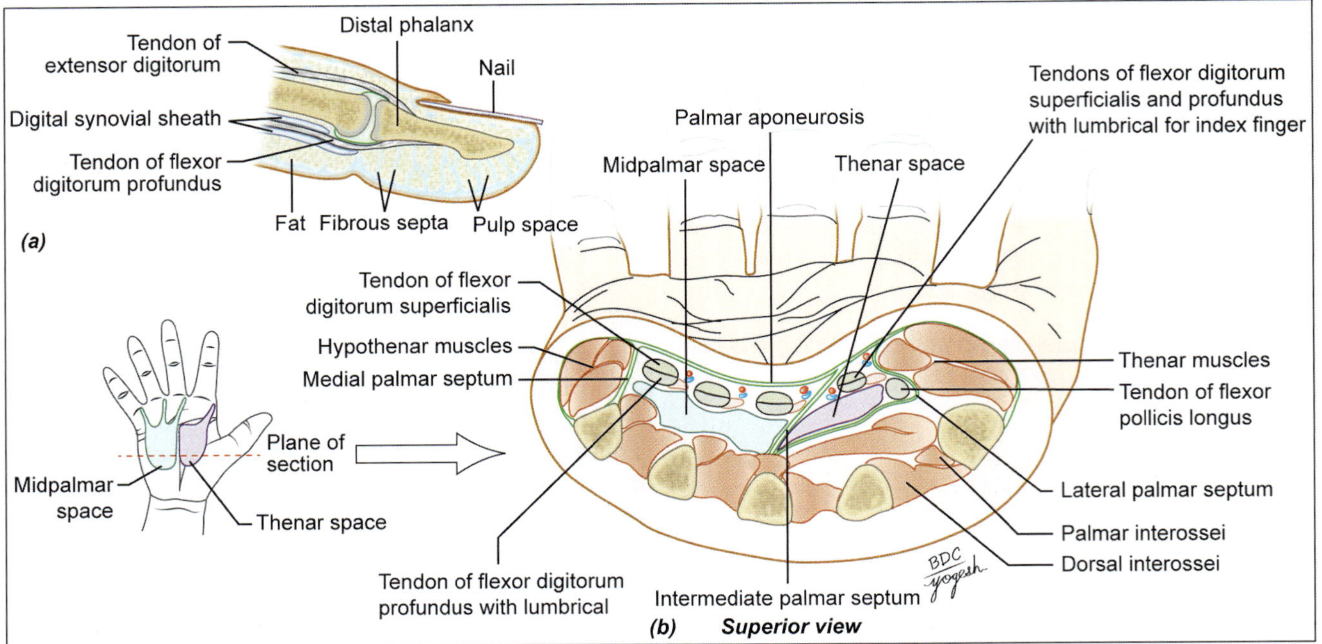

Palmar Spaces

Pulp Space of the Fingers

The tips of the fingers and thumb contain subcutaneous fat arranged in tight compartments formed by fibrous septa, which pass from the skin to the periosteum of the terminal phalanx. Infection of this space is known as ***whitlow***. The rising tension in the space gives rise to severe throbbing pain.

Clinical significance

1. Infections in the pulp space (whitlow) can be drained by a lateral incision, which opens all compartments and avoids damage to the tactile tissue in front of the finger.
2. If neglected, a whitlow may lead to necrosis of the distal 4/5th of the terminal phalanx due to occlusion of the vessels by the tension. The proximal 1/5th (epiphysis) escapes because its artery does not traverse the fibrous septa (Fig. 9.42).

Midpalmar and Thenar Spaces

Midpalmar and thenar spaces are shown in Table 9.7, Fig. 9.19 and Plate 9.17.

TABLE 9.7: Midpalmar and thenar spaces (Fig. 9.19)

Features	*Midpalmar space*	*Thenar space*
1. Shape	Triangular	Triangular
2. Situation	Under the inner half of the hollow of the palm	Under the outer half of the hollow of the palm
3. *Extent*:		
Proximal	Distal margin of the flexor retinaculum	Distal margin of the flexor retinaculum
Distal	Distal palmar crease	Proximal transverse palmar crease
4. *Communications*:		
Proximal	Forearm space of Parona	Forearm space of Parona
Distal	Fascial sheaths of the 3rd and 4th lumbricals	Fascial sheath of the first lumbrical
5. *Boundaries*:		
Anterior	• Palmar aponeurosis • Flexor tendons of 3rd, 4th and 5th digits • 2nd, 3rd and 4th lumbricals	• Palmar aponeurosis • Short muscles of thumb • Flexor tendons of the index finger • First lumbrical
Posterior	Fascia covering interossei and metacarpals	Transverse head of adductor pollicis
Lateral	Intermediate palmar septum	• Tendon of flexor pollicis longus with radial bursa • Lateral palmar septum
Medial	Medial palmar septum	Intermediate palmar septum
6. Drainage	Incision in either the 3rd or 4th web space	Incision in the 1st web posteriorly

Dorsal Spaces

The *dorsal subcutaneous space* lies immediately deep to the loose skin of the dorsum of the hand. The *dorsal subaponeurotic space* lies between the metacarpal bones and the extensor tendons, which are united to one another by a thin aponeurosis.

Forearm Space of Parona

Forearm space of Parona is a rectangular space situated deep in the lower part of the forearm just above the wrist. It lies in front of the pronator quadratus and deep to the long flexor tendons.

Superiorly, the space extends up to the oblique origin of the flexor digitorum superficialis. Inferiorly, it extends up to the flexor retinaculum and communicates with the midpalmar space. The proximal part of the flexor synovial sheath protrudes into the forearm space.

Clinical significance

The forearm space may be infected through infections in the related synovial sheaths, especially of the ulnar bursa. Pus points at the margins of the distal part of the forearm where it may be drained by giving incision along the lateral margin of forearm.

SYNOVIAL SHEATHS

Many of the tendons entering the hand are surrounded by synovial sheaths. The extent of these sheaths is of surgical importance as they can be infected (Fig. 9.6).

Digital Synovial Sheaths

The synovial sheaths of the 2nd, 3rd and 4th digits are independent and terminate proximally at the levels of the heads of the metacarpals. The synovial sheath of the little finger is continuous proximally with the ulnar bursa and that of the thumb with the radial bursa. Therefore, infections of the little finger and thumb are more dangerous because they can spread into the palm and even up to 2.5 cm above the wrist (Fig. 9.6).

Ulnar Bursa

Infection of this bursa is usually secondary to the infection of the little finger, and this, in turn, may spread to the forearm space of the Parona. It results in an ***hourglass swelling*** (so-called because there is one swelling in the palm and another in the distal part of the forearm, the two being joined by a constriction in the region of the flexor retinaculum). It is also called ***compound palmar ganglion***.

Radial Bursa

Infection of the thumb may spread to the radial bursa.

CLINICAL ANATOMY

Surgical incisions

The surgical incisions of the hand are shown in Fig. 9.43.

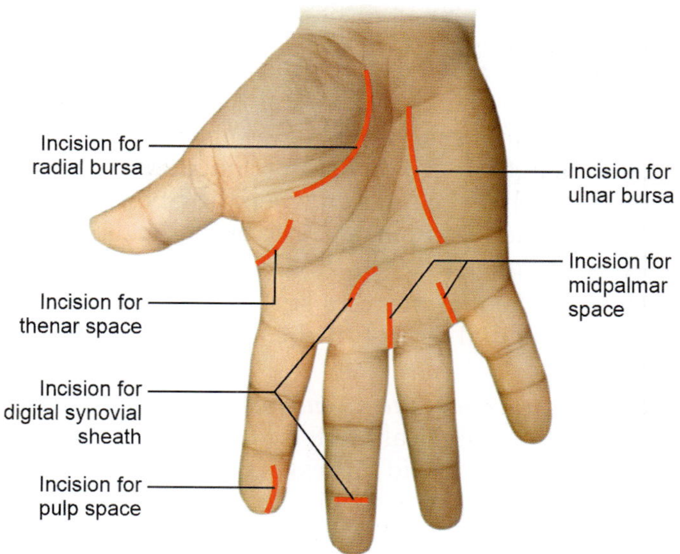

Fig. 9.43: Surgical incisions of the hand

BACK OF FOREARM AND HAND

This section deals mainly with the extensor retinaculum of the wrist, muscles of the back of the forearm, the deep terminal branch of the radial nerve and the posterior interosseous artery.

SURFACE LANDMARKS

1. ***Olecranon process*** of the ulna is the most prominent bony point on the back of a flexed elbow (Fig. 9.44). Normally, it forms a straight horizontal line with the two epicondyles of the humerus when the elbow is extended and a triangle when the elbow is flexed to a right angle. The relative position of the three bony points is disturbed when the elbow is dislocated.

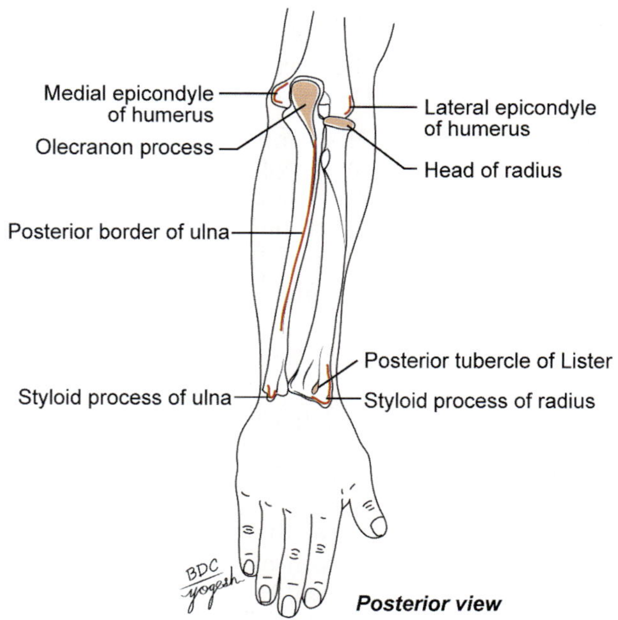

Fig. 9.44: Surface landmarks of the back of forearm

2. ***Head of the radius*** can be palpated in a depression on the posterolateral aspect of an extended elbow just below the lateral epicondyle of the humerus. Its rotation can be felt during pronation and supination of the forearm.
3. ***Posterior border of the ulna*** is subcutaneous in its entire length. It can be felt in a longitudinal groove on the back of the forearm when the elbow is flexed and the hand is supinated. The border ends distally in the ***styloid process of the ulna***.
4. ***Head of the ulna*** forms a surface elevation on the posteromedial aspect of the wrist in a pronated forearm.
5. ***Styloid process of the radius*** can be felt in the upper part of the anatomical snuffbox. It projects down 1 cm lower than the styloid process of the ulna. The relative position of the two styloid processes is disturbed in fractures at the wrist and is a clue to the proper realignment of fractured bones.
6. ***Dorsal tubercle of the radius*** (***Lister's tubercle***) can be palpated on the dorsal surface of the lower end of the radius in line with the cleft between the index and middle fingers. It is grooved on its medial side by the tendon of the extensor pollicis longus.
7. The heads of the metacarpals form the ***knuckles***.

DORSUM OF HAND

1. ***Skin:*** It is loose on the dorsum of hand. It can be pinched off from the underlying structures.
2. ***Superficial fascia:*** The fascia contains dorsal venous plexus, cutaneous nerves and dorsal carpal arch.
   a. ***Dorsal venous plexus or arch:*** The digital veins from adjacent sides of index, middle, ring and little fingers form 3 ***dorsal metacarpal veins*** (*see* Fig. 7.7). These join with each other on dorsum of hand. The lateral end of this arch is joined by one digital vein from index finger and two digital veins from thumb to form ***cephalic vein***. It runs proximally in the *anatomical snuffbox*, curves and a round the lateral border of wrist to come to front of forearm. In a similar manner, the medial end of the arch joins with one digital vein only from medial side of little finger to form ***basilic vein***. It also curves around the medial side of wrist to reach front of forearm. These metacarpal veins may unite in different ways to form a ***dorsal venous plexus***.
   b. ***Cutaneous nerves***: These are *superficial branch of radial nerve* and *dorsal branch of ulnar nerve*. The nail beds and skin of distal phalanges of 3½ lateral nails are supplied by median nerve and 1½ medial nails by ulnar nerve.

      The superficial branch of radial nerve supplies lateral half of dorsum of hand with lateral 3½ digits except their nail beds. The dorsal branch of ulnar supplies medial half of dorsum of hand with medial 1 ½ digits without their nail beds.
   c. ***Dorsal carpal arch:*** It is formed by dorsal carpal branches of radial and ulnar arteries and lies close to the wrist joint. The arch gives three dorsal metacarpal arteries, which supply adjacent sides of index, middle, ring and little fingers. One digital artery goes to medial side of little finger. The arch also gives branches to the dorsum of hand.
3. ***Spaces on dorsum of hand:*** There are two spaces on the dorsum of hand:
   a. ***Dorsal subcutaneous space***, lying just subjacent to skin. Skin of dorsum of hand is loose can be pinched and lifted off.
   b. ***Dorsal subtendinous space*** lies deep to the extensor tendons, between the tendons and the metacarpal bones.
4. ***Deep fascia:*** The deep fascia is modified at the back of hand to form extensor retinaculum.

ANATOMICAL SNUFFBOX

The *anatomical snuffbox* (Fig. 9.45) is a triangular depression on the posterolateral side of the wrist. It is seen best when the thumb is extended.

Boundaries

- *Medial border* (*ulnar side*): Tendon of extensor pollicis longus
- *Lateral border* (*radial side*): Tendons of extensor pollicis brevis and abductor pollicis longus
- *Proximal border*: Styloid process of radius
- *Apex*: Approximation of medial and lateral borders
- *Floor*: Trapezium and scaphoid
- *Roof*: Skin, superficial branch of radial nerve, cephalic vein.

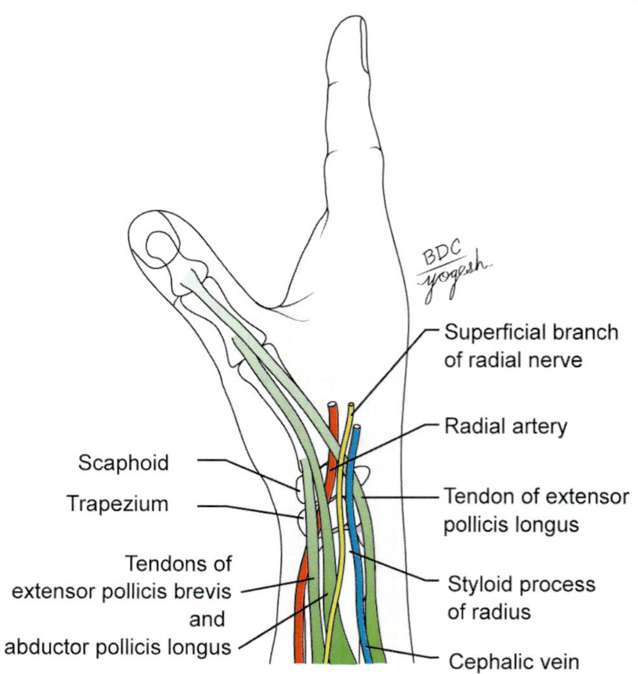

Fig. 9.45: Anatomical snuffbox

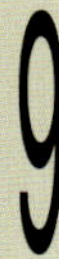

Contents

The radial artery is deep while the superficial branch of radial nerve and cephalic vein are superficial.

Clinical Significance

- The pulsations of radial artery can be felt in the anatomical snuff box.
- The tenderness in the anatomical box indicates fracture of scaphoid bone.
- The cephalic vein at the anatomical box can be used for giving intravenous fluids.

Competency:
AN12.14 Identify and describe compartments deep to extensor retinaculum and describe the boundaries and contents of anatomical snuff box.

Extensor Retinaculum

The deep fascia on the back of the wrist is thickened to form the extensor retinaculum, which holds the extensor tendons in place. It is an oblique band directed downwards and medially. It is about 2 cm broad vertically (Plate 9.18, Fig. 9.46).

Attachments

Laterally: Lower part of the sharp *anterior* (crest-like) border of the radius.
Medially:
1. Triquetral
2. Pisiform.

Note: The extensor retinaculum is not attached to the ulna medially, as the distance between the radius and ulna varies with supination and pronation of the forearm.

Compartments

The retinaculum sends down septa, which are attached to the longitudinal ridges on the posterior surface of the lower end of radius. In this way, ***6 osseofascial compartments*** are formed on the back of the wrist. The structures passing through each compartment, from lateral to the medial side, are listed in Table 9.8 and Fig. 9.46.

Each compartment is lined by a synovial sheath, which is reflected in the contained tendons.

TABLE 9.8: Structures in various compartments under extensor retinaculum

Compartment	*Structure*
I	• Abductor pollicis longus • Extensor pollicis brevis
II	• Extensor carpi radialis longus • Extensor carpi radialis brevis
III	• Extensor pollicis longus
IV	• Extensor digitorum • Extensor indicis • Posterior interosseous nerve • Anterior interosseous artery
V	• Extensor digiti minimi
VI	• Extensor carpi ulnaris

DISSECTION

Make the incision in the centre of dorsum of hand. Reflect the skin of dorsum of hand till the respective borders. Reflect the skin of dorsum of middle finger on each side. Look for nerves on the back of forearm and hand. These are superficial branch of radial nerve and dorsal branch of ulnar nerve.

The dorsal venous network is the most prominent component of the superficial fascia of dorsum of hand. (Identify the beginning of cephalic and basilic veins by tying a tourniquet on the forearm and exercising the closed fist on oneself.)

The deep fascia at the back of wrist is thickened to form extensor retinaculum. Define its margins and attachments. Identify the structures traversing its six compartments.

Clear the deep fascia over the back of forearm. Define the attachment of triceps brachii muscle on the olecranon process of ulna. Define the attachments of the seven superficial muscles of the back of the forearm.

Separate the anterolateral muscles, i.e. brachioradialis, extensor carpi radialis longus and brevis from the extensor digitorum lying in the centre and extensor digiti minimi and extensor carpi ulnaris situated on the medial aspect of the wrist (Plates 9.18 and 9.19). Anconeus is situated on the posterolateral aspect of the elbow joint. Dissect all these muscles and trace their nerve supply.

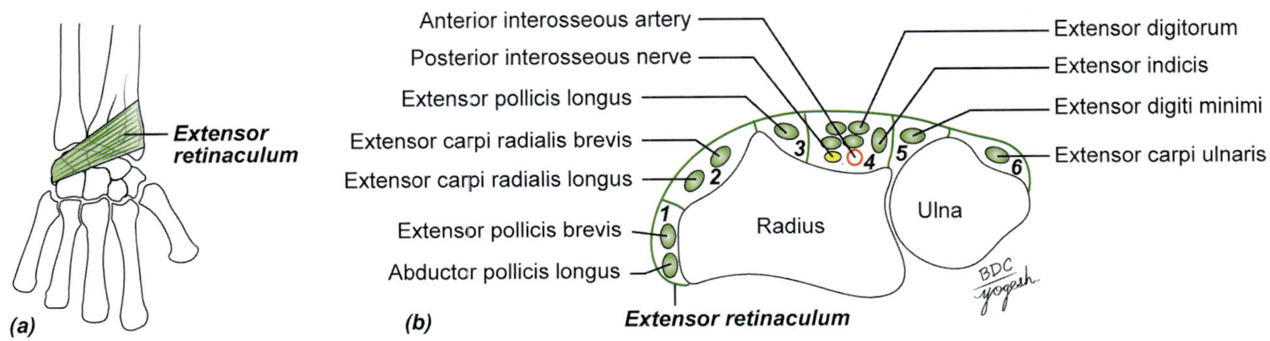

Figs 9.46a and b: (a) Attachments of extensor retinaculum, (b) transverse section passing just above the wrist showing structures passing through 1–6 compartments deep to the extensor retinaculum

Plate 9.18: Extensor retinaculum of forearm

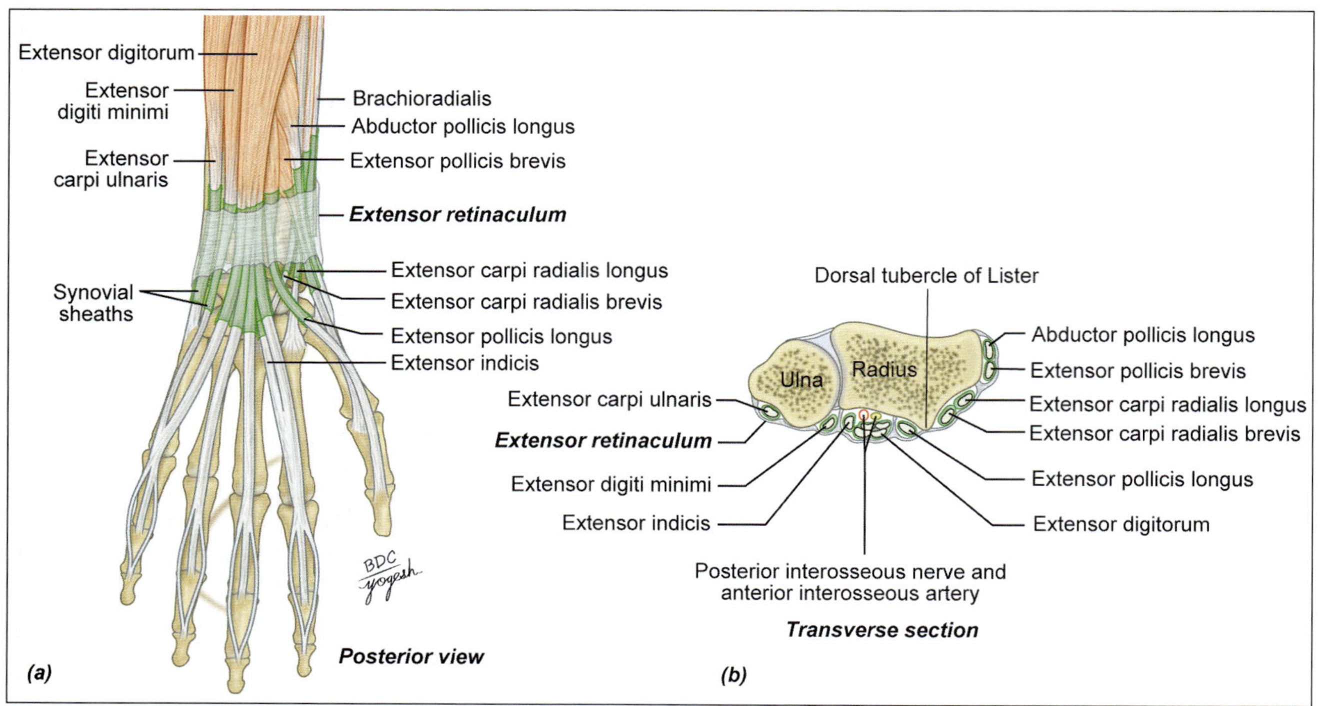

Competency:

AN12.11 Identify, describe and demonstrate important muscle groups of dorsal forearm with attachments, nerve supply and actions.

MUSCLES OF BACK OF FOREARM

SUPERFICIAL MUSCLES

There are seven superficial muscles on the back of the forearm as follows (Plate 9.19, Figs 9.47 and 9.48):

1. Anconeus
2. Brachioradialis
3. Extensor carpi radialis longus
4. Extensor carpi radialis brevis
5. Extensor digitorum
6. Extensor digiti minimi
7. Extensor carpi ulnaris.

All the seven muscles cross the elbow joint. Most of them take origin (entirely or in part) from the tip of the lateral epicondyle of the humerus.

These muscles, with their nerve supply and actions, are described in Tables 9.9 and 9.10.

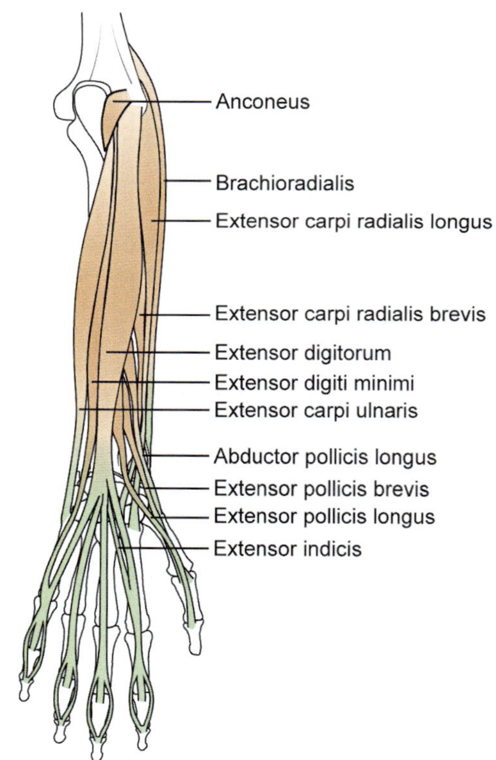

Fig. 9.47: Muscles of the back of forearm

Additional Points

1. The extensor digitorum and extensor indicis pass through the same compartment of the extensor retinaculum, and have a common synovial sheath.
2. The four tendons of the extensor digitorum emerge from under cover of the extensor retinaculum and fan out over the dorsum of the hand. The tendon to the index finger is joined on its medial side by the tendon of the extensor indicis, and the tendon to the little finger is joined on its medial side by the two tendons of the extensor digiti minimi.
3. On the dorsum of the hand, adjacent tendons are variably connected together by three intertendinous connections directed obliquely downwards and laterally. The medial connection is strong; the lateral connection is weakest and may be absent.

The four tendons and three intertendinous connections are embedded in deep fascia and together form the roof of the subtendinous (subaponeurotic) space on the dorsum of the hand.

Plate 9.19: Muscles of back of forearm

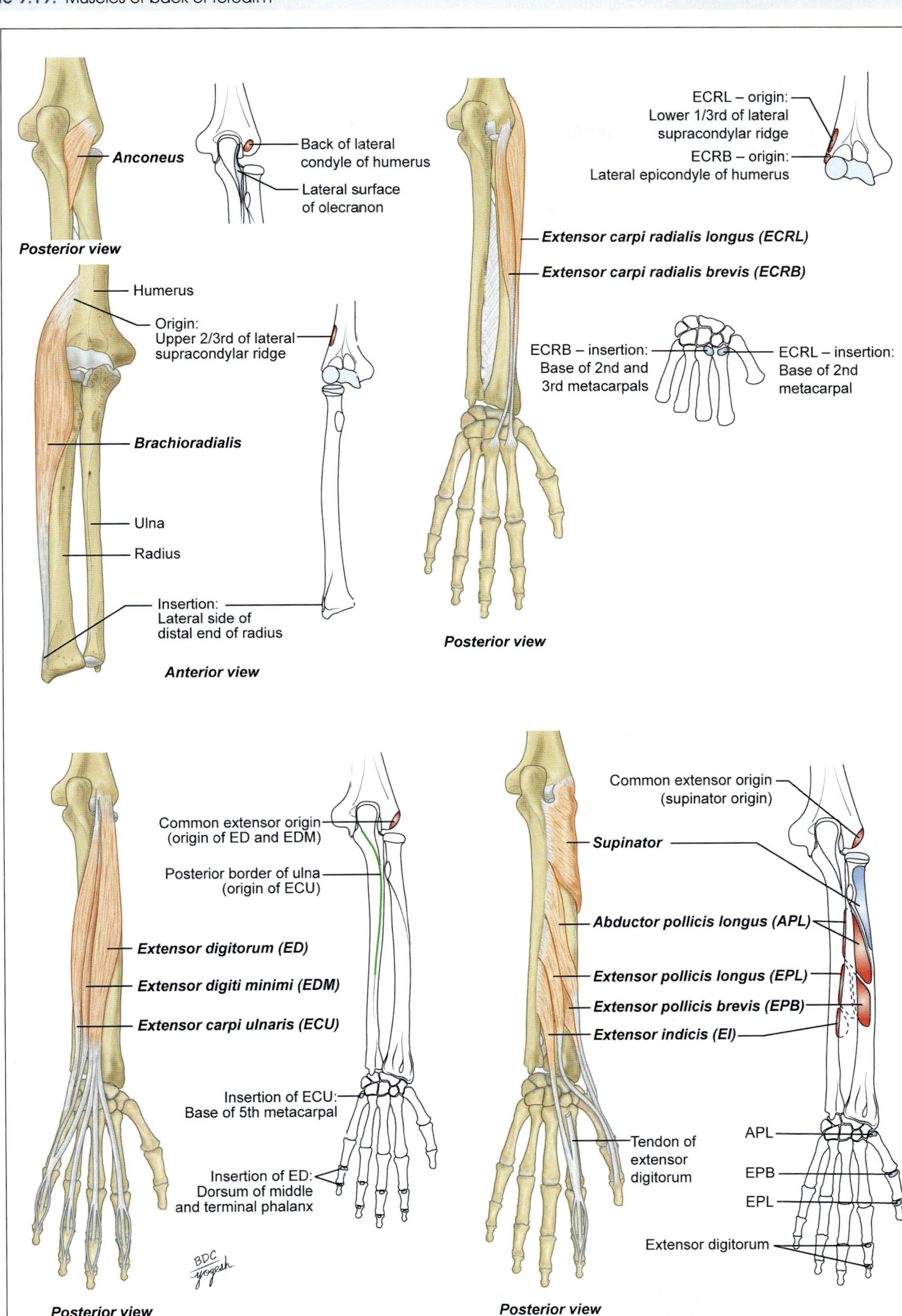

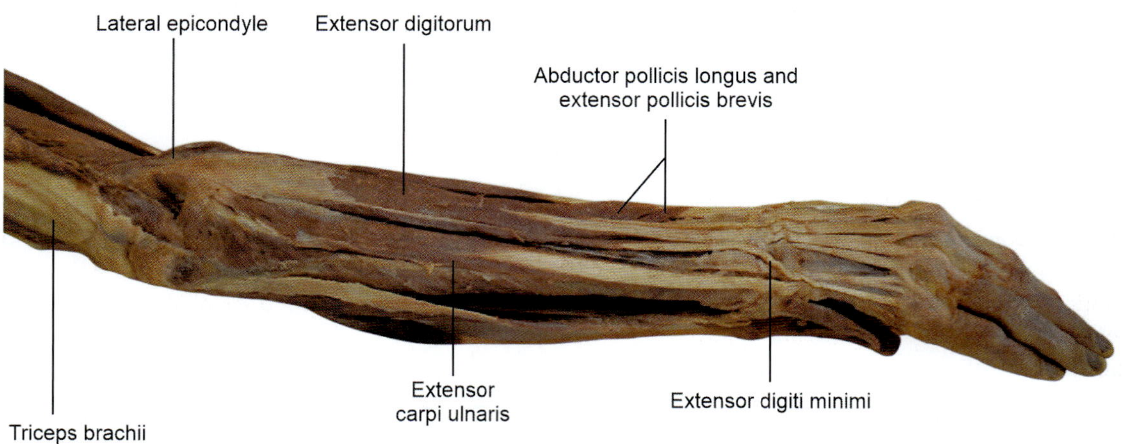

Fig. 9.48: Dissection of back of forearm

TABLE 9.9: Origin and insertion of superficial muscles of back of forearm (Plate 9.19, Figs 9.47 and 9.48)

Muscle	*Origin*	*Insertion*
1. **Anconeus**	Lateral epicondyle of humerus	Lateral surface of olecranon process and upper 1/4th of posterior surface of ulna
2. **Brachioradialis**	Upper 2/3rd of lateral supracondylar ridge of humerus	Lateral surface of radius just above the styloid process
3. **Extensor carpi radialis longus**	Lower 1/3rd of lateral supracondylar ridge of humerus	Posterior surface of base of 2nd metacarpal bone
4. **Extensor carpi radialis brevis**	Lateral epicondyle of humerus	Posterior surface of base of 3rd metacarpal
5. **Extensor digitorum**	Lateral epicondyle of humerus	Bases of middle and distal phalanges of the 2nd–5th digits
6. **Extensor digiti minimi**	Lateral epicondyle of humerus	Extensor expansion of little finger
7. **Extensor carpi ulnaris**	Lateral epicondyle of humerus	Base of 5th metacarpal bone

TABLE 9.10: Nerve supply and actions of superficial muscles of back of forearm

Muscle	*Nerve supply*	*Actions*
1. **Anconeus**	Radial nerve	Extends elbow joint
2. **Brachioradialis**	Radial nerve	Flexes forearm at elbow joint Brings forearm to the midprone position from supine or prone positions
3. **Extensor carpi radialis longus**	Radial nerve	Extends and abducts hand at wrist joint
4. **Extensor carpi radialis brevis**	Deep branch of radial nerve	Extends and abducts hand at wrist joint
5. **Extensor digitorum**	Deep branch of radial nerve	Extends fingers of hand
6. **Extensor digiti minimi**	Deep branch of radial nerve	Extends metacarpophalangeal joint of little finger
7. **Extensor carpi ulnaris**	Deep branch of radial nerve	Extends and adducts hand at wrist joint

DEEP MUSCLES

Features

These are as follows (Plate 9.19, Figs 9.47 and 9.48):
1. Supinator
2. Abductor pollicis longus
3. Extensor pollicis brevis
4. Extensor pollicis longus
5. Extensor indicis

In contrast to the superficial muscles, none of the deep muscles cross the elbow joint. These have been tabulated in Tables 9.11 and 9.12.

Competency:
AN12.15 Identify and describe extensor expansion formation.

Dorsal Digital Expansion/Extensor Expansion

The dorsal digital expansion (extensor expansion) is a small triangular aponeurosis (related to each tendon of the extensor digitorum) covering the dorsum of the proximal phalanx. Its base, which is proximal, covers the metacarpophalangeal (MP) joint. The main tendon of the extensor digitorum occupies the central part of the extension and is separated from the MP joint by a bursa.

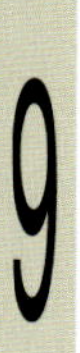

TABLE 9.11: Origin and insertion of deep muscles of back of forearm (Plate 9.19, Figs 9.47 and 9.48)

Muscle	*Origin*	*Insertion*
1. **Supinator**	Lateral epicondyle of humerus Annular ligament of superior radioulnar joint Supinator crest of ulna and depression anterior to it	Neck and upper 1/3rd of lateral surface of shaft of radius
2. **Abductor pollicis longus**	Posterior surface of shafts of radius and ulna	Lateral side of base of 1st metacarpal bone
3. **Extensor pollicis brevis**	Posterior surface of shaft of radius and adjoining part of interosseous membrane	Base of proximal phalanx of thumb
4. **Extensor pollicis longus**	Posterior surface of shaft of ulna and adjoining part of interosseous membrane	Base of distal phalanx of thumb
5. **Extensor indicis**	Posterior surface of shaft of ulna and adjoining	Extensor expansion of index finger

TABLE 9.12: Nerve supply and actions of deep muscles of back of forearm

Muscle	*Nerve supply*	*Actions*
1. **Supinator**	Deep branch of radial nerve	Supination of forearm when elbow is extended
2. **Abductor pollicis longus**	Deep branch of radial nerve	Abducts and extends thumb
3. **Extensor pollicis brevis**	Deep branch of radial nerve	Extends metacarpophalangeal joint of thumb
4. **Extensor pollicis longus**	Deep branch of radial nerve	Extends distal phalanx of thumb
5. **Extensor indicis**	Deep branch of radial nerve	Extends metacarpophalangeal joint of index finger

The posterolateral corners of the extensor expansion are joined by tendons of the interossei and lumbrical muscles. The corners are attached to the deep transverse metacarpal ligament. The points of attachment of the interossei (proximal) and lumbrical (distal) are often called *'wing tendons'* (Fig. 9.49).

Near the proximal interphalangeal joint, the extensor tendon divides into a central slip and two collateral slips. The ***central slip*** is joined by some fibres from the margins of the expansion, crosses the proximal interphalangeal joint and is inserted on the dorsum of the base of the middle phalanx. The ***two collateral slips*** are joined by the remaining thick margin of the extensor expansion. They then join each other and are inserted on the dorsum of the base of the distal phalanx.

At the metacarpophalangeal and interphalangeal joints, the extensor expansion forms the dorsal part of the fibrous capsule of the joints.

The retinacular ligaments (link ligaments) extend from the side of the proximal phalanx and form its fibrous flexor sheath to the margins of the extensor expansion to reach the base of the distal phalanx.

Muscles Inserted on Dorsal Expansion

- *Index finger:* 1st dorsal interosseous, 2nd palmar interosseous, 1st lumbrical, extensor digitorum slip and extensor indicis (Fig. 9.49).
- *Middle finger:* 2nd and 3rd dorsal interossei, 2nd lumbrical, extensor digitorum slip.

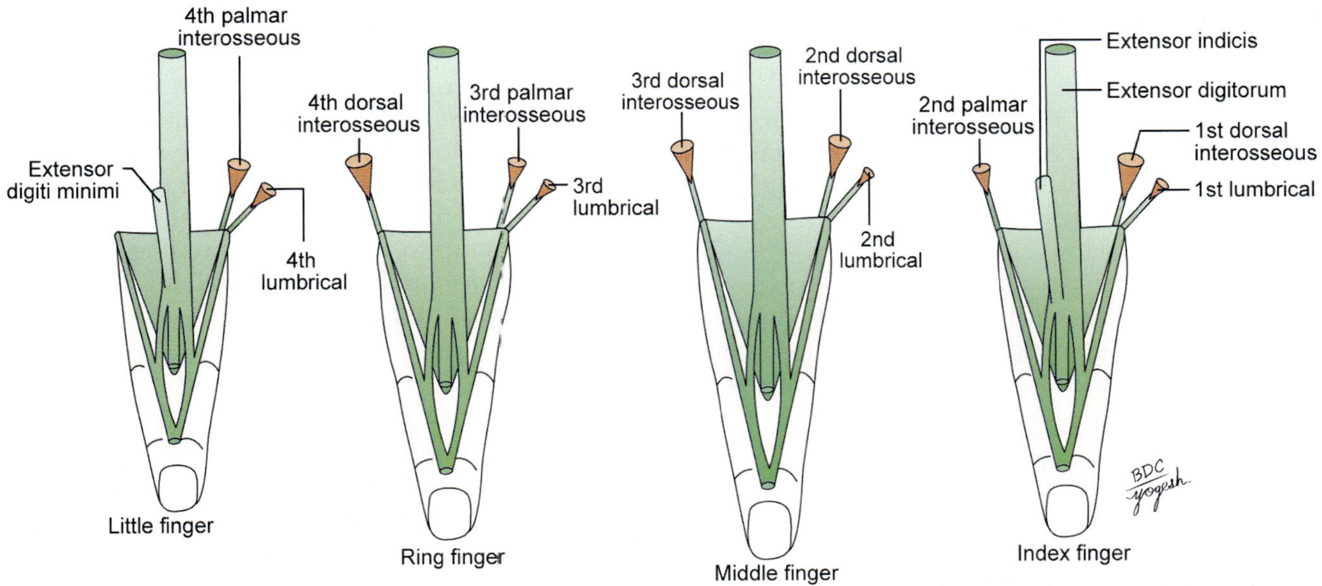

Fig. 9.49: The dorsal digital expansion of right little, ring, middle and index fingers. Note the insertions of the lumbricals and interossei into it

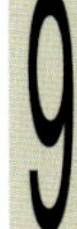

- *Ring finger:* 4th dorsal interosseous, 3rd palmar interosseous, 3rd lumbrical and extensor digitorum slip.
- *Little finger:* 4th palmar interosseous, 4th lumbrical, extensor digitorum slip and extensor digiti minimi.

Functions

1. Dorsal digital expansion is a functional unit that splits the action of muscles, combines the action of muscles and changes the direction of muscles.
2. It helps in flexion at MP joint, extension at IP joint by lumbricals, and also in isolated flexion of proximal and distal IP joints by extensor digitorum.

Clinical Aspects

- *Mallet finger* (baseball finger, cricketers finger or hammer finger): In Mallet finger, a forceful hit over the tip of finger causes sudden, strong flexion of the phalanx that results in avulsion of extensor digitorum tendon from terminal phalanx and inability to do the extension of terminal phalanx.
- *Busch fracture*: Avulsion of base of distal phalanx with tendon of extensor digitorum.

DISSECTION

Separate extensor carpi radials brevis from extensor digitorum and identify deeply placed supinator muscle.

Just distal to supinator is abductor pollicis longus. Other three muscles: Extensor pollicis longus, extensor pollicis brevis and extensor indicis are present distal to abductor pollicis longus. Identify them all.

Competency:

AN12.12 Identify and describe origin, course, relations, branches (or tributaries), termination of important nerves and vessels of back of forearm.

POSTERIOR INTEROSSEOUS NERVE

Features

It is the chief nerve of the back of the forearm. It is a branch of the radial nerve given off in the cubital fossa, just below the level of the lateral epicondyle of the humerus (Plate 9.20, Figs 9.50 and 9.51).

Course

It begins in cubital fossa. It passes through supinator muscle to reach back of forearm, where it descends downwards. It ends in a pseudoganglion in the 4th compartment of extensor retinaculum.

Relations

1. Posterior interosseous nerve leaves the cubital fossa and enters the back of the forearm by passing between the two planes of fibres of the supinator. Within the muscle, it winds backwards around the lateral side of the radius (Fig. 9.50).

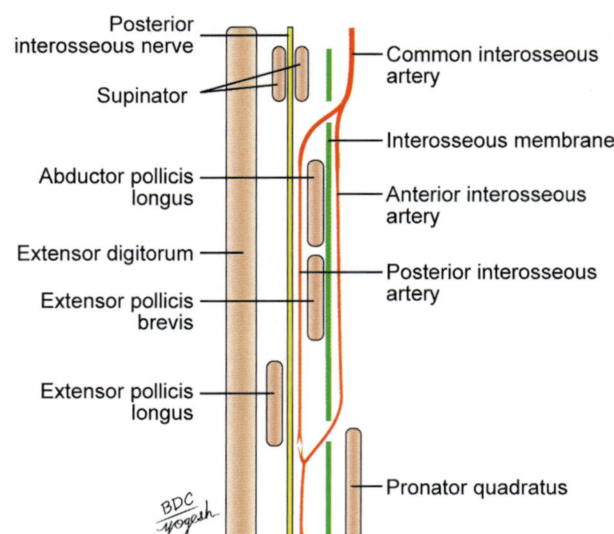

Fig. 9.50: Course and relations of the posterior interosseous nerve and the interosseous arteries

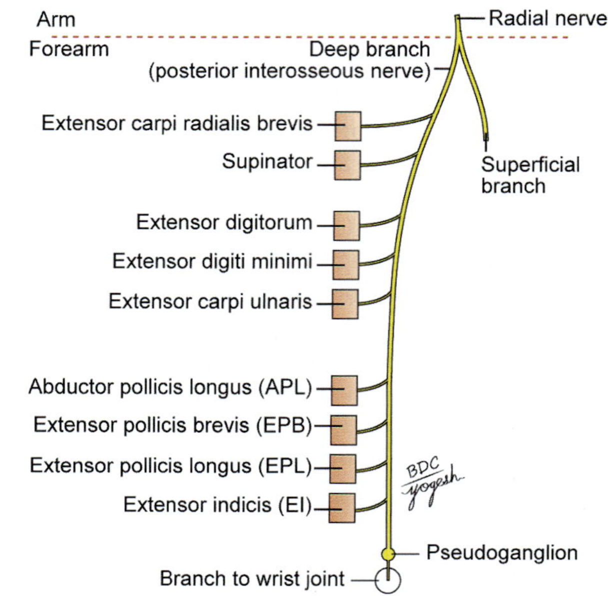

Fig. 9.51: Branches of the posterior interosseous nerve

2. It emerges from the supinator on the back of the forearm. Here, it lies between the superficial and deep muscles. At the lower border of the extensor pollicis brevis, it passes deep to the extensor pollicis longus. It then runs on the posterior surface of the interosseous membrane up to the wrist, where it enlarges into a *pseudoganglion* and ends by supplying the wrist and intercarpal joints.

Branches

The posterior interosseous nerve gives muscular, articular and sensory branches (Fig. 9.51).

A. ***Muscular branches***
   - Before piercing the supinator, branches are given to the extensor carpi radialis brevis and to the supinator.
   - While passing through the supinator, another branch is given to the supinator.

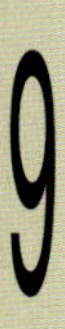

Plate 9.20: Branches of radial nerve in forearm

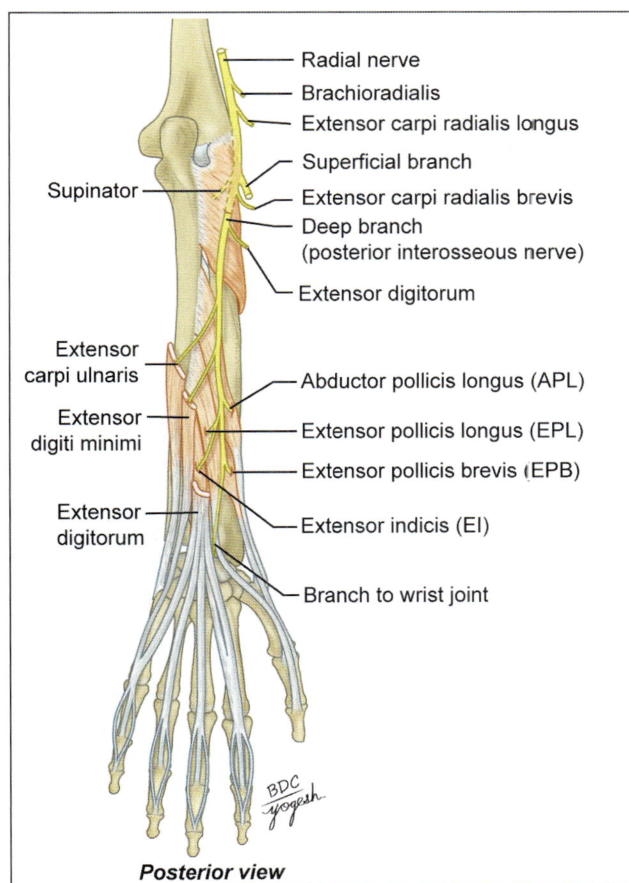

- After emerging from the supinator, the nerve gives three short branches to:
  1. Extensor digitorum (Fig. 9.51)
  2. Extensor digiti minimi
  3. Extensor carpi ulnaris
- It also has two long branches:
  1. A lateral branch supplies the abductor pollicis longus and the extensor pollicis brevis.
  2. A medial branch supplies the extensor pollicis longus and the extensor indicis.

B. ***Articular branches:*** Articular branches are given to:
  1. Wrist joint
  2. Distal radioulnar joint
  3. Intercarpal and intermetacarpal joints

C. ***Sensory branches:*** Sensory branches are given to the interosseous membrane, the radius and the ulna.

DISSECTION

The deep terminal branch of radial nerve/posterior interosseous nerve and posterior interosseous artery: Identify the posterior interosseous nerve at the distal border of exposed supinator muscle. Trace its branches to the various muscles.

Look for the radial nerve in the lower lateral part of front of arm between the brachioradialis, extensor carpi radialis longus laterally and brachialis muscle medially. Trace the two divisions of this nerve in the lateral part of the cubital fossa. The deep branch (posterior interosseous nerve) traverses between the two planes of supinator muscle and reaches the back of the forearm where it is already identified.

The nerve runs amongst the muscles of the back of the forearm, and ends at the level of the wrist in a pseudoganglion (Fig. 9.51).

This nerve is accompanied by posterior interosseous artery distal to the supinator muscle. This artery is supplemented by anterior interosseous artery in lower one-fourth of the forearm.

POSTERIOR INTEROSSEOUS ARTERY

Course

Posterior interosseous artery is the smaller terminal branch of the common interosseous, given off in the cubital fossa.

It enters the back of the forearm and lies in between the muscles there. It terminates by anastomosing with the anterior interosseous artery.

Relations

1. It is the smaller terminal branch of the common interosseous artery in the cubital fossa.
2. It enters the back of the forearm by passing between the oblique cord and the upper margin of the interosseous membrane (Fig. 9.50).
3. It appears on the back of the forearm in the interval between the supinator and the abductor pollicis longus and thereafter accompanies the posterior interosseous nerve. At the lower border of the extensor indicis, the artery becomes markedly reduced and ends by anastomosing with the anterior interosseous artery, which reaches the posterior compartment by piercing the interosseous membrane at the upper border of the pronator quadratus. Thus, in its lower 1/4th, the back of the forearm is supplied by the anterior interosseous artery.
4. The posterior interosseous artery gives off an ***interosseous recurrent branch***, which runs upwards and takes part in the anastomosis on the back of the lateral epicondyle of the humerus (*see* Fig. 8.11).

VIDEO

Video 1.9.1 Forearm: Superficial and deep muscles of front of forearm, Nerves and blood vessels of forearm, Back of forearm.

Video 1.9.2 Palm: Flexor retinaculum, muscles of thenar and hypothenar eminence, Blood vessels and nerves of the palm, Ulnar artery, Ulnar nerve, Median nerve, Muscles and tendons in the palm.

Facts to Remember

- Median nerve exits the cubital fossa by passing between two heads of pronator teres while ulnar artery passes deep to both the heads of pronator teres.

- Anterior interosseous branch of median nerve supplies 2½ muscles of front of the forearm, i.e. flexor pollicis longus, pronator quadratus and lateral half of flexor digitorum profundus.
- Flexor retinaculum has a superficial slip medially and a deep slip laterally. Deep to superficial slip course ulnar nerve and vessels and superficial to the deep slip passes the tendon of flexor carpi radialis.
- Thenar eminence *does not* include the adductor pollicis muscle. It comprises abductor pollicis brevis, flexor pollicis brevis and opponens pollicis.
- Median nerve supplies 5 muscles in the palm, three muscles of thenar eminence and 1st and 2nd lumbricals. It is called *'labourer's nerve'*. Median nerve is also the *'Eye of the hand or peripheral eye'*.
- Ulnar nerve is called *'Musician's nerve'*. It supplies 15 intrinsic muscles of the hand.
- There are 12 muscles on the back of forearm, two are smaller (supinator and anconeus) lying in upper 1/4th of the forearm, five are inserted close to the wrist (BR, APL, ECRL, ECRB and ECU); five get inserted into the phalanges (EPB, EPL, EI, ED and EDM). All are supplied by radial or posterior interosseous nerve. Injury to the nerve causes *'wrist drop'*.
- Lateral 3½ nail beds are supplied by median nerve and medial 1½ nail beds by ulnar nerve.

BDC's Anatomy *e*-book

1. Arches of hand
2. Kanavel's sign
3. Cleland and Grayson ligament
4. Handlebar neuropathy
5. Froment's sign
6. Movements of thumb
7. Muscles of posterior compartment of forearm
8. Dorsal digital expansion and mallet finger
9. Sectional anatomy of the forearm and palm
10. Nerves and vessels of forearm and palm
11. Further reading
12. Viva voce questions

Right axilla

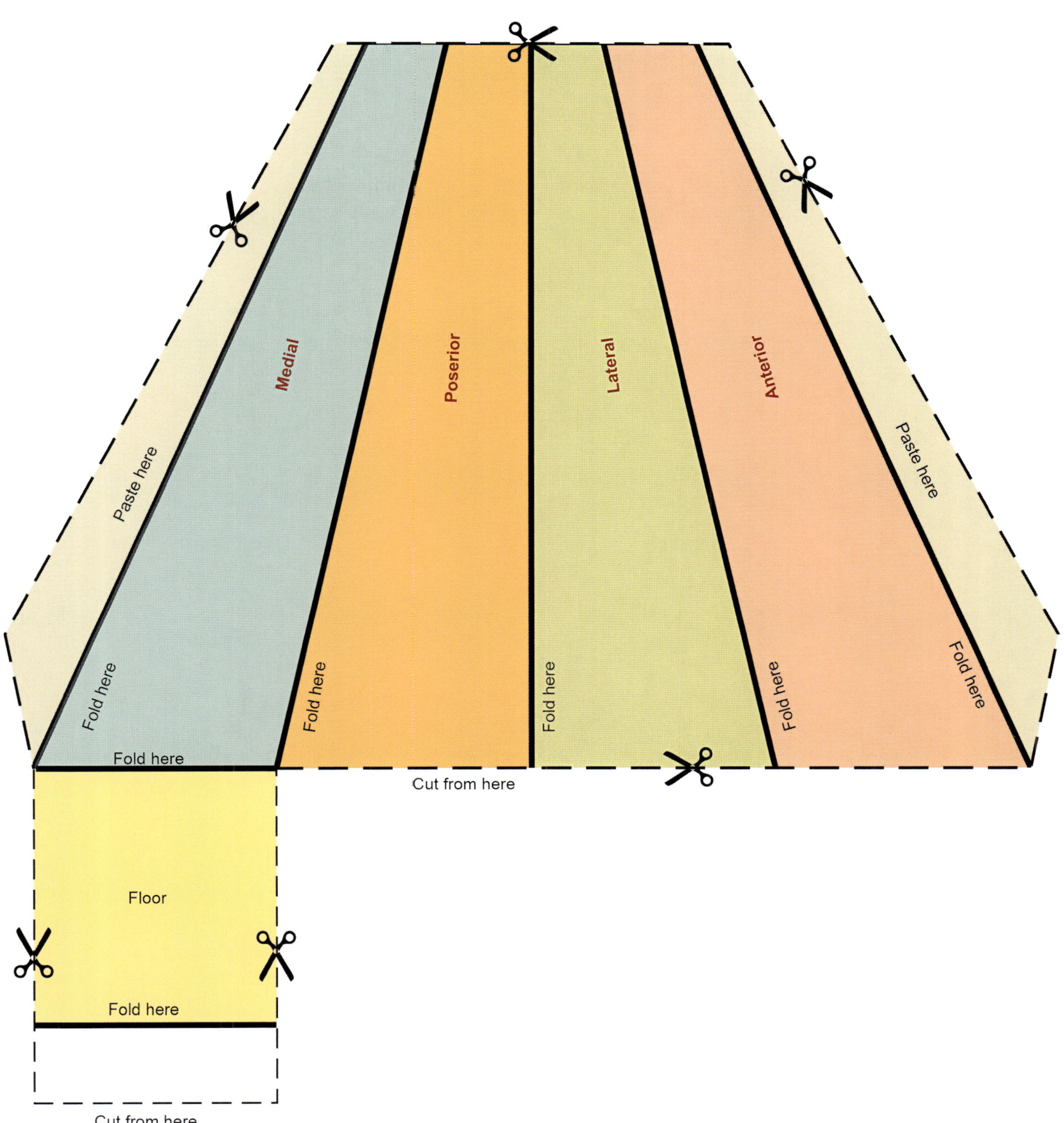

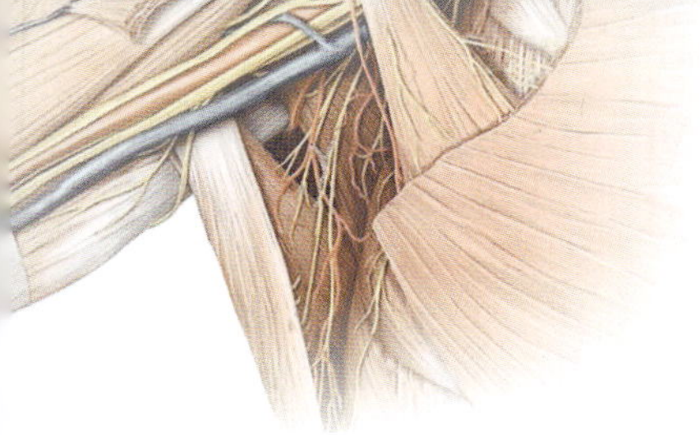

Chapter

10

Joints of Upper Limb

Joints are sites where two or more bones or cartilages articulate. The bones of upper limb form the following joints:

1. Sternoclavicular joint
2. Acromioclavicular joint
3. Shoulder joint
4. Elbow joint
5. Radioulnar joints (superior, middle and inferior)
6. Wrist joint
7. Intercarpal joints
8. Carpometacarpal joints
9. Metacarpophalangeal joints
10. Interphalangeal joints (proximal and distal).

Shoulder joint is the most freely mobile joint. Shoulder joint gets excessive mobility at the cost of its own stability. The carrying angle in relation to elbow joint is to facilitate carrying objects like buckets without hitting the pelvis.

Supination and pronation are basic movements for the survival of human being. During pronation, the food is picked and by supination it is put at the right place—the mouth. The first carpometacarpal joint allows movements of opposition of thumb with the fingers for picking up or holding things.

SHOULDER GIRDLE

The shoulder girdle connects the upper limb to the axial skeleton. It consists of the clavicle and the scapula. Anteriorly, the clavicle reaches the sternum and articulates with it at the *sternoclavicular joint*. The clavicle and the scapula are united to each other at the *acromioclavicular joint*. The scapula is not connected to the axial skeleton directly, but is attached to it through muscles.

Competency:
AN13.4 Describe sternoclavicular joint, acromioclavicular joint, carpometacarpal joints and metacarpophalangeal joint.

STERNOCLAVICULAR JOINT

Features

Type

The sternoclavicular joint is a *synovial joint of saddle variety*. It is a *compound joint* as there are three elements taking part in it; namely the medial end of the clavicle, the clavicular notch of the manubrium sterni, and the upper surface of the first costal cartilage. It is a *complex joint* as its cavity is subdivided into two compartments—superomedial and inferolateral by an intra-articular disc (Fig. 10.1).

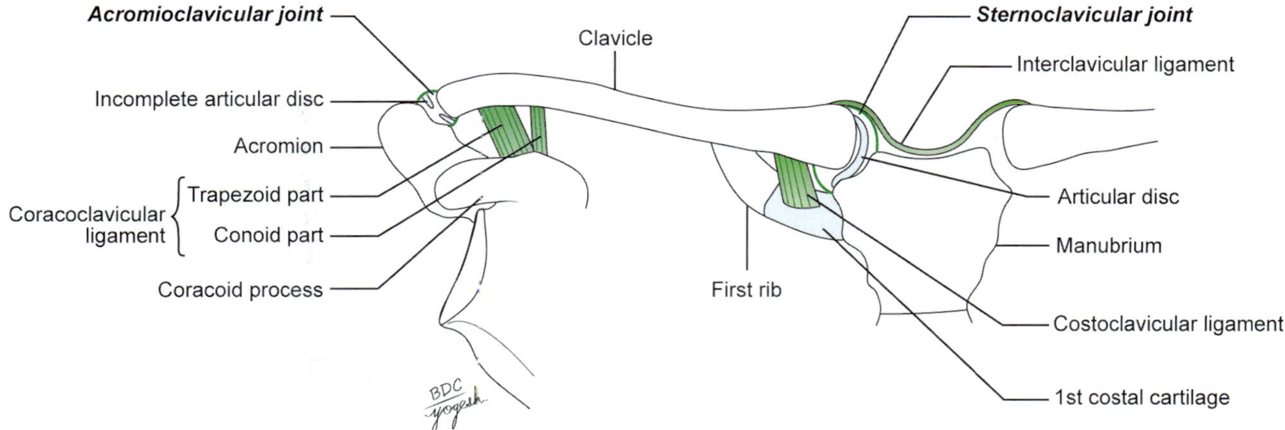

Fig. 10.1: The sternoclavicular and acromioclavicular joints

Articular Surfaces

The *articular surface* of the clavicle is covered with fibrocartilage (as the clavicle is a membrane bone). The surface is convex from above downwards and slightly concave from front to back. The sternal surface is smaller than the clavicular surface. It has a reciprocal convexity and concavity. Due to the concavo-convex shape of the articular surfaces, the joint can be classified as a saddle joint.

Ligaments

1. The *capsular ligament* is attached laterally to the margins of the clavicular articular surface and medially to the margins of the articular areas on the sternum and on the first costal cartilage.
2. The capsular ligament is strong anteriorly and posteriorly where it constitutes the ***anterior and posterior sternoclavicular ligaments***.
3. The ***interclavicular ligament*** passes between the sternal ends of the right and left clavicles, some of its fibres being attached to the upper border of the manubrium sterni (Plate 10.1, Fig. 10.1).
4. The ***costoclavicular ligament*** is attached above to the rough area on the inferior aspect of the medial end of the clavicle. Inferiorly, it is attached to the first costal cartilage and to the first rib. It consists of anterior and posterior laminae.

Note: The main bond of union at this joint is the ***articular disc***. The disc is attached laterally to the clavicle on a rough area above and posterior to the articular area for the sternum. Inferiorly, the disc is attached to the sternum and to the first costal cartilage at their junction. Anteriorly and posteriorly, the disc fuses with the capsule.

Blood Supply

Internal thoracic and suprascapular arteries.

Nerve Supply

Medial supraclavicular nerve.

Movements

Movements of the sternoclavicular joint are elevation/depression, protraction/retraction, and anterior and posterior rotation of the clavicle. The anterior and posterior rotation of clavicle is utilised in overhead movements of the shoulder girdle.

DISSECTION

Remove the subclavius muscle from 1st rib at its attachment with its costal cartilage. Identify the costoclavicular ligament. Define the sternoclavicular joint and clean the anterior and superior surfaces of the capsule of this joint. Cut carefully through the joint to expose the intra-articular disc positioned between the clavicle and the sternum. The fibrocartilagenous disc divides the joint cavity into superomedial and inferolateral compartments.

ACROMIOCLAVICULAR JOINT

Features

Type

The acromioclavicular joint is a *plane synovial joint*.

Articular Surfaces

It is formed by articulation of small facets present:

1. At the lateral end of the clavicle.
2. On the medial margin of the acromion process of the scapula.

The facets are covered with fibrocartilage. The cavity of the joint is subdivided by an articular disc, which may have perforation in it (Plate 10.1, Fig. 10.1).

Ligaments

1. The bones are held together by a *fibrous capsule* and by the articular disc.
2. The main bond of union between the scapula and the clavicle is the *coracoclavicular ligament* (Fig. 10.1). The ligament consists of two parts—conoid and trapezoid. The *trapezoid part* is attached below to the upper surface of the coracoid process and above to the trapezoid line on the inferior surface of the lateral part of the clavicle. The *conoid part* is attached, below to the root of the coracoid process just lateral to the scapular notch. It is attached above to the inferior surface of the clavicle on the conoid tubercle.

Blood Supply

Suprascapular and thoracoacromial arteries.

Nerve Supply

Lateral supraclavicular nerve.

Movements

The movements of the acromioclavicular joints permit the movements of the shoulder joint specially the overhead abduction at shoulder.

Ligaments of the Scapula

1. ***Coracoacromial ligament*** (Fig. 10.1): It is a triangular ligament, the apex of which is attached to the tip of the acromion process, and the base to the lateral border of the coracoid process.

   The acromion process, the coracoacromial ligament, and the coracoid process together form the *coracoacromial arch,* which is known as the secondary socket of the joint and protects the head of the humerus.
2. ***Suprascapular ligament:*** It converts the scapular notch into a foramen. The suprascapular nerve passes below the ligament, and the suprascapular artery and vein above the ligament (Fig. 10.2).
3. ***Spinoglenoid ligament:*** It is a weak band that bridges the spinoglenoid notch. The suprascapular nerve and vessels pass beneath the arch to enter the infraspinous fossa (Fig. 10.2).

Plate 10.1: Sternoclavicular and acromioclavicular joints

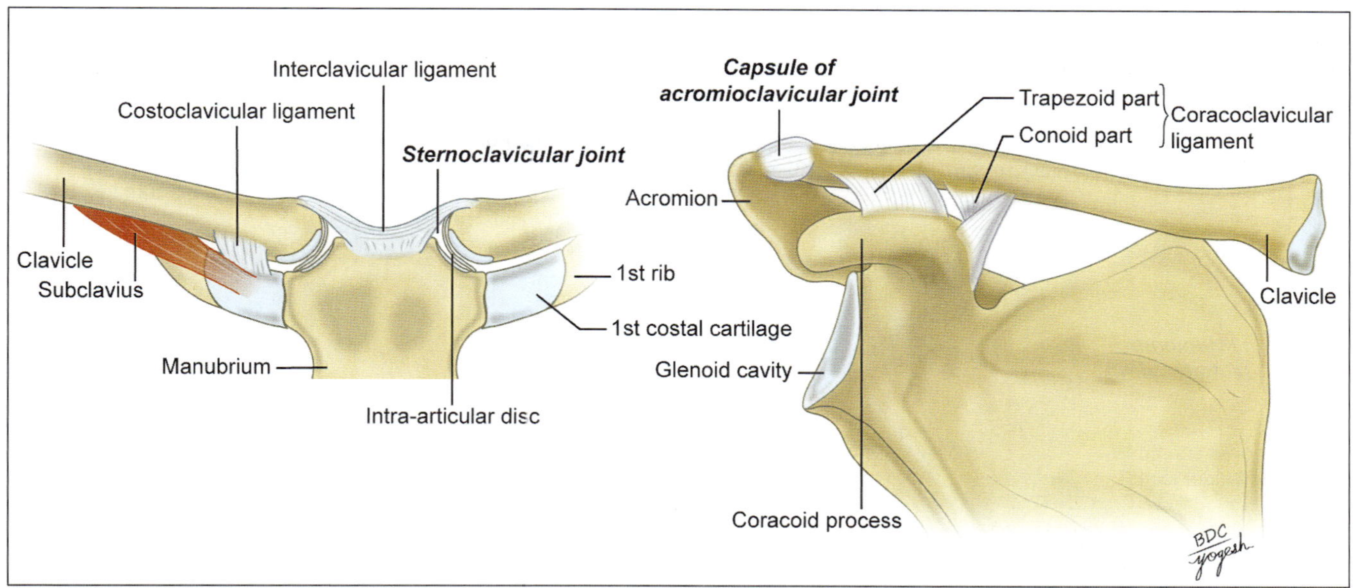

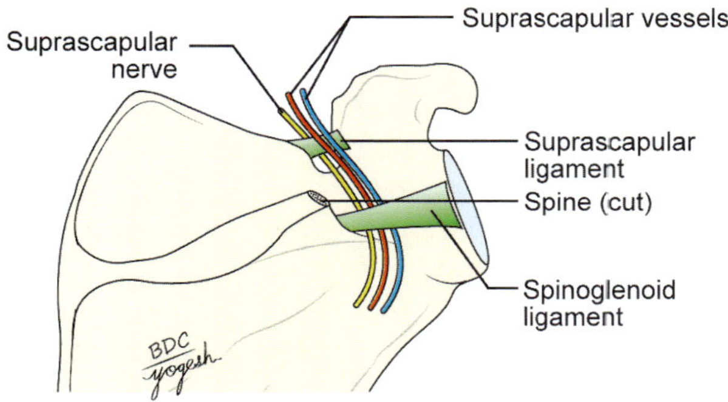

Fig. 10.2: The suprascapular and spinoglenoic ligaments

DISSECTION

Remove the muscles attached to the lateral end of clavicle and acromial process of scapula. Define the articular capsule surrounding the joint. Cut through the capsule to identify the intra-articular disc. Look for the strong coracoclavicular ligament.

Competency:

AN10.12 Describe and demonstrate shoulder joint for—type, articular surfaces, capsule, synovial membrane, ligaments, relations, movements, muscles involved, blood supply, nerve supply and applied anatomy.

CLINICAL ANATOMY

- ***Dislocation of clavicle***: The clavicle may be dislocated at either of its ends. At the medial end, it is usually dislocated forwards. Backward dislocation is rare as it is prevented by the costoclavicular ligament.

  The main bond of union between the clavicle and the manubrium is the articular disc. Apart from its attachment to the joint capsule, the disc is also attached above to the medial end of the clavicle, and below to the manubrium. This prevents the sternal end of the clavicle from tilting upwards when the weight of the arm depresses the acromial end (Fig. 10.1).

  The clavicle dislocates upwards at the acromioclavicular joint because the clavicle overrides the acromion process.
- ***Weight transmission***: The weight of the limb is transmitted from the scapula to the clavicle through the coracoclavicular ligament, and from the clavicle to the sternum through the sternoclavicular joint. Some of the weight also passes to the first rib by the costoclavicular ligament. The clavicle usually fractures between these two ligaments (Fig. 10.1).

SHOULDER JOINT

Type

The shoulder joint is a synovial joint of ball and socket variety.

Articular Surface

The joint is formed by articulation of the ***glenoid cavity of scapula*** and the ***head of the humerus*** (Plate 10.2, Fig. 10.3, Flowchart 10.1). Therefore, it is also known as the *glenohumeral articulation*. Structurally, it is a weak joint because the glenoid cavity is too small and shallow to hold the head of the humerus in place (the head is four times the size of the glenoid cavity). However, this arrangement permits great mobility.

Factors Maintaining Stability of Shoulder Joint

Stability of the joint is maintained by the following factors.

1. The coracoacromial arch or secondary socket for the head of the humerus.
2. The musculotendinous cuff of the shoulder formed by expansions from tendons of subscapularis (anteriorly);

Plate 10.2: Shoulder joint: Articular surfaces, ligaments and synovial membrane

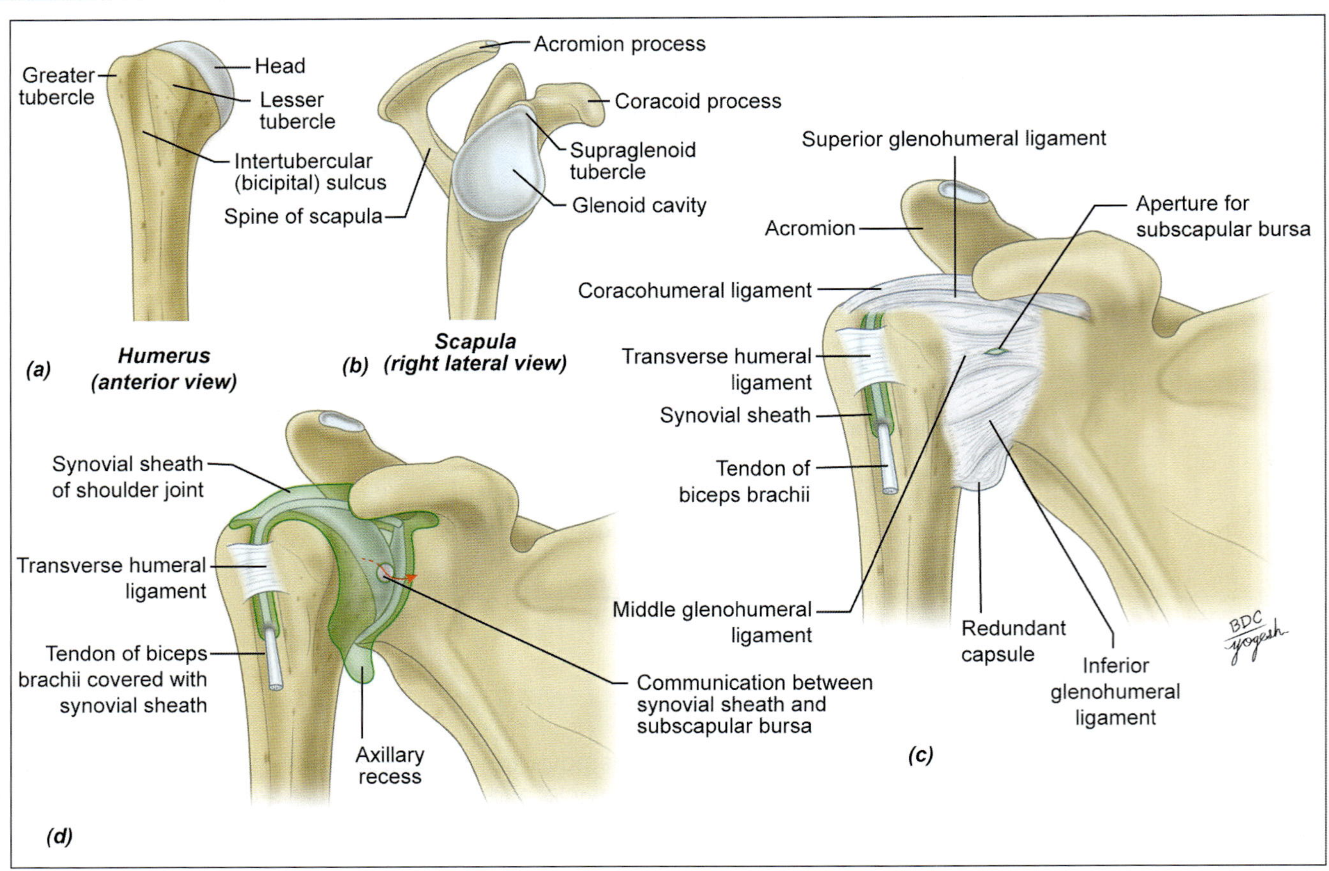

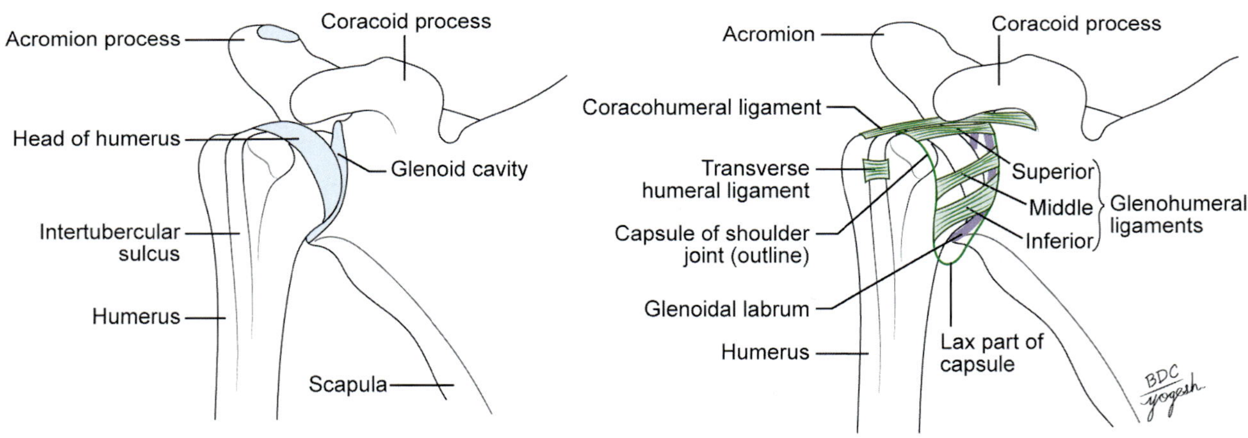

Fig. 10.3: Articular surfaces and ligaments of shoulder joint

supraspinatus (above) and infraspinatus and teres minor (posteriorly).

3. The glenoidal labrum (Latin *lip*) helps in deepening the glenoid fossa.
4. Stability is also provided by the muscles attaching the humerus to the pectoral girdle, the long head of the biceps brachii, and the long head of the triceps brachii.
5. Atmospheric pressure also stabilises the joint.

Ligaments

1. ***Capsular ligament:*** It is very loose and permits free movements. It is least supported inferiorly where dislocations are common. Such a dislocation may damage the closely related axillary nerve.
   - Medially, the capsule is attached to the scapula beyond the supraglenoid tubercle and the margins of the labrum.
   - Laterally, it is attached to the anatomical neck of the humerus with the following exceptions.
     - Inferiorly, the attachment extends down to the surgical neck.
     - Superiorly, it is deficient for passage of the tendon of the long head of the biceps brachii (Plate 10.2).

Flowchart 10.1: Shoulder joint

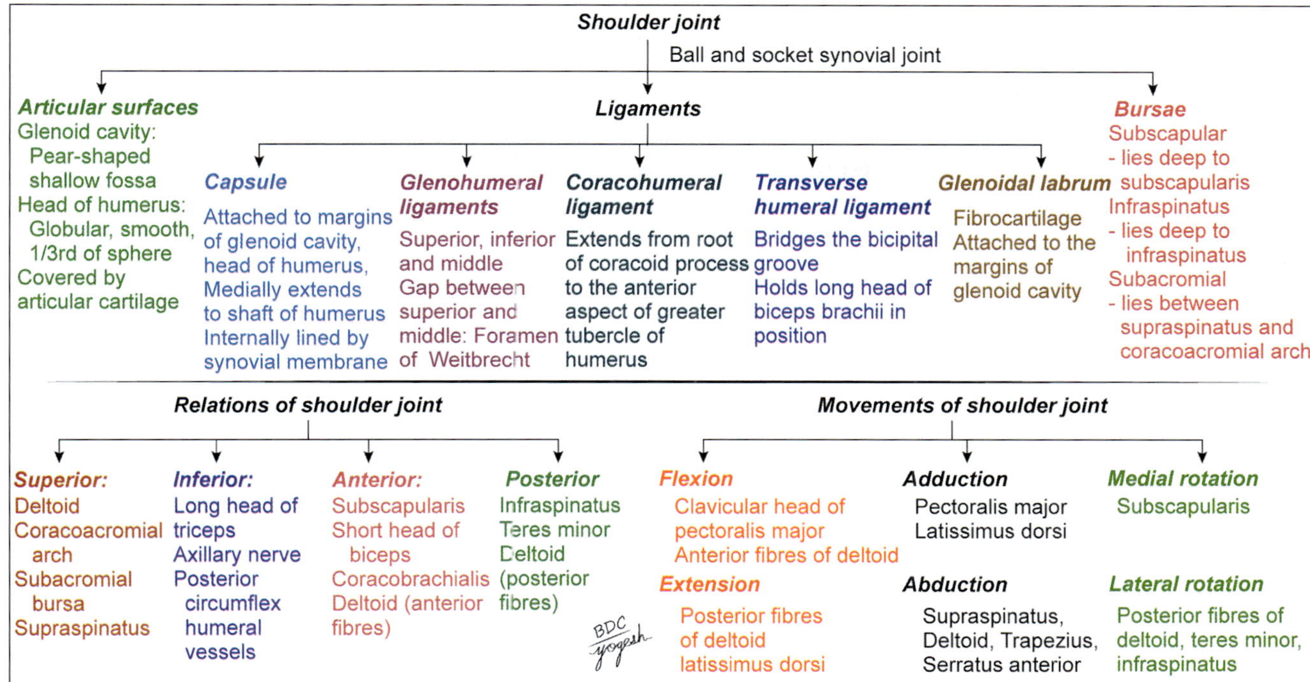

- Anteriorly, the capsule is reinforced by supplemental bands called the superior, middle, and inferior glenohumeral ligaments (Fig. 10.3). The area between the superior and middle glenohumeral ligament is a point of weakness in the capsule (foramen of Weitbrecht) which is a common site of anterior dislocation of humeral head.
- The capsule is lined with *synovial membrane*. An extension of this membrane forms a tubular sheath for the tendon of the long head of the biceps brachii.

2. ***Coracohumeral ligament:*** It extends from the root of the coracoid process to the neck of the humerus opposite the greater tubercle. It gives strength to the capsule.
3. ***Transverse humeral ligament:*** It bridges the upper part of the bicipital groove of the humerus (between the greater and lesser tubercles). The tendon of the long head of the biceps brachii passes deep to the ligament.
4. ***Glenoidal labrum:*** It is a fibrocartilaginous rim which covers the margins of the glenoid cavity, thus increasing the depth of the cavity.

Bursae Related to the Joint

1. The *subacromial (subdeltoid) bursa* (Plate 10.3, Fig. 10.4).
2. The *subscapular bursa*—communicates with the joint cavity.
3. The *infraspinatus bursa*—may communicate with the joint cavity.

The subacromial and the subdeltoid bursae are commonly continuous with each other but may be

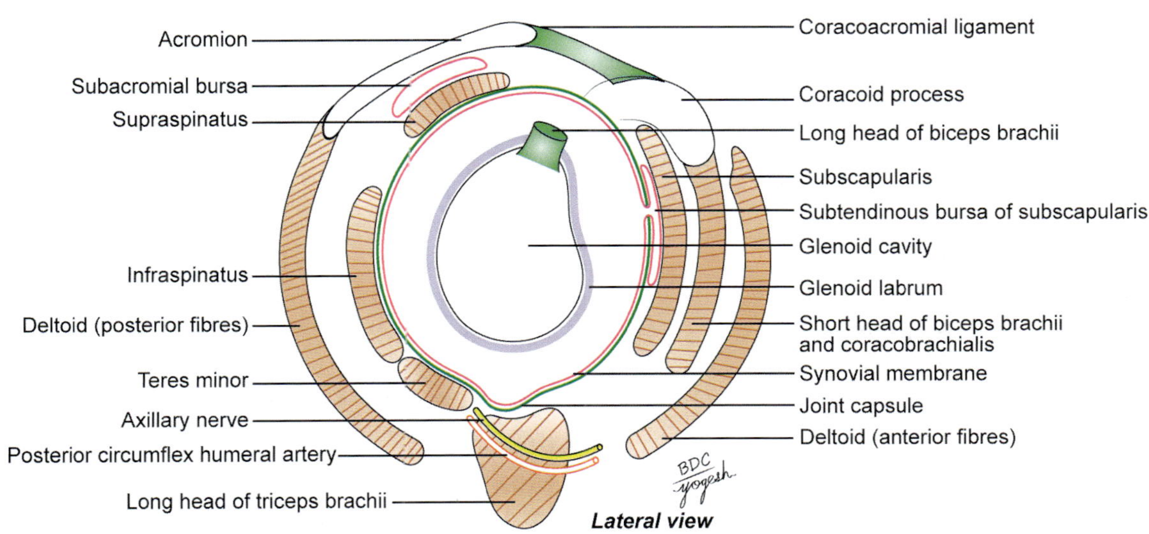

Fig. 10.4: Relations of shoulder joint (sagittal section)

Plate 10.3: Relations of shoulder joint

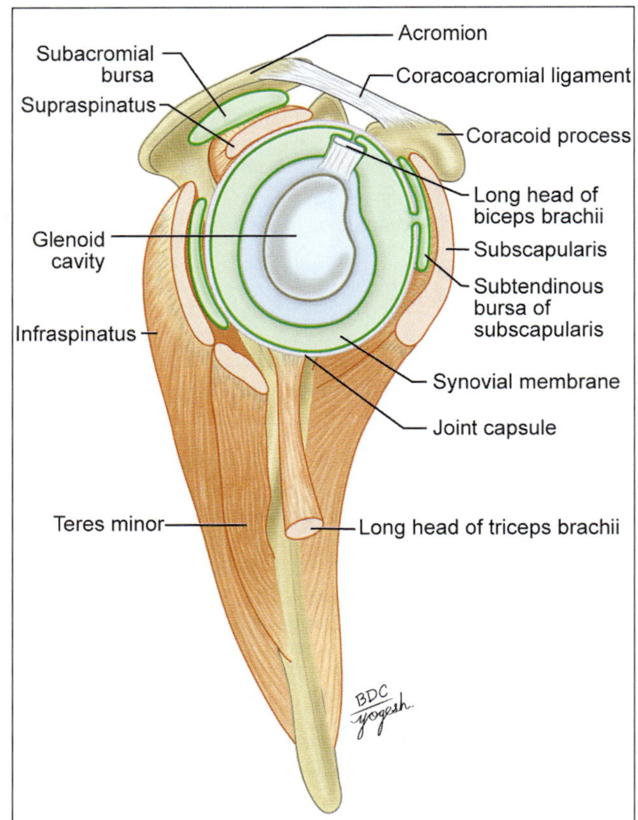

separate. Collectively they are called the subacromial bursa, which separates the acromion process and the coracoacromial ligaments from the supraspinatus tendon and permits smooth motion. Any failure of this mechanism can lead to inflammatory conditions of the supraspinatus tendon.

Relations

Superiorly:	Coracoacromial arch, subacromial bursa, supraspinatus and deltoid (Plate 10.3, Fig. 10.4).
Inferiorly:	Long head of the triceps brachii, axillary nerve and posterior circumflex humeral artery.
Anteriorly:	Subscapularis, coracobrachialis, short head of biceps brachii and deltoid.
Posteriorly:	Infraspinatus, teres minor and deltoid.
Within the joint:	Tendon of the long head of the biceps brachii.

Blood Supply

1. Anterior circumflex humeral vessels
2. Posterior circumflex humeral vessels
3. Suprascapular vessels
4. Subscapular vessels.

Nerve Supply

1. Axillary nerve
2. Musculocutaneous nerve
3. Suprascapular nerve.

Movements of Shoulder Joint

The shoulder joint enjoys great freedom of mobility at the cost of stability. The following movements take place at the shoulder joint (Figs 10.5 and 10.6):

1. ***Flexion and extension:*** During flexion, the arm moves forwards and medially, and during extension, the arm moves backwards and laterally. Thus, flexion and extension take place in a plane parallel to the surface of the glenoid cavity (Fig. 10.5).
2. ***Abduction and adduction*** take place at right angles to the plane of flexion and extension, i.e. approximately midway between the sagittal and coronal planes. In abduction, the arm moves anterolaterally away from the trunk. This movement is in the same plane as that of the body of the scapula (Fig. 10.5).
3. ***Medial and lateral rotations*** are best demonstrated with a mid-flexed elbow. In this position, the hand is moved medially across the chest either in front or behind the chest in medial rotation, and laterally in lateral rotation of the shoulder joint (Fig. 10.5).
4. ***Circumduction*** is a combination of different movements as a result of which the hand moves along a circle. The range of any movement depends on the availability of an area of free articular surface on the head of the humerus.
5. ***Scapulohumeral rhythm:*** In abduction of arm, two movements take place simultaneously as follows:
   a. Abduction of glenohumeral (shoulder) joint,
   b. Rotation of scapula. For every 2° abduction of shoulder joint, 1° rotation of scapula takes place. This is called scapulohumeral rhythm.

Muscles bringing about movements at shoulder joint are shown in Table 10.1.

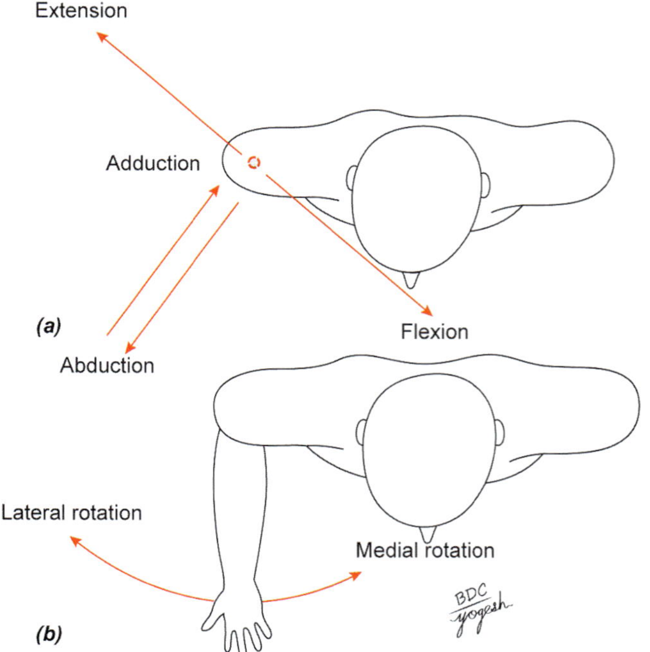

Figs 10.5a and b: Planes of movements of the shoulder joint: (a) Flexion, extension, abduction, adduction and (b) medial and lateral rotations

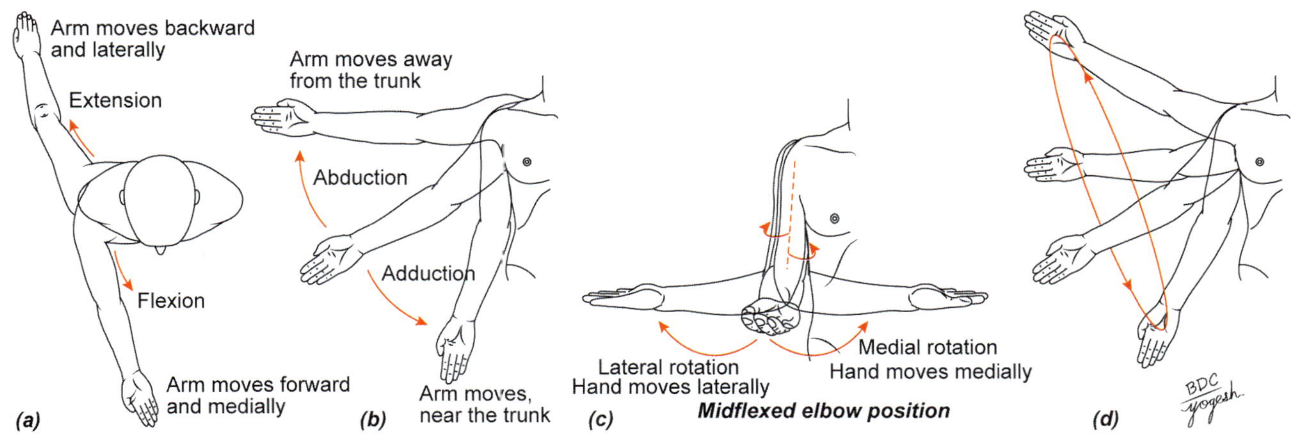

Figs 10.6a to d: Movements of the shoulder joint: (a) Flexion and extension, (b) abduction and adduction, (c) medial rotation and lateral rotation, and (d) circumduction

TABLE 10.1: Muscles bringing about movements at the shoulder joint

Movements	*Main muscles*	*Accessory muscles*
1. Flexion	• Clavicular head of the pectoralis major • Anterior fibres of deltoid	• Coracobrachialis • Short head of biceps brachii
2. Extension	• Posterior fibres of deltoid • Latissimus dorsi	• Teres major • Long head of triceps brachii • Sternocostal head of the pectoralis major
3. Adduction	• Pectoralis major • Latissimus dorsi	• Teres major • Coracobrachialis • Short head of biceps brachii • Long head of triceps brachii
4. Abduction	• Both supraspinatus and deltoid muscles initiate abduction and are involved throughout the range of abduction from 0°–90°. • Serratus anterior 90°–180° • Upper and lower fibres of trapezius 90°–180°	—
5. Medial rotation	• Subscapularis	• Pectoralis major • Anterior fibres of deltoid • Latissimus dorsi • Teres major
6. Lateral rotation	• Posterior fibres of deltoid	• Infraspinatus • Teres minor
7. Circumduction	• Combination of most of the above muscles	

DISSECTION

Identify the muscles attached to the greater, and lesser tubercles of humerus. Deep to the acromion process look for the subacromial bursa.

Identify coracoid process, acromion process and triangular coracoacromial arch binding these two bones together

Trace the supraspinatus muscle from supraspinous fossa of scapula to the greater tubercle of humerus. On its way, it is intimately fused to the capsule of the shoulder joint. In the same way, tendons of infraspinatus and teres minor also fuse with the posterior part of the capsule.

Inferiorly, trace the tendon of long head of triceps brachii from the infraglenoid tubercle of scapula.

Cut through the subscapularis muscle at the neck of scapula. It also gets fused with the anterior part of capsule of the shoulder joint as it passes to the lesser tubercle of humerus. Having studied the structures related to shoulder joint, the capsule of the joint is to be opened. A vertical incision is given in the posterior part of the capsule of the shoulder joint. The arm is rotated medially and laterally. This helps in head of humerus getting separated from the shallow glenoid cavity.

Inside the capsule, the shining tendon of long head of biceps brachii is visible as it traverses the intertubercular sulcus to reach the supraglenoid tubercle of scapula. This tendon also gets continuous with the labrum glenoidale attached to the rim of glenoid cavity.

CLINICAL ANATOMY

- ***Dislocation of shoulder joint:*** The shoulder joint is more prone to dislocation than any other joint. This is due to laxity of the capsule and the disproportionate area of the articular surfaces. Dislocation may be anterior or posterior. Anterior dislocation is more common and usually occurs when the arm is abducted. In this position, the head of the humerus presses against the lower unsupported part of the capsular ligament. Thus, almost always, the dislocation is primarily subglenoid. Dislocation endangers the axillary nerve, which is closely related to the lower part of the joint capsule (Fig. 10.7).
- ***Optimum attitude:*** In order to avoid ankylosis, many diseases of the shoulder joint are treated in an optimum position of the joint. In this position, the arm is abducted by 45°–90°.
- ***Aspiration of shoulder joint:*** The shoulder joint is most commonly approached (surgically) from the front. However, for aspiration, the needle may be introduced either anteriorly through the deltopectoral triangle (closer to the deltoid) or laterally just below the acromion process (Fig. 10.8).
- ***Frozen shoulder:*** This is a common occurrence. Pathologically, there is fibroelastic proliferation in the capsule that leads to formation of adhesions and consequent stiffness and pain on attempted movements. Clinically, the patient (usually 40–60 years of age) complains of progressively increasing pain in the shoulder, stiffness in the joint, and restriction of all movements, particularly external rotation, abduction, and medial rotation.
- The surrounding muscles show disuse atrophy. The disease is self-limiting and the patient may recover spontaneously in about two years and much earlier by physiotherapy.
- ***Calcific tendinitis of shoulder:*** It results from:
  a. inflammation and calcification of subacromial bursa —called calcific *scapulohumeral bursitis*
  b. calcified supraspinatus tendon causing *subacromial bursitis*.
- ***Glenoidal labrum tears:*** It occurs commonly in athletes with shoulder instability. It results in painful movements of the shoulder joint.

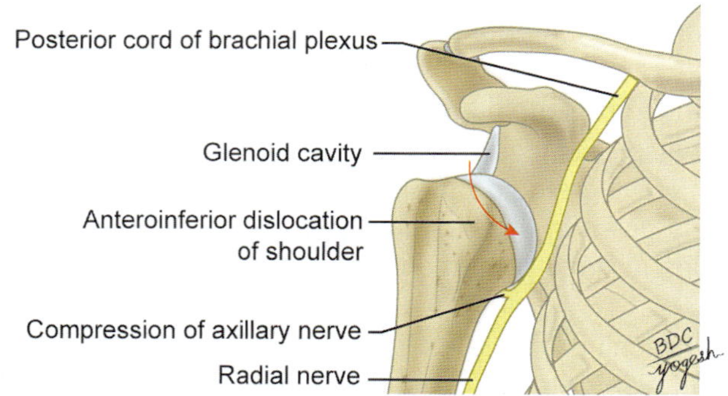

Fig. 10.7: Dislocation of shoulder joint (right, anterior view)

- ***Shoulder tip pain:*** Irritation of the peritoneum underlying diaphragm from any surrounding pathology causes referred pain in the shoulder. This is so because the phrenic nerve carrying impulses from peritoneum and the supraclavicular nerves (supplying the skin over the shoulder) both arise from spinal segments C3, C4 (Fig. 10.9).

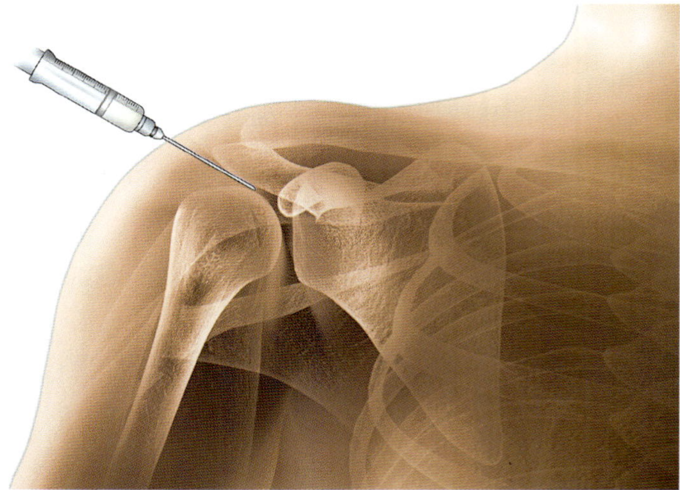

Fig. 10.8: Site of aspiration of shoulder joint

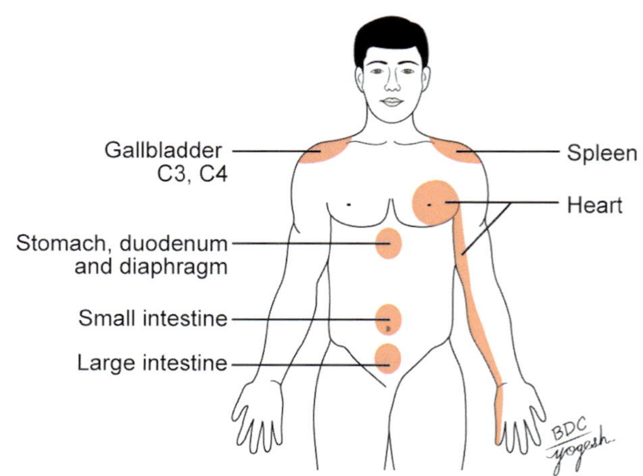

Fig. 10.9: Shoulder tip pain. Other sites of referred pain

Competency:

AN13.3 Identify and describe the type, articular surfaces, capsule, synovial membrane, ligaments, relations, movements, blood and nerve supply of elbow joint, proximal and distal radioulnar joints, wrist joint and first carpometacarpal joint.

ELBOW JOINT

The elbow joint is a joint between the lower end of humerus and the upper ends of radius and ulna bones. Elbow joint is the term used for *humeroradial* and *humeroulnar joints*. The term elbow complex also includes the superior radioulnar joint also (Plate 10.4, Fig. 10.10, Flowchart 10.2).

Plate 10.4: Elbow joint: Articular surfaces and capsular ligament

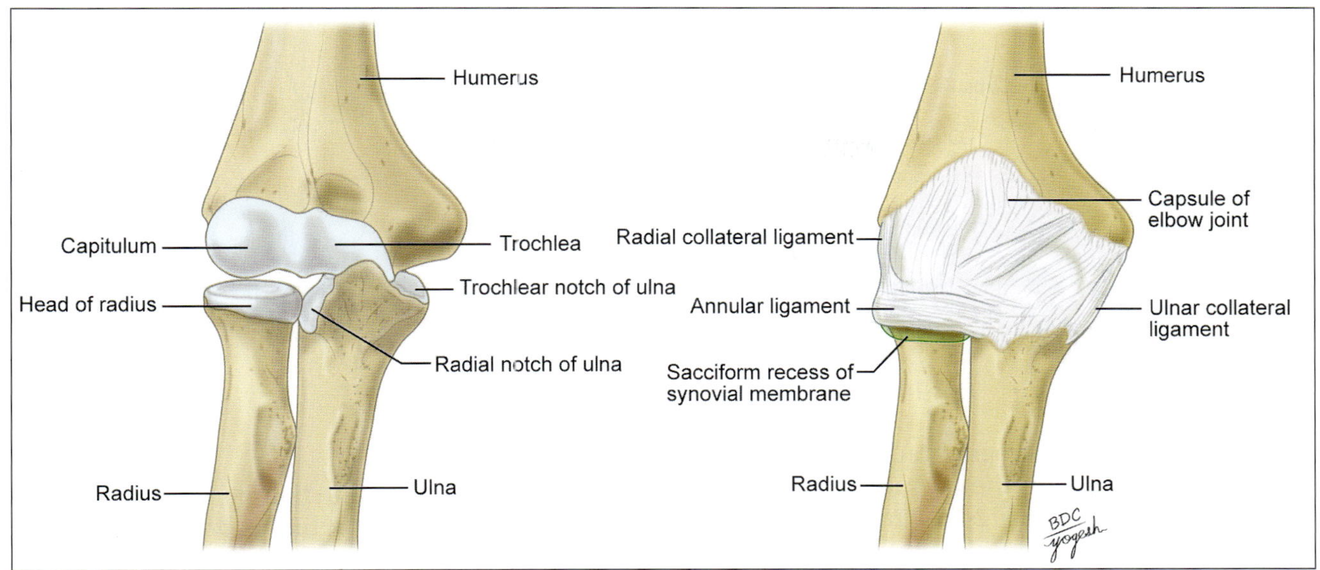

Flowchart 10.2: Elbow joint

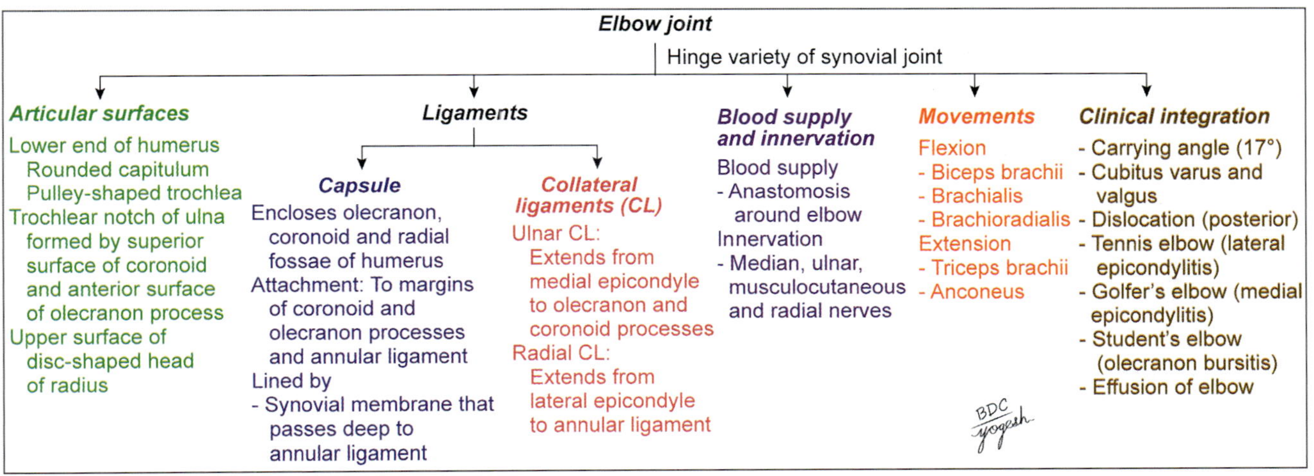

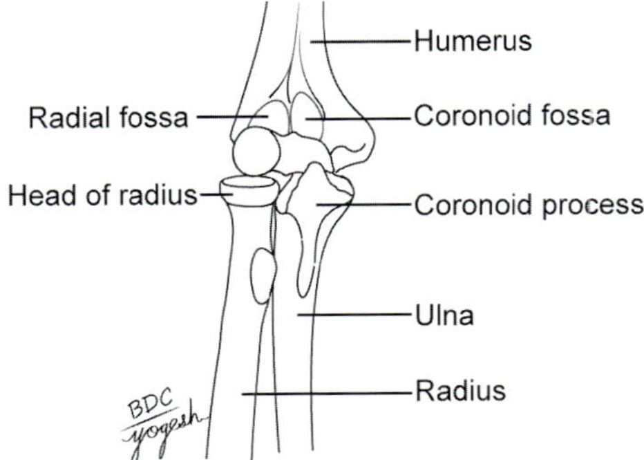

Fig. 10.10: Elbow joint: Articular surfaces

Type

The elbow joint is a *hinge* variety of synovial joint. It is also a *compound joint* as more than one bone participate in the joint formation (humerus, radius, and ulna).

Articular Surfaces

Upper

The ***capitulum and trochlea of the humerus***. The *coronoid fossa* lies just above the trochlea and is designed in a manner that the coronoid process of ulna fits into it in extreme flexion. Similarly, the *radial fossa* just above the capitulum allows for radial head fitting in the radial fossa in extreme flexion.

Lower

1. Upper surface of the ***head of the radius*** articulates with the capitulum.
2. ***Trochlear notch of the ulna*** articulates with the trochlea of the humerus.

The elbow joint is continuous with the superior radioulnar joint. The humeroradial, the humeroulnar, and the superior radioulnar joints are together known as ***cubital articulations***.

Ligaments

1. ***Capsular ligament:*** *Superiorly*, it is attached to the lower end of the humerus in such a way that the capitulum, the trochlea, the radial fossa, the coronoid fossa, and the olecranon fossa are intracapsular. *Inferomedially*, it is attached to the margin of the trochlear notch of the ulna except laterally; *inferolaterally*, it is attached to the

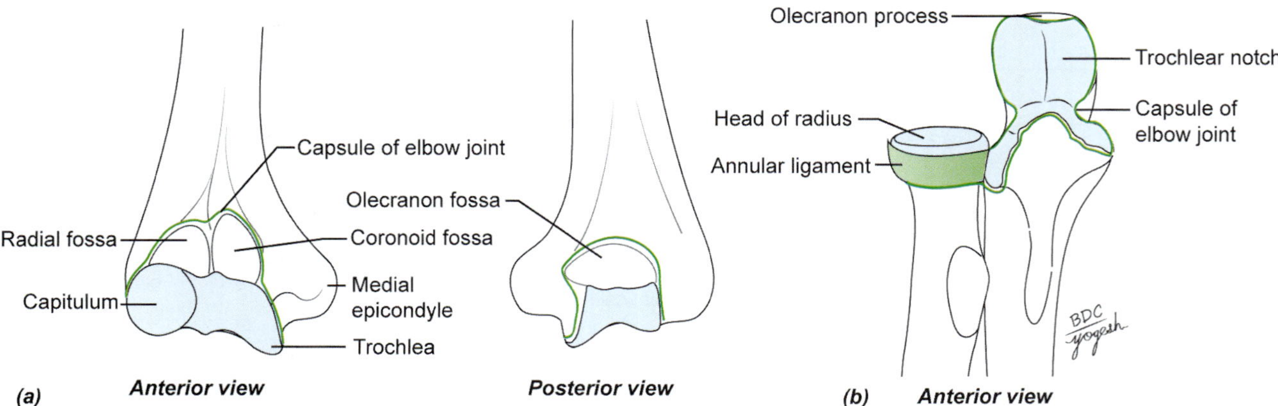

Figs 10.11a and b: Attachment of the capsular ligament

annular ligament of the superior radioulnar joint. The synovial membrane lines the capsule and the fossae, named above (Plate 10.4, Figs 10.11a and b).

The *anterior ligament* and the *posterior ligament* are thickenings of the capsule.

2. ***Ulnar collateral ligament*** is triangular in shape (Fig. 10.12a). Its apex is attached to the medial epicondyle of the humerus, and its base to the ulna. The ligament has thick anterior and posterior bands: These are attached below to the coronoid process and the olecranon process, respectively. Their lower ends are joined to each other by an oblique band which gives attachment to the thinner intermediate fibres of the ligament. The ligament is crossed by the *ulnar nerve* and it gives origin to the flexor digitorum superficialis.
3. ***Radial collateral or lateral ligament****:* It is a fan-shaped band extending from the lateral epicondyle to the annular ligament. It gives origin to the supinator and to the extensor carpi radialis brevis (Fig. 10.12b).

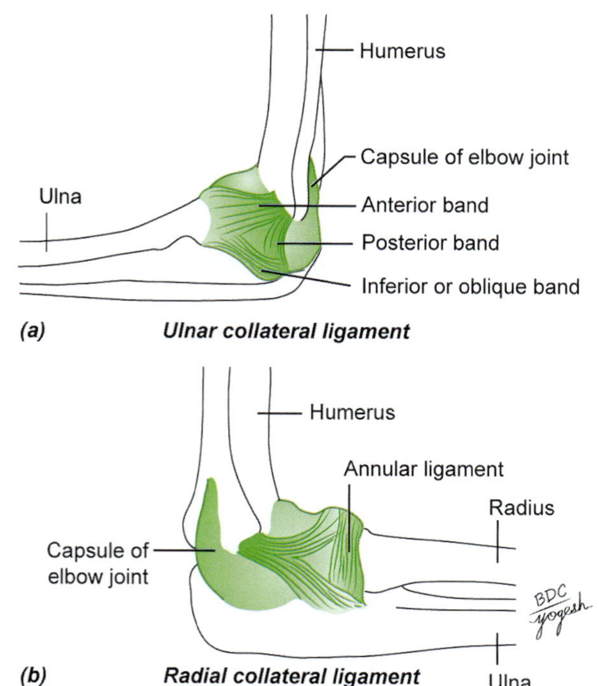

Figs 10.12a and b: (a) Ulnar collateral ligament, (b) radial collateral ligament

Relations

Anteriorly: Brachialis, median nerve, brachial artery, and tendon of biceps brachii (Fig. 10.13).

Posteriorly: Triceps brachii and anconeus.

Medially: Ulnar nerve, flexor carpi ulnaris and common flexors.

Laterally: Supinator, extensor carpi radialis brevis and other common extensors.

Bursae Related to Elbow Joint

- Elbow joint is supported with the following bursae (Fig. 10.14):
  1. ***Olecranon bursae:***
     a. *Subcutaneous olecranon bursa:* It lies between skin and posterior triangular surface of the olecranon.
     b. *Subtendinous olecranon bursa*: It lies between the tendon of triceps brachii and superior surface of olecranon process of ulna.
  2. ***Bicipitoradial bursa:*** It lies between the tendon of biceps brachii and anterior smooth part of radial tuberosity.

Blood Supply

From anastomoses around the elbow joint (*see* Fig. 8.11).

Nerve Supply

The joint receives branches from the following nerves:
1. Ulnar nerve
2. Median nerve
3. Radial nerve
4. Musculocutaneous nerve through its branch to the brachialis.

Movements

1. Flexion is brought about by:
   - Brachialis
   - Biceps brachii
   - Brachioradialis.

[*Mnemonics:* Busy Bees Buzz: **B**rachialis, **B**iceps brachii, **B**rachioradialis.]

2. Extension is produced by:
   - Triceps brachii
   - Anconeus.

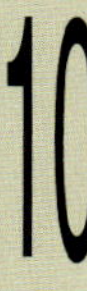

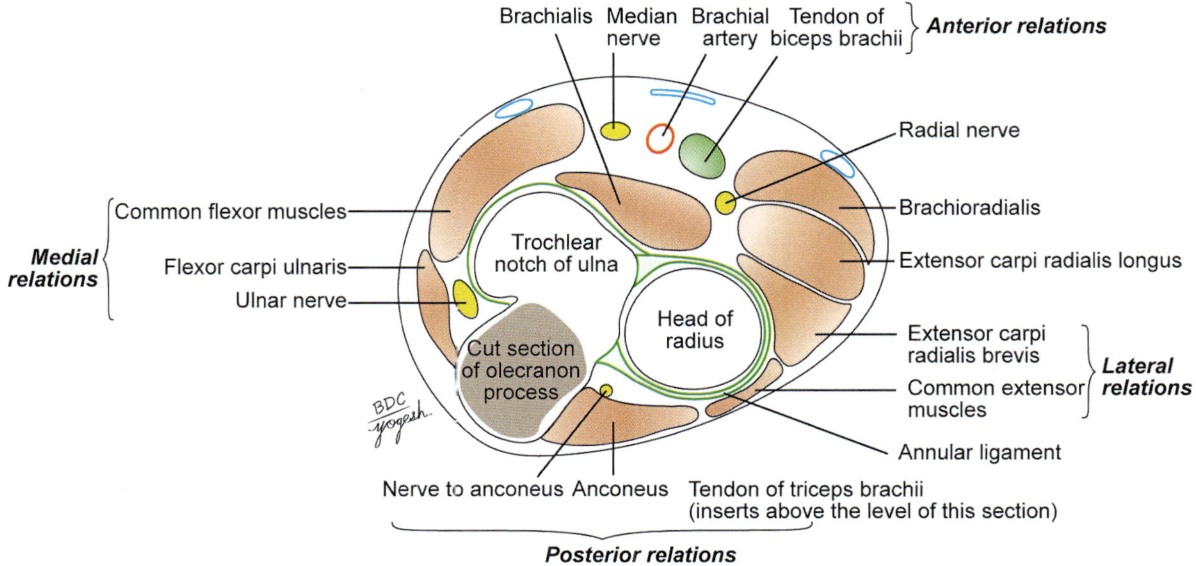

Fig. 10.13: Relations of elbow joint (superior view, section passing through the cavity of elbow joint)

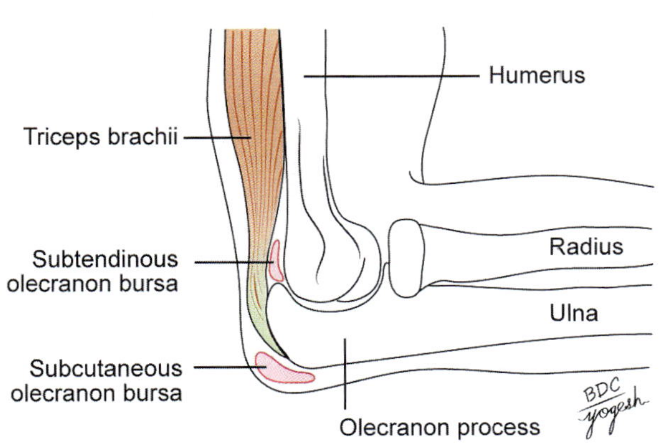

Fig. 10.14: Bursae related to elbow joint

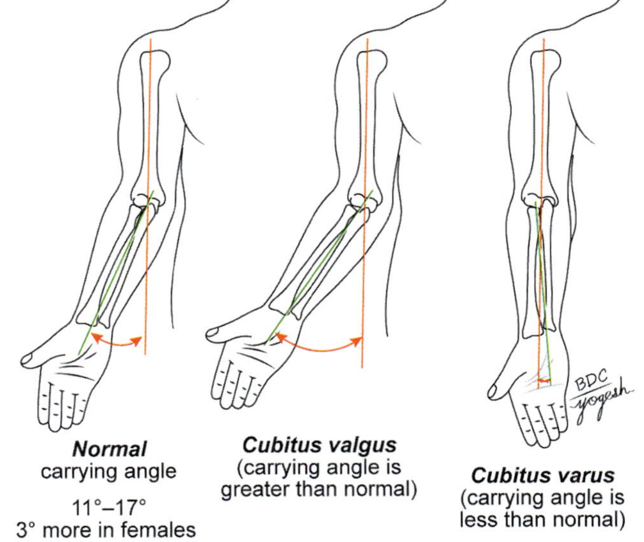

Fig. 10.15: Carrying angle, cubitus varus and cubitus valgus

Carrying Angle

Definition: In extended forearm, carrying angle is the angle of deviation of long axis of forearm from the long axis *of arm* (Fig. 10.15).

Anatomical basis: The transverse axis of the elbow joint is directed medially and downwards. Because of this, the extended forearm is not in straight line with the arm, but makes an angle of about 13° with it. This is known as the *carrying angle.*

The factors responsible for formation of the carrying angle are as follows:

1. The medial flange of the trochlea is 6 mm deeper than the lateral flange.
2. The superior articular surface of the coronoid process of the ulna is placed oblique to the long axis of the bone.

Normal carrying angle is 11°–17°. Carrying angle varies from individual to individual. It is 3° more in females than in males.

The carrying angle disappears in full flexion of the elbow, and also during pronation of the forearm. The forearm comes in line with the arm in the midprone position, and this is the position in which the hand is mostly used. This arrangement of gradually increasing carrying angle during extension of the elbow increases the precision with which the hand (and objects held in it) can be controlled.

DISSECTION

Cut through the muscles arising from the lateral and medial epicondyles of humerus and reflect them distally, if not already done. Also cut through biceps brachii, brachialis, and triceps brachii 3 cm proximal to the elbow joint and reflect them distally. Remove all the muscles fused with the fibrous capsule of the elbow joint and define its attachments.

CLINICAL ANATOMY

- ***Elbow effusion:*** Distension of the elbow joint by an effusion occurs posteriorly because here the capsule is weak and the covering deep fascia is thin. Aspiration is done posteriorly on any side of the olecranon process (Fig. 10.16).
- ***Dislocation* of the elbow** is usually posterior, and is often associated with fracture of the coronoid process. The triangular relationship between the olecranon process and the two humeral epicondyles is lost.
- ***Pulled elbow***: *Subluxation* of the head of the radius (pulled elbow) occurs in children when the forearm is suddenly pulled in pronation. The head of the radius slips out from the annular ligament (*see* Fig. 2.21).
- ***Tennis elbow*** usually occurs in tennis players. It affects individuals whose work profile involves repetitive wrist extension against resistance and twisting activities (Fig. 10.17). This is possibly due to:
  1. Sprain of radial collateral ligament.
  2. Tearing of fibres of the extensor carpi radialis brevis.
  3. Recent researches have pointed out that it is more of a degenerative condition rather than inflammatory condition.
- ***Student's (miner's) elbow*** is characterised by effusion into the bursa over the subcutaneous posterior surface of the olecranon process. Students during lectures support their head (for sleeping) with their hands with flexed elbows. The bursa on the olecranon process gets inflamed (Fig. 10.18).
- ***Golfer's elbow*** is the microtrauma of medial epicondyle of humerus, occurs commonly in golf players. The common flexor origin undergoes repetitive strain and results in a painful condition on the medial side of the elbow (Fig. 10.19).
- ***Cubitus valgus and varus:*** If carrying angle (normal is 11°–17°) is more, the condition is *cubitus valgus*, ulnar nerve may get stretched leading to weakness of intrinsic muscles of hand. If the angle is less, it is called *cubitus varus* (Fig. 10.20).
- *Under* ***optimal position*** *of the elbow*: Generally elbow flexion between 30° and 40° is sufficient to perform common activities of daily living such as eating, combing, dressing, etc. Because of this flexion or extension after a fracture/trauma are able to accomplish these personal tasks without much problems.

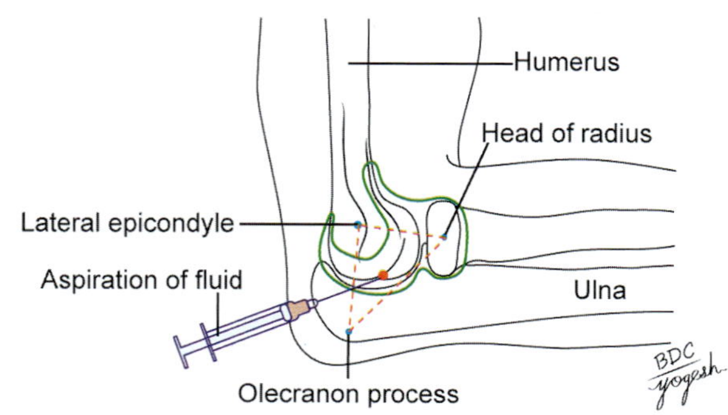

Fig. 10.16: Aspiration of elbow joint

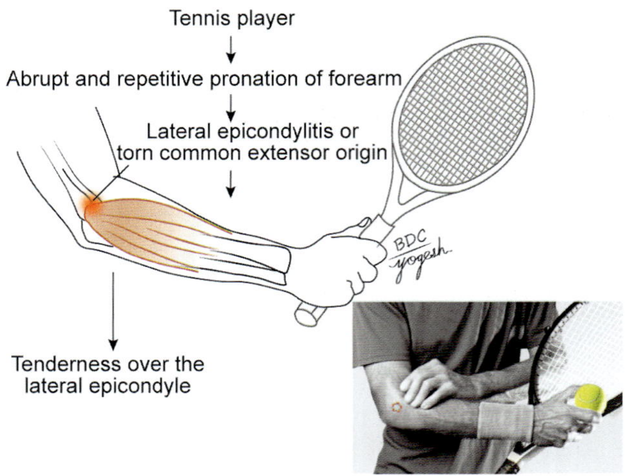

Fig. 10.17: Tennis elbow

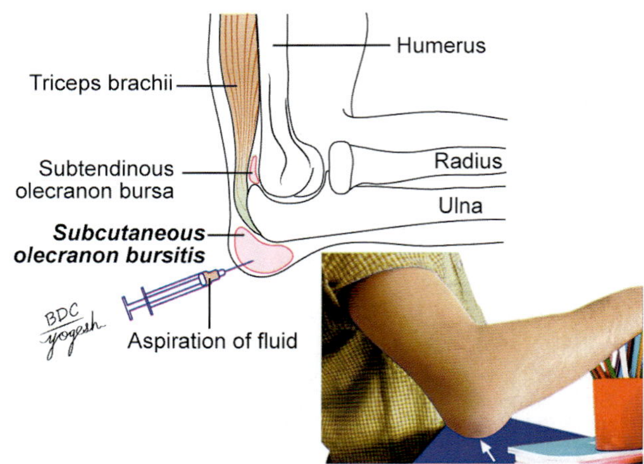

Fig. 10.18: Student's elbow

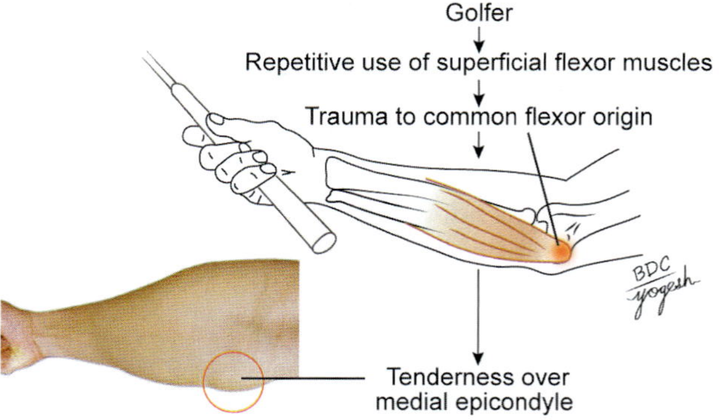

Fig. 10.19: Golfer's elbow

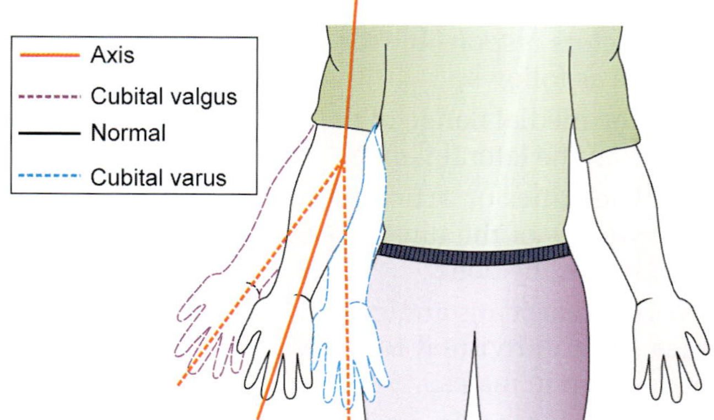

Fig. 10.20: Normal, cubitus valgus, and cubitus varus

RADIOULNAR JOINTS

Features

Radius and ulna articulate with each other at three junctions as follows (Plate 10.5, Flowchart 10.3):

1. *Superior radioulnar joint* (Table 10.2).
2. *Middle radioulnar joint* – formed by interosseous membrane.
3. *Inferior radioulnar joint* (Table 10.2).

INTEROSSEOUS MEMBRANE

The interosseous membrane connects the shafts of the radius and ulna. It is attached to the interosseous borders of these bones. The fibres of the membrane run downwards and medially from the radius to ulna (Plate 10.5, Fig. 10.21).

The two bones are also connected by the ***oblique cord*** which extends from the tuberosity of the ulna to the tuberosity of the radius. The direction of its fibres is opposite to that in the interosseous membrane. The oblique cord represents degenerated part of the flexor pollicis longus muscle.

Features

1. Superiorly, the interosseous membrane begins 2–3 cm below the radial tuberosity. Between the oblique cord and the interosseous membrane, there is a gap for passage of the posterior interosseous vessels to the back of the forearm.
2. Inferiorly, a little above its lower margin, there is an aperture for the passage of the anterior interosseous vessels to the back of the forearm.
3. The anterior surface is related to the flexor pollicis longus, the flexor digitorum profundus, the pronator quadratus, and to the anterior interosseous vessels and nerve.
4. The posterior surface is related to the supinator, the abductor pollicis longus, the extensor pollicis brevis, the extensor pollicis longus, the extensor indicis, the anterior interosseous artery, and the posterior interosseous nerve.

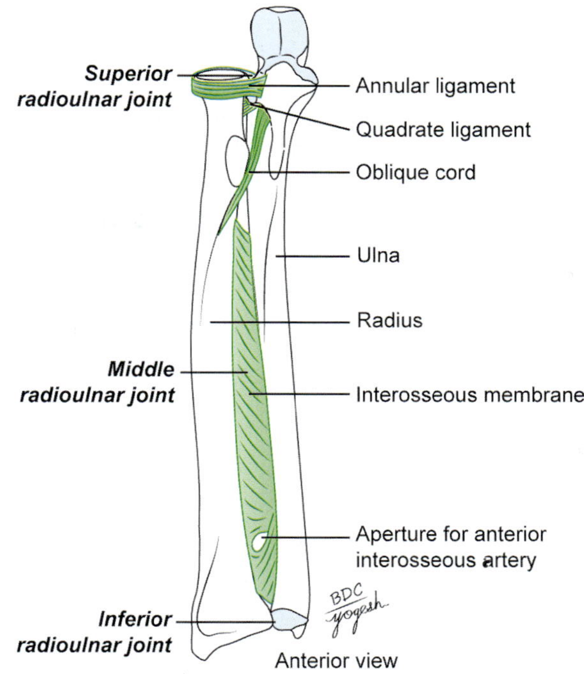

Fig. 10.21: Ligaments of radioulnar joints

Flowchart 10.3: Superior and inferior radioulnar joints

Radioulnar joints	*Superior radioulnar joint*	*Inferior radioulnar joint*
Type	Uniaxial pivot synovial joint	Uniaxial pivot synovial joint
Articular surfaces	Head of radius Radial notch of ulna Annular ligament	Capsular ligament Triangular fibrocartilage
Ligaments	Capsular ligament Quadrate ligament	Head of ulna Ulnar notch of radius
Prime stabiliser	Annular ligament	Triangular articular disc
Movements	Supination and pronation	Supination and pronation

TABLE 10.2: Radioulnar joints (Fig. 10.19)

Features	*Superior radioulnar joint*	*Inferior radioulnar joint*
Type	Pivot type of synovial joint	Pivot type of synovial joint
Articular surfaces	• Circumference of head of radius • Osseofibrous ring, formed by the radial notch of the ulna and the annular ligament	• Head of ulna • Ulnar notch of radius
Ligaments	• The annular ligament forms four-fifths of the ring within which the head of the radius rotates. It is attached to the margins of the radial notch of the ulna, and is continuous with the capsule of the elbow joint above • The quadrate ligament extends from the neck of the radius to the lower margin of the radial notch of the ulna	• The capsule surrounds the joint. The weak upper part is evaginated by the synovial membrane to form a recess (recessus sacciformis) in front of the interosseous membrane • The apex of triangular fibrocartilaginous articular disc is attached to the base of the styloid process of the ulna, and the base to the lower margin of the ulnar notch of the radius (Fig. 10.20)
Blood supply	Anastomoses around the lateral side of the elbow joint	Anterior and posterior interosseous arteries
Nerve supply	Musculocutaneous, median, and radial nerves	Anterior and posterior interosseous nerves
Movements	Supination and pronation	Supination and pronation

Plate 10.5: Radioulnar joint

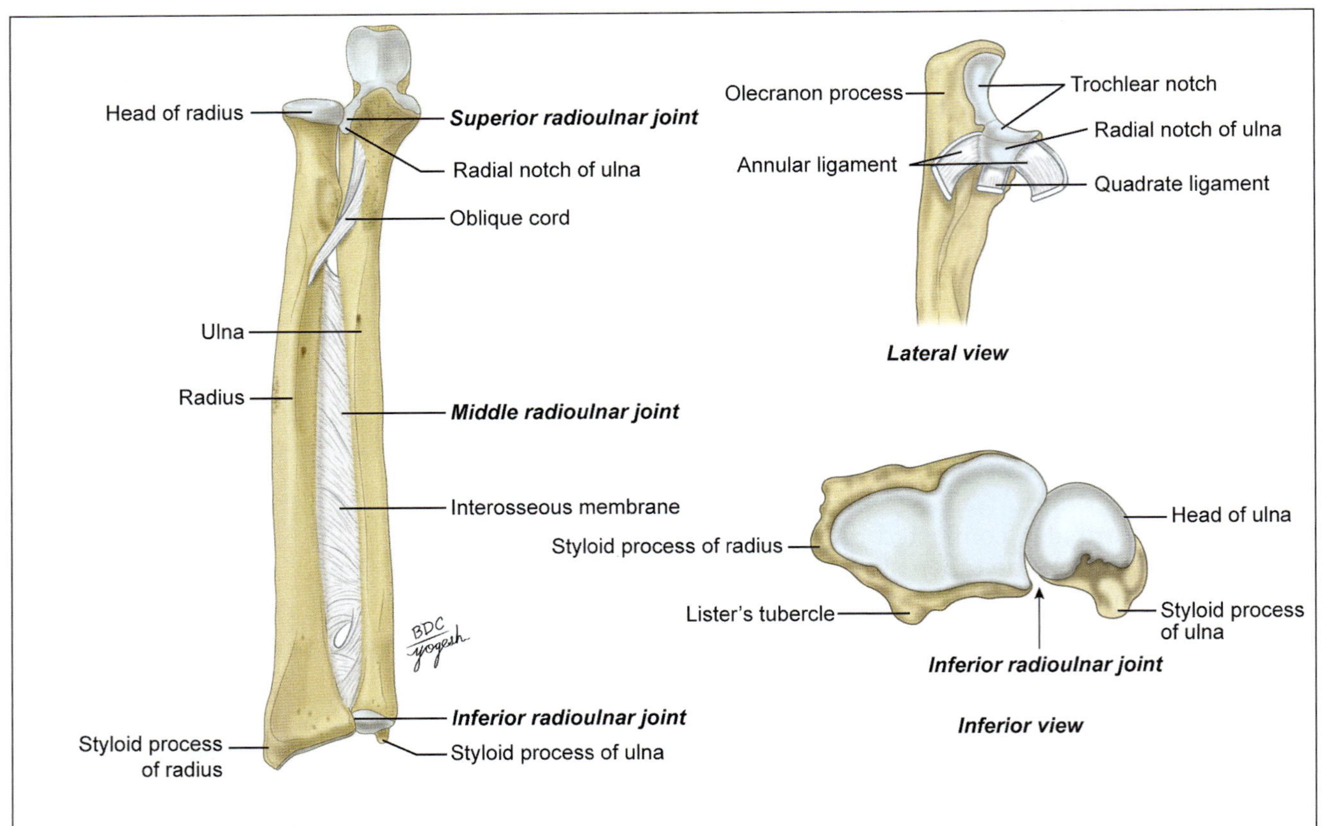

Functions

The interosseous membrane performs the following functions.

1. It binds the radius and ulna to each other.
2. It provides attachments to many muscles.
3. It transmits forces (including weight) applied to the radius (through the hand) to the ulna. This transmission is necessary as radius is the main bone taking part in the wrist joint, while the ulna is the main bone taking part in the elbow joint.
4. Separates the forearm into flexor and extensor compartments.

MIDDLE RADIOULNAR JOINT

Type: Syndesmosis, joined by interosseous membrane attached to interosseous borders of radius and ulna. It is attached to posterior border of medial surface at lower end of radius.

SUPINATION AND PRONATION

Definition: Supination and pronation are rotatory movements of the forearm/hand around a vertical axis. In a semiflexed elbow, the palm is turned upwards in supination, and downwards in pronation (*kings pronate, beggars supinate*).

Involved joints: The movements are permitted at the superior and inferior radioulnar joints. During pronation, head of radius spins within annular ligament. As radius with the hand comes medially across the lower part of ulna, the interosseous membrane is spiralised. During supination, the membrane is despiralised.

Axis: The vertical axis of movement of the radius passes through the centre of the head of the radius above, and through the ulnar attachment of the articular disc below (Fig. 10.22). However, this axis is not stationary because the lower end of the ulna is not fixed: It moves backwards and laterally during pronation, and forwards and medially during supination. As a result of this movement, the axis (defined above) is displaced laterally in pronation, and medially in supination.

Muscles Responsible

1. Around 50° of supination and 50° of pronation are generally required to perform many of the routine activities, brought about by brachioradialis.
2. *Pronation is brought about* chiefly by the pronator quadratus. It is aided by the pronator teres when the movement is rapid and against resistance. Gravity also helps.
3. *Supination is brought about* by the supinator muscle and the biceps brachii. Slow supination, with elbow extended, is done by the supinator. Rapid supination with the elbow flexed, and when performed against resistance, is done mainly by the biceps brachii. Both the pronators and both the supinators are "inserted into radius". Even brachioradialis performing halfway pronation and supination is "inserted into radius".

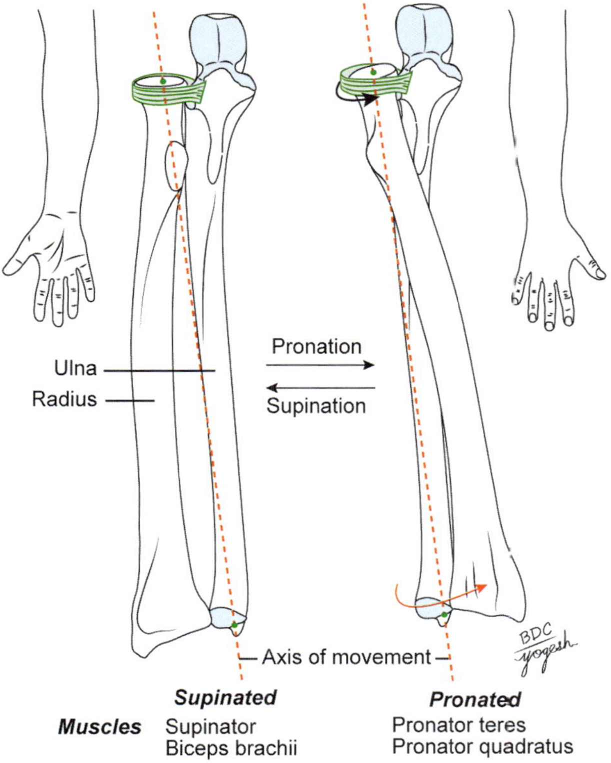

Fig. 10.22: Supination and pronation

Functional utility: Supination is more powerful than pronation because it is an antigravity movement. Supination movements are responsible for all screwing movements of the hand, e.g. as in tightening nuts and bolts. Morphologically, pronation and supination were evolved for picking up food and taking it to the mouth.

CLINICAL ANATOMY

Supination and pronation: During supination, the radius and ulna are parallel to each other. During pronation, radius crosses over the ulna (Fig. 10.22). In synostosis (fusion) of upper end of radius and ulna, pronation is not possible.

DISSECTION

Remove all the muscles covering the adjacent sides of radius, ulna and the intervening interosseous membrane. This will expose the superior and inferior radioulnar joints including the interosseous membrane. Cut through the annular ligament to see the superior radioulnar joint.

Clean and define the interosseous membrane. Lastly cut through the capsule of inferior radioulnar joint to locate the intra-articular fibrocartilaginous disc of the joint. Learn the movements of supination and pronation on dry bones and on yourself.

WRIST (RADIOCARPAL) JOINT

Wrist joint is a joint between lower end of radius and articular disc of inferior radioulnar joint proximally and three lateral bones of proximal row of carpus, i.e. scaphoid, lunate and triquetral distally (Plate 10.6, Flowchart 10.4).

Note: The pisiform does not play a role in the radiocarpal articulation. It is a sesamoid bone acting as a pulley for flexor carpi ulnaris.

Type

Wrist joint is a synovial joint of the ellipsoid variety (biaxial joint). It is *compound* synovial joint as more than two bones participate in the joint formation.

Articular Surfaces

Upper

1. Inferior surface of the lower end of the radius (Fig. 10.23).
2. Articular disc of the inferior radioulnar joint (Fig. 10.23).

Lower

1. Scaphoid
2. Lunate
3. Triquetral bones.

Ligaments (Fig. 10.24)

1. The ***articular capsule*** surrounds the joint. It is attached above to the lower ends of the radius and ulna, and below to the proximal row of carpal bones.
2. The ***palmar radiocarpal ligament*** is a broad band. It begins above from the anterior margin of the lower end of the radius and its styloid process, runs downwards and medially, and is attached below to the anterior surfaces of the scaphoid, the lunate, and triquetral bones.
3. The ***palmar ulnocarpal ligament*** is a rounded fasciculus. It begins above from the base of the styloid process of the ulna and the anterior margin of the articular disc, runs downwards and laterally, and is attached to the lunate and triquetral bones. Both the palmar carpal ligaments are considered to be intracapsular.
4. The ***dorsal radiocarpal ligament*** is weaker than the palmar ligaments. It begins above from the

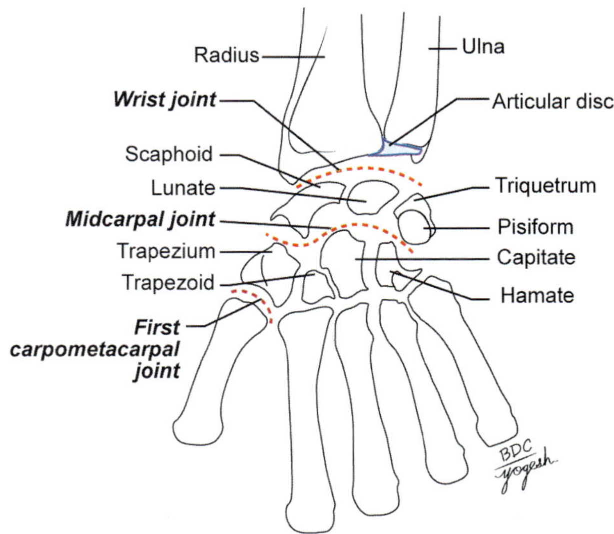

Fig. 10.23: Wrist, midcarpal and 1st carpometacarpal joints

Plate 10.6: Wrist joint: Articular surface and ligaments (Fig. 10.24)

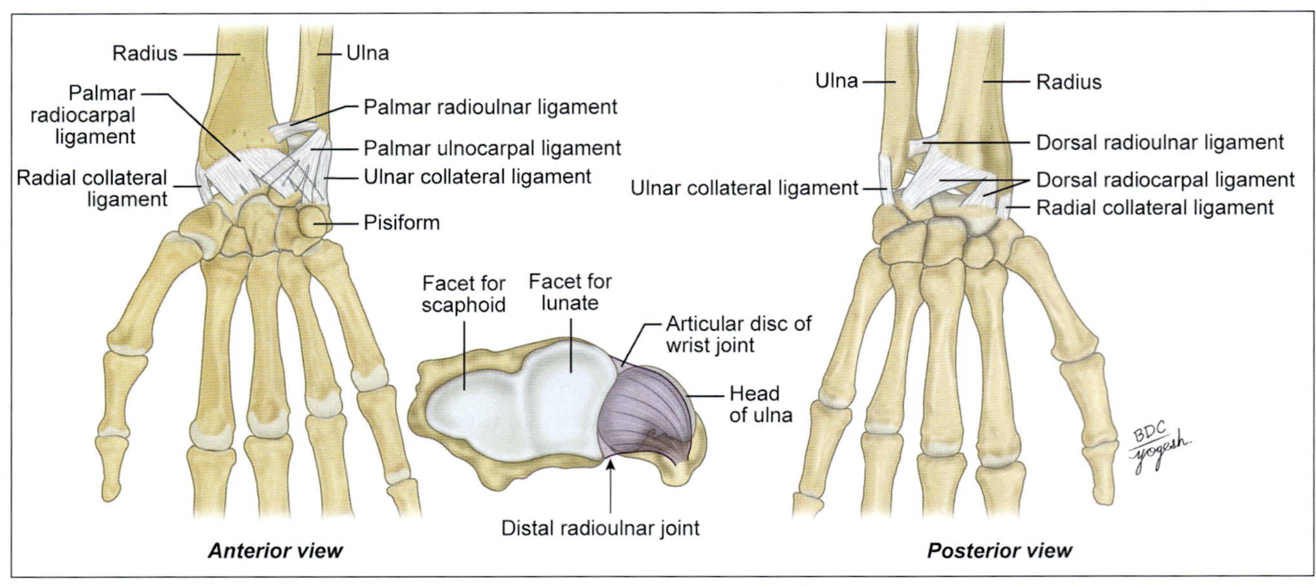

Flowchart 10.4: Wrist joint

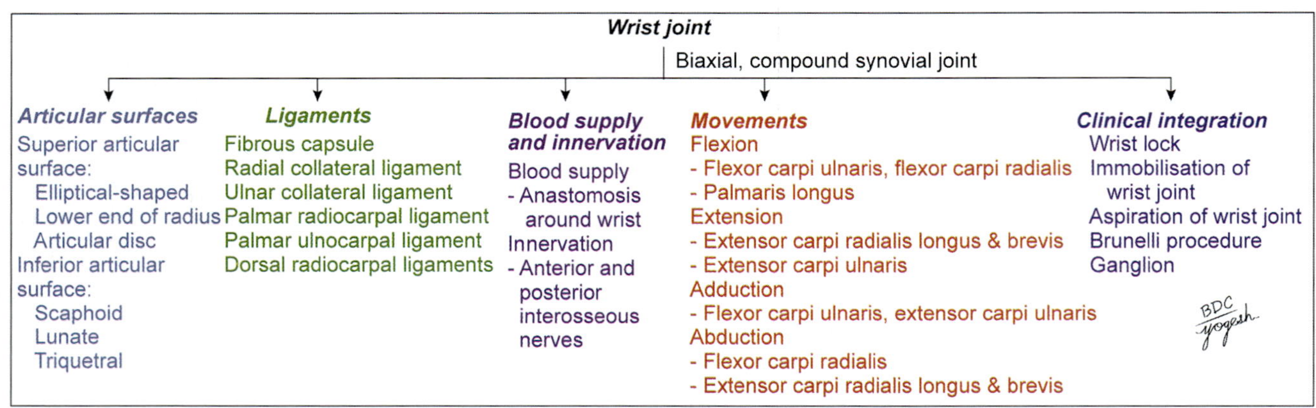

posterior margin of the lower end of the radius, runs downwards and medially, and is attached below to the dorsal surfaces of the scaphoid, lunate and triquetral bones (Plate 10.6).

5. The ***radial collateral ligament*** extends from the tip of the styloid process of the radius to the lateral side of the scaphoid bone. It is related to the radial artery.

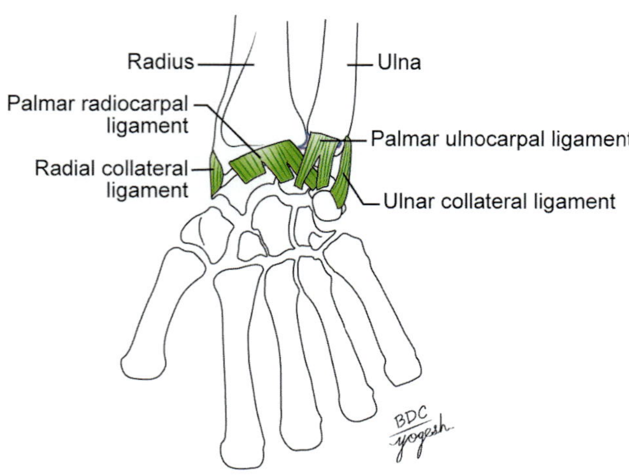

Fig. 10.24: Ligaments of wrist joint

6. The ***ulnar collateral ligament*** extends from the tip of the styloid process of the ulna to the triquetral and pisiform bones. Both the collateral ligaments are poorly developed.

Note: A protrusion of synovial membrane, called the ***recessus sacciformis***, lies in front of the styloid process of the ulna and in front of the articular disc. It is bounded inferiorly by a small meniscus projecting inwards from the ulnar collateral ligament between the styloid process and the triquetral bone.

Relations

Anterior: Long flexor tendons with their synovial sheaths, and median nerve (Fig. 10.25).

Posterior: Extensor tendons of the wrist and fingers with their synovial sheaths (Fig. 10.25).

Lateral: Radial artery (Fig. 10.25).

Blood Supply

Anterior and posterior carpal arches.

Nerve Supply

Anterior and posterior interosseous nerves.

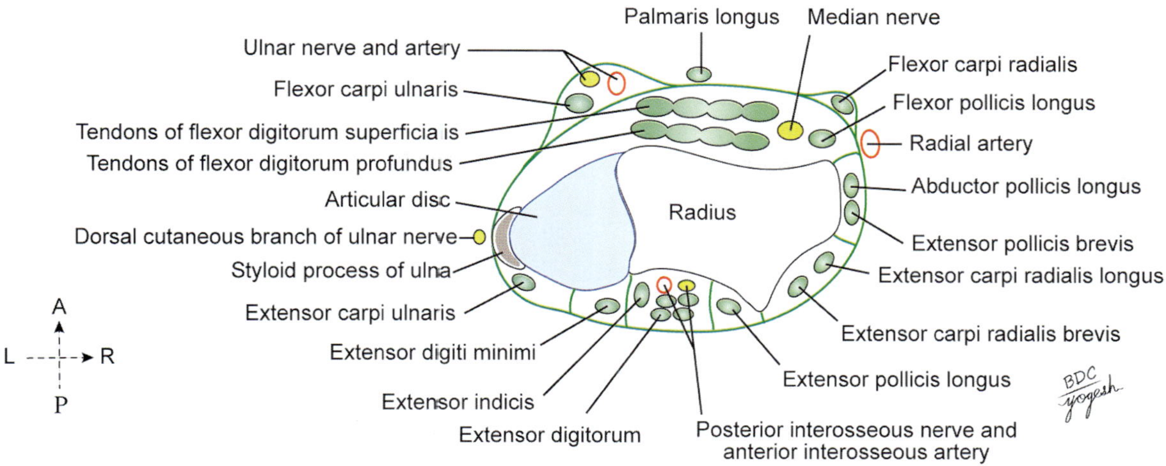

Fig. 10.25: Relations of wrist joint: transverse section passing through the wrist joint

Movements

The wrist joint has the following movements (Fig. 10.26):

1. *Flexion:* It takes place more at the midcarpal than at the wrist joint. The main flexors are:
   - Flexor carpi radialis
   - Flexor carpi ulnaris
   - Palmaris longus.

   The movement is assisted by long flexors of the fingers and thumb (Figs 10.35a and b), and abductor pollicis longus.
2. *Extension:* It takes place mainly at the wrist joint. The main extensors are:
   - Extensor carpi radialis longus
   - Extensor carpi radialis brevis
   - Extensor carpi ulnaris.

   It is assisted by the extensors of the fingers and thumb.
3. *Abduction (radial deviation):* It occurs mainly at the midcarpal joint. The main abductors are:
   - Flexor carpi radialis
   - Extensor carpi radialis longus and extensor carpi radialis brevis
   - Abductor pollicis longus and extensor pollicis brevis.
4. *Adduction (ulnar deviation):* It occurs mainly at the wrist joint. The main adductors are:
   - Flexor carpi ulnaris
   - Extensor carpi ulnaris.
5. *Circumduction:* It is a combination of movements in sequence. All the muscles work in co-ordination. The range of flexion is more than that of extension. Similarly, the range of adduction is greater than abduction (due to the shorter styloid process of ulna).

Note: Movements at the radiocarpal joints are accompanied by movements at the midcarpal joint. The midcarpal joint is anatomically separate from radiocarpal joint.

The joint between the two rows of carpal bones does not have smooth joint line because of multiple small joints. However, it still behaves as a functional unit in all movements of the wrist joint.

In addition to the congruency and the shape of the articular surfaces of radius and carpal bones, the length of the ulna can also affect the amount of motion available at the wrist joint. In the ulnar negative variance, the distal end of ulna is shorter than the radius and vice versa in ulnar positive variance.

CLINICAL ANATOMY

- ***Rheumatoid arthritis***: It is a chronic autoimmune disease that mostly affects joints, causing pain, swelling, stiffness, and loss of function. The wrist joint, metacarpophalangeal joints, and interphalangeal joints are commonly involved in rheumatoid arthritis (Fig. 10.27).
- ***Ganglion***: The back of the wrist is the common site for a ganglion. It is a cystic swelling resulting from mucoid degeneration of synovial sheaths around the tendons (Fig. 10.28).
- ***Aspiration of wrist joint***: The wrist joint can be aspirated from the posterior surface between the tendons of the extensor pollicis longus and the extensor digitorum (Fig. 10.29).
- ***Optimum position:*** The joint is immobilised in optimum position of 30° dorsiflexion (extension).
- Because of the complex nature of the joint and the multiple articulations, any injury to the ligaments attached to the proximal or the distal row of carpal bones may cause subluxation of the carpals ventrally or dorsally, leading to painful condition of the wrist.

DISSECTION

Cut through the thenar and hypothenar muscles from their origins and reflect them distally.

Separate the flexor and extensor retinacula of the wrist from the bones.

Cut through flexor and extensor tendons (if not already done) and reflect them distally.

Define the capsular attachments and ligaments and relations of the wrist joint.

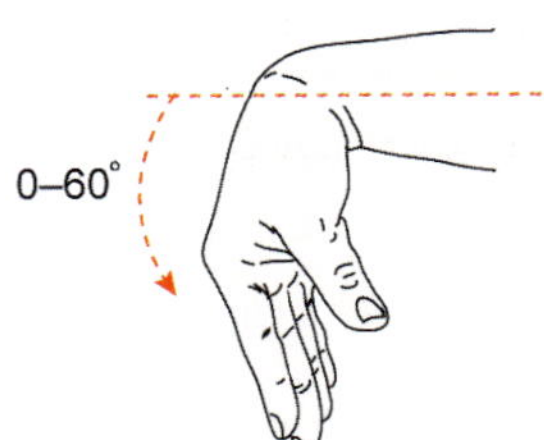

Flexion
Flexor carpi radialis
Flexor carpi ulnaris
Palmaris longus

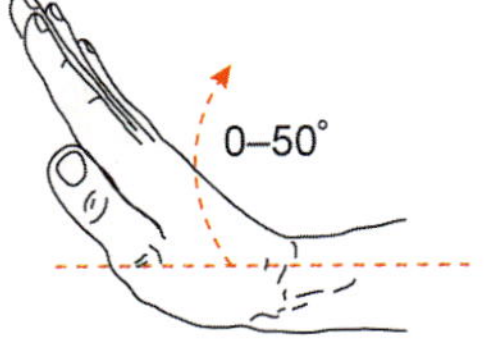

Extension
Extensor carpi radialis longus
Extensor carpi radialis brevis
Extensor carpi ulnaris

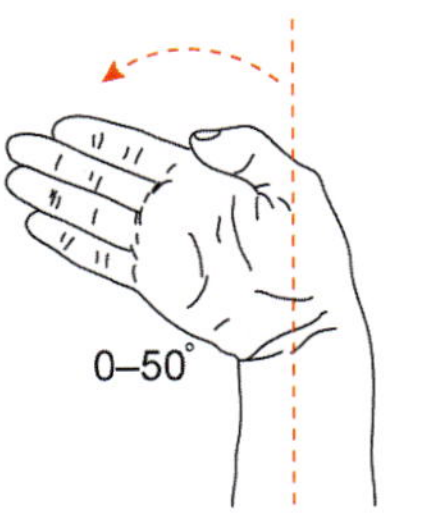

Adduction
Flexor carpi ulnaris
Extensor carpi ulnaris

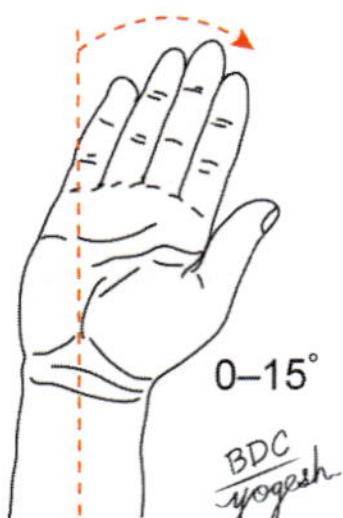

Abduction
Flexor carpi radialis
Extensor carpi radialis longus
Extensor carpi radialis brevis
Abductor pollicis longus
Extensor pollicis brevis

Fig. 10.26: Movements of wrist joint

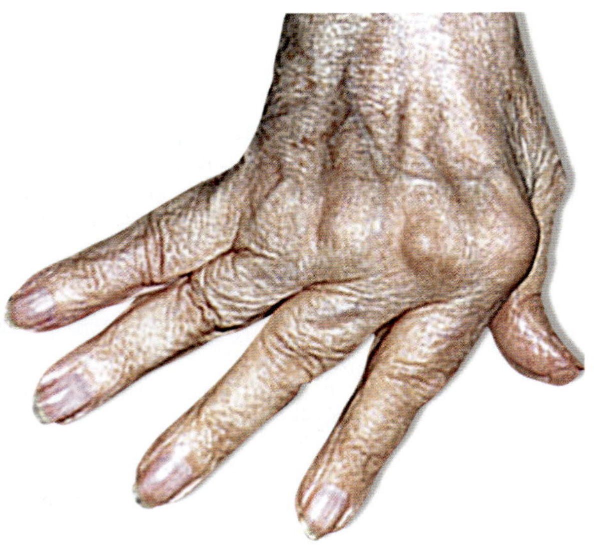

Fig. 10.27: Rheumatoid arthritis leads to deformities of the tendons (Fig. 10.29).

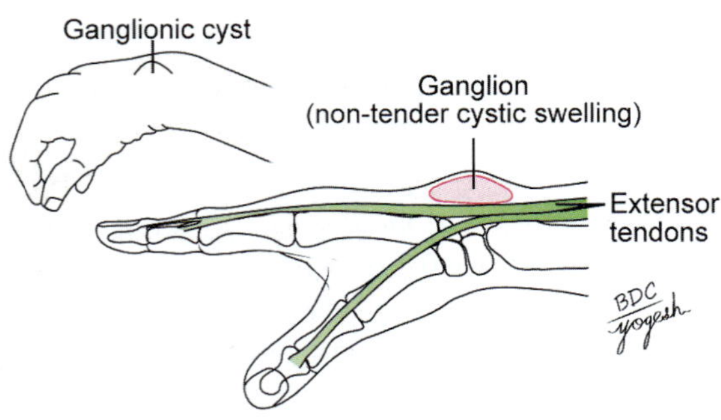

Fig. 10.28: Ganglion cyst at the back of wrist

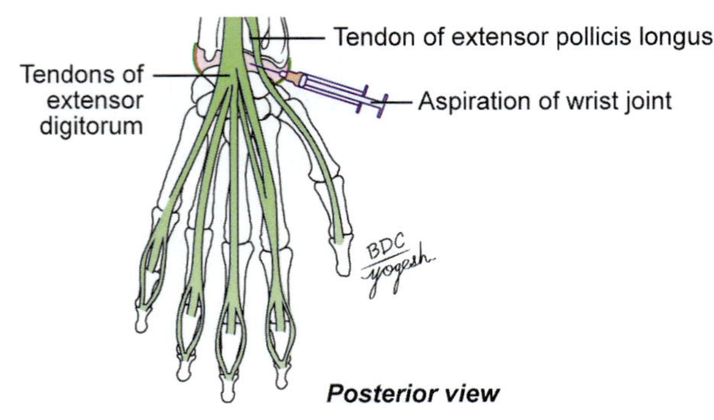

Fig. 10.29: Aspiration of the wrist joint

Competencies:

AN13.4 Describe sternoclavicular joint, acromioclavicular joint, carpometacarpal joints, and metacarpophalangeal joint.

AN12.6 Describe and demonstrate movements of thumb and muscles involved.

JOINTS OF HAND

INTERCARPAL, CARPOMETACARPAL AND INTERMETACARPAL JOINTS

There are three joint cavities among the intercarpal, carpometacarpal and intermetacarpal joints, which are:

1. Pisotriquetral,
2. First carpometacarpal, and
3. A common cavity for the rest of the joints. The common cavity may be described as the ***midcarpal (transverse intercarpal) joint*** between the proximal and distal rows of the carpus, which communicates with intercarpal joints superiorly, and with intercarpal, carpometacarpal and intermetacarpal joints inferiorly (Fig. 10.23).

The midcarpal joint permits movements between the two rows of the carpus as already described with the wrist joint.

FIRST CARPOMETACARPAL/ TRAPEZIO-METACARPAL JOINT (JOINT OF THUMB)

First carpometacarpal joint is only carpometacarpal joint which has a separate joint cavity. Movements at this joint are, therefore, much more free than at any other corresponding joint.

Type

Saddle variety of synovial joint (because the articular surfaces are concavo-convex).

Articular Surfaces

1. The distal surface of the ***trapezium***
2. The proximal surface of the ***base of the 1st metacarpal*** bone.

The articulating surface of trapezium is concave in the sagittal plane and convex in the frontal plane.

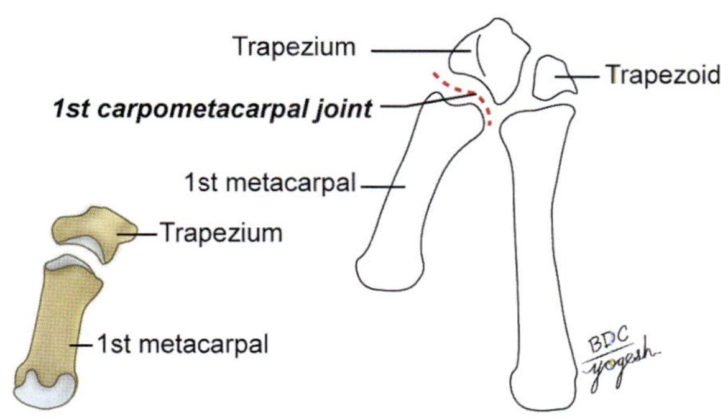

Fig. 10.30: First carpometacarpal (trapezio-metacarpal) joint

The concavo-convex nature of the articular surfaces permits a wide range of movements (Fig. 10.30).

Ligaments

1. Capsular ligament surrounds the joint. In general, it is thick but loose, and is thickest dorsally and laterally.
2. Lateral ligament is broad band which strengthens the capsule laterally.
3. The anterior ligament
4. The posterior ligaments are oblique bands running downwards and medially.

Relations

Anteriorly: The joint is covered by the muscles of the thenar eminence.

Posteriorly: Long and short extensors of the thumb.

Medially: First dorsal interosseous muscle, and the radial artery (passing from the dorsal to the palmar aspect of the hand through the interosseous space).

Laterally: Tendon of the abductor pollicis longus.

Blood Supply

Radial vessels.

Nerve Supply

1st digital branch of median nerve.

Movements

Flexion and extension of the thumb take place in the plane of the palm, and abduction and adduction at right angles to the plane of the palm. In opposition, the thumb crosses the palm and touches other fingers. Flexion is associated with medial rotation and extension with lateral rotation at the joint.

The following muscles bring about the movements (Fig. 10.31):

Flexion:	Flexor pollicis brevis Opponens pollicis
Extension:	Extensor pollicis brevis Extensor pollicis longus
Abduction:	Abductor pollicis brevis Abductor pollicis longus
Adduction:	Adductor pollicis
Opposition:	Opponens pollicis Flexor pollicis brevis
Circumduction:	Combination of different movements mentioned above

Note: The ***opposition*** is a sequential movement of abduction, flexion, adduction of the 1st metacarpal with simultaneous rotation. Opposition is unique to human beings and is one of the most important movements of the hand considering that this motion is used in almost all types of gripping actions. The adductor pollicis and the flexor pollicis longus exert pressure on the opposed fingers.

CLINICAL ANATOMY

- The 1st carpometacarpal joint can undergo degenerative changes with age which is a painful condition of the base of the thumb.
- The synovial lining of the tendons of extensor pollicis brevis and abductor pollicis longus can get inflamed due to repetitive strain and can lead to a painful condition called ***De Quervain's tenosynovitis***. Movement of the thumb can aggravate pain in this condition.

DISSECTION

Out of these, the most important joint with a separate joint cavity is the first carpometacarpal joint. This is the joint of the thumb and a wide variety of functionally useful movements take place here. Identify the distal surface of trapezium and base of first metacarpal bone.

Define the metacarpophalangeal and interphalangeal joints.

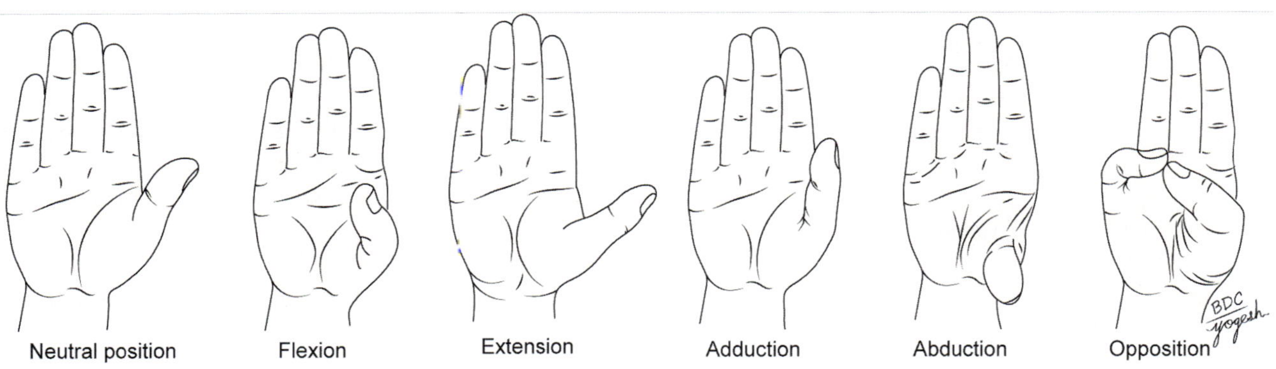

Fig. 10.31: Movements of the thumb

For their dissection, remove all the muscles and tendons from the anterior and posterior aspects of any two metacarpophalangeal joints. Define the articular capsule and ligaments. Do the same for proximal and distal interphalangeal joints of one of the fingers and define the ligaments.

METACARPOPHALANGEAL JOINTS

Type

Metacarpophalangeal joints are synovial joints of the ellipsoid variety.

Ligaments

Each joint has the following ligaments.

1. ***Capsular ligament:*** This is thick in front and thin behind.
2. ***Palmar ligament:*** This is a strong fibrocartilaginous plate (volar plate) which replaces the anterior part of the capsule. It is more firmly attached to the phalanx than to the metacarpal. The various palmar ligaments of the metacarpophalangeal joints are joined to one another by the deep transverse metacarpal ligament.
3. ***Medial and lateral collateral ligaments:*** These are oblique bands placed at the sides of the joint. Each runs downwards and forwards from the head of the metacarpal bone to the base of the phalanx. These are taut in flexion and relaxed in extension.

Movements at 1st Joint and Muscles Producing Them

Flexion: Flexor pollicis longus and flexor pollicis brevis.

Extension: Extensor pollicis longus and extensor pollicis brevis.

Abduction: Abductor pollicis brevis.

Adduction: Adductor pollicis.

Movements at 2nd to 5th Joints and Muscles Producing Them

Flexion: Interossei and lumbricals

Extension: Extensors of the fingers

Abduction: Dorsal interossei

Adduction: Palmar interossei

Circumduction: Above muscles in sequence.

INTERPHALANGEAL JOINTS (PROXIMAL AND DISTAL)

Type

Hinge variety of synovial joints (Fig. 10.32).

Ligaments

Similar to the metacarpophalangeal joints, that is one palmar fibrocartilaginous ligament and two collateral bands running downwards and forwards.

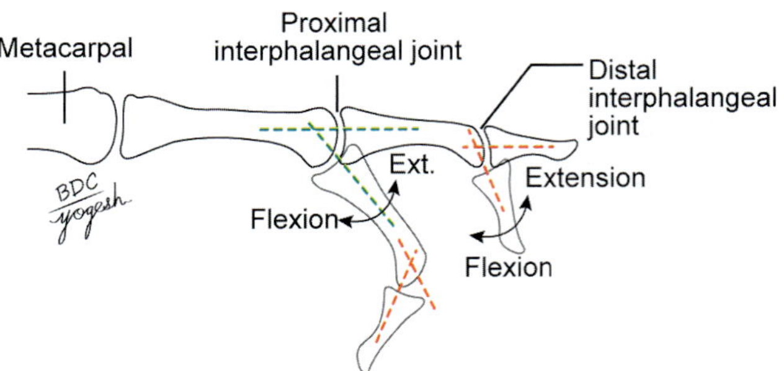

Fig. 10.32: Joints of the fingers

Movements at Interphalangeal Joint of Thumb

Flexion: Flexor pollicis longus.

Extension: Extensor pollicis longus.

Movements at 2nd to 5th Digits

Flexion: Flexor digitorum superficialis at the proximal interphalangeal joint, and the flexor digitorum profundus at the distal joint.

Extension: Interossei and lumbricals.

CLINICAL ANATOMY

***Position of immobilization of hand*:** The collateral ligaments of the metacarpophalangeal are full stretched only when the joint is fully flexed to 90°. The collateral ligaments of interphalangeal joint are stretched only when the joint is fully extended. In the immobilizing of the hand, contracture/shortening of the ligaments occurs within two weeks in the situation where the joints are immobilized with lax ligaments. Therefore, the hand should be mobilized with fully flexed metacarpophalangeal joints and fully extended interphalangeal joints.

Segmental Innervation of Movements of Upper Limb

In Figure 10.33 shows the segments of the spinal cord responsible for movements of the various joints of the upper limb.

The proximal muscles of upper limb are supplied by proximal nerve roots forming brachial plexus and distal muscles by the distal or lower nerve roots. In shoulder, abduction is done by muscles supplied by C5 spinal segment and adduction by muscles innervated by C6, C7 spinal segments.

Elbow joint is flexed by C5, C6 and extended by C7, C8 innervated muscles. Supination is caused by muscle innervated by C6 spinal segment even pronation is done through C6 spinal segment.

Extension and flexion of wrist is done through C6, C7 spinal segments. Both the palmar and dorsal interossei are innervated by T1 spinal segment.

The interphalangeal joints also are flexed and extended by same spinal segments, i.e. C7, C8.

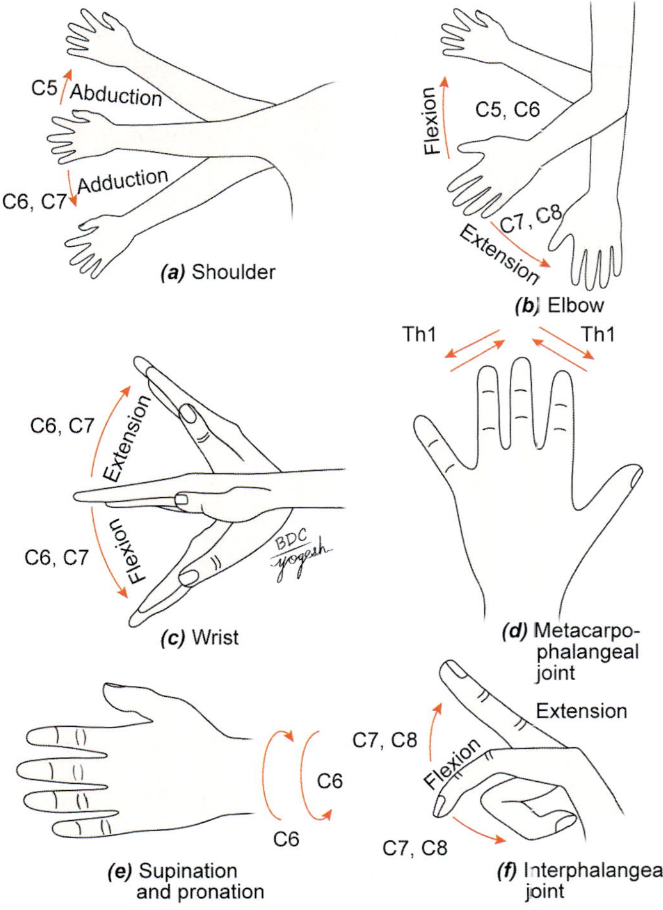

Figs 10.33a to f: Segmental innervation of movements of the upper limb

VIDEO

Video 1.10 Joints of Upper Limb.

Facts to Remember

- Sternoclavicular joint is a saddle variety of synovial joint. Its cavity is divided into two parts by an articular disc.
- Coracoclavicular ligament is the strongest ligament of the upper limb.
- Movements of shoulder girdle help the movements of shoulder joint during 90°–180° abduction.
- Shoulder joint is the most freely movable joint and most commonly dislocated joint in the body. It commonly undergoes recurrent dislocations.
- Shoulder joint commonly dislocates antero-inferiorly.
- Subacromial bursa is the largest synovial bursa of the body.
- Rotator cuff is the most important factor for maintaining the stability of the shoulder joint.
- Ulnar nerve lies behind medial epicondyle. It is not a content of the cubital fossa.
- Carrying angle separates the wrist from the hip joint while carrying buckets, etc.
- Biceps brachii is an important supinator of forearm when the elbow is flexed.
- Kings pronate, while beggars supinate.
- Movements of pronation and supination are not occurring at the elbow or wrist joints.
- First carpometacarpal joint is the most important joint as it permits the thumb to oppose the palm fingers for holding things.
- Ulnar nerve lies behind medial epicondyle, pressing the nerve cause tingling sensation. That is why the bone is named 'humerus'.
- Wrist joint complex = Radiocarpal joint + Mid carpal joint
- In midprone position, the bones of the forearm are most stable.
- Axis of movements of abduction and adduction of fingers is through the centre of the middle finger.

BDC's Anatomy *e*-book

1. Movements of the shoulder girdle
2. Mobility of shoulder joint
3. Analysis of the overhead movement of the shoulder
4. Dancing shoulder
5. Exclusion of shoulder joint disease
6. Anatomical basis of referred pain at shoulder tip
7. Classification of movements of the hand
8. Functional components of hand
9. Position of arthrodesis
10. Further reading
11. Viva voce questions

Chapter

11

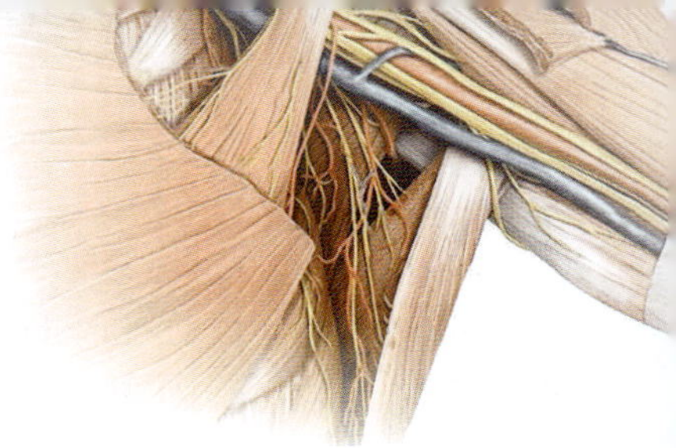

Surface Marking and Radiological Anatomy of Upper Limb

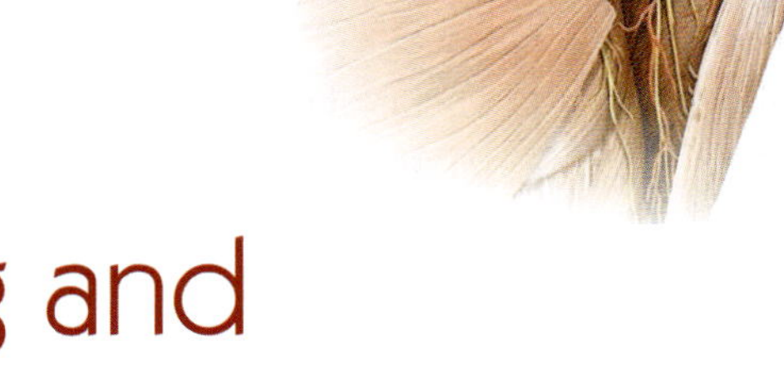

Surface marking is the projection of the deeper structures on the surface. Its importance lies in various medical and surgical procedures. It is a useful guide for the location and palpation of organs and arteries, for the percussion, and the auscultation.

SURFACE MARKING

Bony landmarks have been shown in Fig. 11.1. The surface marking of important structures is given below.

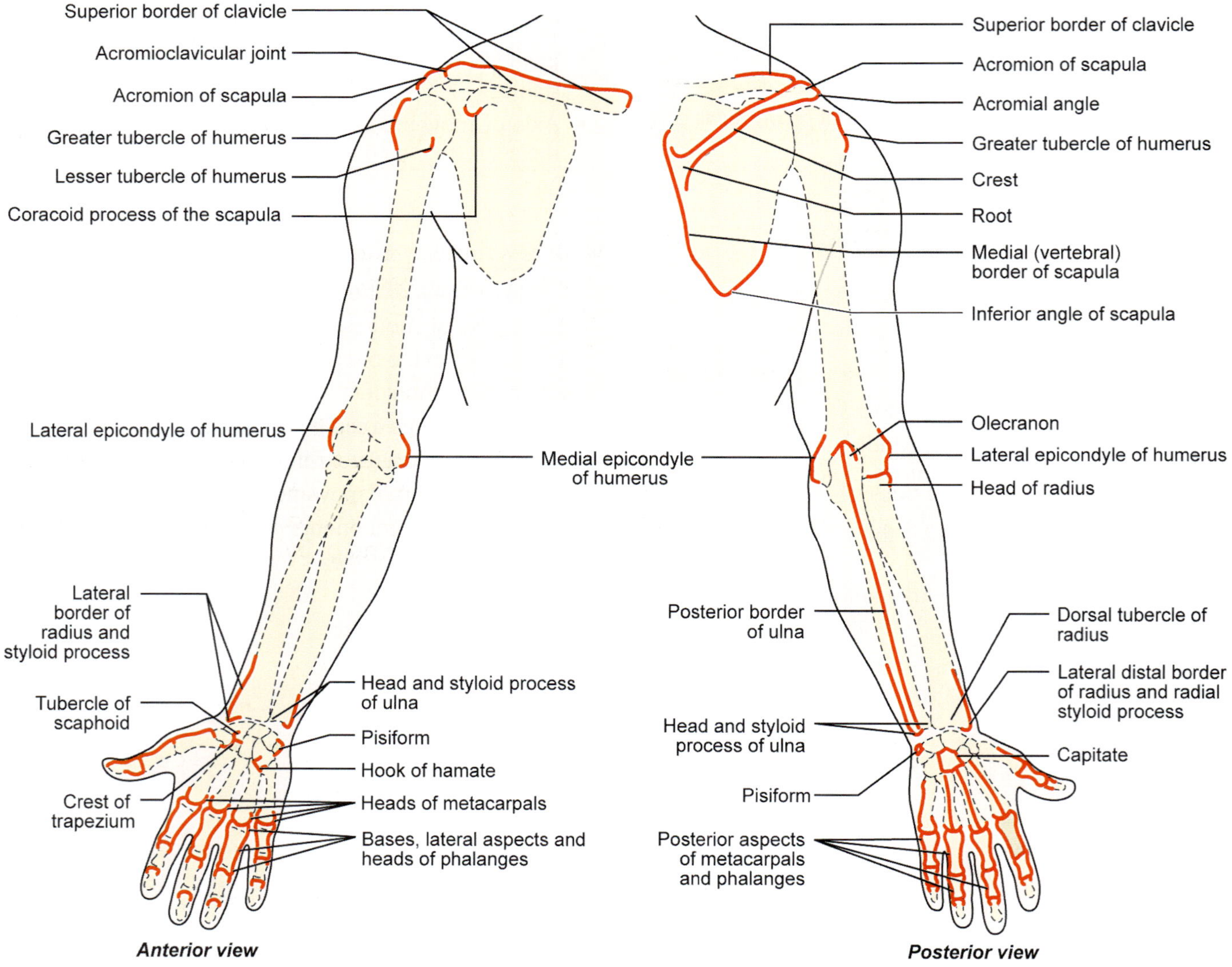

Superior border of clavicle
Acromioclavicular joint
Acromion of scapula
Greater tubercle of humerus
Lesser tubercle of humerus
Coracoid process of the scapula
Lateral epicondyle of humerus
Medial epicondyle of humerus
Lateral border of radius and styloid process
Tubercle of scaphoid
Crest of trapezium
Head and styloid process of ulna
Pisiform
Hook of hamate
Heads of metacarpals
Bases, lateral aspects and heads of phalanges
Anterior view

Superior border of clavicle
Acromion of scapula
Acromial angle
Greater tubercle of humerus
Crest
Root
Medial (vertebral) border of scapula
Inferior angle of scapula
Olecranon
Lateral epicondyle of humerus
Head of radius
Posterior border of ulna
Dorsal tubercle of radius
Lateral distal border of radius and radial styloid process
Head and styloid process of ulna
Capitate
Pisiform
Posterior aspects of metacarpals and phalanges
Posterior view

Fig. 11.1: Bony landmarks/palpable features of upper limb bones

MAMMARY GLAND

1. Point at margin of sternum opposite manubriosternal joint.
2. Point of the sternal end of 6th costal cartilage (Fig. 11.2).
3. Line along 6th costal cartilage.
4. Mid-axillary line.
5. Point at the pulsation of axillary artery deep to anterior axillary fold.
6. Line along anterior part of 2nd rib and its cartilage.

Draw a circle joining points 1, 2, 3, 4 with projection upwards towards point 5 and continue along 6 to reach back at point 1. Nipple is projection of 1 cm below the centre of this circle. Areola is circle of 1.5 cm around the nipple.

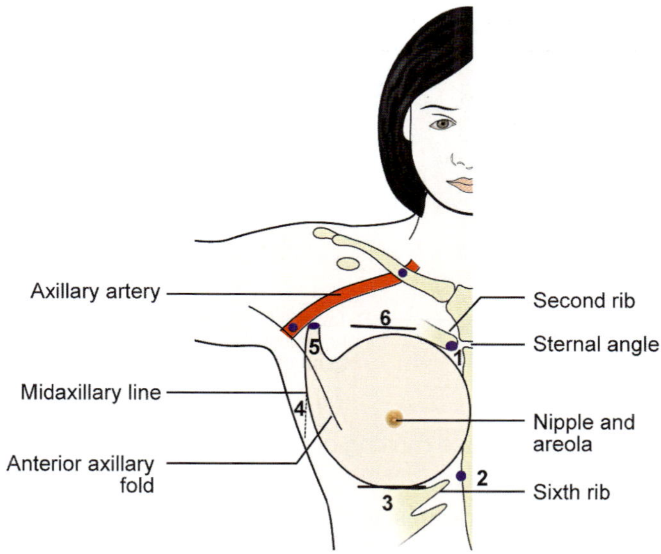

Fig. 11.2: Mammary gland

Competency:
AN13.7 Identify and demonstrate surface projection of—cephalic and basilic vein, palpation of brachial artery, radial artery; testing of muscles—trapezius, pectoralis major, serratus anterior, latissimus dorsi, deltoid, biceps brachii, brachioradialis.

ARTERIES AND NERVES IN ARM

Axillary Artery

Hold the arm at right angles to the trunk and mark the following points:

- *Point 1*: Midpoint of the clavicle (Fig. 11.3).
- *Point 2*: On the lower part of axillary artery present in the groove behind coracobrachialis muscle posteromedial to biceps brachii in front of posterior axillary fold.

These points are joined by a broad curved line.

Clinical utility: Pulsation of this artery can be felt in the living.

Brachial Artery

- *Point 2:* Point on the lower part of axillary artery presents in the groove behind coracobrachialis muscle (posteromedial to biceps brachii) in front of the posterior axillary fold. Pulsation of the artery can be felt in living (Fig. 11.3).
- *Point 3:* At the level of the neck of the radius medial to the tendon of the biceps on the medial side of the upper part of the forearm.

Join points 3 and 4 by a line that runs downwards and slightly laterally to end in front of the elbow. At its termination, it bifurcates into radial and ulnar arteries.

Clinical utility: Surface anatomy of the brachial artery is important:

- To feel the pulsation of the brachial artery: Pulsation of brachial artery can be felt in the cubital fossa, medial to the tendon of biceps brachii.
- For auscultation of brachial artery during measurement of blood pressure.

Median Nerve

Mark the brachial artery. Mark median nerve lateral to the artery in upper half and medial to the artery in lower half. The nerve crosses the artery anteriorly in the middle of the arm (Fig. 11.3).

Musculocutaneous Nerve

Hold the arm at right angles to the trunk

- *Point A:* Just lateral to axillary artery 5 cm below coracoid process (Fig. 11.4).
- *Point B:* Lateral to tendon of biceps brachii muscle 2 cm above the bend of below. Here, it pierces deep

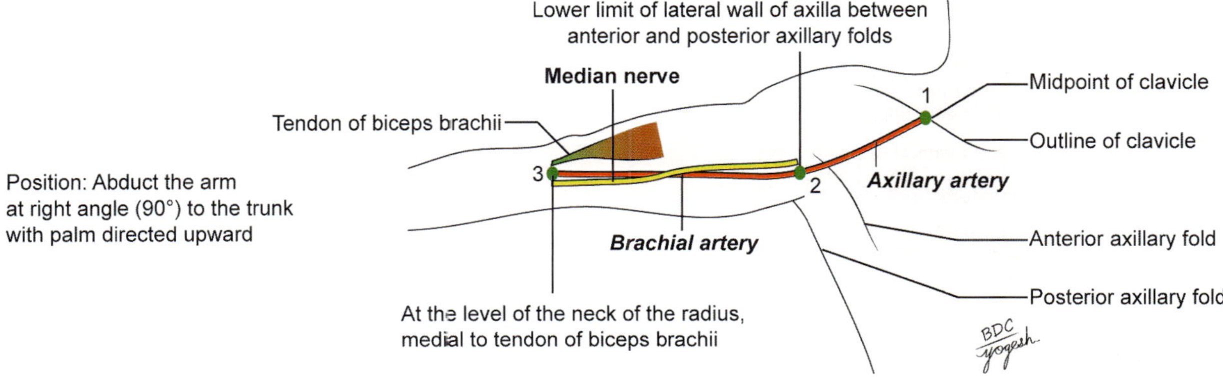

Fig. 11.3: Surface marking of axillary and brachial arteries and median nerve

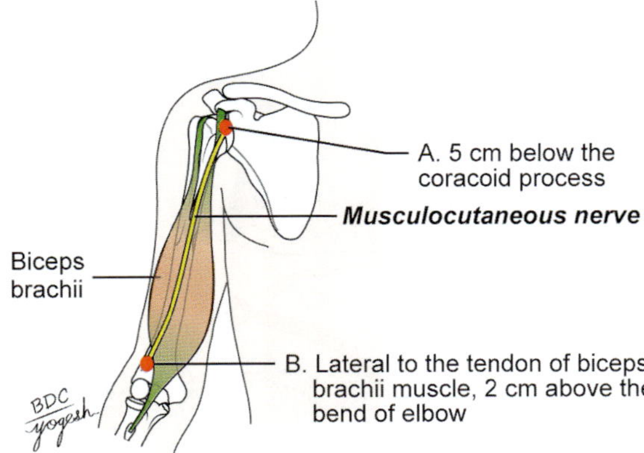

Fig. 11.4: Surface marking of musculocutaneous nerve

fascia and continues as the lateral cutaneous nerve of the forearm.

The musculocutaneous nerve lies lateral to axillary artery, crosses deep to the bulge formed by biceps brachii to reach the lateral side of tendon of biceps brachii.

Radial Nerve

Arm is kept on the side of trunk. Radial nerve is marked both on anterior and posterior aspects of the arm (Fig. 11.5).

- *Point A:* At the lateral wall of axilla at its lower limit.
- *Point B:* Junction of point of upper 1/3rd and lower 2/3rd of line joining deltoid tuberosity to lateral epicondyle of humerus.
- *Point C:* Infront of the elbow, just below the lateral epicondyle of humerus, where it divides into superficial and posterior interosseous (deep) branch. Join points A and B across back of arm and points B and C on front of arm.

Axillary Nerve

- *Point A:* At tip of acromion process of scapula (Fig. 11.6).
- *Point B:* At the insertion of deltoid muscle.
- Join points A and B.
- *Point C:* Midpoint of the line A–B.
- *Point D:* 2 cm above point C.

Draw a horizontal line of 3 cm along point D. This line represents the axillary nerve.

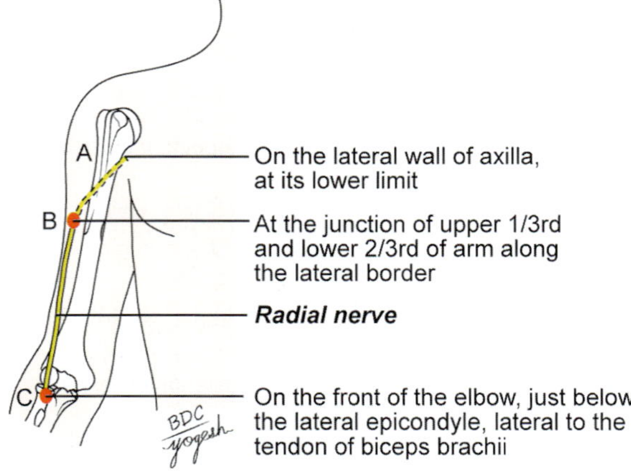

Fig. 11.5: Surface marking of radial nerve in arm

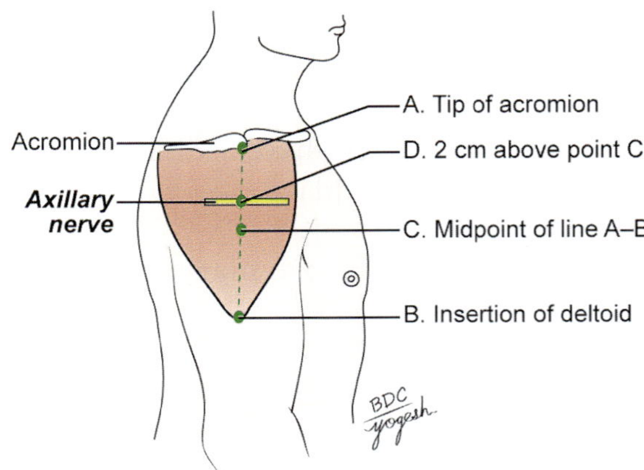

Fig. 11.6: Surface marking of axillary nerve

Ulnar Nerve

- *Point A:* On the posterior wall of axilla at its lower limit where pulsations of axillary artery are felt in the living (Fig. 11.7).
- *Point B:* At the middle of the medial border of the arm.
- *Point C:* Behind the base of the medial epicondyle of the humerus.

Join points A and B on anterior aspect of arm.

Join points B and C on posterior aspect of arm.

ARTERIES AND NERVES IN FOREARM AND HAND

Radial Artery

In the Forearm

Radial artery is marked by joining the following points:

- *Point A:* In front of the elbow at the level of the neck of the radius medial to the tendon of the biceps brachii (Fig. 11.8).
- *Point B:* At the wrist between the anterior border of the radius and the tendon of the flexor carpi radialis (Fig. 11.8).

Its course is curved with a gentle convexity to the lateral side.

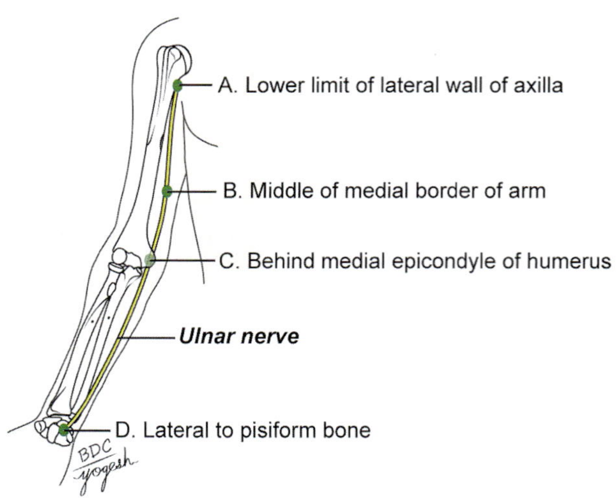

Fig. 11.7: Surface marking of ulnar nerve

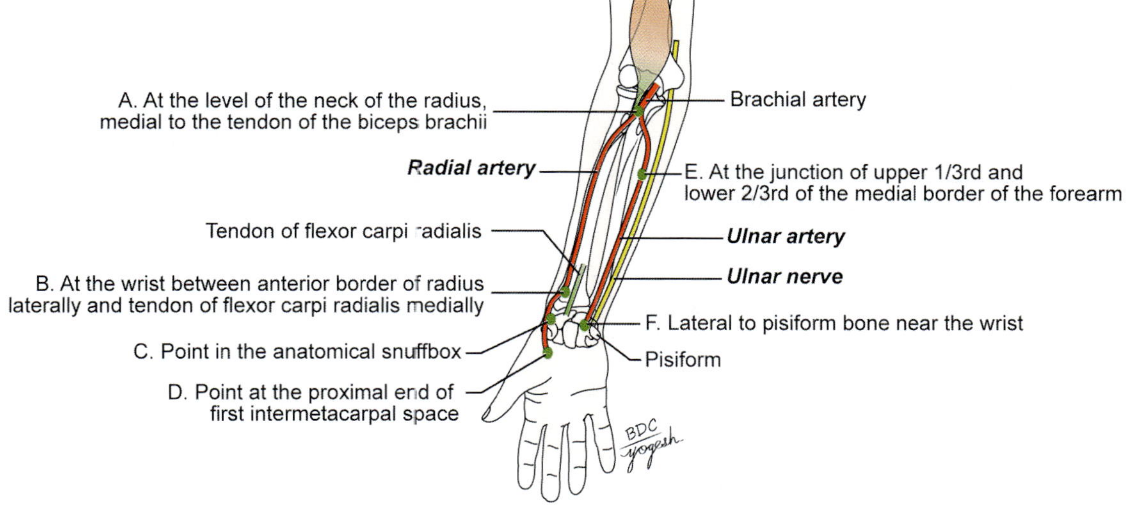

Fig. 11.8: Surface marking of radial and ulnar arteries

At the Wrist

Radial artery is marked by joining the following points (Fig. 11.8):

- *Point C:* Point in the anatomical snuffbox
- *Point D*: Point at the proximal end of the first intermetacarpal space.
- Joint point C and D with lateral convexity to mark the radial artery.
- *Clinical utility*:
  - Radial artery pulsation: Radial artery is palpated in the lower part of forearm against the anterior surface of lower end of radius lateral to the tendon of flexor carpi radialis.
  - Incision to dissect out radial artery for coronary artery bypass grafting (CABG): Radial artery is useful to bypass the blockage site of coronary artery.
  - Arterial blood sample: The radial artery may be used to draw arterial blood for blood gas analysis.

Ulnar Artery

Ulnar artery is marked by joining the following three points.

- *Point A:* In front of the elbow at the level of the neck of the radius medial to the tendon of the biceps brachii (Fig. 11.6).
- *Point E:* At the junction of the upper one-third and lower two-thirds of the medial border of the forearm (lateral to the ulnar nerve) (Fig. 11.6).
- *Point F:* Lateral to the pisiform bone (Fig. 11.6). Thus, the course of the ulnar artery is oblique in its upper 1/3rd, and vertical in its lower 2/3rd. The ulnar nerve lies just medial to the ulnar artery in the lower 2/3rd of its course. The ulnar artery continues in the palm as the superficial palmar arch (Fig. 11.8).

Superficial Palmar Arch

- *Point 1:* Just lateral to pisiform bone (Fig. 11.9).
- *Point 2:* Medial to hook of hamate.
- *Point 3:* Distal border of thenar eminence.

The convexity of arch is directed towards the finger.

Deep Palmar Arch

Deep palmar arch is formed as the direct continuation of the radial artery. It has a slight convexity towards the fingers.

- *Point 4:* At proximal part of 1st dorsal intermetacarpal space (Fig. 11.9).
- *Point 5:* Just distal to hook of hamate. It is marked by a slightly convex line, 4 cm long, just distal to the hook of the hamate bone.

The deep palmar arch lies 1.2 cm proximal to the superficial palmar arch across the metacarpals, immediately distal to their bases. The deep branch of ulnar nerve lies in its concavity.

Ulnar Nerve

Ulnar nerve is marked by joining the following two points.

- *Point C:* On the back of the base of the medial epicondyle of the humerus (Fig. 11.7).
- *Point D:* Lateral to the pisiform bone.

In the lower two-thirds of the forearm, the ulnar nerve lies medial to the ulnar artery (Fig. 11.7).

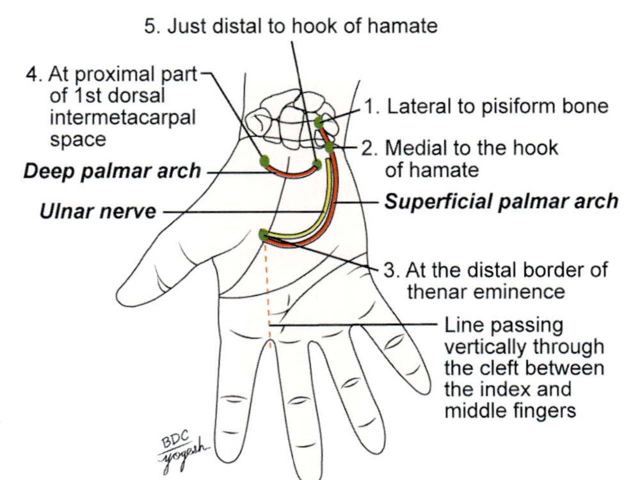

Fig. 11.9: Surface marking of superficial and deep palmar arches

In the Hand

Ulnar nerve lies superficial to the medial part of flexor retinaculum and medial to ulnar vessels where it divides into superficial and deep branches (Fig. 11.7).

The superficial branch supplies medial 1½ digits, including their nail beds. The deep branch passes backwards between pisiform and hook of hamate to lie in the concavity of the deep palmar arch.

Median Nerve

In the Forearm

Median nerve is marked by joining the following two points.

- *Point 1:* Medial to the brachial artery at the bend of the elbow (Fig. 11.10).
- *Point 2:* In front of the wrist (over the tendon of the palmaris longus) or 1 cm medial to the tendon of the flexor carpi radialis (Fig. 11.10).

In the Hand

Median nerve enters the palm by passing deep to flexor retinaculum, immediately below which it divides into lateral and medial branches. Lateral branch supplies the three muscles of thenar eminence and gives two branches to the thumb, and one to lateral side of index finger including 1st lumbrical muscle. Medial branch gives branches for the adjacent sides of index, middle, and ring fingers including 2nd lumbrical muscle. The lateral 3½ nail beds are also supplied.

Radial Nerve

In the Forearm

Superficial branch of radial nerve is marked by joining the following three points.

- *Point 1:* 1 cm lateral to the biceps tendon just below the level of the lateral epicondyle (Fig. 11.11).
- *Point 2:* At the junction of the upper two-thirds and lower one-third of the lateral border of the forearm just lateral to the radial artery.
- *Point 3:* At the anatomical snuffbox.

The nerve is vertical in its course between points *1* and 2. At the second point, it inclines backwards to reach the snuffbox. The nerve is closely related to the lateral side of the radial artery only in the middle one-third of the forearm. The nerve turns towards the back of forearm. Then it lies in the anatomical snuffbox to descend on the back of hand.

Posterior Interosseous Nerve/Deep Branch of Radial Nerve

It is marked by joining the following three points.

- *Point 1:* 1 cm lateral to the biceps brachii tendon just below the level of the lateral epicondyle (Fig. 11.12).
- *Point 2:* At the junction of the upper 1/3rd and lower 2/3rd of a line joining the middle of the posterior aspect of the head of the radius to the dorsal tubercle at the lower end of the radius (Lister's tubercle).

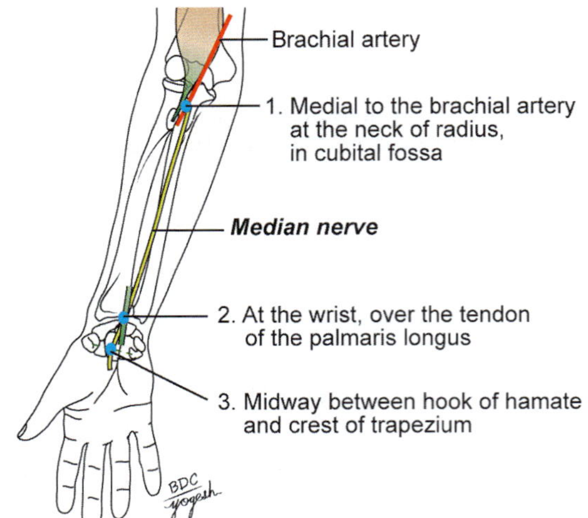

Fig. 11.10: Surface marking of median nerve in forearm and hand

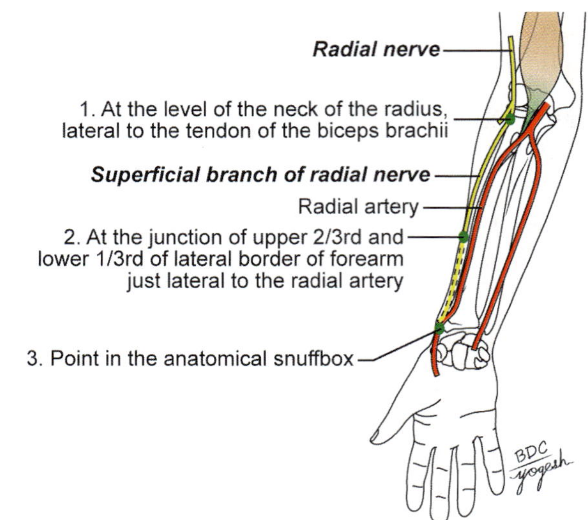

Fig. 11.11: Surface marking of superficial branch of radial nerve

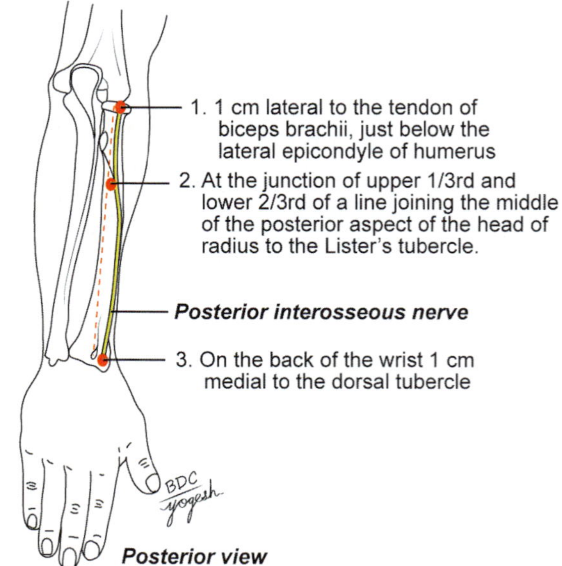

Fig. 11.12: Surface marking of posterior interosseous nerve

- *Point 3:* On the back of the wrist 1 cm medial to the dorsal tubercle.

Posterior interosseous nerve supplies the muscles of posterior aspect of the forearm.

JOINTS

Shoulder Joint

The anterior margin of the glenoid cavity corresponds to the lower half of the shoulder joint. It is marked by a line 3 cm long drawn downwards from a point just lateral to the tip of the coracoid process. The line is slightly concave laterally.

Elbow Joint

The joint line is situated 2 cm below the line joining the two epicondyles, and slopes downwards and medially.

This slope is responsible for the carrying angle.

Wrist Joint

The joint line is concave downwards and is marked by joining the styloid processes of the radius and ulna.

RETINACULA

Flexor Retinaculum

Flexor retinaculum is marked by joining the following four points.

1. Pisiform bone
2. Tubercle of the scaphoid bone
3. Hook of the hamate bone (Fig. 11.13)
4. Crest of the trapezium.

The upper border is obtained by joining the first and second points, and the lower border by joining the third and fourth points. The upper border is concave upwards, and the lower border is concave downwards.

Clinical utility: Flexor retinaculum and carpal bones together form carpal tunnel. It holds the long flexor tendons in place. Compression of median nerve in this tunnel causes carpal tunnel syndrome.

Extensor Retinaculum

Extensor retinaculum is an oblique band directed downwards and medially, and is about 2 cm broad (vertically) (Fig. 11.14). Laterally, it is attached to the lower salient part of the anterior border of the radius, and medially to the medial side of the carpus (pisiform and triquetral bones) and to the various ridges on the back of lower end of radius. It is not attached to ulna.

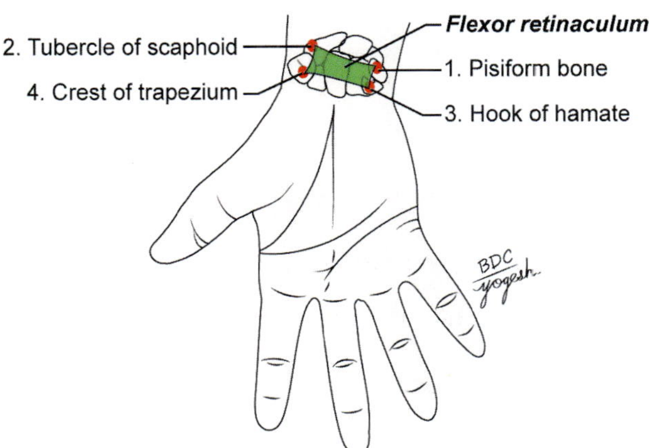

Fig. 11.13: Surface marking of flexor retinaculum of upper limb

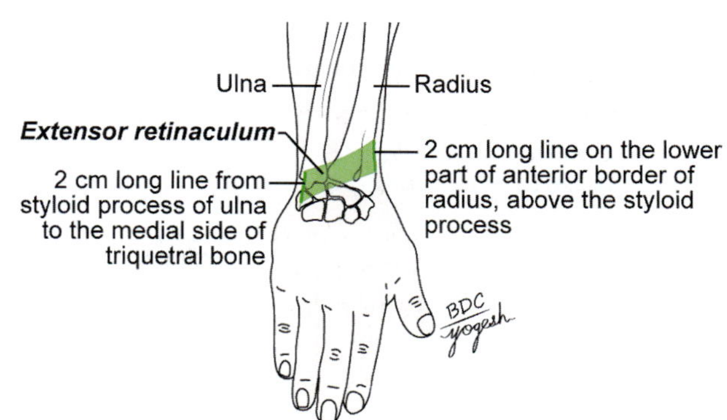

Fig. 11.14: Surface marking of extensor retinaculum of upper limb

Clinical utility: Extensor retinaculum holds the long extensor tendons and their synovial sheaths in place. It needs to be excised to release the pressure of inflamed synovial sheaths in De Quervain's tenosynovitis.

SYNOVIAL SHEATHS OF THE FLEXOR TENDONS

Common Flexor Synovial Sheath (Ulnar Bursa)

Above the flexor retinaculum (or lower transverse crease of the wrist), it extends into the forearm for about 2.5 cm. Here its medial border corresponds to the lateral edge of the tendon of the flexor carpi ulnaris, and its lateral border corresponds roughly to the tendon of the palmaris longus.

Ulnar bursa becomes narrower behind the flexor retinaculum and broadens out below it.

Most of it terminates at the level of the upper transverse crease of the palm, but the medial part is continued up to the distal transverse crease of the little finger.

Synovial Sheaths for the Tendon of Flexor Pollicis Longus (Radial Bursa)

Radial bursa is a narrow tube which is coextensive with the ulnar bursa in the forearm and wrist. Below the flexor retinaculum, it is continued into the thumb up to its distal crease.

Digital Synovial Sheaths

The synovial sheaths of the flexor tendons of the index, middle, and ring fingers extend from the necks of the metacarpal bones (corresponding roughly to the lower transverse crease of the palm) to the bases of the terminal phalanges.

Competency:

AN13.5 Identify the bones and joints of upper limb seen in anteroposterior and lateral view radiographs of shoulder region, arm, elbow, forearm, and hand.

RADIOLOGICAL ANATOMY OF UPPER LIMB

In the case of the limbs, plain radiography is mainly required. For complete information, it is always advisable to have anteroposterior (AP) as well as lateral views; and as far as possible radiographs of the opposite limb should be available for comparison. The skeleton, owing to its high radiopacity, forms the most striking feature in plain skiagrams. In general, the following information can be obtained from plain skiagrams of the limbs.

1. *Fractures* are seen as breaks in the surface continuity of the bone. A fracture line is usually irregular and asymmetrical. An epiphyseal line of an incompletely ossified bone, seen as a gap, should not be mistaken for a fracture: It has regular margins and is bilaterally symmetrical. Supernumerary or accessory bones are also symmetrical.
2. *Dislocations* are seen as deranged or distorted relations between the articular bony surfaces forming a joint.
3. Below the age of 25 years, the age of a person can be determined from the knowledge of ossification of the bones.
4. Certain *deficiency diseases* like rickets and scurvy can be diagnosed.
5. *Infections* (osteomyelitis) and growths (osteoma, osteoclastoma, osteosarcoma, etc.) can be diagnosed. A localised rarefaction of a bone may indicate an infection.
6. *Congenital absence or fusion* of bones can be seen.

Reading Plain Skiagrams of Limbs

1. Identify the view of the picture, anteroposterior (AP) or lateral. Each view shows a specific shape and arrangement of the bones.
2. Identify the region and the side (right, left).
3. Identify all the bones and their different parts visible in the given radiogram. Normal overlapping and 'end-on' appearances of bones in different views should be carefully studied.
4. Study the normal relations of the bones forming joints. The articular cartilage is radiolucent and does not cast any shadow. The radiological 'joint space' indicates the size of the articular cartilages. Normally, the joint space is about 2–5 mm in adults.
5. Study the various epiphyses visible in young bones and try to determine the age of the person concerned.

Shoulder

A. The following are seen in an AP view of the shoulder (Fig. 11.15).
   1. The upper end of the humerus, including the head, greater and lesser tubercles and intertubercular sulcus.
   2. The scapula, including the glenoid cavity, coracoid (seen end-on), acromion process, its lateral, medial and superior borders, and the superior and inferior angles. The suprascapular notch may be seen.
   3. The clavicle, except for its medial end.
   4. Upper part of the thoracic cage, including the upper ribs.

B. Study the normal appearance of the following joints.
   1. *Shoulder joint:* The glenoid cavity articulates only with the lower half of the head of the humerus (when the arm is in the anatomical position). The upper part of the head lies beneath the acromion process. The greater tuberosity forms the lateral most bony point in the shoulder region.
   2. Acromioclavicular joint.

C. Note the epiphyses, if any, and determine the age with the help of ossifications described with individual bones.

Elbow

A. Identify the following bones in an AP and lateral views of the elbow (Figs 11.16a and b).
   1. The lower end of humerus, including the medial and lateral epicondyles, the medial and lateral supracondylar ridges, trochlea, the capitulum and the olecranon fossa.

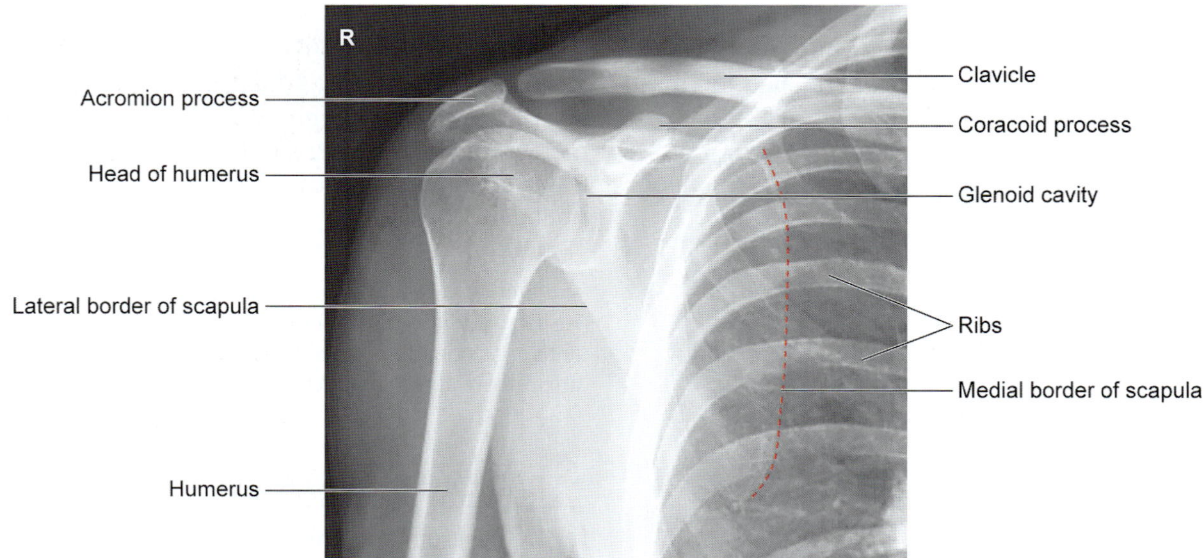

Fig. 11.15: Anteroposterior view of the shoulder joint

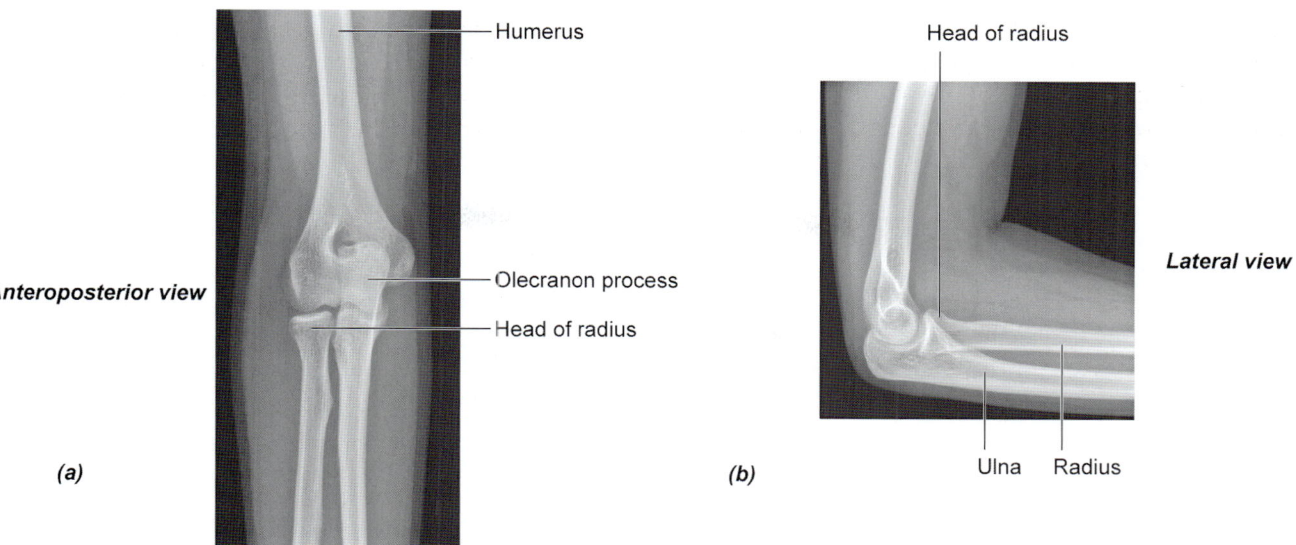

Figs 11.16a and b: Radiographs of elbow region: (a) AP view and (b) lateral view

2. The upper end of the ulna, including the olecranon and coronoid processes.
3. The upper end of the radius including its head, neck, and tuberosity.

B. Study the normal appearance of the following joints in AP view.
   1. Elbow joint
   2. Superior radioulnar joint

C. Note the olecranon and coronoid processes in a lateral view of the elbow (Figs 11.16a and b).

D. Note the epiphyses (if any) and determine the age with the help of ossifications described with individual bones.

Hand

A. Identify the following bones in an AP skiagram (Fig. 11.17).
   1. The lower end of the radius with its styloid process.
   2. The lower end of the ulna with its styloid process.
   3. The eight carpal bones. Note the overlapping of the triquetral and pisiform bones; and of the trapezium with the trapezoid. Also, identify the tubercle of the scaphoid and the hook of the hamate.
   4. The five metacarpal bones
   5. The fourteen phalanges
   6. The sesamoid bones present in relation to the thumb, and occasionally in relation to the other fingers.

B. Study the normal appearance of these joints.
   1. The wrist joint
   2. The inferior radioulnar joint
   3. The intercarpal, carpometacarpal, metacarpophalangeal, and interphalangeal joints.

C. Note the following bones in a lateral skiagram.
   1. Lunate
   2. Scaphoid
   3. Capitate
   4. Trapezium

D. Note the epiphyses and other incomplete ossifications and determine the age with the help of ossifications described with individual bones.

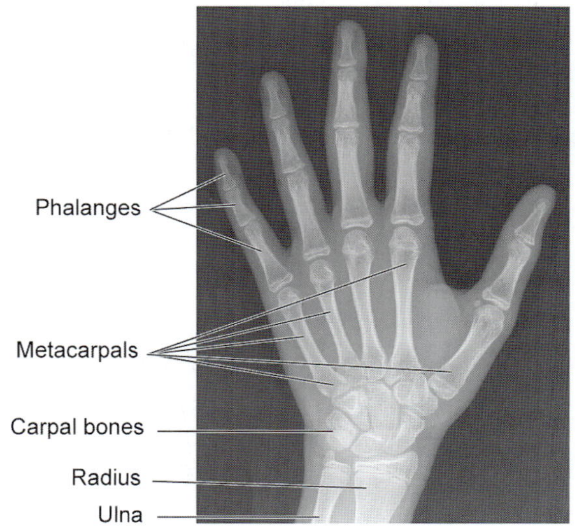

Fig. 11.17: Anteroposterior view of the hand

BDC's Anatomy *e*-book

1. Clinical testing of muscles of upper limb
2. Tracings of radiographs of upper limb
3. Clinical integration of radiographs of upper limb
4. Age determination using radiograph of hand
5. Comparison of upper and lower limbs
6. Further reading

Appendix

1

Major Nerves and Arteries of Upper Limb

MAJOR NERVES OF UPPER LIMB

The upper limb is supplied by major five nerves arising from the brachial plexus in addition to other smaller nerves:

1. Axillary nerve
2. Musculocutaneous nerve
3. Radial nerve
4. Median nerve
5. Ulnar nerve.

Most of the nerves course through different regions of the upper limb and have been described in parts in the respective regions. The course of the entire nerve, branches and clinical aspects has been described briefly in this annexure (Fig. A1.1a).

MUSCULOCUTANEOUS NERVE

Musculocutaneous nerve is so named as it supplies muscles of front of arm and skin of lateral side of forearm. This nerve rarely gets injured.

Root Value

Ventral rami of C5–C7 segments of spinal cord.

Course

Axilla and Arm

Musculocutaneous nerve is a branch of the lateral cord of brachial plexus, lies lateral to axillary and upper part of brachial artery. It supplies coracobrachialis, pierces the muscle to lie in the intermuscular septum between biceps brachii and brachialis muscles, both of which are supplied by this nerve (*see* Plate 8.3 and A1.1).

Forearm

About 2.5 cm above the crease of elbow, it becomes cutaneous by piercing the deep fascia. The nerve is called the lateral cutaneous nerve of forearm which supplies skin of lateral side of forearm both on the front and back.

Branches

Muscular: Coracobrachialis
Biceps brachii
Brachialis (large medial part) (Fig. A1.1)

Cutaneous: Lateral side of forearm (both on the front and the back).

Articular: Elbow joint.

Features of the musculocutaneous nerve injury are described in Fig. A1.2.

AXILLARY OR CIRCUMFLEX NERVE

Axillary nerve is called axillary as it runs through the upper part of axilla though it does not supply any structure there. It is called ***circumflex nerve*** as it courses around the surgical neck of humerus (*see* Fig. 6.3) to supply the prominent deltoid muscle.

Root Value

Ventral rami of C5, C6 segments of spinal cord.

Course

Axilla

Axillary or circumflex nerve is the smaller terminal branch of posterior cord seen in the axilla (*see* Fig. 4.14).

Quadrangular Space

The nerve passes backwards through the quadrangular space (bounded by subscapularis above, teres major below, long head of triceps brachii medially and surgical neck of humerus laterally) (*see* Fig. 6.9). Here it lies below the capsule of the shoulder joint.

Surgical Neck of Humerus

Then it passes behind the surgical neck of humerus where it divides into anterior and posterior divisions (Fig. A1.1).

Branches

The branches of axillary nerve are presented in Table A1.1.

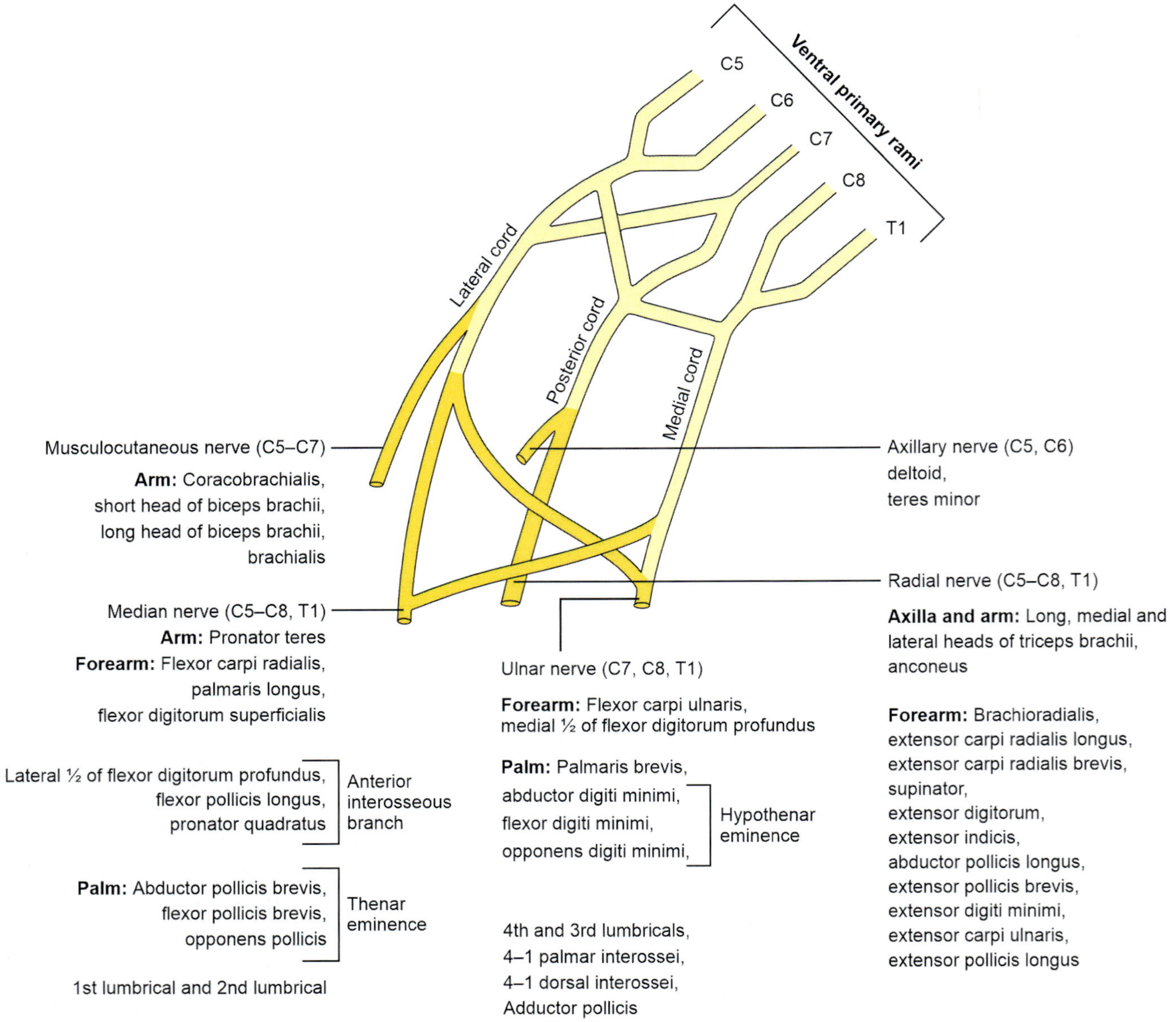

Ventral primary rami
C5
C6
C7
C8
T1
Lateral cord
Posterior cord
Medial cord

Musculocutaneous nerve (C5–C7)
Arm: Coracobrachialis, short head of biceps brachii, long head of biceps brachii, brachialis

Axillary nerve (C5, C6)
deltoid, teres minor

Radial nerve (C5–C8, T1)
Axilla and arm: Long, medial and lateral heads of triceps brachii, anconeus

Forearm: Brachioradialis, extensor carpi radialis longus, extensor carpi radialis brevis, supinator, extensor digitorum, extensor indicis, abductor pollicis longus, extensor pollicis brevis, extensor digiti minimi, extensor carpi ulnaris, extensor pollicis longus

Median nerve (C5–C8, T1)
Arm: Pronator teres
Forearm: Flexor carpi radialis, palmaris longus, flexor digitorum superficialis

Lateral ½ of flexor digitorum profundus, flexor pollicis longus, pronator quadratus — Anterior interosseous branch

Palm: Abductor pollicis brevis, flexor pollicis brevis, opponens pollicis — Thenar eminence

1st lumbrical and 2nd lumbrical

Ulnar nerve (C7, C8, T1)
Forearm: Flexor carpi ulnaris, medial ½ of flexor digitorum profundus

Palm: Palmaris brevis,
abductor digiti minimi, flexor digiti minimi, opponens digiti minimi, — Hypothenar eminence

4th and 3rd lumbricals,
4–1 palmar interossei,
4–1 dorsal interossei,
Adductor pollicis

Fig. A1.1: Brachial plexus and muscular branches of the main nerves

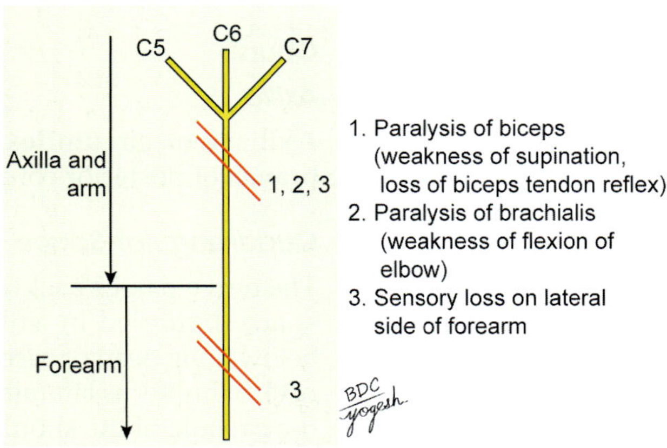

Fig. A1.2: Musculocutaneous nerve injury

TABLE A1.1: Branches of axillary nerve

	Trunk	*Anterior division*	*Posterior division*
Muscular	—	Deltoid (most part)	Deltoid (posterior part) and teres minor. The nerve to teres minor is characterised by the presence of a *pseudoganglion*
Cutaneous	—	—	Upper lateral cutaneous nerve of arm
Articular and vascular	Shoulder joint	—	To posterior circumflex humeral artery

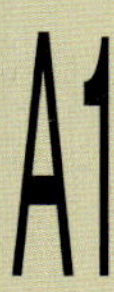

CLINICAL ANATOMY

Axillary nerve injury:

Paralysis of deltoid (Weakness of abduction of arm up to 90° and loss of rounded contour of shoulder)

Sensory loss over lower half of deltoid—Regimental badge anaesthesia

RADIAL NERVE

Radial nerve is the thickest branch of brachial plexus.

Root Value

Ventral rami of C5–C8, T1 segments of spinal cord (*see* Fig. 4.14).

Course

Axilla

Radial nerve lies against the muscles forming the posterior wall of axilla, i.e. subscapularis, teres major distance in arm behind brachial artery. Then, it enters in the lower triangular space between teres major, long head of triceps brachii and shaft of humerus. It gives two muscular and one cutaneous branches in the axilla (Fig. A1.1).

Radial Groove

Radial nerve enters through the lower triangular space into the radial groove/sulcus, where it lies between the lateral and medial heads of triceps brachii along with profunda brachii vessels (*see* Plate 6.4). Long and lateral heads form the roof of the radial sulcus. It leaves the sulcus by piercing the lateral intermuscular septum. In the sulcus, it gives three muscular and two cutaneous branches.

Front of Arm

The radial nerve descends on the lower and lateral side of front of arm deep in the interval between brachialis on medial side and brachioradialis with extensor carpi radialis longus on the lateral side to reach capitulum of humerus.

Cubital Fossa

The nerve enters the lateral side of cubital fossa. There the radial nerve terminates by dividing into ***superficial and deep branches*** (*see* Fig. 8.16). The deep branch supplies extensor carpi radialis, brevis and supinator. Then, it courses between two heads of supinator to reach back of forearm.

Front of Forearm

The superficial branch leaves the cubital fossa to enter lateral side of front of forearm, accompanied by the radial vessels in its upper 2/3rd. At the junction of upper 2/3rd and lower 1/3rd, the superficial branch turns laterally to reach the posterolateral aspect of forearm.

Wrist and Dorsum of Hand

The superficial branch descends till the "anatomical snuffbox" to reach dorsum of hand, where it supplies skin of lateral half of dorsum of hand and lateral 3½ digits till distal interphalangeal joints (*see* Figs 7.1b and 9.45).

Back of Forearm and Wrist

The deep branch of radial nerve enters the back of forearm, where it supplies the muscles mentioned in Table A1.2. Lower down it passes through the 4th compartment under the extensor retinaculum to reach the back of wrist where it ends in a ***pseudoganglion***, branches of which supply the neighbouring joints (*see* Fig. 9.51).

Branches of Radial Nerve

The branches of radial nerve are presented in Table A1.2.

Branches of deep division of radial nerve are shown in Table A1.3.

Branches of superficial division of radial nerve are shown in Table A1.4.

Features of the radial nerve injury are described in Fig. A1.3.

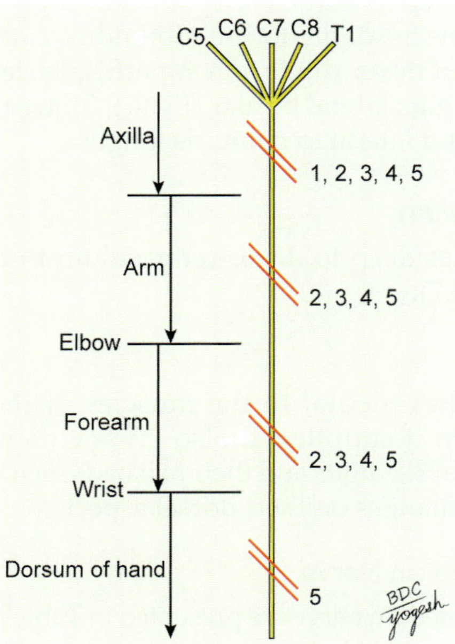

1. Paralysis of triceps brachii (loss of extension of elbow)*
2. Paralysis of extensor group of muscles in forearm (wrist drop)**
3. Paralysis of extensor pollicis longus (loss of extension at metacarpophalangeal and interphalangeal joints of thumb)
4. Paralysis of extensor digitorum, extensor indicis, and extensor digiti minimi (finger drop)***
5. Sensory loss (in lateral and posterior aspect of arm, posterior aspects, forearm, hand, and lateral 3½ fingers)

*When injured at arm, elbow extension is possible though it is weak as motor branches to long and medial head of triceps arise in the lower triangular space of axilla

**When injured at forearm, wrist drop may not be very pronounced as extensor carpi radialis longus is not involved

***Metacarpophalangeal joints cannot be extended but interphalangeal joints can be extended due to the action of lumbricals innervated by the median and ulnar nerves

Fig. A1.3: Radial nerve injury

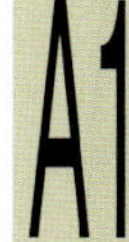

TABLE A1.2: Branches of radial nerve

	Axilla	*Radial sulcus*	*Lateral side of arm*
Muscular	Long head of triceps brachii Medial head of triceps brachii	Lateral head of triceps brachii Medial head of triceps brachii Anconeus	Brachioradialis Extensor carpi radialis longus Lateral part of brachialis (proprioceptive)
Cutaneous	Posterior cutaneous nerve of arm	Posterior cutaneous nerve of forearm Lower lateral cutaneous nerve of arm	—
Vascular		To profunda brachii artery	—
Terminal	—	—	Superficial and deep or posterior interosseous branches

TABLE A1.3: Branches of deep division of radial nerve

	Cubital fossa	*Back of forearm*	*Wrist*
Muscular	Extensor carpi radialis brevis Supinator	Abductor pollicis longus Extensor pollicis brevis Extensor pollicis longus Extensor digitorum Extensor indicis Extensor digiti minimi Extensor carpi ulnaris	—
Articular	—	—	To inferior radioulnar, wrist and intercarpal joints

TABLE A1.4: Branches of superficial division of radial nerve

	Forearm	*Anatomical snuffbox and dorsum of hand*
Cutaneous and vascular	Lateral side of forearm and radial vessels	Skin over anatomical snuffbox, lateral half of dorsum of hand and lateral 3½ digits till their distal interphalangeal joints
Articular	—	To wrist joint, 1st carpometacarpal joint, metacarpophalangeal and interphalangeal joints of the thumb, index and middle fingers

MEDIAN NERVE

Median nerve is called median as it runs in the median plane of the forearm.

Root Value

Ventral rami of C5–C8, T1 segments of spinal cord.

Course

Axilla

Median nerve is formed by two roots, lateral root from lateral cord (C5–C7) and medial root from medial cord (C8, T1) of brachial plexus. Medial root crosses the axillary artery to join the lateral root. The median nerve runs on the lateral side of axillary artery (*see* Plate 8.4).

Arm

Median nerve continues to run on the lateral side of brachial artery till the middle of arm, where it crosses in front of the artery, passes anterior to elbow joint into the cubital fossa (*see* Plate 8.4 and A1.1).

Cubital Fossa

Median nerve lies most medial in the cubital fossa. It gives three branches to flexor muscles of the forearm. It leaves the fossa by passing between two heads of pronator teres (*see* Figs 8.16 and 8.17).

Forearm

Median nerve enters the forearm and lies in the centre of forearm. It lies deep to fibrous arch of flexor digitorum superficialis on the flexor digitorum profundus. Adheres to deep surface of flexor digitorum superficialis, leaves the muscle, along its lateral border (Plate 9.3). Lastly, it is placed deep and lateral to palmaris longus.

Flexor Retinaculum

Median nerve lies deep to flexor retinaculum to enter palm (*see* Plate 9.7).

Palm

Median nerve lies medial to the muscles of thenar eminence, which it supplies. It also gives cutaneous branches to lateral 3½ digits and their nail beds including skin of distal phalanges on their dorsal aspect.

Branches of Median Nerve

The branches of median nerve are presented in Table A1.5.

Features of the median nerve injury are described in Fig. A1.4.

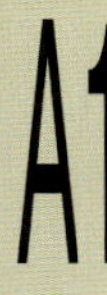

TABLE A1.5: Branches of median nerve

	Axilla and arm	*Cubital fossa*	*Forearm*	*Palm*
Muscular	Pronator teres in lower part of arm	Flexor carpi radialis Flexor digitorum superficialis Palmaris longus	Anterior interosseous which supplies: Lateral half of flexor digitorum profundus, pronator quadratus, and flexor pollicis longus	Recurrent branch for abductor pollicis brevis, flexor pollicis brevis, opponens pollicis. 1st and 2nd lumbricals from the digital nerves
Cutaneous	—	—	Palmar cutaneous branch for lateral 2/3rd of palm	Two digital branches to lateral and medial sides of thumb One to lateral side of index finger Two to adjacent sides of index and middle fingers Two to adjacent sides of middle and ring fingers. These branches also supply dorsal aspects of distal phalanges of lateral 3½ digits including nail beds (Fig. A1.2)
Articular and vascular	Gives sympathetic fibres to axillary and brachial arteries	Elbow joint	Gives sympathetic fibres to radial and ulnar arteries	Gives articular branches to joints of hand

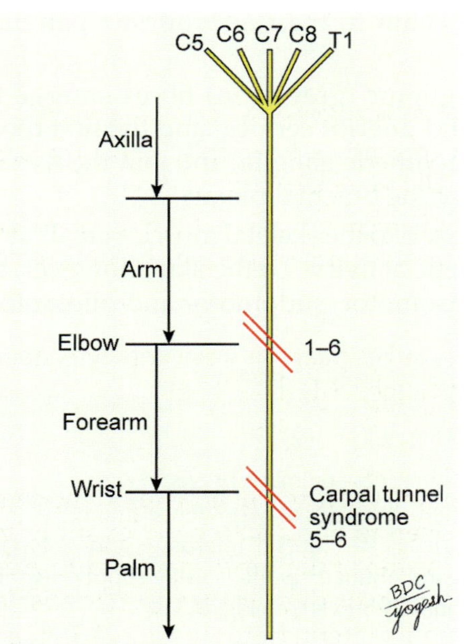

1. Paralysis of all flexors of wrist except flexor carpi ulnaris and medial half of flexor digitorum profundus (weak flexion of wrist. The wrist deviates to ulnar side on flexion)
2. Paralysis of pronator teres and pronator quadratus (loss of pronation of forearm)
3. Paralysis of flexor digitorum superficialis and lateral half of flexor digitorum profundus and paralysis of 1st and 2nd lumbricals (when the patient is asked to close his hands and make a fist, he is able to close the ring and little finger as these have functioning flexor digitorum profundus, supplied by ulnar nerve. The middle finger also closes partially as FDPs are partially interlinked, but index finger remains open [pointing finger sign]).
4. Paralysis of flexor pollicis longus (loss of flexion at interphalangeal joint of thumb)
5. Paralysis of thenar muscles (loss of thenar eminence, Ape-like thumb)
6. Sensory, trophic and vasomotor changes over lateral 3½ fingers including their nails beds.

Fig. A1.4: Median nerve injury

ULNAR NERVE

Ulnar nerve is named so as it runs along the medial or ulnar side of the upper limb.

Root Value

Ventral rami of C8 and T1. It also gets fibres of C7 from the lateral root of median nerve (*see* Fig. 4.14).

Course

Axilla

Ulnar nerve lies in the axilla between the axillary vein and axillary artery on a deeper plane.

Arm

Ulnar nerve lies medial to brachial artery. Runs downwards with the brachial artery in its proximal part (*see* Fig. 8.7). At the middle of arm, it pierces the medial intermuscular septum to lie on its back and descends on the back of medial epicondyle of humerus where it can be palpated. Palpation causes tingling sensations (*see* Fig. 8.12a). That is why humerus is called 'funny bone'.

Forearm

Ulnar nerve enters the forearm by passing between two heads of flexor carpi ulnaris. There it lies on medial part

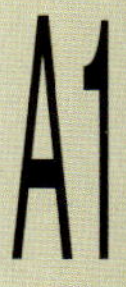

of flexor digitorum profundus. *Ulnar nerve is not a content of cubital fossa.*

It is accompanied by the ulnar artery in lower 2/3rd of forearm.

It gives two muscular and two cutaneous branches (Table A1.4 and Fig. A1.1).

Flexor Retinaculum

Finally, it lies on the medial part of flexor retinaculum to enter palm. At the distal border of retinaculum, the nerve divides into its superficial and deep branches.

Palm

Superficial branch supplies palmaris brevis and gives digital branches to medial 1½ digits including medial 1½ nail beds till the distal interphalangeal joints (Fig. A1.2).

Deep branch supplies most of the intrinsic muscles of the hand. At first, it supplies three muscles of hypothenar eminence. Running in the concavity of deep palmar arch, it gives branches to 3rd and 4th lumbricals from deep aspect; all dorsal and palmar interossei to end in adductor pollicis (Table A1.5). Since it supplies intrinsic muscles of hand responsible for finer movements, this nerve is called 'musician's nerve'.

Branches

The branches of ulnar nerve are presented in Table A1.6 and Fig. A1.1.

CLINICAL ANATOMY

- Features of the ulnar nerve injury are described in Fig. A1.5.
- ***Ulnar paradox***: If ulnar nerve is injured at the elbow, the clawing of the fingers is less, because medial half of flexor digitorum profundus (flexor of proximal and distal interphalangeal joints) also gets paralysed. If ulnar nerve is injured at wrist, the clawing of the fingers is more as intact flexor digitorum profundus flexes the digits more. Thus, if lesion is proximal (near elbow), clawing is less. On the contrary, if lesion is distal (near wrist), clawing is more. This is called 'action of paradox'/ulnar paradox.
- ***Complete claw hand:*** If both ulnar and median nerves get paralysed, there is complete claw hand (*see* Fig. 9.40).
- Table A1.7 shows the comparison between injuries of median and ulnar nerves at the wrist.

SYMPATHETIC INNERVATION

1. The sympathetic innervation of the upper limb is derived from the upper six thoracic segments of the spinal cord. The fibres arise from the lateral horn cells and come out with the ventral roots as preganglionic (white rami) fibres. These fibres ascend in the sympathetic chain to their appropriate ganglia for relay.
2. The postganglionic (grey rami) fibres emerge from the middle and inferior cervical and the first thoracic (stellate) sympathetic ganglia, and join the five roots (C5–C8, T1) of the brachial plexus.
3. The blood vessels to the skeletal muscles are dilated by the sympathetic activity. To the skin, however, these nerves are vasomotor, sudomotor and pilomotor.

TABLE A1.6: Branches of ulnar nerve

	Forearm	***Hand*** (*see* Fig. 9.31)
Muscular	Medial half of flexor digitorum profundus Flexor carpi ulnaris	Superficial branch—palmaris brevis Deep branch—muscles of hypothenar eminence, medial two lumbricals, 4–1 dorsal interossei and 4–1 palmar interossei and adductor pollicis. May supply deep head of flexor pollicis brevis (*see* Fig. 9.31)
Cutaneous/digital	Dorsal cutaneous branch for medial half of dorsum of hand. Palmar cutaneous branch for medial one-third of palm. Digital branches to medial 1½ fingers, nail beds and dorsal aspects of distal phalanges	—
Vascular/articular	Also supplies digital vessels and joints of medial side of hand	

TABLE A1.7: Comparison of injury of median and ulnar nerves at wrist

Injury to median nerve at wrist	***Injury to ulnar nerve at wrist***
Loss of thenar eminence	Loss of hypothenar eminence
Normal fist making by 4th, 5th digits	Clawing of 4th and 5th digits
Lagging behind of 2nd and 3rd digits in fist making	Slight clawing of 2nd and 3rd digits Gutters seen in palm
Sensory loss over lateral 3½ digits	Sensory loss over medial 1½ digits
Loss of pronation of forearm	Loss of adduction of 2nd, 4th and 5th digits
Loss of opposition of thumb	Loss of abduction of 2nd–4th digits

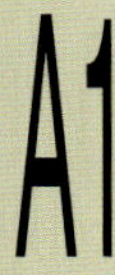

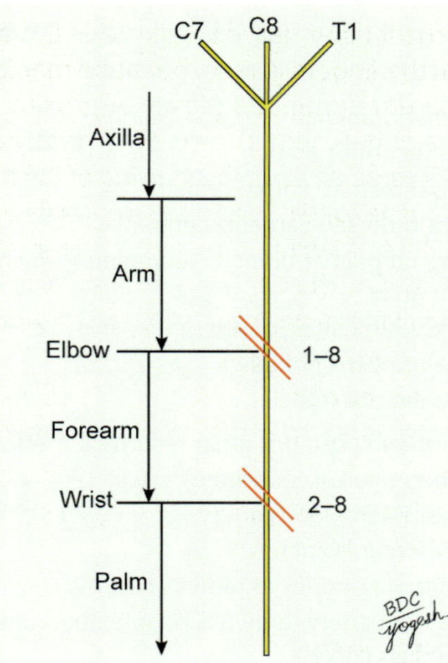

1. Paralysis of flexor carpi ulnaris and medial ½ of flexor digitorum profundus (flattening of medial border of forearm, loss of flexion at distal interphalangeal joints of 4th and 5th digits, weak flexion of the wrist*)
2. Paralysis of hypothenar muscles (loss of hypothenar eminence)
3. Paralysis of adductor pollicis (loss of adduction of thumb)
4. Paralysis of palmar interossei (loss of abduction of all fingers except little finger)
5. Paralysis of dorsal interossei (loss of adduction of 2nd, 4th and 5th digits)
6. Paralysis of interossei (slight clawing of 2nd and 3rd digits [intactness of median nerve supply to lateral ½ of flexor digitorum profundus])
7. Paralysis of 3rd and 4th lumbricals (marked clawing of 4th and 5th digits)
8. Sensory, trophic and vasomotor changes (Fig. A1.2)

* The wrist deviates to radial side due to lack of pull by paralysed flexor carpi ulnaris.

Fig. A1.5: Ulnar nerve injury

MAJOR ARTERIES OF UPPER LIMB

The upper limb is supplied by the axillary artery. The brief of the major arteries of the upper limb and their branches have been tabulated in Table A1.6. For the detailed course, relations and applied aspects of these arteries, refer corresponding chapters.

BDC's Anatomy *e*-book

1. Embryology of the upper limb
2. Clinical terms
3. Further reading
4. Viva voce questions

TABLE A1.6: Arteries of upper limb

Artery	*Origin, course and termination*	*Branches*
Axillary artery (*see* Figs 4.6 and A1.3)	Starts at the outer border of first rib as continuation of subclavian artery, runs through axilla and continues as brachial artery at the lower border of teres major muscle	*1st part*: Superior thoracic artery *2nd part*: Thoracoacromial trunk a. Pectoral b. Acromial c. Clavicular d. Deltoid branches Lateral thoracic artery 3rd part: Subscapular artery a. Circumflex scapular artery Anterior circumflex humeral artery a. Ascending branch Posterior circumflex humeral artery
Brachial artery (*see* Fig. 8.8)	Starts at the lower border of teres major as continuation of axillary artery. Runs on anterior aspect of arm and ends by dividing into radial and ulnar arteries at neck of radius in the cubital fossa	1. Profunda brachii artery a. Deltoid (ascending) branch b. Nutrient artery to humerus c. Numerous muscular branches d. Anterior descending (radial collateral) artery e. Posterior descending (middle collateral) artery 2. Superior ulnar collateral artery 3. Inferior ulnar collateral artery 4. Nutrient artery to humerus 5. Unnamed muscular arteries 6. Ulnar artery 7. Radial artery

(Contd.)

TABLE A1.6: Arteries of upper limb *(Contd.)*

Artery	*Origin, course and termination*	*Branches*
Radial artery (*see* Fig. 9.8):	Starts as smaller branch of brachial artery, lies on the lateral side of forearm, then in the anatomical snuffbox to reach the palm, where it continues as deep palmar arch	1. Muscular branches 2. Radial recurrent branch 3. Anterior (palmar) carpal branch 4. Posterior (dorsal) carpal branch 5. Superficial palmar branch – completes superficial palmar arch 6. First dorsal metacarpal artery 7. Arteria princeps pollicis 8. Arteria radialis indicis
Ulnar artery (*see* Plate 9.7)	Originates as the larger terminal branch of brachial artery at neck of radius. Courses first obliquely in upper one-third and then vertically in lower two-thirds of forearm. Lies superficial to flexor retinaculum and ends by dividing into superficial and deep branches	1. Anterior and posterior ulnar recurrent arteries 2. Common interosseous artery Anterior interosseous artery a. Muscular branches b. Nutrient arteries to radius and ulna c. Median artery (only 8% people) that runs with median nerve Posterior interosseous artery 3. Anterior and posterior ulnar carpal branches 4. Terminal branches – Superficial branch – continues as superficial palmar arch – Deep branch – completes deep palmar arch
Superficial palmar arch (*see* Plate 9.15)	Superficial palmar arch is the continuation of superficial branch of ulnar artery. It begins over the muscles of hypothenar eminence just below the flexor retinaculum. In palm, it runs laterally with downward convexity. It is completed by superficial palmar branch of radial artery	1–3. Three common palmar digital arteries for adjacent sides of medial 3½ digits 4. One proper digital artery for medial side of little finger 5. Cutaneous branches of the skin of palm
Deep palmar arch (*see* Plate 9.15)	Deep palmar arch is the continuation of radial artery after it emerges in the palm between transverse and oblique heads of adductor pollicis muscle. It is completed medially by deep palmar branch of ulnar artery at the base of 5th metacarpal bone	1–3. Three palmar metacarpal arteries 4–6. Three perforating arteries 7. Recurrent branch to superficial palmar arch

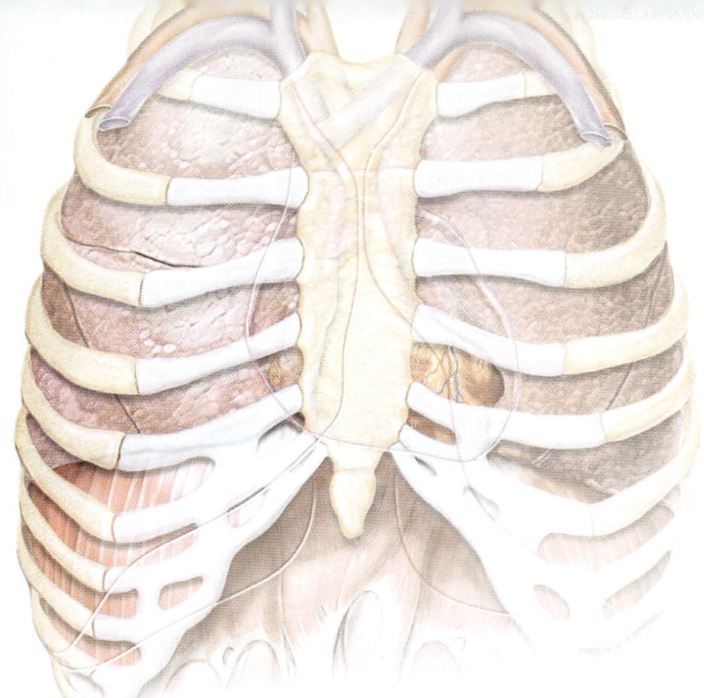

Section 2

Thorax

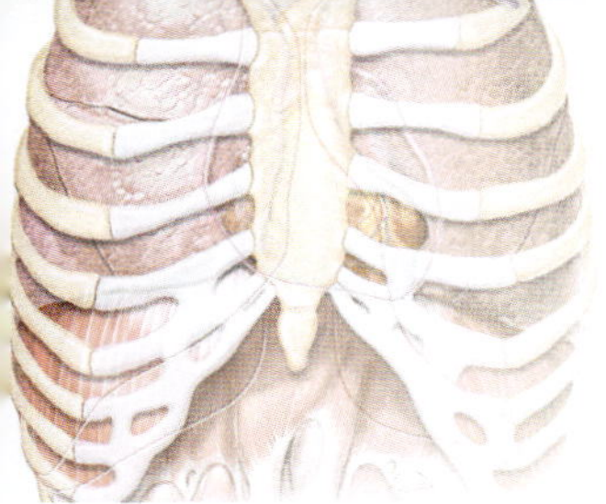

Chapter

12

Introduction

Thorax (Latin *chest*) forms the upper part of the trunk of the body. It not only permits boarding and lodging of the thoracic viscera, but also provides necessary shelter to some of the abdominal viscera.

The trunk of the body is divided by the *diaphragm* into an upper part, called the *thorax,* and a lower part, called the *abdomen.* The thorax is supported by a skeletal framework, *thoracic cage.* The thoracic cavity contains the lungs (the principal organs of respiration) and the heart (of circulation), both of which are vital for life.

SURFACE LANDMARKS OF THORAX

Bony Landmarks

1. ***Suprasternal or jugular notch*** (Fig. 12.1)**:** It is felt just above the superior border of the manubrium between the sternal ends of the clavicles. It lies at the level of the lower border of the body of the second thoracic vertebra. The trachea can be palpated in this notch.
2. ***Sternal angle/angle of Louis:*** It is felt as a transverse ridge about 5 cm below the suprasternal notch. It marks the manubriosternal joint, and lies at the level of the second costal cartilage anteriorly, and the disc between the fourth and fifth thoracic vertebrae posteriorly. *This is an important landmark for the following reasons.*
   a. The ribs are counted from this level. The second costal cartilage and second rib lie at the level of the sternal angle or angle of Louis (French physician, 1787–1872).
   b. It lies at the level of the disc between the 4th and 5th thoracic vertebrae.
   c. It marks the plane which separates the superior mediastinum from the inferior mediastinum.
   d. The ascending aorta ends at this level. The arch of the aorta begins and also ends at this level. The descending aorta begins at this level. The trachea divides into two principal bronchi.
   e. The azygos vein arches over the root of the right lung and opens into the superior vena cava.

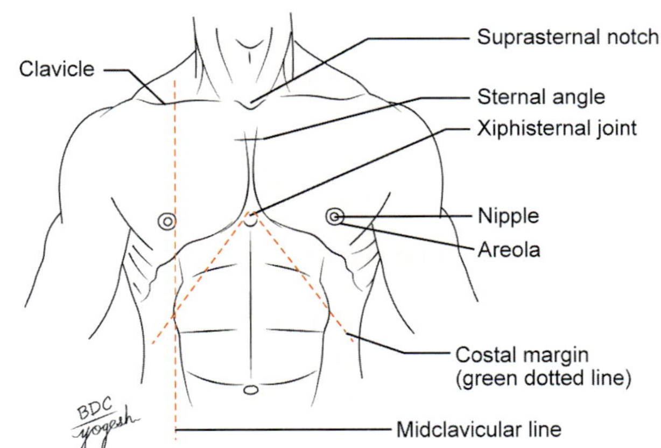

Fig. 12.1: Surface anatomy of thoracic region (anterior view)

   f. The pulmonary trunk divides into two pulmonary arteries just below this level.
   g. The thoracic duct crosses from the right to the left side at the level of the fifth thoracic vertebra and reaches the left side at the level of the sternal angle.
   h. It marks the upper limit of the base of the heart.
3. ***Xiphisternal joint:*** The costal margin on each side is formed by the 7th to 10th costal cartilages. Between the two costal margins, there lies the ***infrasternal*** or ***subcostal angle***. The depression in the angle is also known as the ***epigastric fossa***. The xiphoid (Greek *sword*) process lies in the floor of the epigastric fossa. At the apex of the angle, the xiphisternal joint may be felt as a short transverse ridge. It lies at the level of the upper border of the 9th thoracic vertebra (Fig. 12.1).
4. ***Costal cartilages:*** The 2*nd* costal (Latin *rib*) cartilage is attached to the sternal angle. The 7*th* costal cartilage bounds the upper part of the infrasternal angle. The 10th costal cartilage forms the lower part of the costal margin (Fig. 12.1 and Plate 12.1).
5. ***Ribs:*** The scapula overlies the 2nd to 7th ribs on the posterolateral aspect of the chest wall. The 10th rib is the lowest point, lies at the level of the 3rd lumbar vertebra.
6. ***Thoracic vertebral spines:*** The 1st prominent spine felt at the lower part of the back of the neck is that of the

Plate 12.1: Thoracic cage

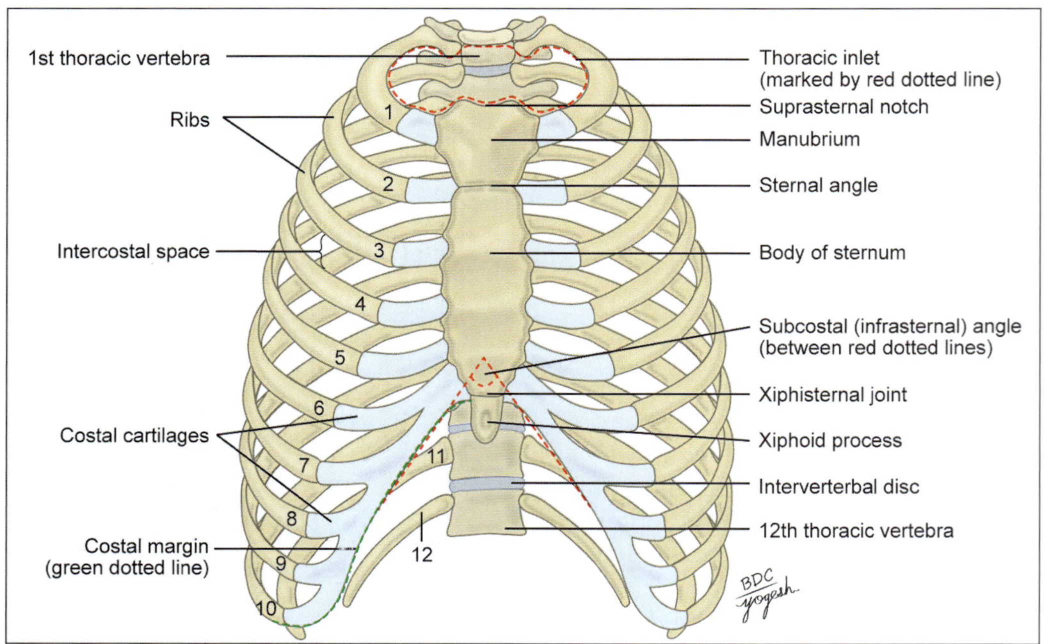

7th cervical vertebra or *vertebra prominens.* Below this spine, all the thoracic spines can be palpated along the posterior median line. The 3rd thoracic spine lies at the level of the roots of the spines of the scapulae. The 7th thoracic spine lies at the level of the inferior angles of the scapulae.

Soft Tissue Landmarks

1. ***Nipple:*** The position of the nipple varies considerably in females, but in males it usually lies in the 4th intercostal space about 10 cm from the midsternal line (Fig. 12.1).
2. ***Apex beat:*** It is a visible and palpable cardiac impulse in the left 5th intercostal space, 9 cm from the midsternal line, or medial to the midclavicular line and nipple.
3. ***Trachea:*** It is palpable in the suprasternal notch midway between the two clavicles.

SKELETON OF THORAX (THORACIC CAGE)

- The skeleton of thorax is also known as the ***thoracic cage***. It is an osseocartilaginous elastic cage which is primarily designed for increasing and decreasing the intrathoracic pressure, so that air is sucked into the lungs during inspiration and expelled during expiration.

FORMATION

Anteriorly: Sternum (Greek *chest*) (Plate 12.1).

Posteriorly: 12 thoracic vertebrae and the intervening intervertebral discs.

On each side: 12 ribs with their cartilages.

Note: The ribs articulate as follows:

Posteriorly: Each rib articulates posteriorly with the vertebral column.

Anteriorly:

a. The upper seven ribs articulate with the sternum through their cartilages and these are called ***true or vertebrosternal ribs***.

b. The costal cartilages of the next three ribs, i.e. the 8th, 9th, and 10th end by joining the next higher costal cartilage. These ribs are, therefore, known as ***vertebrochondral ribs***.

c. The anterior ends of the 11th and 12th ribs are free. These are called ***floating or vertebral ribs***.

The vertebrochondral and vertebral ribs, i.e. the last five ribs, are also called ***false ribs*** because they do not articulate with the sternum.

CLINICAL ANATOMY

The chest wall of the child is highly elastic, and fractures of the ribs are, therefore, rare. In adults, the ribs may be fractured by direct or indirect violence (Fig. 12.2). In indirect violence, like crush injury, the rib fractures at its weakest point located at the angle. The upper two ribs which are protected by the clavicle, and the lower two ribs which are free to swing are least commonly injured.

SHAPE

- The thorax resembles a ***truncated cone*** which is narrow above and broad below (Fig. 12.3). The ***narrow upper end*** is continuous with the root of the neck from which it is partly separated by the suprapleural membrane or Sibson's fascia. The ***broad lower end*** is almost completely separated from the abdomen by the ***diaphragm*** which is deeply concave downwards.

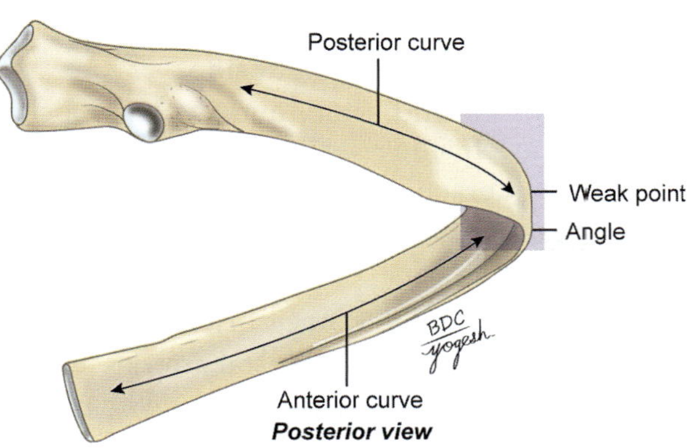

Fig. 12.2: Vulnerable site of fracture of the rib

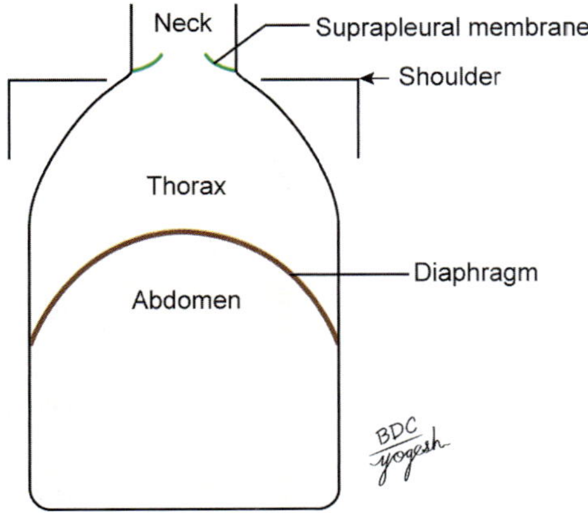

Fig. 12.3: Scheme to show how the size of the thoracic cavity is reduced by the upward projection of the diaphragm, and by the inward projection of the shoulders

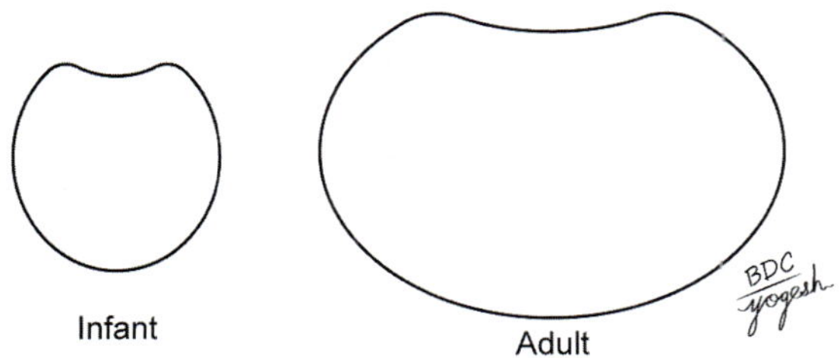

Fig. 12.4: The shape of the thorax as seen in transverse section in: Human infant and adult

- The thoracic cavity is actually much smaller than what it appears to be because the narrow upper part appears broad due to the shoulders, and the lower part is greatly encroached upon by the abdominal cavity due to the upward convexity of the diaphragm.
- In transverse section, the thorax is reniform (bean-shaped, or kidney-shaped) (Fig. 12.4). The transverse diameter is greater than the anteroposterior diameter. However, in infants below the age of two years, it is circular.
- In infants, the ribs are horizontal and as a result the respiration is purely ***abdominal respiration*** by the action of the diaphragm. In adults, the thorax is oval. The ribs are oblique and their movements alternately increase and decrease the diameters of the thorax. This results in the drawing in of air into the thorax called *inspiration* and its expulsion is called *expiration*. This is called ***thoracic respiration***. Therefore, in the adult, there is ***abdominothoracic respiration***.

CLINICAL ANATOMY

- Diaphragm descends during inspiration to increase the vertical diameter of thoracic cage.
- ***Hiccups***: These occur due to spasmodic involuntary contractions of the diaphragm accompanied by closed glottis. These usually occur due to gastric irritation. Hiccups may also be due to phrenic nerve irritation, uraemia, or hysteria.
- ***Postoperative pneumonia in children***: In children up to the age of 2 years, respiration is abdominal (because ribs are horizontal). In postoperative period of abdominal surgeries, the child resists abdominal breathing and lung secretions accumulate causing pneumonia.

Competency:
AN21.3 Describe and demonstrate the boundaries of thoracic inlet, cavity and outlet along with its applied aspect (thoracic inlet syndrome).

SUPERIOR APERTURE (INLET OF THORAX)

The narrow upper end of the thorax, which is continuous with the neck, is called the *inlet of the thorax* (Fig. 12.5) (*Note*: Clinicians refer the superior thoracic aperture as the *thoracic outlet*). It is kidney-shaped. Its transverse diameter is 10–12 cm. The anteroposterior diameter is about 5 cm.

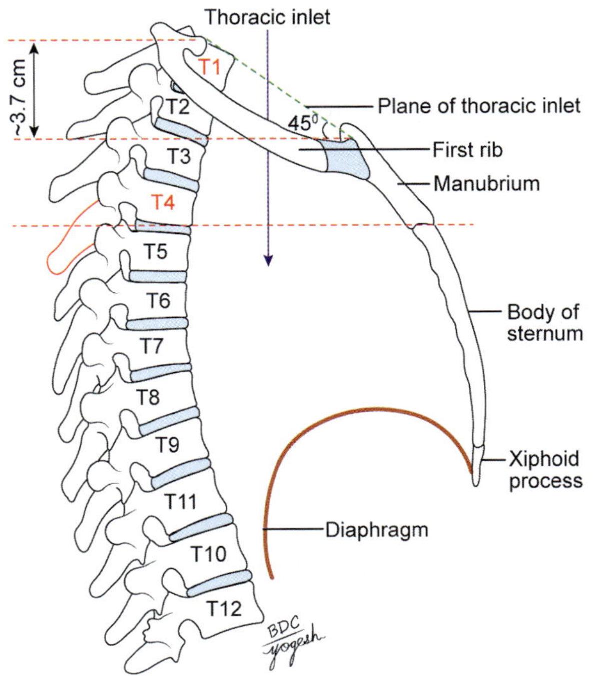

Fig. 12.5: Orientation of thoracic cage and plane of thoracic inlet

Boundaries

Anteriorly: Upper border of the manubrium sterni.
Posteriorly: Superior surface of the body of the first thoracic vertebra.
On each side: 1st rib with its cartilage.

Plane of Inlet

The plane of the inlet is directed downwards and forwards with an obliquity of about 45°. The anterior part of the inlet lies 3.7 cm below the posterior part, so that the upper border of the manubrium sterni lies at the level of the upper border of the 3rd thoracic vertebra.

Suprapleural Membrane or Sibson's Fascia

- The thoracic inlet is partitioned into two halves—right and left, with a cleft in-between. Each half is covered by a fascia, known as *Sibson's fascia or suprapleural membrane*. It partly separates the thorax from the neck.
- The membrane is triangular in shape.
- ***Attachments:*** Its *apex* is attached to the tip of the transverse process of the 7th cervical vertebra and the *base* to the inner border of the 1st rib and its cartilage.
- Morphologically, Sibson's fascia is regarded as the flattened tendon of the scalenus minimus (pleuralis) muscle. It is thus formed by scalenus minimus and endothoracic fascia.
- ***Relations:*** The inferior surface of the membrane is fused to the cervical pleura, beneath which lies the apex of the lung. Its superior surface is related to the subclavian vessels and other structures at the root of the neck (Figs 12.6a and b).
- ***Function:*** Functionally, it provides rigidity to the thoracic inlet, so that the root of the neck is not puffed up and down during respiration.

Structures Passing through the Inlet of Thorax

Viscera

Trachea, oesophagus, apices of the lungs with pleura, remains of the thymus (Fig. 12.7).

Large Vessels

1. Brachiocephalic artery on right side
2. Left common carotid artery and the left subclavian artery on the left side
3. Right and left brachiocephalic veins.

Smaller Vessels

1. Right and left internal thoracic arteries
2. Right and left superior intercostal arteries
3. Right and left first posterior intercostal veins
4. Inferior thyroid veins.

Nerves

1. Right and left phrenic nerves
2. Right and left vagus nerves
3. Right and left sympathetic trunks
4. Right and left first thoracic nerves as they ascend across the first rib to join the brachial plexus.

Muscles

Sternohyoid, sternothyroid, and longus colli.

CLINICAL ANATOMY

- A ***cervical rib*** is a rib attached to vertebra C7. It occurs in about 0.5–2% of subjects (Fig. 12.8). Such a rib may exert traction on the lower trunk of the brachial plexus. Such a person complains of paraesthesia or abnormal sensations along the ulnar border of the forearm, and wasting of the small muscles of the hand supplied by segment T1.
- ***Thoracic inlet syndrome***: Clinically it is called *thoracic outlet syndrome.* Two structures arch over the first rib—the subclavian artery and first thoracic nerve. These structures may be pulled or pressed by a cervical rib or by variations in the insertion of the scalenus anterior. The symptoms may, therefore, be vascular, neural, or both.

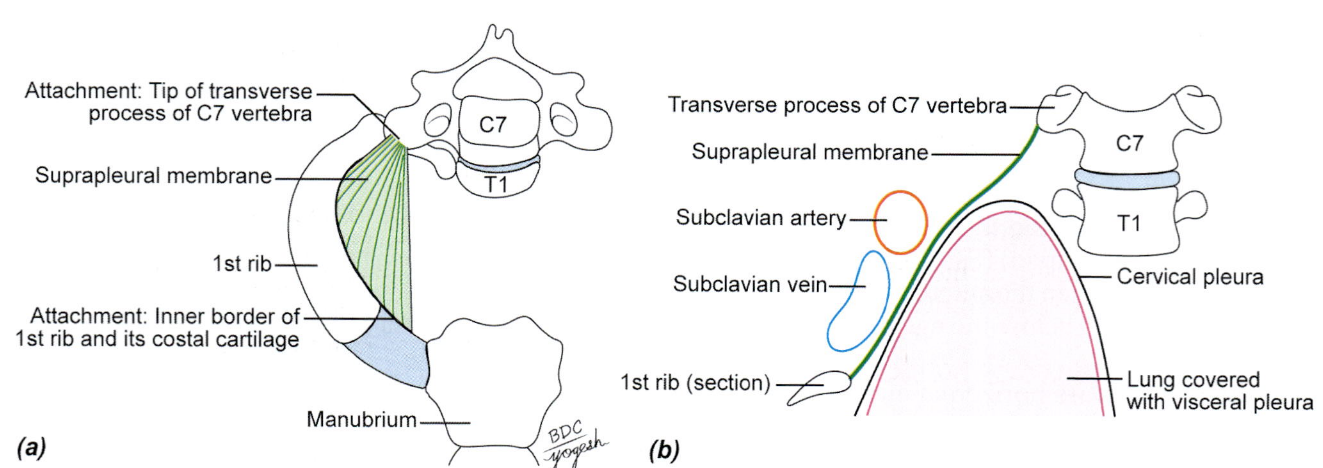

Figs 12.6a and b: The suprapleural membrane: (a) Surface view and (b) sectional view

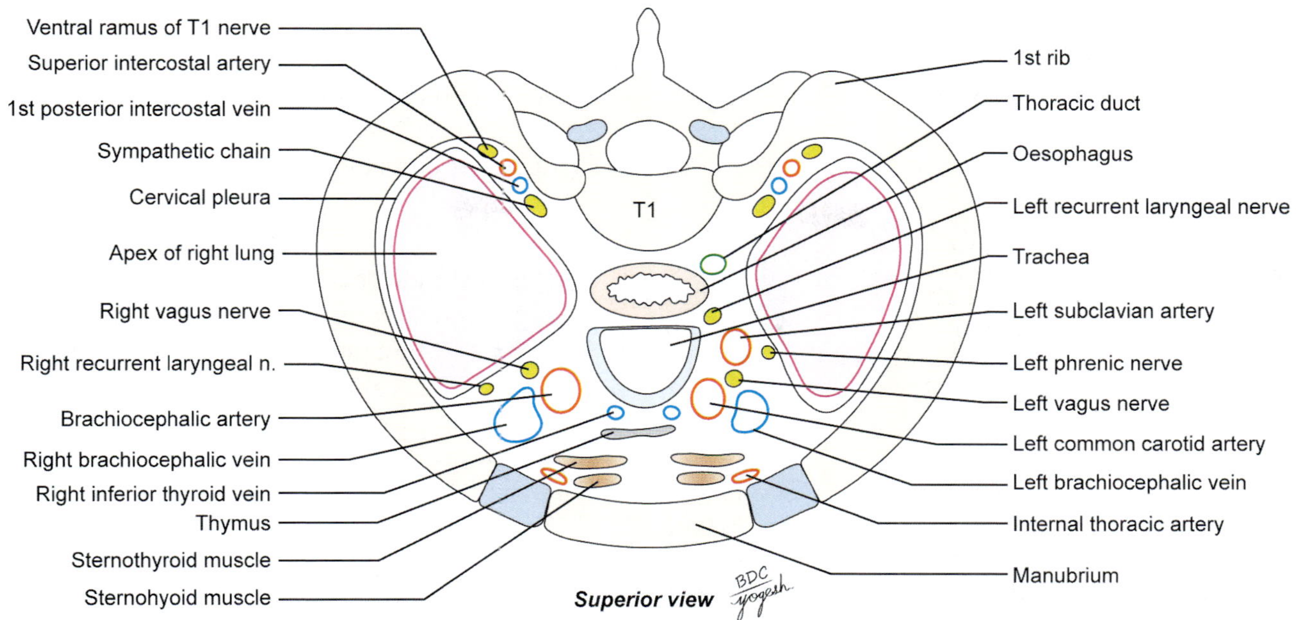

Fig. 12.7: Structures passing through the inlet of the thorax

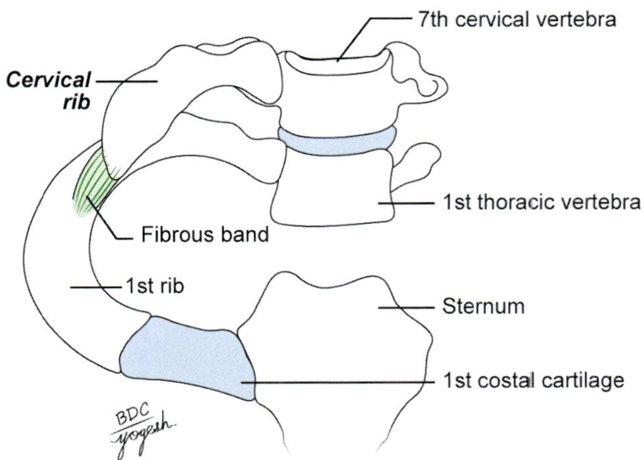

Fig. 12.8: Cervical rib

INFERIOR APERTURE (OUTLET OF THORAX)

- The inferior aperture is the broad end of the thorax which surrounds the upper part of the abdominal cavity, but is separated from it by the diaphragm (Greek *across fence*).

Boundaries

Anteriorly: Infrasternal angle between the two costal margins.

Posteriorly: Inferior surface of the body of the twelfth thoracic vertebra.

On each side: Costal margin formed by the cartilages of seventh to twelfth ribs.

DIAPHRAGM AT THE OUTLET OF THORAX

- The outlet is closed by a large musculotendinous partition, called the diaphragm—the ***thoracoabdominal diaphragm***—which separates the thorax from the abdomen (Figs 12.9 and 12.10).

Origin

- The domes of diaphragm project into thoracic cavity. It has three groups of fibres (Fig. 12.9):
  1. Sternal part: It consists of two fleshy slips that arise from back of xiphoid process.
  2. Costal part: It arises from inner surface of lower six ribs and their costal cartilages.
  3. Vertebral part: It consists of right and left crura and five arcuate ligaments (Fig. 12.10).
- ***Crura*** are elongated muscular slips. ***Right crus*** arises from right side of anterior surface of L1–L3 vertebrae and corresponding intervertebral discs. ***Left crus*** is smaller than the right. It arises from left side of anterior surface of L1 and L2 vertebrae and corresponding intervertebral disc.
- ***Arcuate ligaments:*** There are 5 arcuate ligaments.
  - One ***median arcuate ligament*** arches between upper ends of right and left crura.
  - Two ***medial arcuate ligaments*** arch between L2 vertebra to the tip of transverse process of L1 vertebra.
  - Two ***lateral arcuate ligaments*** arch between tip of transverse process of L1 vertebra and the 12th rib.

Insertion

- All the fibers converge and insert into central tendon. It is an aponeurotic sheet. It is ***trifoliate-shaped***: Has a single triangular median/anterior leaflet and two tongue-shaped posterior leaflets (right and left). It is fused superiorly with fibrous pericardium.

Nerve Supply

- *Motor supply:* Phrenic nerve (C3, C4, C5)
- *Sensory supply:* Central part of diaphragm by phrenic nerve. Peripheral part by lower 6–7 intercostal nerves.

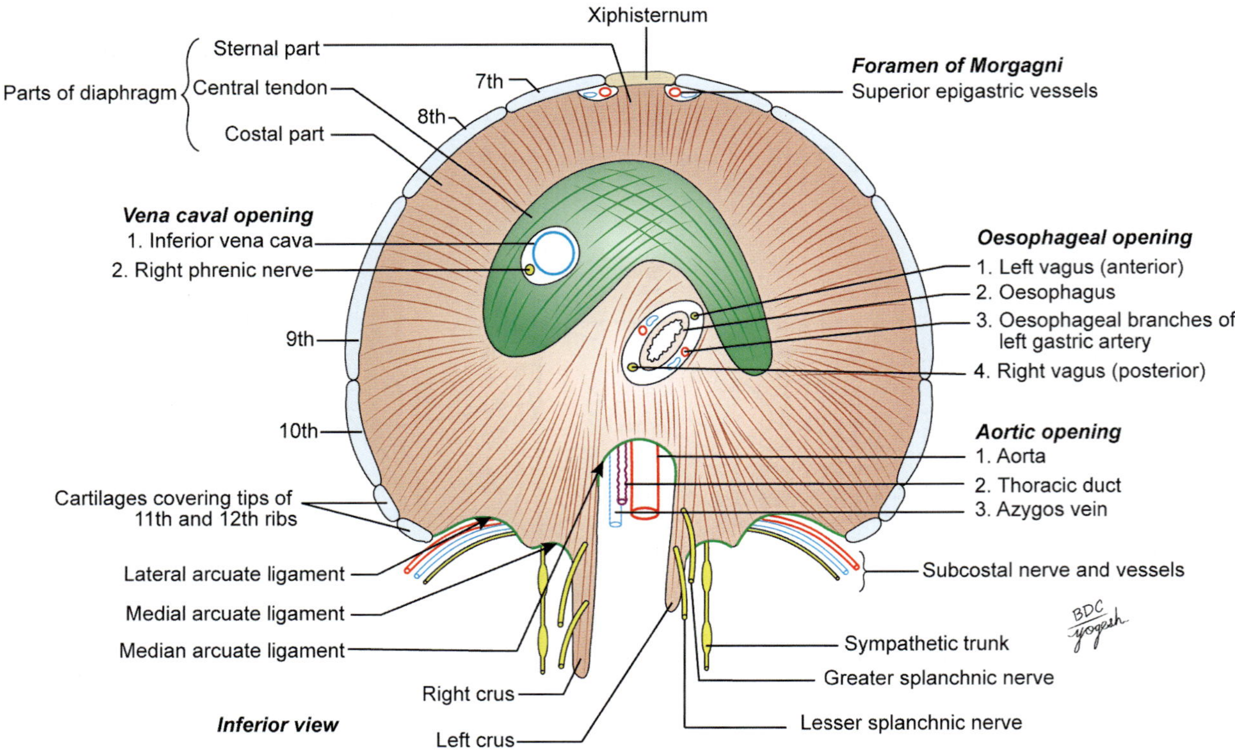

Fig. 12.9: Openings in the diaphragm and structures passing through these openings

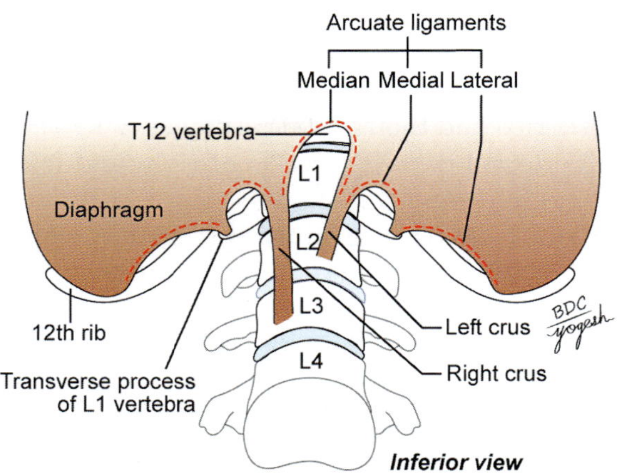

Fig. 12.10: Arcuate ligaments and crura of diaphragm

Structures Passing through the Diaphragm

- There are three large and several small openings in the diaphragm which allow passage to structures from thorax to abdomen or *vice versa* (Fig. 12.9).

Large openings:

1. Vena caval opening in the central tendon
2. Oesophageal opening in the right crus of diaphragm
3. Aortic opening behind the median arcuate ligament.

The structures passing through large openings are put in Table 12.1.

Small openings:

1. ***Superior epigastric artery*** passes in ***space of Larrey*** present between slip of xiphoid process and 7th costal cartilaginous slip of the diaphragm. When foramen is enlarged it is known as ***foramen of Morgagni***. Musculophrenic artery perforates diaphragm at the level of 9th costal cartilage.
2. ***Lower 5 intercostal vessels and nerves*** pass between costal origins of diaphragm and transversus abdominis.
3. ***Subcostal vessels and nerves*** pass behind lateral arcuate ligament.
4. ***Sympathetic trunk*** passes behind medial arcuate ligament.

TABLE 12.1: Large openings in thoracoabdominal diaphragm

Opening	*Location*	*Shape*	*Structures passing*	*Effect on contraction*
Vena caval	T8, right part of central tendon	Quadrilateral	IVC Right phrenic nerve Lymphatic of liver	Dilation
Oesophageal	T10, splitting of right crus	Elliptical	Oesophagus Both vagal trunks Left gastric vessels	Constriction
Aortic	T12, behind median arcuate ligament	Rounded	Aorta Thoracic duct Azygos vein	No change

5. *Greater and lesser splanchnic nerves* pierce each crus.
6. *Left phrenic nerve* pierces left cupola.

CLINICAL ANATOMY

- ***Paralysis of diaphragm***: Damage to the nerve supply (phrenic nerve) leads to paralysis of diaphragm. In ***unilateral paralysis of diaphragm***, the paralysed dome of diaphragm remains elevated during inspiration and moves downward in expiration. This is called ***paradoxical movements*** (Fig. 12.11). It can be observed on radiological fluoroscopy (real-time viewing). Bilateral paralysis may lead to respiratory failure.
- ***Hiccups***: Irritation of diaphragm may cause spasmodic involuntary contraction of diaphragm and produce hiccups.
- ***Diaphragmatic hernia***: It is the protrusion of abdominal contents into the chest through a defective diaphragm. It may be congenital or acquired.
- ***Congenital diaphragmatic hernia*** (CDH) occurs due to failure of proper formation of the diaphragm (Fig. 12.12).

  Congenital diaphragmatic hernia has three types:

  a. ***Bochdalek hernia (posterolateral hernia)***: About 95% cases of CDH are Bochdalek hernia. It occurs due to the failure of contribution of pleuroperitoneal membrane to the diaphragm.

  b. ***Morgagni hernia (retrosternal or parasternal hernia)***: It occurs through foramen of Morgagni or space of Larry.

  c. ***Diaphragmatic eventration***: It refers to abnormal contour of diaphragmatic dome because of paralysis, aplasia, or atrophy to varying degrees of muscle fibres.
- ***Acquired diaphragmatic hernia*** may be (traumatic hernia) sliding hiatal hernia or rolling hiatal hernia (Fig. 12.13).

  a. In ***sliding hernia***, a part of stomach protrudes into thoracic cavity through esophageal opening of the diaphragm. It occurs due to old age, obesity, chronic cough, and so on. It may result in *gastroesophageal reflux disease* (*GERD*) and gastric ulcers. Sliding hernia is the commonest of all the internal hernias.

  b. ***Rolling hiatal hernia***: In this, paraoesophageal junction remains within the abdominal cavity and fundus of stomach bulges into the thoracic cavity.

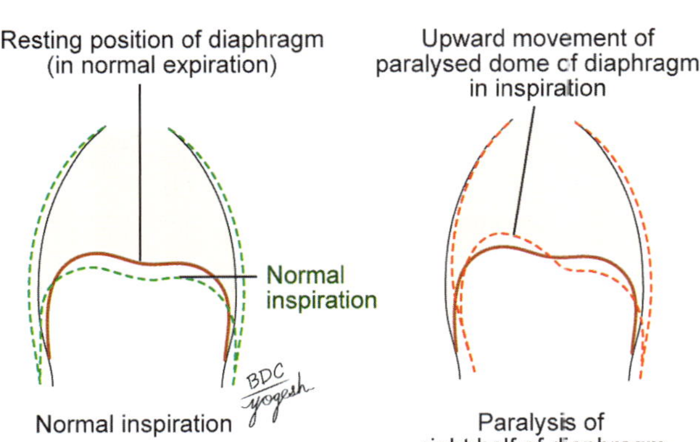

Fig. 12.11: Normal and paradoxical movement of diaphragm

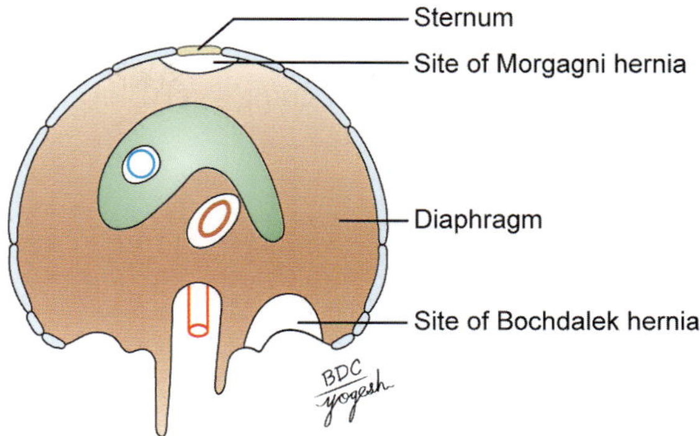

Fig. 12.12: Sites of Bochdalek and Morgagni hernia

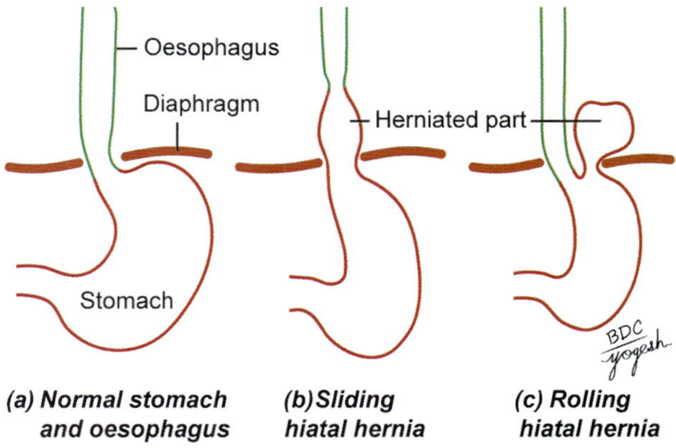

Figs 12.13a to c: Acquired diaphragmatic hernia; (a) Normal stomach and oesophagus; (b) Sliding hiatal hernia; (c) Rolling hiatal hernia

Facts to Remember

- Thoracic cavity houses a single heart with pericardium, two lungs with pleurae, blood vessels, nerves and lymphatics.
- Ribs may be present in relation to cervical seven and lumbar one vertebrae.
- Ribs are weak at their angles and are vulnerable to injury at that area.
- Ribs are horizontal in children up to 2 years of age.
- Manubriosternal angle is used for counting the intercostal spaces.
- 1–7 ribs with costal cartilages reach the sternum, costal cartilages of 8–10 ribs form the costal margin, while 11th and 12th ribs do not reach the front at all.
- Diaphragm is the principal muscle of inspiration.
- Right dome of diaphragm lies higher than left due to location of liver.
- About 95% cases of congenital diaphragmatic hernia are Bochdalek hernia.
- Levels
  - 2nd costal cartilage — sternal angle
  - Suprasternal notch — lower border of T2 vertebra

- Root of spine of scapula — spine of T3 vertebra
- Inferior angle of scapula — spine of T7 vertebra
- Apex beat — below and medial to the normally placed left nipple.
- Openings in diaphragm — vena caval opening – T8 level, oesophageal opening – T10 level, aortic opening – T12 level.

BDC's Anatomy *e*-book

1. Construction of the thoracic cage
2. Soft tissue landmarks
3. Surface marking of midclavicular and midaxillary lines
4. Cervical rib
5. Rib notching in coarctation of aorta
6. Further reading
7. Viva voce questions

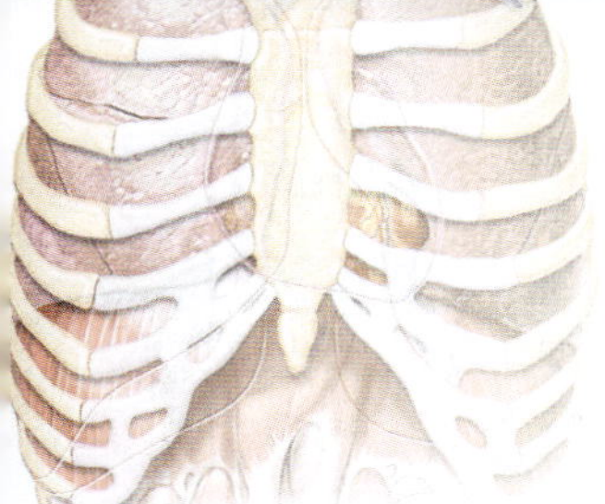

Chapter

13

Bones and Joints of Thorax

The thorax is an osseocartilaginous cavity or cage for various viscera, providing them due support and protection. This cage is not static but dynamic, as it moves at its various joints, increasing or decreasing the various diameters of the cavity for an extremely important process of respiration, which is life for all of us.

Competency:

AN21.1 Identify and describe the salient features of sternum, typical rib and typical thoracic vertebra.

BONES OF THORAX

STERNUM

The sternum is a flat bone, forming the anterior median part of the thoracic skeleton.

Shape and parts

In shape, it resembles a dagger or short sword and has the following three parts:

1. The upper part, corresponding to the handle, is called the ***manubrium***.
2. The middle part, resembling the blade, is called the ***body***.
3. The lowest tapering part forming the point of the sword is the ***xiphoid process*** or *xiphisternum*.

Length: The sternum is about 17 cm long. It is longer in males than in females (Plate 13.1, Fig. 13.1, Flowchart 13.1).

Anatomical Position

Hold the sternum in such a way so that:

1. Rough convex surface face anteriorly.
2. Broad manubrium lies superiorly and pointed xiphoid process lies inferiorly.
3. Anterior surface of sternum is slightly inclined forward.

Manubrium

The manubrium is quadrilateral in shape. It is the thickest and strongest part of the sternum.

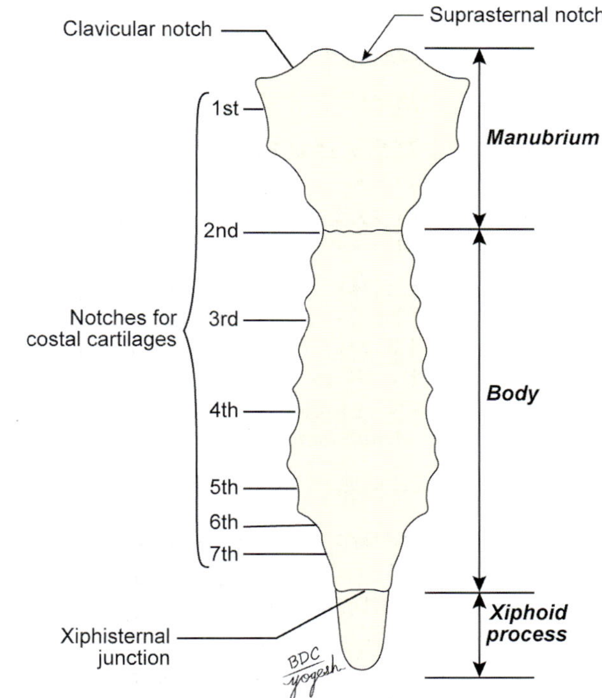

Fig. 13.1: Sternum: Anterior aspect

It has:

Two surfaces: Anterior and posterior

Four borders: Superior, inferior, and two lateral.

1. ***Anterior surface*** is convex from side-to-side and concave from above downwards (*see* Fig. 13.1).
2. ***Posterior surface*** is concave and forms the anterior boundary of the superior mediastinum.
3. ***Superior border*** is thick, rounded, and concave. It is marked by the *suprasternal notch* or jugular notch or interclavicular notch in the median part, and by the *clavicular notch* on each side. The clavicular notch articulates with the medial end of the clavicle to form the *sternoclavicular joint* (*see* Fig. 13.1).
4. ***Inferior border*** forms a secondary cartilaginous joint with the body of the sternum. The manubrium makes a slight angle with the body, convex forwards, called the ***sternal angle of Louis***. Events at the sternal angle. It is marked by a transverse ridge on the anterior aspect of the sternum.

Plate 13.1: Sternum

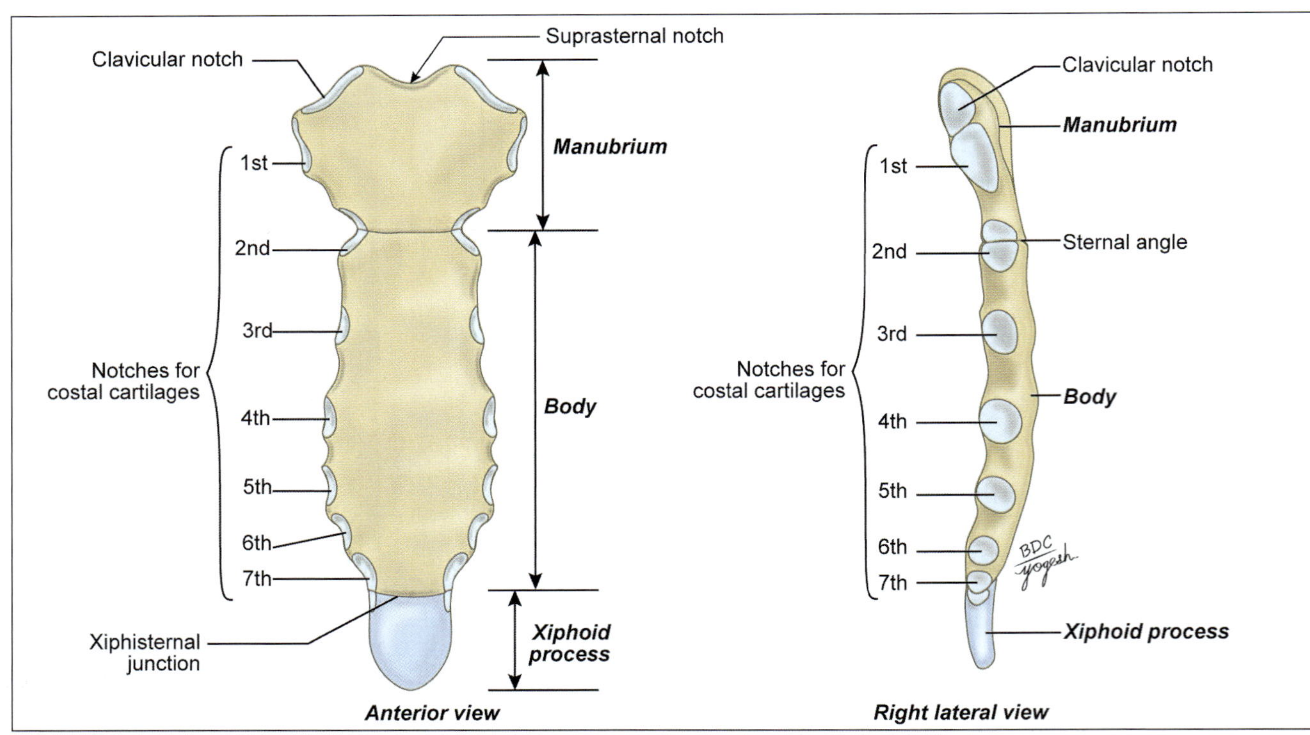

Flowchart 13.1: Sternum

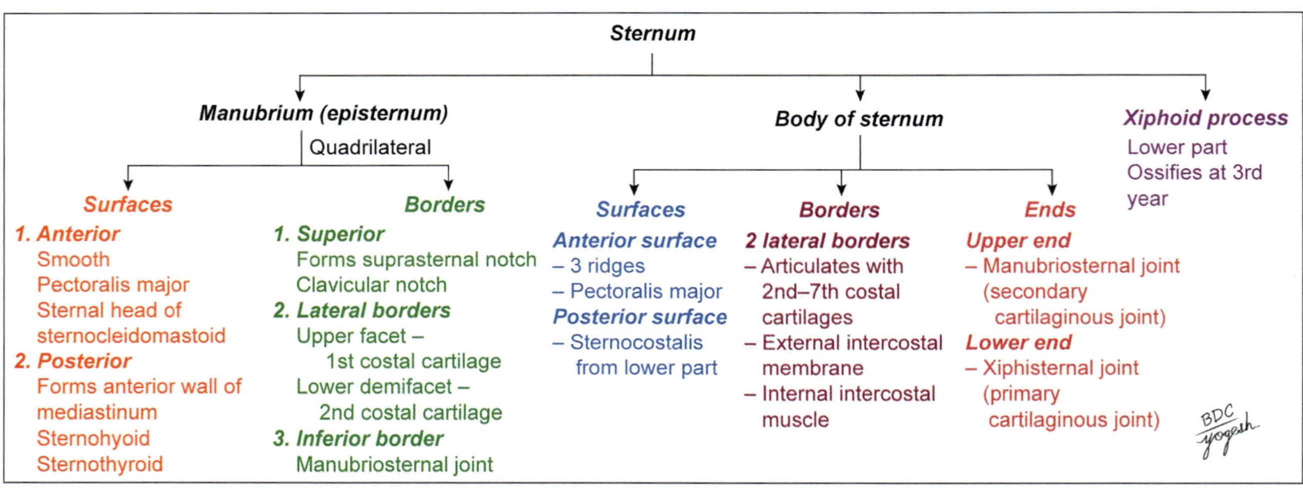

5. Each *lateral border* forms a primary cartilaginous joint with the first costal cartilage, and presents a demifacet for synovial articulation with the upper part of the 2nd costal cartilage.

Attachments

1. *Anterior surface* gives origin on either side to:
   a. Pectoralis major.
   b. Sternal head of the sternocleidomastoid (Fig. 13.2).
2. *Posterior surface* gives origin to:
   a. Sternohyoid in upper part (Fig. 13.2).
   b. Sternothyroid in lower part.
   c. The lower half of this surface is related to the arch of the aorta.
   d. The upper half is related to the left brachiocephalic vein, the brachiocephalic artery, the left common carotid artery, and the left subclavian artery. The lateral portions of the surface are related to the corresponding lung and pleura.
3. *Suprasternal notch*—Lower fibres of the interclavicular ligament and investing layer of cervical fascia.
4. Margins of each *clavicular notch* — Capsule of the sternoclavicular joint (*see* Chapter 10, page 142).

Body of the Sternum

The body is longer, narrower, and thinner than the manubrium. It is widest close to its lower end opposite the articulation with the fifth costal cartilage.

It has:

Two surfaces: Anterior and posterior
Two lateral borders
Two ends: Upper and lower.

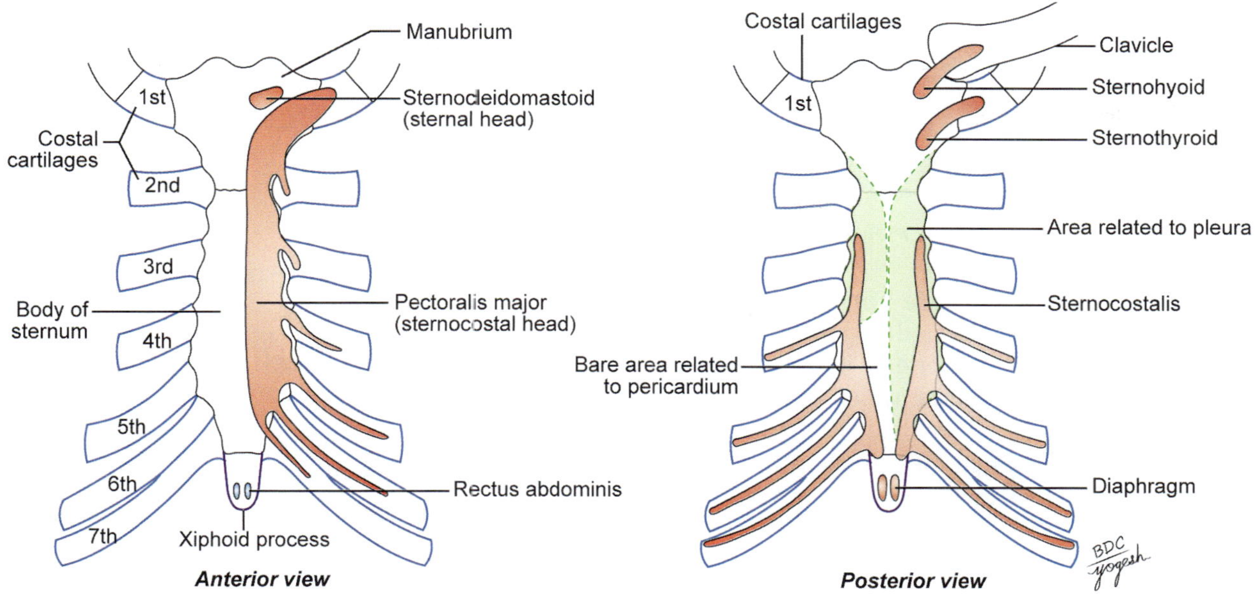

Fig. 13.2: Attachments on the sternum

1. The ***anterior surface*** is nearly flat and directed forwards and slightly upwards. It is marked by three ill-defined transverse ridges, indicating the lines of fusion of the four small segments called *sternebrae*.
2. The ***posterior surface*** is slightly concave and is marked by less distinct transverse lines.
3. The ***lateral borders*** form synovial joints with the lower part of the 2nd costal cartilage, the 3rd to 6th costal cartilages, and the upper half of the 7th costal cartilage (Fig. 13.11).
4. The ***upper end*** forms a secondary cartilaginous joint with the manubrium at the sternal angle.
5. The ***lower end*** is narrow and forms a primary cartilaginous joint with the xiphisternum.

Attachments

1. *Anterior surface*
   - Pectoralis major muscle origin on either side (Fig. 13.2).
2. *Posterior surface*
   - The lower part of the posterior surface including that of xiphoid process gives origin on either side to the sternocostalis muscle.
   - On the right side of the median plane, the posterior surface is related to the anterior border of the right lung and pleura.
   - On the left side, the upper two pieces of the body are related to the left lung and pleura, and the lower two pieces to the pericardium (Fig. 13.2).
3. *Lateral borders*
   - Between the facets for articulation with the costal cartilages, the lateral borders provide attachment to the external intercostal membranes and to the internal intercostal muscles.

Xiphoid Process

The xiphoid process is the smallest part of the sternum. Initially, it is cartilaginous, but in the adult it becomes ossified near its upper end. It varies greatly in shape and may be bifid or perforated. It lies in the floor of the epigastric fossa (Fig. 13.1).

Attachments

1. The anterior surface provides insertion to the medial fibres of the rectus abdominis, and to the aponeuroses of the external and internal oblique muscles of the abdomen.
2. The posterior surface gives origin to the diaphragm and sternocostalis. It is related to the anterior surface of the liver.
3. The lateral borders of the xiphoid process give attachment to the aponeuroses of the internal oblique and transversus abdominis muscles.
4. The upper end forms a primary cartilaginous joint with the body of the sternum.
5. The lower end affords attachment to the linea alba.

DEVELOPMENT AND OSSIFICATION

The sternum develops by the fusion of two sternal plates formed on either side of the midline. The fusion of the two plates takes place in a craniocaudal direction.

Sternum ossifies from the following centres of ossification (Figs 13.3a and b):

- Manubrium — one centre — appears in 5th month of IUL
- *Body*

  1st sternebrae — one centre — 5th month of IUL

  2nd sternebrae — one centre — 5th month of IUL

  3rd sternebrae — one pair of centres — 5th–6th month of IUL

  4th sternebrae — one pair of centres — 5th–6th month of IUL
- Xiphoid process — one centre — 3rd year of life.

These ossified 4 sternebrae fuse with each other during and after puberty.

Fusion is completed by 25 years of age (Figs 13.3a and b). The xiphoid process fuses with the body at about 40 years (Figs 13.3a and b).

The manubriosternal joint is a secondary cartilaginous joint and usually persists throughout life.

CLINICAL ANATOMY

- ***Sternal puncture:*** Sample for bone marrow examination is usually obtained by manubriosternal puncture (Fig. 13.4). It is done in its upper half to prevent injury to arch of aorta, which lies behind its lower half.
- The slight movements that take place at the manubriosternal joint are essential for movements of the ribs.
- ***Funnel chest*:** In the anomaly called 'funnel chest', the sternum is depressed (Fig. 13.5a).
- ***Pigeon chest:*** In 'pigeon chest', there is forward projection of the sternum like the keel of a boat, and flattening of the chest wall on either side (Fig. 13.5b).
- ***Mid-sternectomy:*** For cardiac surgery, the manubrium and/or body of sternum need to be splitted in midline and the incision is closed with stainless steel wires.
- Sternum is protected from injury by attachment of elastic costal cartilages. Indirect violence may lead to fracture of sternum.
- ***Sternal foramina, bifid xiphoid:*** Non-fusion of the sternal plates causes *ectopia cordis*, where the heart lies uncovered on the surface. Partial fusion of the plates may lead to the formation of *sternal foramina*, *bifid xiphoid process*, etc.

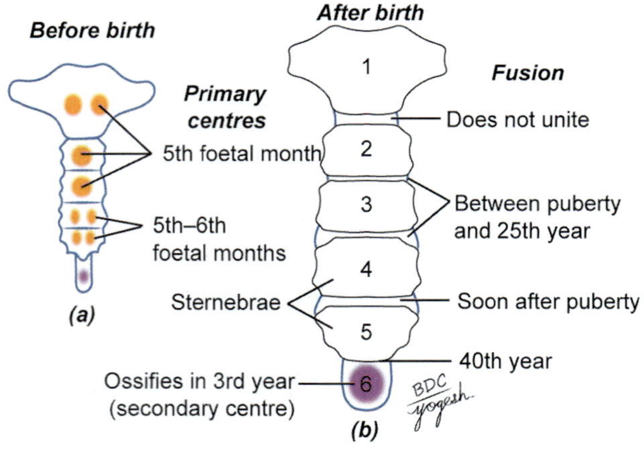

Figs 13.3a and b: Ossification of sternum

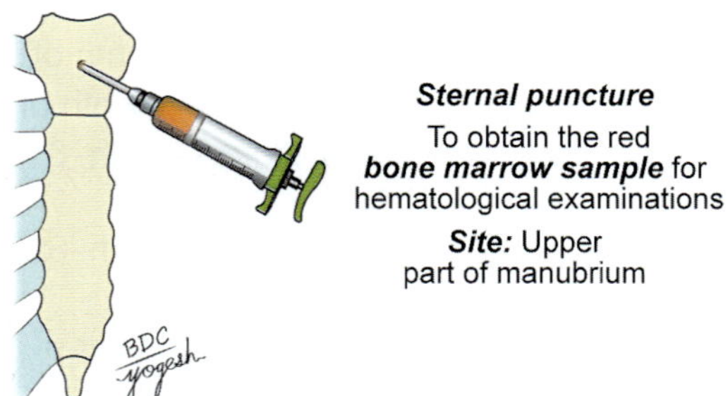

Fig. 13.4: Sternal puncture for bone marrow biopsy

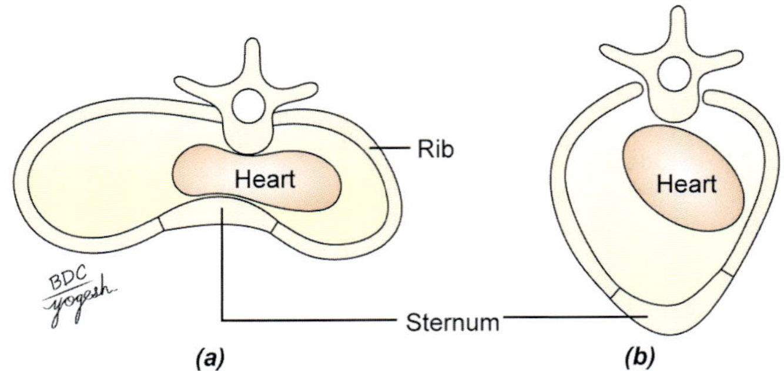

Figs 13.5a and b: (a) Funnel chest and (b) pigeon chest

RIBS OR COSTAE

The ribs are also called costae (costa = rib in Latin). They are flat, elongated, and curved bones.

Number

1. There are 12 ribs on each side forming the greater part of the thoracic skeleton.
2. The number may be increased by development of a cervical or a lumbar rib; or the number may be reduced to 11 by the absence of the 12th rib.

Arrangements of Ribs

1. The ribs are bony arches arranged one below the other (Plate 13.2, Flowchart 13.2, Fig. 13.6).
2. The gaps between the ribs are called ***intercostal spaces***. The spaces are deeper in front than behind, and deeper between the upper than between the lower ribs.
3. The ribs are placed obliquely, the upper ribs being less oblique than the lower. The obliquity reaches its maximum at the ninth rib, and thereafter it gradually decreases to the 12th rib.

Length and Width

1. The length of the ribs increases from the 1st to the 7th ribs, and then gradually decreases from the 8th to 12th ribs.
2. The breadth of the ribs decreases from above downwards. In the upper 10 ribs, the anterior ends are broader than the posterior ends.

Flowchart 13.2: Classification of ribs

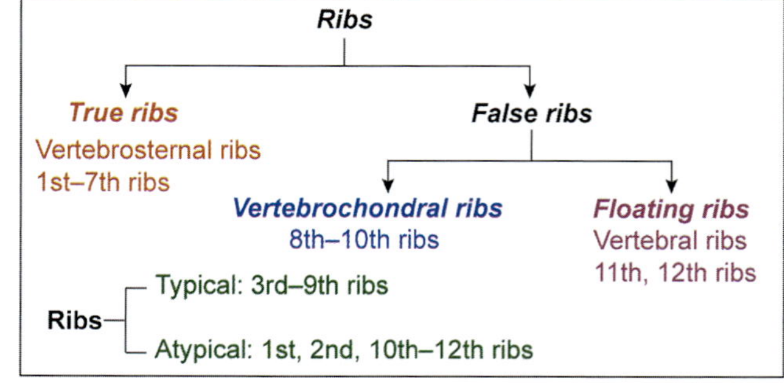

Plate 13.2: Typical rib

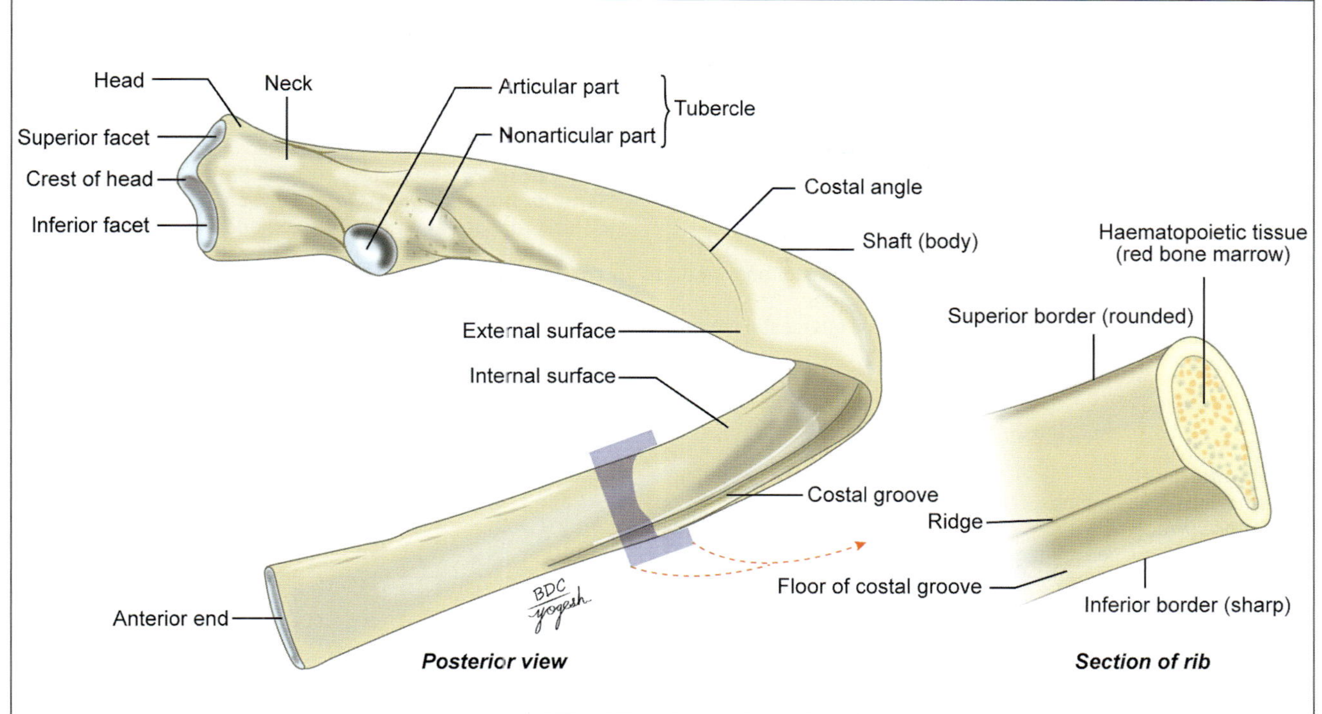

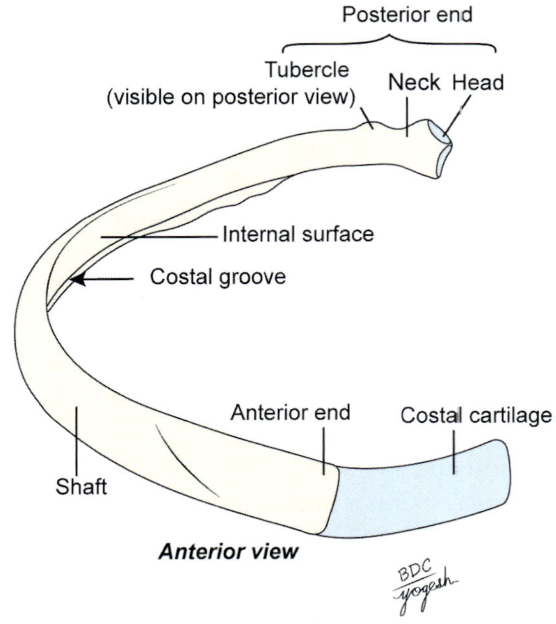

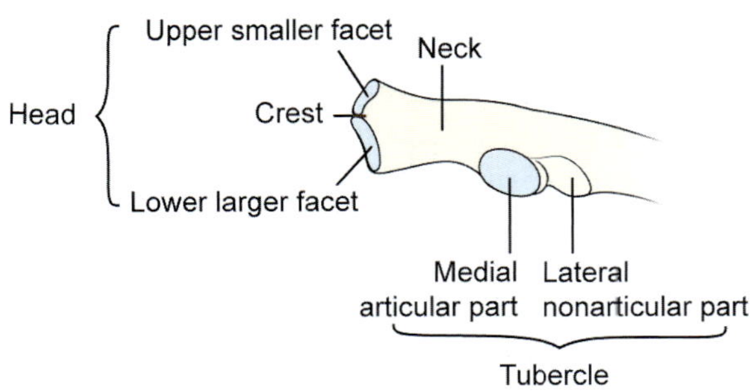

Posterior view of posterior end of the rib

Fig. 13.6: A typical rib

Classification

A. ***According to articulations with sternum*** (Flowchart 13.2):

True ribs: 1st–7th ribs. These are connected through their cartilages to the sternum are called true ribs, or ***vertebrosternal ribs***.

False ribs: 8th–12th ribs.

Vertebrochondral ribs: The cartilages of the 8th–10th ribs are joined to the next higher cartilage and are known as *vertebrochondral ribs*.

Vertebral ribs: The anterior ends of the 11th and 12th ribs are free and are called ***floating ribs*** or *vertebral ribs*.

B. ***According to morphological features***

Typical ribs: 3rd–9th ribs. They have same general features.

Atypical ribs: 1st, 2nd, 10th–12th ribs. They have special features. The 3rd–9th ribs are typical ribs.

TYPICAL RIBS

These ribs have common general features. For example, 3rd–9th ribs (Flowchart 13.3).

Side Determination

Hold the rib in such a way that

1. Its anterior end has a concave depression and posterior end has a globular head.
2. Shaft is flat and convex outward.
3. Costal groove and sharp inferior border lie downwards.

The convexity of the shaft is directed toward the side of the rib. Tilt the rib so that the posterior end lies at higher level than the anterior end.

Flowchart 13.3: Typical rib

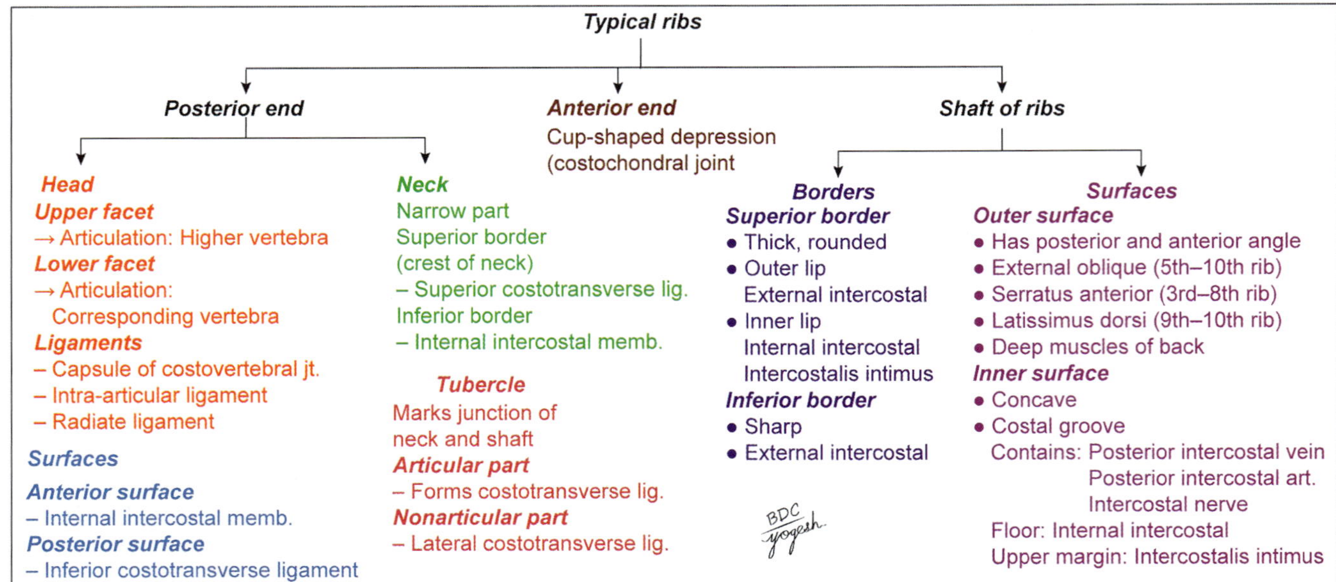

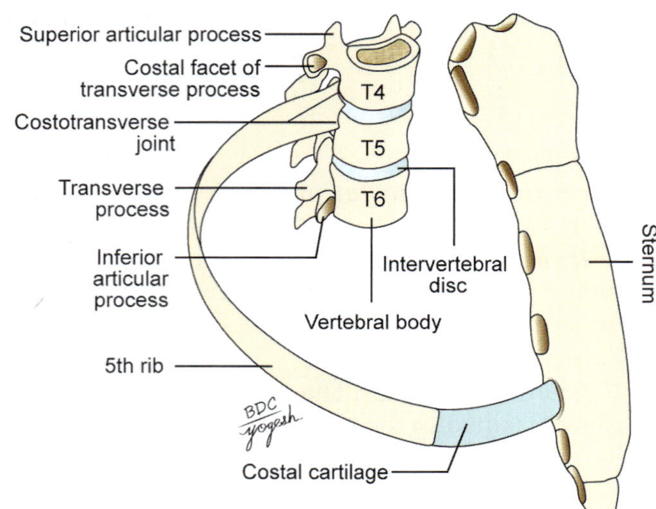

Fig. 13.7: Articulations of the 5th rib

Features

Each rib has two ends: Anterior and posterior. Its shaft comprises upper and lower borders and outer and inner surfaces.

Anterior or Sternal End

- It is oval and concave for articulation with its costal cartilage.

Posterior or Vertebral End

- The posterior end has head, neck, and tubercle.

Head

- It has two facets that are separated by a crest.
- The ***lower larger facet*** articulates with the body of the numerically corresponding vertebra while the ***upper smaller facet*** articulates with the next higher vertebra (Figs 13.6 and 13.7).

Neck

- It lies in front of the transverse process of its own vertebra, and has ***two surfaces***: Anterior and posterior; and ***two borders***: Superior and inferior.
- The anterior surface of the neck is smooth. The posterior surface is rough.
- The superior border or ***crest of the neck*** is thin. The inferior border is rounded.

Tubercle

- It is placed on the outer surface of the rib at the junction of the neck and shaft.
- Its medial part is articular and forms the *costotransverse joint* with the transverse process of the corresponding vertebra. The lateral part is non-articular (Fig. 13.6).

Shaft

- It is flattened so it has:
  Two surfaces: Outer and inner
  Two borders: Upper and lower
- The shaft is curved with its convexity outwards (Fig. 13.6). It is bent at the ***angle*** which is situated about 5 cm lateral to the tubercle. It is also twisted at the angle.
- **Outer surface***:* The angle is marked by an oblique line on the outer surface, directed downwards and laterally.
  Posterior angle of rib is marked by an oblique ridge and lies about 5 cm lateral to the tubercle.
  Anterior angle of rib is a faint oblique line, about 5 cm from anterior end.
- ***Inner surface*** is smooth and covered by the pleura. This surface is marked by a ridge which is continuous behind with the lower border of the neck.
  The ***costal groove*** lies between this ridge and the inferior border.

The costal groove lodges the following structures from above downward:

1. Posterior intercostal **V**ein
2. Posterior intercostal **A**rtery
3. Intercostal **N**erve.

[*Mnemonic*: VAN]

- ***Upper border*** is thick and has outer and inner lips.
- ***Lower border*** is sharp and forms the lower border of the costal groove.

Attachments and Relations of a Typical Rib

Head

1. Anteriorly, the head provides attachment to the triradiate ligament (Plate 13.3, Fig. 13.6) and is related to the sympathetic chain and to the costal pleura.
2. The crest of the head provides attachment to the intra-articular ligament of the costovertebral joint.

Neck

1. The inferior costotransverse ligament connects the posterior surface of rib to the transverse process of corresponding vertebra (Fig. 13.5).
2. The two laminae of the superior costotransverse ligament connect superior border (crest of neck) with the transverse process of the vertebra above (Fig. 13.6).

Tubercle

The lateral non-articular part of the *tubercle* gives attachment to the lateral costotransverse ligament that extends to the to the tip of transverse process of the corresponding vertebra.

Shaft

1. *Superior border*: The external intercostal muscle inserts on the outer lip of superior border. The internal intercostal muscle and intercostalis intimus muscle insert into the inner lip of superior border (Plate 13.4).
2. *Inferior border*: The external intercostal muscle arises from the inferior border of rib.
3. *Costal groove*: The internal intercostal muscle arises from the floor of costal groove. The intercostalis intimus muscle arises from the middle 2/4th of the ridge above the groove.
4. The subcostalis is attached to the inner surfaces of the lower ribs.
5. The *thoracolumbar fascia* and the lateral fibres of the sacrospinalis muscle (iliocostalis) are attached to the posterior angle.
6. Medial to the posterior angle, the levator costae and the sacrospinalis (longissimus) are attached.
7. *Anterior angle* separates the origins of the external oblique from serratus anterior in case of 5th–8th ribs. The anterior angle also separates the origin of external oblique from that of latissimus dorsi in case of 9th and 10th ribs.

Competency:
AN21.2 Identify and describe the features of atypical ribs and atypical thoracic vertebrae.

First Rib

Identification

1. It is the shortest, broadest, and most curved rib (Plate 13.5, Flowcharts 13.4 and 13.5).
2. Its shaft is flat and has superior and inferior surfaces, and inner and outer borders.
3. Head has only one small facet.
4. Tubercle has only articular facet (no nonarticular area).
5. There is no costal groove.
6. Anterior end is very broad and thick.
7. Upper surface shows two grooves separated by scalene tubercle.

Side Determination

Hold the bone in such a way that

1. Upper surface with two grooves facing upward and forward making an angle of 45° with horizontal plane.
2. Rounded head lies posteriorly, and broad anterior end lies anteriorly at lower level than posterior end.
3. Convex outer border faces the side of the bone.

Note: Keep the 1st rib on the table in correct position, its both ends should touch the table surface. If it is placed wrongly, only anterior end will touch the table.

Features of First Rib

- ***Anterior end*** is larger and thicker than that in the other ribs. It is continuous with the first costal cartilage (Plate 13.5, Flowchart 13.4).
- ***Posterior end*** comprises the following.
  - ***Head*** is small and rounded. It articulates with the body of first thoracic vertebra.
  - ***Neck*** is rounded directed laterally, upwards and backwards.

Flowchart 13.4: First rib

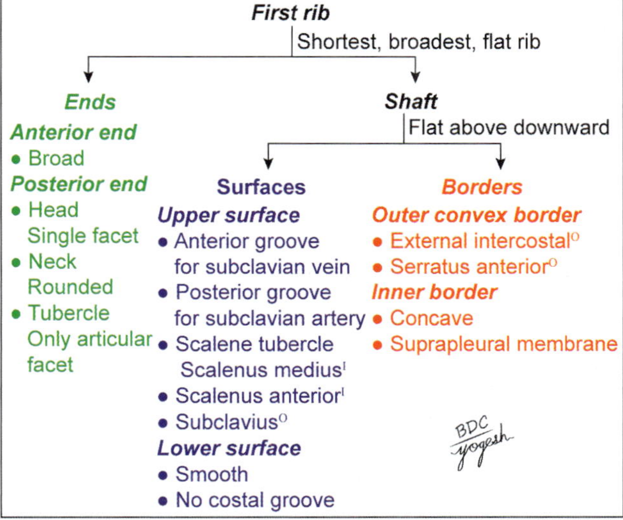

Plate 13.3: Ligaments between vertebrae and rib

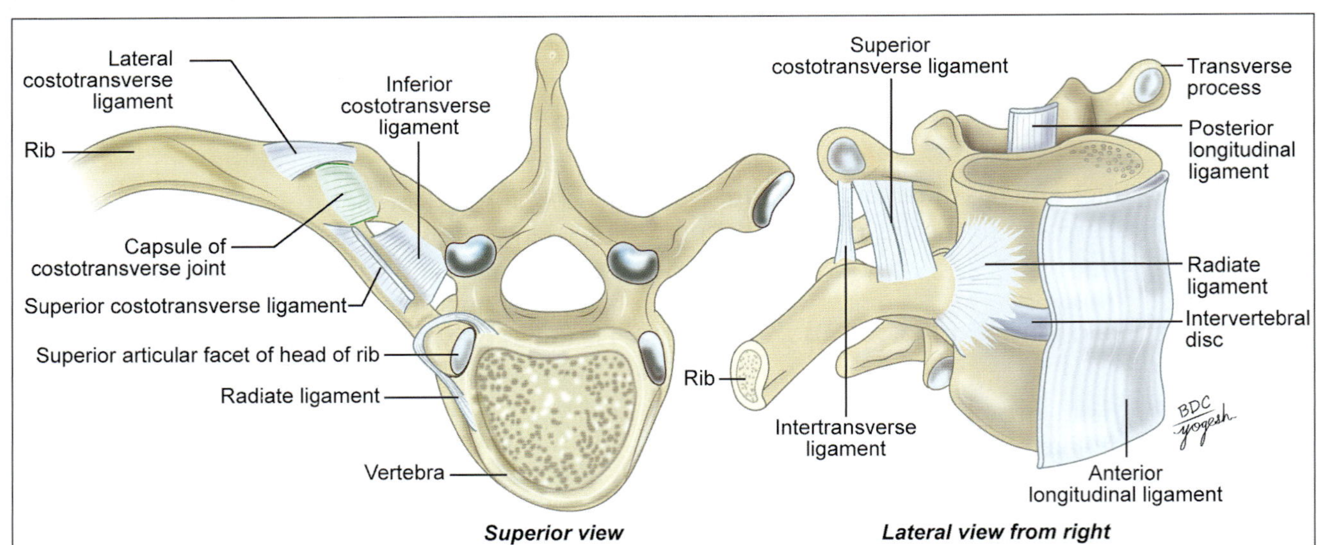

Plate 13.4: Contents of costal groove and intercostal muscles

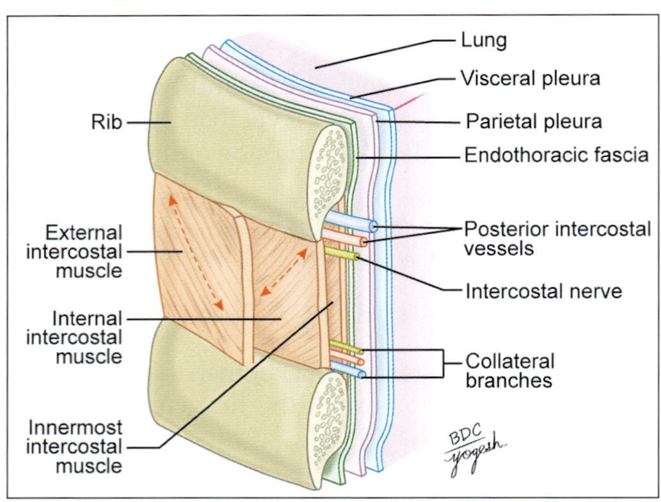

Plate 13.5: First rib

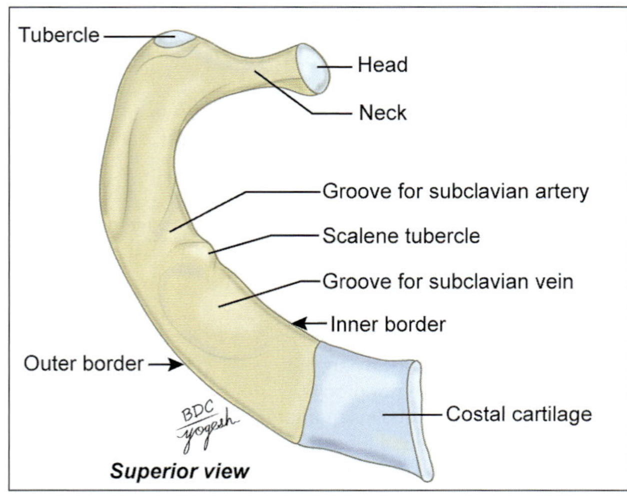

- *Tubercle* is large. It coincides with the angle of the rib. It articulates with the transverse process of first thoracic vertebra to form the costotransverse joint.

- ***Shaft*** *(body)* has two surfaces—upper and lower; and two borders—outer and inner.
  - *Upper surface* is marked by two shallow grooves, separated near the inner border by the ***scalene tubercle***.
  - *Lower surface* is smooth and has no costal groove.
  - *Outer border* is convex, thick behind and thin in front.
  - *Inner border* is concave.

Attachments and Relations

1. ***Neck:*** Anteriorly, the neck is related from medial to lateral side to (Fig. 13.8):
   a. Sympathetic **chain**
   b. First posterior intercostal **v**ein
   c. Superior intercostal **a**rtery
   d. Ventral ramus of first thoracic **n**erve.

[*Mnemonic*: **Chain** pulling a **VAN**].

2. *Superior surface*: Anterior groove on the superior surface of the shaft lodges the subclavian vein, and the posterior groove lodges the subclavian artery and the lower trunk of the brachial plexus.

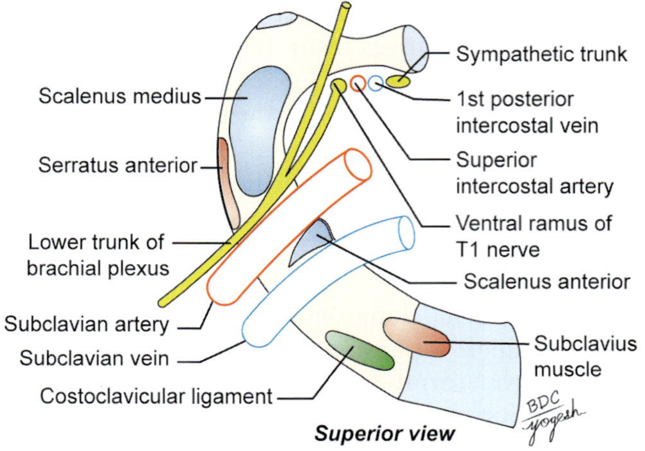

Fig. 13.8: Superior view of the first rib

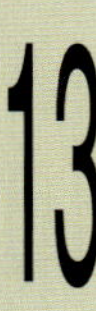

Flowchart 13.5: Atypical rib

Atypical ribs	1st rib	2nd rib	10th rib	11th rib	12th rib
Length	Shortest rib	—	—	—	Smaller rib
Head	Single facet	Two facets	Single facet	Single facet	Single facet
Neck	Present	Present	Present	Absent	Absent
Tubercle	No nonarticular part	Small nonarticular part	Present	Absent	Absent
Costal groove	Absent	Small	Present	Faint	Absent
Angle	Coincide with tubercle	—	—	Faint	Absent
Ossification centres One primary for shaft	Present	Present	Present	Present	Present
Secondary centres	1 for head 1 for tubercle	1 for head 2 for tubercles	1 for head 2 for tubercles	1 for head —	1 for head —

The structures attached to the upper surface of the shaft are:

a. Origin of the subclavius muscle at the anterior end.
b. Attachment of the costoclavicular ligament at the anterior end in front of subclavius.
c. Insertion of the scalenus anterior on the scalene tubercle.
d. Insertion of the scalenus medius on the elongated rough area behind the groove for the subclavian artery.

3. *Lower surface*: The lower surface of the shaft is covered by costal pleura and is related near its outer border to the small first intercostal nerve which is very small.
4. Outer border — gives origin to:
   a. External intercostal muscle, and
   b. The upper part of the first digitation of the serratus anterior, just behind the groove for the subclavian artery.
5. Inner border — gives attachment to the suprapleural membrane.
6. Tubercle — gives attachment to the lateral costotransverse ligament.

Second Rib

Features

The features of the second rib are:

1. *Length*: The length is twice that of the first rib.
2. *Shaft*: The shaft is sharply curved, like that of the first rib (Fig. 13.9).
3. *Tubercle*: The non-articular part of the tubercle is small.
4. The angle is slight and is situated close to the tubercle.
5. The shaft has no twist. The outer surface is convex and faces more upwards than outwards. Near its middle, it is marked by a large rough tubercle (Fig. 13.9). This tubercle is a unique feature of the second rib. The inner surface of the shaft is smooth and concave. It faces more downwards than inwards. There is a short costal groove on the posterior part of this surface.

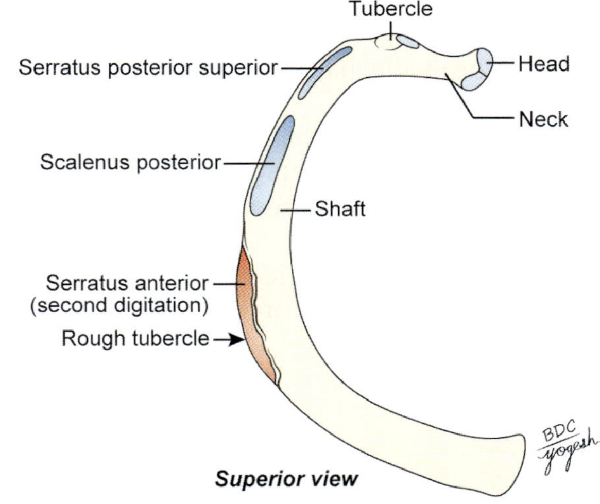

Fig. 13.9: Superior surface of 2nd rib

Attachments

1. The rough tubercle on the outer surface gives origin to 1½ digitations of the serratus anterior muscle.
2. The rough part of the upper border receives the insertion of the scalenus posterior.

Tenth Rib

The tenth rib closely resembles a typical rib, but is:

1. Shorter.
2. Has only a single facet on the head, for the body of the tenth thoracic vertebra.

Eleventh Rib

Identification features

- Head — single large articular facet.
- Neck — absent.

- Tubercle — absent.
- Anterior end — pointed.
- Angle — faintly marked angle on the outer surface.

Twelfth Ribs

Identification features
- Head — single facet
- Anterior end — pointed
- Neck, tubercle, angle, costal groove — absent.

Side Determination and Anatomical Position

Hold the bone in such a way that
1. Its pointed end is directed forward and laterally.
2. Sharp border is directed inferiorly.
3. Its concave inner surface is directed inward and slightly upward.

- Its convex outer surface faces the side of the bone and will determine the side to which bone belongs.

Attachments and Relations of the 12th Rib

1. *Inner surface*
   a. Quadratus lumborum is inserted on the lower part of the medial half to two-thirds of this surface (Fig. 13.10a).
   b. The fascia covering the quadratus lumborum is also attached to this part of the rib.
   c. The internal intercostal muscle is inserted near the upper border.
   d. The costodiaphragmatic recess of the pleura is related to the medial three-fourths of the costal surface.
   e. The diaphragm takes origin from the anterior end of this surface.
2. *Outer surface*
   a. *Attachments on the medial half*
      - Costotransverse ligament (Fig. 13.10b)
      - Lumbocostal ligament
      - Lowest levator costae
      - Iliocostalis and longissimus parts of sacrospinalis.
   b. *Attachments on the lateral half*
      - Insertion of serratus posterior inferior
      - Origin of latissimus dorsi
      - Origin of external oblique muscle of abdomen.
3. *Upper border*
   a. Internal intercostal muscle is originated.
   b. External intercostal muscle is inserted.
4. *Lower border*
   c. Middle layer of thoracolumbar fascia.
   d. Lateral arcuate ligament, at the lateral border of the quadratus lumborum.
   e. Lumbocostal ligament near the head, extending to the transverse process of first lumbar vertebra.

OSSIFICATION OF RIBS

All the ribs ossify in cartilage as follows, except 1st, 11th, and 12th ribs:

a. ***One primary centre*** (for the shaft) which appears, near the angle, at about the 8th week of intrauterine life.
b. ***Three secondary centres***, one for the head and two for the tubercle, which appear at puberty and unite with the rest of the bone after 20 years.

First rib

The 1st rib ossifies from one primary centre for the shaft at 8th week of intrauterine life.

For the posterior end there are only two secondary centres, one for the head and the other for the tubercle. These secondary centres appear at puberty and unite with rest of bone after 20 years.

Eleventh and twelfth rib

The 11th and 12th ribs ossify from one primary centre for the shaft and one secondary centre for the head.

CLINICAL ANATOMY

- ***Fracture of rib***: Weakest area of rib is the region of its angle. This is the commonest site of fracture.
- ***Cervical rib*** occurs in 0.5–2% of persons. It may articulate with first rib or may have a free end. It may cause pressure on lower trunk of brachial plexus and the subclavian artery.
- ***Lumbar rib***: It is also called ***gorilla rib***. It develops from costal element of L1 vertebra.
- In ***rickets***, there is inadequate mineralisation of bone matrix at the growth plates due to increased bone

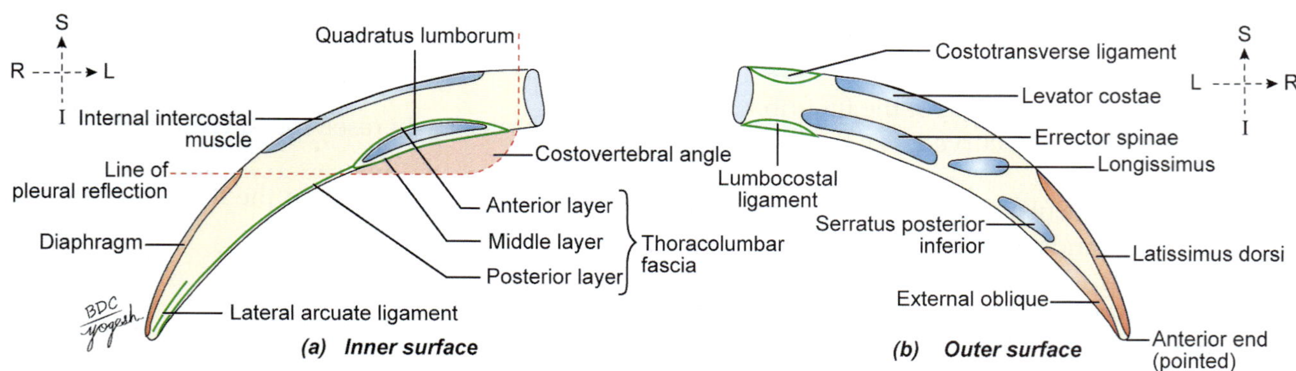

Figs 13.10a and b: Twelfth rib: (a) Inner surface (anterior aspect); (b) Outer surface (posterior aspect)

resorption. Due to deposition of unmineralized matrix, there is widening of the wrist and rachitic rosary, i.e. prominent costochondral junctions in thoracic cage and Harrison's sulcus.

- ***Flail chest (stove-in chest)***: In case of multiple fractures of a rib, a segment of rib moves freely and paradoxically (moves inside during inspiration and outward during expiration). This segment is called flail segment. It should be treated surgically with plates or wires.
- ***Rib excision***: Ribs are excised to access the thoracic structures in surgeries such as pulmonectomy (removal of lungs).

COSTAL CARTILAGES

The costal cartilages represent the unossified anterior parts of the ribs. They are made up of hyaline cartilage. They contribute materially to the elasticity of the thoracic wall.

Features

Each cartilage has
Two surfaces—anterior and posterior
Two borders—superior and inferior
Two ends—lateral and medial.

Articulation

Medial End

- The medial ends of the costal cartilages of the first seven ribs are attached directly to the sternum.
- The 1st cartilage forms a primary cartilaginous joint with the manubrium.
- The 2nd to seventh cartilages form synovial joints with the sternum.
- The 8th and 9th cartilages are connected to the next higher cartilage by synovial joints.
- The 10th cartilage is united to 9th cartilage by fibrous tissue.
- The cartilages of the 11th and 12th ribs are small, pointed, and free.

Lateral End

- The lateral end of each cartilage forms a primary cartilaginous joint with the rib concerned.

THORACIC VERTEBRAE

- There are 12 thoracic vertebrae.
- ***Identification:*** The thoracic vertebrae are identified by the presence of ***costal facets*** on the sides of the vertebral bodies. The costal facets may be two or only one on each side (Flowchart 13.6, Plate 13.6, Fig. 13.11).
- The thoracic vertebrae are grouped as:
  1. *Typical vertebrae*: T2–T8 vertebrae
  2. *Atypical vertebrae*: T1, T9–T12 vertebrae.

Typical Thoracic Vertebrae

Parts: The typical thoracic vertebra has:

a. Body
b. Vertebral arch: It consists of pedicle, transverse process, vertebral foramen, and spine.

1. **Body:** The body is heart-shaped with roughly the same measurements from side-to-side and antero-posteriorly.
   On each side, it bears two costal demifacets. The ***superior costal demifacet*** is larger and placed on the upper border of the body near the pedicle. It articulates with the head of the numerically corresponding rib.
   The ***inferior costal demifacet*** is smaller and placed on the lower border in front of the inferior vertebral notch. It articulates with the next lower rib (Fig. 13.11).
2. ***Vertebral foramen:*** It is comparatively small and circular.
3. ***Vertebral arch***: It shows:
   a. The ***pedicles*** are directed straight backwards. The *superior vertebral notch* is shallow, while the *inferior vertebral notch* is deep and conspicuous.
   b. The ***laminae*** overlap each other from above.
   c. The ***superior articular processes*** project upwards from the junction of the pedicles and laminae. The articular facets are flat and are directed backwards. This direction permits rotatory movements of the spine.
   d. The ***inferior articular processes*** are fused to the laminae. Their articular facets are directed forwards.
   e. The ***transverse processes*** are large, and are directed laterally and backwards from the junction of the pedicles and laminae. The anterior surface of each process bears a facet near its tip, for articulation with the tubercle of the corresponding rib.
   f. The ***spine*** is long, and is directed downwards and backwards. The 5th to 9th spines are the longest, more vertical and overlap each other. The upper and lower spines are less oblique in direction.

Note: In the upper six vertebrae, the costal facets on the transverse processes are concave, and face forwards and laterally. In lower four, the facets are flat and face upwards, laterally and slightly forwards (Plate 13.7). In the last two vertebrae, the articular facets are absent (*see* costotransverse joints below).

Flowchart 13.6: Typical thoracic vertebra

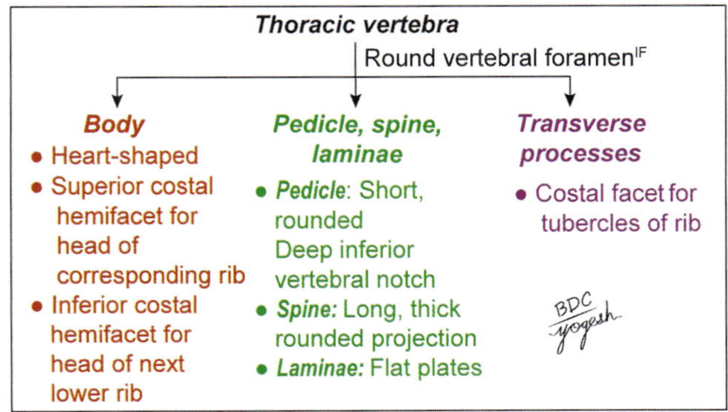

Plate 13.6: Typical thoracic vertebra

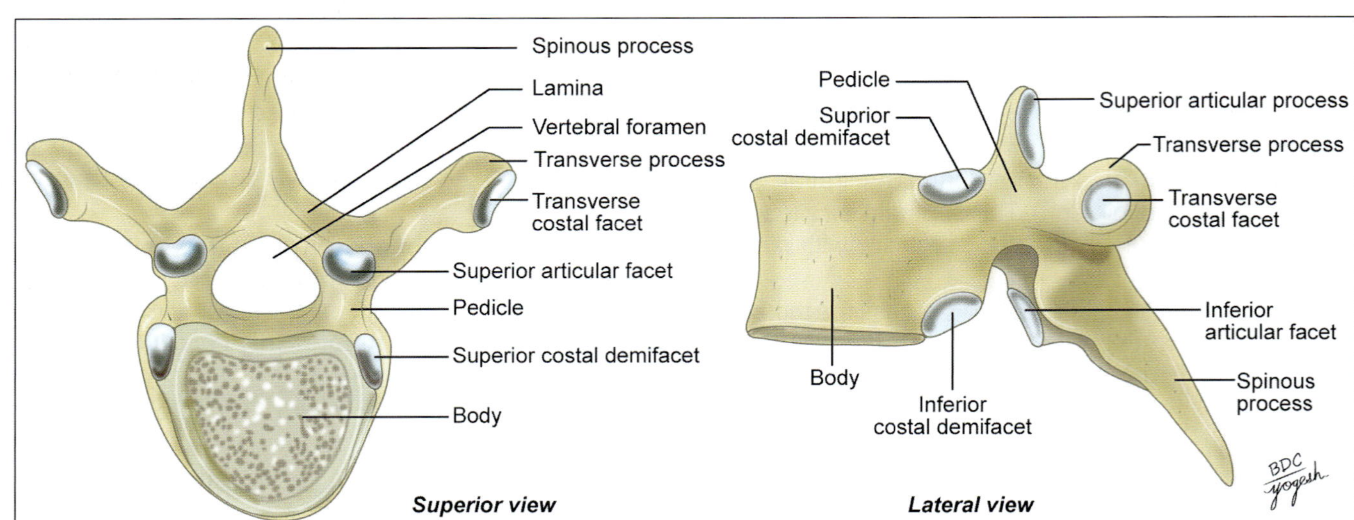

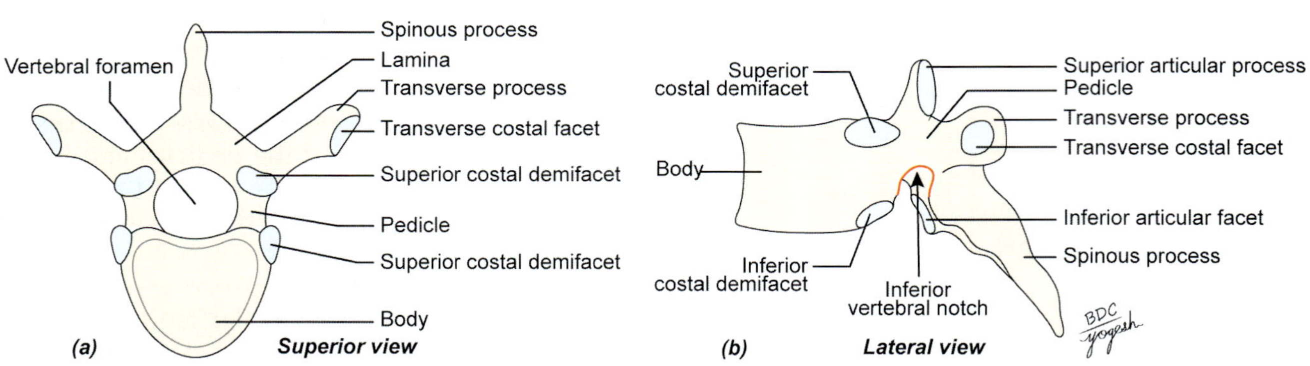

Figs 13.11a and b: Typical thoracic vertebra: (a) Superior view and (b) lateral view

Attachments

1. *Body*: The upper and lower borders of the body give attachment in front and behind, respectively, to the anterior and posterior longitudinal ligaments (Plate 13.7).
2. *Laminae*: The upper borders and lower parts of the anterior surfaces of the laminae provide attachment to the ligamenta flava.
3. *Transverse process*: The transverse process gives attachment to:
   a. The lateral costotransverse ligament at the tip.
   b. The superior costotransverse ligament along the lower border.
   c. The inferior costotransverse ligament along the anterior surface.
   d. The intertransverse ligaments and muscles to upper and lower borders.
   e. The levator costae on the posterior surface.
4. *Spine*: The spines give attachment to the *supraspinous* and *interspinous ligaments*. They also give attachment to several muscles including the trapezius, the rhomboids, the latissimus dorsi, the serratus posterior superior and the serratus posterior inferior, and many deep muscles of the back.

First Thoracic Vertebra

1. *Body*: The body of this vertebra resembles that of a cervical vertebra. It is broad and not heart-shaped. Its upper surface is lipped laterally and bevelled anteriorly. The superior costal facet on the body is complete (Fig. 13.12). It articulates with the head of the first rib. The inferior costal facet is a 'demifacet' for the second rib.
2. *Spine*: It is thick, long and nearly horizontal.
3. The superior vertebral notches are well marked, as in cervical vertebrae.
4. Facet on transverse process is concave on T1–T6 vertebrae.

Ninth Thoracic Vertebra

The 9th thoracic vertebra resembles a typical thoracic vertebra except that

a. The body has only the superior costal demifacets.
b. The inferior costal facets are absent (Fig. 13.12).

Tenth Thoracic Vertebra

The 10th thoracic vertebra resembles a typical thoracic vertebra except that the body has a single complete superior costal facet on each side, extending onto the root of the pedicle (Fig. 13.12).

Plate 13.7: Attachment of thoracic vertebrae

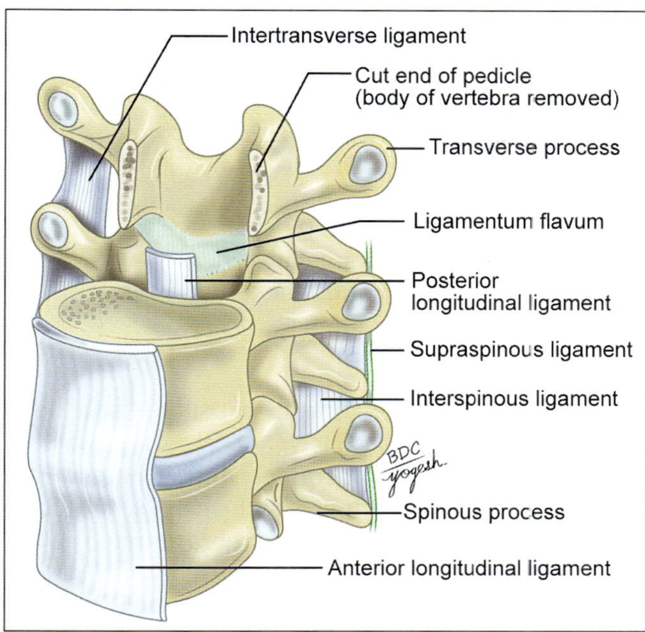

Eleventh Thoracic Vertebra

1. The body has a single large costal facet on each side, extending onto the upper part of the pedicle (Fig. 13.12).
2. The transverse process is small, and has no articular facet.

Sometimes it is difficult to differentiate between tenth and eleventh thoracic vertebrae.

Twelfth Thoracic Vertebra

1. *Body*: The shapes of the body, pedicles, transverse processes and spine are similar to those of a lumbar vertebra. However, the body bears a *single costal facet* on each side, which lies more on the lower part of the pedicle than on the body.
2. The inferior articular facets are lumbar in type. These are everted and are directed laterally, but the superior articular facets are thoracic in type.
3. *Transverse process*: The transverse process is small and has no facet, but has superior, inferior and lateral tubercles (Fig. 13.12).

Note: Three tubercles of transverse process:

a. Superior tubercle corresponds to the mammillary process of lumbar vertebrae.
b. Inferior tubercle corresponds to accessory process of lumbar vertebrae.
c. Lateral tubercle represents the true transverse process.

OSSIFICATION

The ossifications of typical vertebra and a thoracic vertebra are similar.

It ossifies in cartilage from three primary and five secondary centres as follows:

- The three primary centres: 1 for the centrum and 1 for each half of the neural arch, appear during 8th to 9th weeks of IUL.
- At birth, the vertebra consists of three parts, the centrum and two halves of the neural arch. The two halves of the neural arch fuse posteriorly during the 1st year of life. The neural arch is joined with the centrum by the *neurocentral synchondrosis*. Bony fusion occurs here during the 3rd to 6th years of life.
- Five secondary centres: 1 for the upper surface and 1 for the lower surface of the body, 1 for each transverse process, and 1 for the spine appear at about the 15th year and fuse with the rest of the vertebra at about the 25th year (Fig. 13.13).

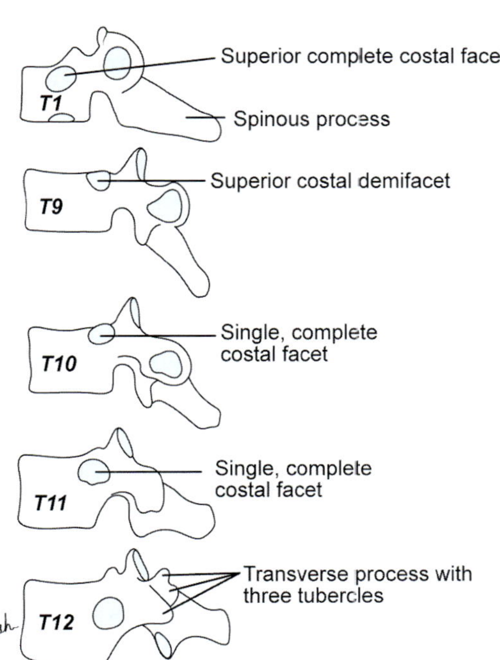

T1 Body — resembles body of cervical vertebrae
Superior costal facet — complete
Inferior costal facet — demifacet
Spine — long and horizontal

T9 Only superior costal demifacet

T10 Costal facet — single circular or oval

T11 Costal facet — single, large circular, extends on to the upper part of the pedicle
No costal facet on transverse process

T12 Body — resembles lumbar vertebrae
Costal facet — single, large oval costal facet
No costal facet on the transverse process
Transverse process with 3 tubercles — superior, lateral, and inferior

Fig. 13.12: Features of atypical thoracic vertebrae

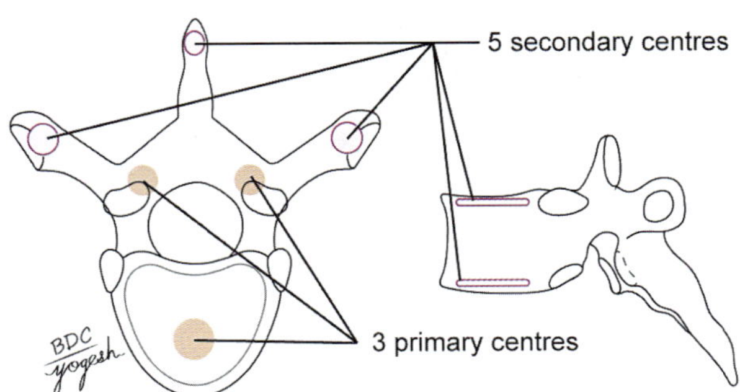

Fig. 13.13: Ossification of a thoracic vertebra

CLINICAL ANATOMY

- ***Spina bifida***: Failure of fusion of the two halves of the neural arch results in 'spina bifida'. Sometimes the body ossifies from two primary centres, and if one centre fails to develop, one half, right or left of the body is missing. This results in a ***hemivertebra*** and lateral bend in the vertebral column or ***scoliosis***.
- ***Disc prolapse***: In young adults, the discs are very strong. However, after the second decade of life, degenerative changes set in resulting in weakness of the annulus fibrosus. When such a disc is subjected to strain, the annulus fibrosus may rupture leading to prolapse of the nucleus pulposus. This is commonly referred to as *disc prolapse* (Fig. 13.14). Disc prolapse is usually posterolateral. The prolapsed nucleus pulposus presses upon adjacent nerve roots and gives rise to pain that radiates along the distribution of the nerve.

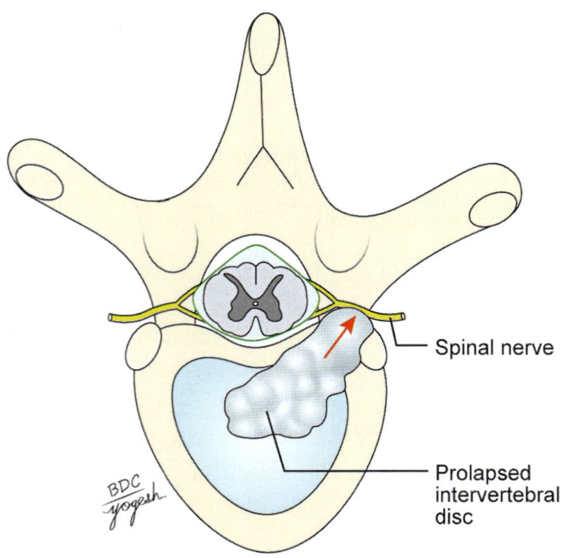

Fig. 13.14: Disc prolapse causing pressure on the spinal nerve

Competency:
AN21.8 Describe and demonstrate type, articular surfaces and movements of manubriosternal, costovertebral, costotransverse and xiphisternal joints.

JOINTS OF THORAX

Manubriosternal Joint

Manubriosternal joint is a ***secondary cartilaginous joint*** (***symphysis***). It permits slight movements of the body of the sternum on the manubrium during respiration (Flowchart 13.7).

Costovertebral Joints

The head of a typical rib articulates with its own vertebra, and also with the body of the next higher vertebra.

Type: Plane synovial joint.

Ligaments:

1. ***Capsular ligament***: A fibrous capsule is attached to the margin of articular facets.
2. ***Triradiate ligament***: It connects anterior margin of head of the rib to vertebra with the help of *three bands*.. The *upper band* is attached to vertebra above. The *lower band* is attached to vertebra below. The *middle band* of the triradiate ligament forms the hypochordal bow, uniting the joints of the two sides.
3. ***Intra-artricular ligament***: It connects the crest of the head (that separates articular facets) with the intra-articular disc. It divides the joint cavity into two parts.

Competency:
AN21.10 Describe costochondral and interchondral joints.

Costotransverse Joints

The tubercle of a typical rib articulates with the facet on anterior surface of transverse process of the corresponding vertebra (Figs 13.15a and b).

Type: Plane synovial joint.

Ligaments:

1. ***Capsular ligament***: It is attached to the margins of articular facets.
2. ***Three costotransverse ligaments***: The capsule is strengthened by three costotransverse ligaments.

The ***superior costotransverse ligament*** has two laminae which extend from the crest on the neck of the rib to the transverse process of the vertebra above.

The ***inferior costotransverse ligament*** passes from the posterior surface of the neck to the transverse process of its own vertebra.

The ***lateral costotransverse ligament*** connects the lateral non-articular part of the tubercle to the tip of the transverse process of its own vertebra (Plate 13.3).

Costochondral Joints

Each rib is continuous anteriorly with its cartilage, to form a ***primary cartilaginous joint***. No movements are permitted at these joints.

Chondrosternal Joints

1. The ***1st chondrosternal joint*** is a ***primary cartilaginous*** joint, it does not permit any movement. This helps in the stability of the shoulder girdle and of the upper limb (Plate 13.8).

Plate 13.8: Joints of costal cartilages

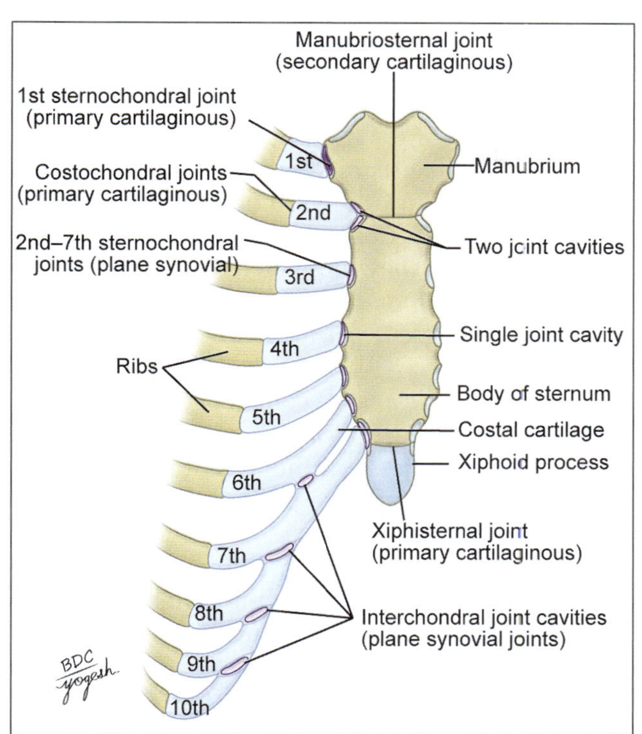

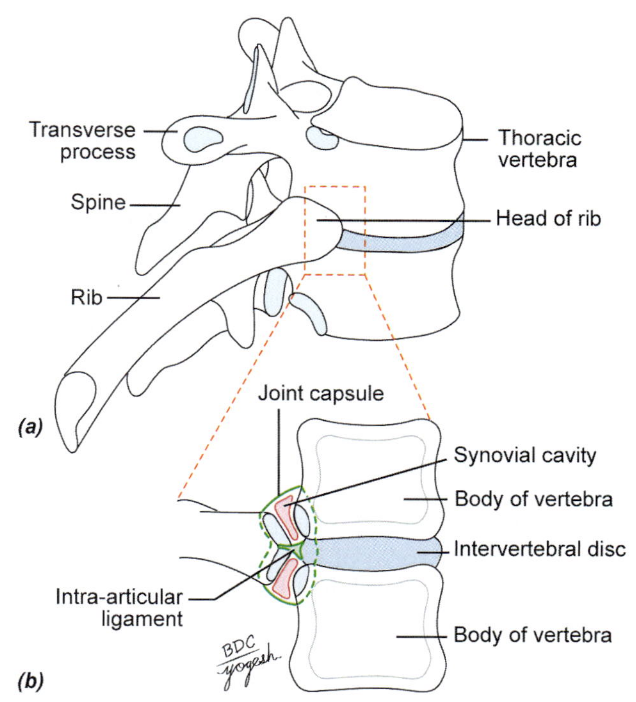

Figs 13.15a and b: (a) Costotransverse joint; (b) A section through the costotransverse joints

Flowchart 13.7: Joints of thoracic cage

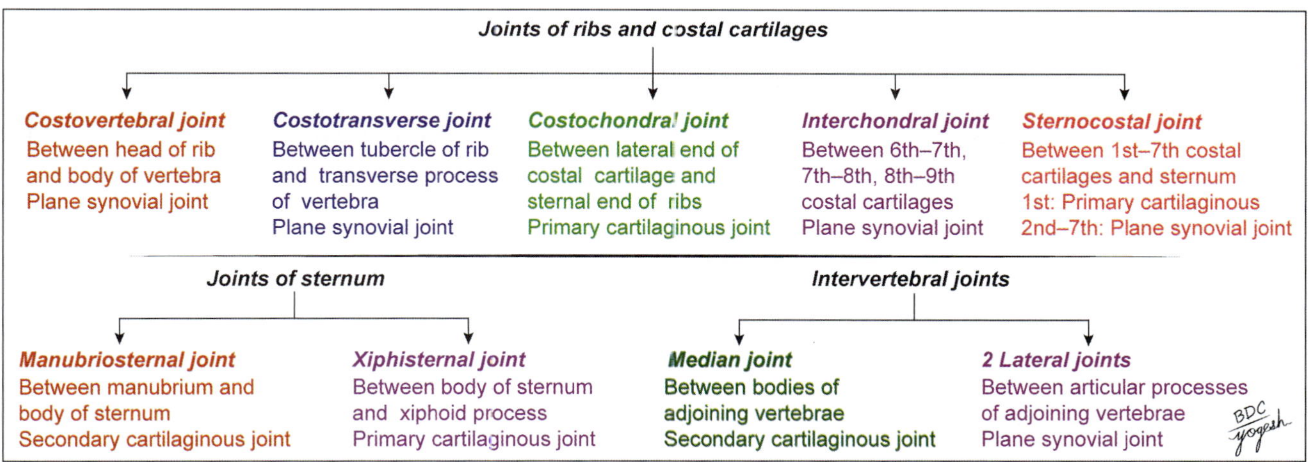

2. The ***2nd to 7th costal cartilages*** articulate with the sternum by ***synovial*** joints. Each joint has a single cavity except in the 2nd joint where the cavity is divided in two parts. The joints are held together by the capsular ligaments (Plate 13.8).

Interchondral Joints

1. The 7th to 9th costal cartilages articulate with one another by ***synovial joints***.
2. The 10th cartilage is united to the 9th by ***fibrous tissue***.

Intervertebral Joints

Adjoining vertebrae (T5 and T6) are connected to each other at three joints.

1. A median joint between the vertebral bodies
   The joint between the vertebral bodies is a *symphysis* (secondary cartilaginous joint).
   The surfaces of the vertebral bodies are lined by thin layers of hyaline cartilage. Between these layers of hyaline cartilage, there is a thick plate of ***fibrocartilage*** which is called the ***intervertebral disc***.
2. Two joints—one on the right side and one on the left side—between the articular processes.
   The joints between the articular processes are ***plane synovial joints***.

Intervertebral Discs

These are *fibrocartilaginous discs* which intervene between the bodies of adjacent vertebrae, and bind them together.

The discs contribute about one-fifth of the length of the vertebral column. The contribution is greater in the cervical and lumbar regions than in the thoracic region.

Shape: Their shape corresponds to that of the vertebral bodies between which they are placed.

Thickness: The thickness of the disc varies in different regions of the vertebral column, and in different parts of the same disc. In the cervical and lumbar regions, the discs are thicker in front than behind, while in the thoracic region they are of uniform thickness. The discs are thinnest in the upper thoracic region, and thickest in the lumbar region.

Structure: Each disc is made up of the following two parts.

1. The ***nucleus pulposus*** is the central part of the disc. It is soft and gelatinous at birth. It is kept under tension and acts as a hydraulic shock absorber. With advancing age, the elasticity of the disc is much reduced (Fig. 13.16).
2. The ***annulus fibrosus*** forms the peripheral part of the disc. It is made up of a narrower outer zone of collagenous fibres and a wider inner zone of fibrocartilage. The fibres form laminae that are arranged in the form of incomplete rings. The rings are connected by strong fibrous bands. The outer collagenous fibres blend.

Functions

1. The intervertebral discs give shape to the vertebral column.
2. They act as a remarkable series of shock absorbers or buffers.
3. Because of their elasticity, they allow slight movement of vertebral bodies on each other, more so in the cervical and lumbar regions. When the slight movements at individual discs are added together, they become considerable.

CLINICAL ANATOMY

- ***Herniation of disc (slipped disc)***: It is protrusion of nucleus pulposus from the damaged or ruptured annulus fibrosus. It may cause pain, numbness, or paralysis.
- ***Degenerative disc disease***: With advancing age, intervertebral disc may show degenerative changes. These changes cause reduced elasticity and shock absorption (annulus/anus = ring in Latin).

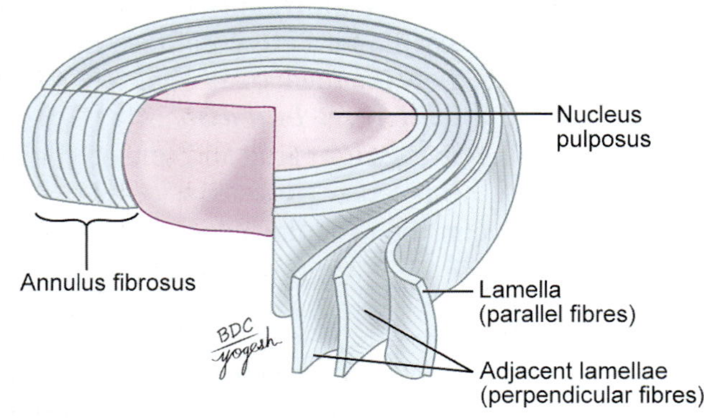

Fig. 13.16: Structure of an intervertebral disc

Ligaments Connecting Adjacent Vertebrae

Apart from the intervertebral discs and the capsules around the joints between the articular processes, adjacent vertebrae are connected by several ligaments which are as follows:

1. The *anterior longitudinal ligament* passes from the anterior surface of the body of one vertebra to another. Its upper end reaches the basilar part of the occipital bone.
2. The *posterior longitudinal ligament* is present on the posterior surface of the vertebral bodies within the vertebral canal. Its upper end reaches the body of the axis vertebra (C2) beyond which it is continuous with the *membrana tectoria*.
3. The *intertransverse ligaments* connect adjacent transverse processes.
4. The *interspinous ligaments* connect adjacent spines.
5. The *supraspinous ligaments* connect the tips of the spines of vertebrae from the seventh cervical to the sacrum. In the cervical region, they are replaced by the ligamentum nuchae.
6. The *ligamenta flava* (singular = ligamentum flavum) connect the laminae of adjacent vertebrae. They are made up mainly of elastic tissue.

Movements of the Vertebral Column

- Movements between adjacent vertebrae occur simultaneously at all the joints connecting them.
- Movement between any two vertebrae is slight. However, when the movements between several vertebrae are added together the total range of movement becomes considerable.
- The movements are those of ***flexion, extension, lateral flexion and a certain amount of rotation*** (Fig. 13.17).
- The range of movement differs in different parts of the vertebral column. This is influenced by the thickness and flexibility of the intervertebral discs and by the orientation of the articular facets.
- ***Flexion*** and ***extension*** occur freely in the cervical and lumbar regions (because the disc is thicker in front part and thin in the back part), but not in the thoracic region.
- ***Rotation*** is free in the thoracic region (because of uniform thickness of the disc) and restricted in the lumbar and cervical regions.

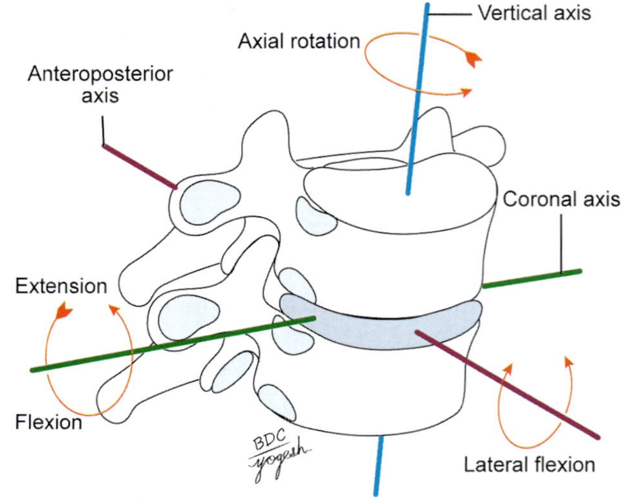

Fig. 13.17: Movements of vertebral column.

Facts to Remember

- Manubrium sterni is the thickest and strongest part of sternum. It is the most preferred site for bone marrow aspiration.
- Sternum forms joints with its own parts:
  - One manubriosternal joint—secondary cartilaginous.
  - Three joints between four sternebrae—primary cartilaginous.
  - One joint between sternum and xiphoid process—primary cartilaginous.
  - Sternum forms two joints with clavicles of the two sides—saddle type of synovial joint.
  - It articulates with 1st–7th costal cartilages on each side forming a total of 14 joints—all plane synovial joints except 1st chondrosternal which is synchondrosis.
- A typical thoracic vertebra forms following joints:
  - Body of one vertebrae with body of vertebra above and body of vertebra below—secondary cartilaginous joint (2 joints).
  - Lower larger part of head of corresponding rib for the demifacet along the upper border of the body on each side (2 cavities, 1 joint).
  - Upper smaller part of head of a lower rib for the demifacet along the lower border of the body on each side (2 cavities, 1 joint).
  - Superior articular processes on each side with the inferior articular processes of the vertebra above (2 joints)
  - Inferior articular processes on each side with the superior articular processes of the vertebra below (2 joints).
  - Transverse process of the vertebra with the articular part of the tubercle of the rib on each side (2 joints).
  - Body/centrum of the vertebra with the neural arch of the vertebra on each side—primary cartilaginous joints (2 joints)/neurocentral synchondrosis.
- The 1st rib is widest and most curved rib, whereas the 12th rib is the narrowest and smallest rib.
- *The ribs are arched bones. Joints formed by a typical rib are:*
  - Posterior end or head of a typical rib articulates with two adjacent vertebrae, corresponding one and one above it and the intervening intervertebral disc.
  - The articular part of the tubercle articulates with transverse process of corresponding vertebra.
  - The anterior part of the shaft of rib continues as the costal cartilage. It is primary cartilaginous joint.
  - A costal cartilage forms plane synovial joint with the side of sternum.

BDC's Anatomy *e*-book

1. Attachments of costal cartilages
2. Vertebral column as a whole
3. Parts of a typical vertebra
4. difference between thoracic and lumbar vertebrae
5. Movements of ribs and sternum
6. Further reading
7. Viva voce questions

Chapter

14

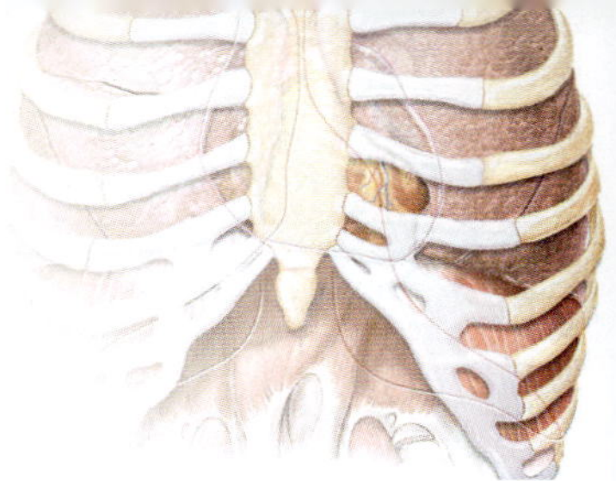

Walls of Thorax

The thorax is covered by muscles of pectoral region of upper limb. In addition, the intercostal muscles and membranes fill up the gaps between adjacent ribs and cartilages. These muscles provide integrity to the thoracic wall.

COVERINGS OF THE THORACIC WALL

The thoracic wall is covered from outside to inside by the following structures:

1. Skin
2. Superficial fascia
3. Deep fascia
4. Extrinsic muscles.

Superficial Fascia

- Superficial fascia in thoracic region contains moderate amount of fat, cutaneous nerves, and vessels.
- In female, superficial fascia contains well-developed mammary gland (rudimentary in males).

Extrinsic Muscles Covering the Thorax

Muscles of the Upper Limb and Back

1. Pectoralis major, pectoralis minor, subclavius
2. Serratus anterior, latissimus dorsi
3. Trapezius, levator scapulae, rhomboid major, rhomboid minor
4. Serratus posterior superior, serratus posterior inferior
5. Erector spinae (sacrospinalis).

Muscles of the Abdomen

1. Rectus abdominis
2. External oblique.

THORACIC WALL PROPER

The thoracic cage forms the skeletal framework of the wall of the thorax. The gaps between the ribs are called ***intercostal spaces***. They are occupied by the intercostal muscles and contain the intercostal nerves, vessels, and lymphatics. There are nine intercostal spaces anteriorly and eleven intercostal spaces posteriorly.

TYPICAL INTERCOSTAL SPACES

Typical intercostal spaces are the spaces whose intercostal nerves and vessels are confined to thoracic wall only. Examples: 3rd to 6th intercostal spaces.

Contents (Plate 14.1)

1. Intercostal muscles
2. Two anterior intercostal arteries and veins
3. Posterior intercostal artery and vein with its collateral branch
4. Intercostal nerve and its collateral branch
5. Intercostal lymphatics and lymph nodes.

> ***Competency:***
> **AN21.4** Describe and demonstrate extent, attachments, direction of fibres, nerve supply, and actions of intercostal muscles.

INTERCOSTAL MUSCLES

These are (Table 14.1, Figs 14.1 and 14.2):

1. External intercostal muscle (superficial layer)
2. Internal intercostal muscle (intermediate layer)
3. Transversus thoracis muscle (deep layer) — divisible into three parts:
   a. Subcostalis (Plate 14.2)
   b. Intercostalis intimi (innermost intercostal)
   c. Sternocostalis (Plate 14.2).

The attachments of these muscles are given in Table 14.1.

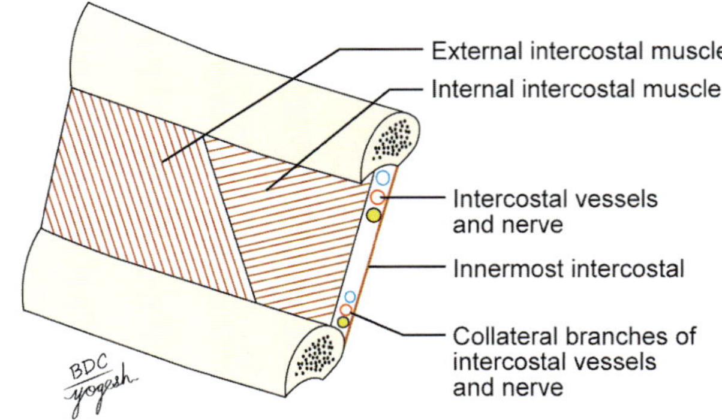

Fig. 14.1: External and internal intercostal muscles with external and internal intercostal membranes

Plate 14.1: Intercostal muscles and content of costal groove

External intercostal muscle
Rib (4th)
T4
T5
Origin: Lower border of rib
Insertion: Outer lip of the upper border of rib
Sternum
Anterior intercostal membrane
Internal intercostal muscle
Rib (4th)
Thoracic vertebra
Origin: Floor of the costal groove
Posterior intercostal membrane
T4
T5
Insertion: Inner lip of the upper border of rib
Sternum
Innermost intercostal muscle
Origin: Middle 2/4th of ridge above the costal groove
T4
T5
Insertion: Inner surface of rib
Content of costal groove
Lung
Visceral pleura
Rib
Parietal pleura
Endothoracic fascia
External intercostal muscle
Posterior intercostal vessels
Intercostal nerve
Internal intercostal muscle
Collateral branches
Innermost intercostal muscle
BDC

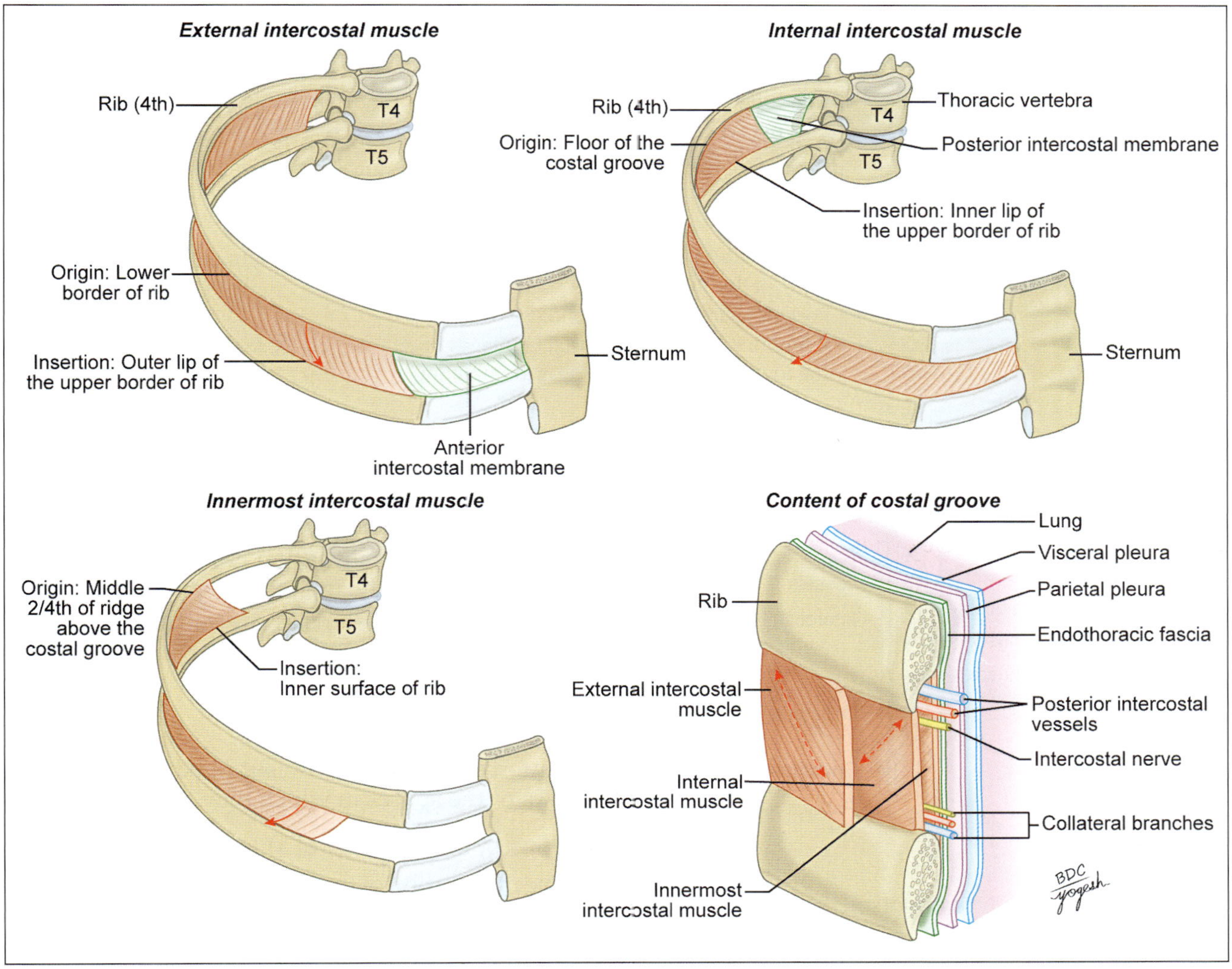

Plate 14.2: Sternocostalis and subcostalis muscles

Costal cartilage
Manubrium
Body of sternum
Sternocostalis
Insertion: Inner surface of 2nd – 6th costal cartilages
Xiphoid process
Costal cartilage
Inner surface of rib
Origin
– Lower 1/3rd of body of sternum
– Xiphoid process
– Costal cartilages of lower 3–4 true ribs
Posterior view
Ribs
7th
8th
9th
10th
11th
12th
T7
T8
T9
T10
T11
T12
Subcostalis
Origin: Inner surface of a rib near its angle
Insertion: Inner surface of second or third rib below
Cut surface of rib
BDC
Anterior view

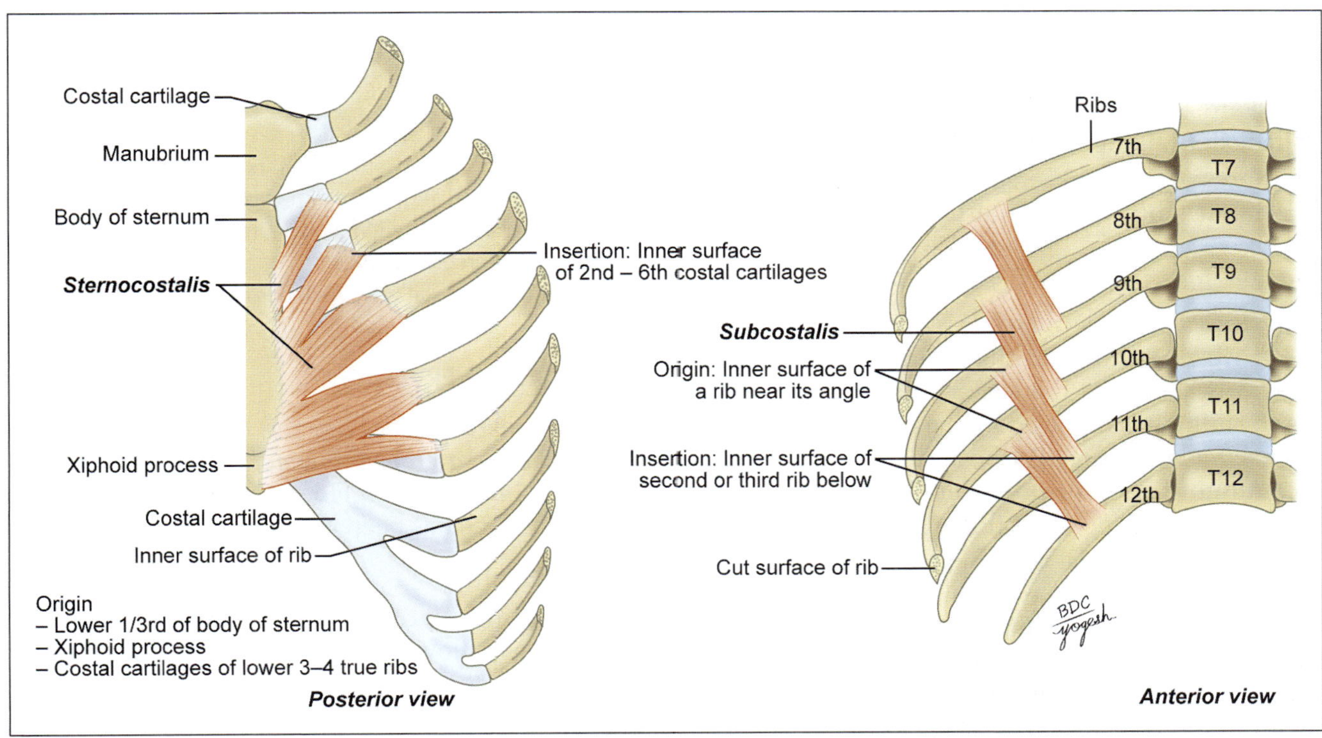

TABLE 14.1: Origin and insertion of the intercostal muscles (Plates 14.1 and 14.2, Figs 14.1 and 14.2)

Muscle	*Origin*	*Insertion*
1. External intercostal	Lower border of the rib above the space	Outer lip of the upper border of the rib below
2. Internal intercostal	Floor of the costal groove of the rib above	Inner lip of the upper border of the rib below
3. Transversus thoracis		
a. Subcostalis	Inner surface of the rib near the angle	Inner surface of two or three ribs below
b. Intercostalis intimi/innermost intercostal	Middle 2/4th of the ridge above the costal groove	Inner lip of the upper border of the rib below
c. Sternocostalis	• Lower 1/3rd of the posterior surface of the body of the sternum • Posterior surface of the xiphoid process • Posterior surface of the costal cartilages of the lower 3 or 4 true ribs near the sternum	Costal cartilages of the 2nd–6th ribs

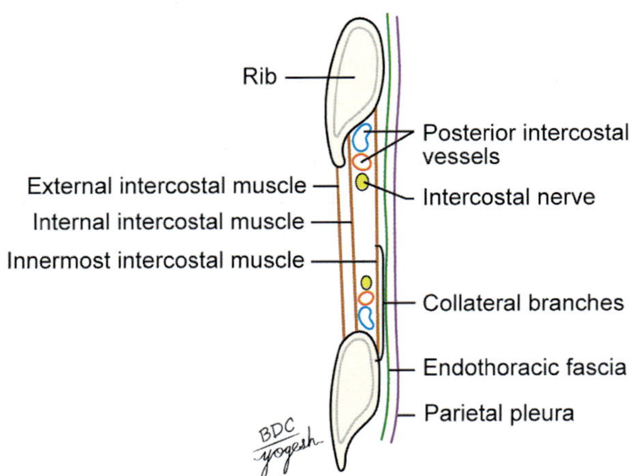

Fig. 14.2: Section of typical intercostal space with neurovascular bundle and its collateral branches

Direction of Fibres

In the anterior part of the intercostal space:

1. The fibres of the external intercostal muscle run downwards, forwards, and medially in front.
2. The fibres of the internal intercostal run downwards, backwards, and laterally, i.e. at right angle to those of the external intercostal.
3. The fibres of the transversus thoracis run in the same direction as those of the internal intercostal.

Extent

1. The *external intercostal muscle* extends from the tubercle of the rib posteriorly to the costochondral junction anteriorly. Between the costochondral junction and the sternum, it is replaced by the external or ***anterior intercostal membrane***. The posterior end of the muscle is continuous with the posterior fibres of the ***superior costotransverse ligament*** (Plate 14.1).
2. The *internal intercostal muscle* extends from the lateral border of the sternum to the angle of the rib. Beyond the angle, it becomes continuous with the ***internal** or **posterior intercostal membrane***, which is continuous with the anterior fibres of the ***superior costotransverse ligament***.
3. Transversus thoracis comprises the following 3 parts:
   a. The subcostalis is confined to the posterior part of the lower intercostal spaces only.
   b. The intercostalis intimi is confined to the middle 2/4th of all the intercostal spaces (Plate 14.2).
   c. The sternocostalis is present in relation to the anterior parts of the upper intercostal spaces (Plate 14.2).

Nerve Supply

All intercostal muscles are supplied by the intercostal nerves of the spaces in which they lie.

Actions of the Intercostal Muscles

1. The main action of the intercostal muscles is to prevent intercostal spaces being drawn in during inspiration and bulging outwards during expiration.
2. The external intercostals, interchondral portions of the internal intercostals, and the levator costae may elevate the ribs during inspiration.
3. The internal intercostals except for the interchondral portions and the transversus thoracis may depress the ribs or cartilages during expiration.

Competencies:

AN21.5 Describe and demonstrate origin, course, relations and branches of a typical intercostal nerve.

AN21.7 Mention the origin, course, relations and branches of:

1. Atypical intercostal nerve.
2. Superior intercostal artery, subcostal artery.

INTERCOSTAL NERVES

The ***intercostal nerves*** are the *ventral primary rami* of thoracic ***one to eleven thoracic spinal nerves*** (Plate 14.3, Figs 14.3 and 14.4, Flowchart 14.1) after the dorsal primary ramus has been given off.

Classification

According to the distribution, intercostal nerves are classified as follows:

Typical intercostal nerves: These are confined to the thoracic wall. *Examples*: 3rd–6th intercostal nerves.

Plate 14.3: Typical intercostal nerve and artery

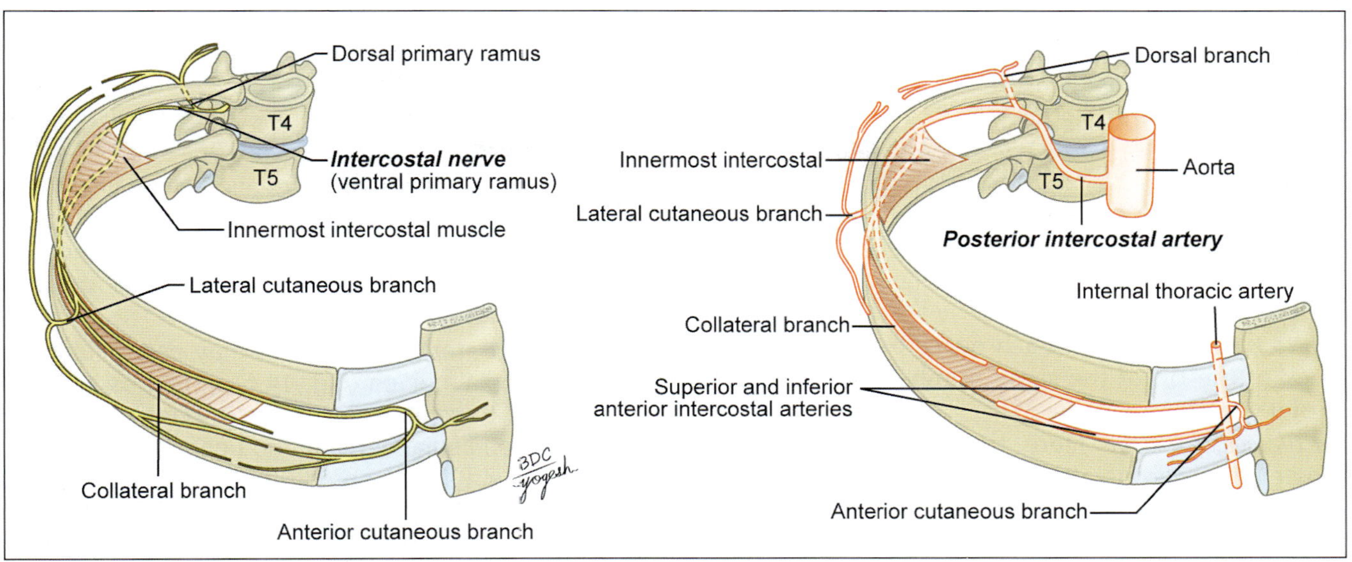

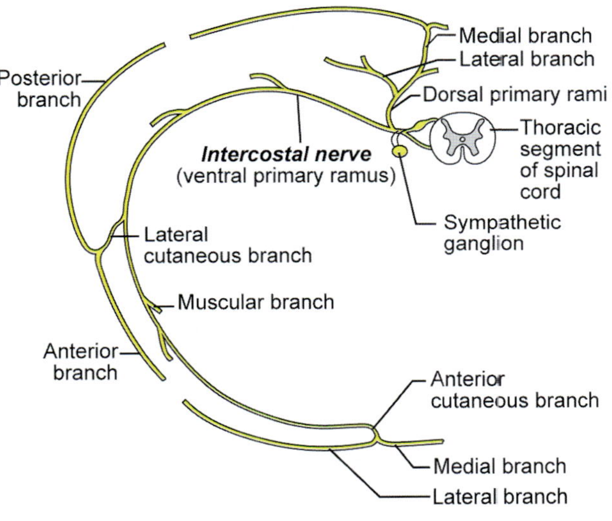

Fig. 14.3: Typical thoracic spinal nerve

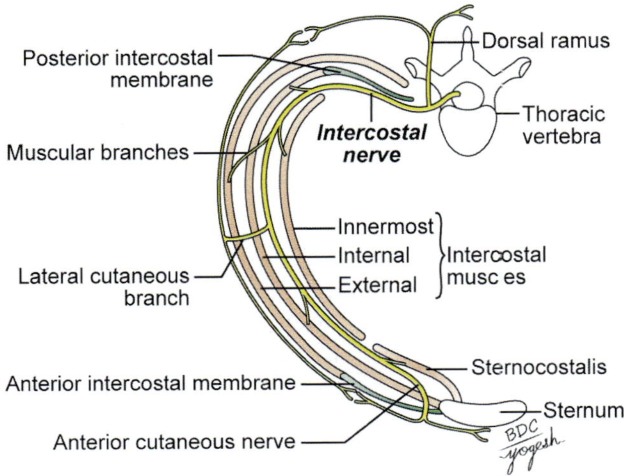

Fig. 14.4: Course and branches of a typical intercostal nerve

***Atypical intercostal nerves*:** These nerves in addition to thoracic wall supply additional structures.

Flowchart 14.1: Intercostal nerve

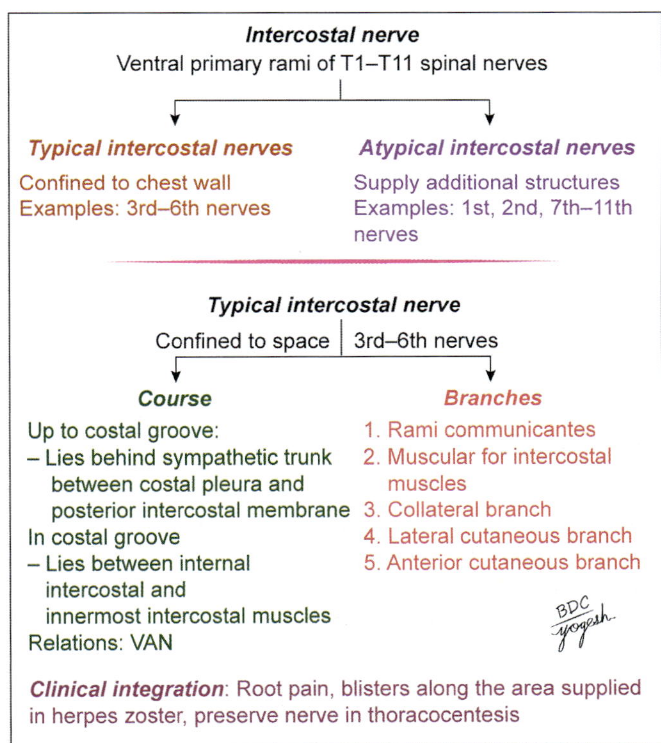

Examples:

- *1st intercostal nerve*: Major part joins with the ventral ramus of 8th cervical spinal nerve to form lower trunk of brachial plexus.
- *2nd intercostal nerve*: It gives lateral cutaneous branch called intercostobrachial nerve. This nerve supplies the skin of the floor of the axilla and upper part of the medial side of the arm through medial cutaneous nerve of the arm.
- *7th–11th intercostal nerves*: These nerves supply the anterior abdominal wall, in addition to the thoracic wall. Hence, they are also called ***thoracoabdominal nerves***.

The anterior primary ramus of the twelfth thoracic nerve forms the ***subcostal nerve***. The ***subcostal nerve*** is distributed to the abdominal wall and to the skin of the buttock.

TYPICAL INTERCOSTAL NERVE

Course

The typical intercostal nerve runs in the costal groove and ends near the sternum (Fig. 14.4).

Relations

1. *Up to the costal groove:* Each nerve passes below the neck of the rib of the same number and enters the costal groove.
2. *In the costal groove*: Here, the nerve lies below the posterior intercostal vessels. The relationship of structures in the costal groove from above downwards is posterior intercostal vein, posterior intercostal artery, and intercostal nerve (**VAN**) (Figs 14.2a and b). In the posterior part of the costal groove, the nerve lies between the pleura, with the endothoracic fascia and the internal intercostal membrane. In the greater part of the space, the nerve lies between the intercostalis intimi and the internal intercostal muscle (Fig. 14.4).
3. *Near the sternum*: The nerve crosses in front of the internal thoracic vessels and the sternocostalis muscle. It then pierces the internal intercostal muscle, the external intercostal membrane and the pectoralis major muscle to terminate as the *anterior cutaneous nerve of the thorax*.

Branches (Fig. 14.3)

Muscular Branches

1. ***Muscular branches:*** They supply the intercostal muscles, the transversus thoracis, and the serratus posterior superior.
2. ***Collateral branch:*** It arises near the angle of the rib and runs in the lower part of the space in the same neurovascular plane. It supplies muscles of the space.

Sensory Branches

1. The main branch and the collateral branch also supply parietal pleura, periosteum of the ribs. The lower nerves in addition supply the parietal peritoneum.
2. ***Lateral cutaneous branch:*** It arises near the angle of the rib and accompanies the main trunk up to the lateral thoracic wall where it pierces the intercostal muscles and other muscles of the body wall along the midaxillary line. It is distributed to the skin after dividing into anterior and posterior branches.
3. ***Anterior cutaneous branch:*** It emerges on the side of the sternum to supply the overlying skin after dividing into medial and lateral branches.

Communicating Branches

1. Each nerve is connected to a thoracic sympathetic ganglion by a distally placed white and a proximally placed ***grey ramus communicans*** (Fig. 14.3).
2. The lateral cutaneous branch of the second intercostal nerve is known as the ***intercostobrachial nerve***. It supplies the skin of the floor of the axilla and of the upper part of the medial side of the arm (*see* Figs 7.1).

CLINICAL ANATOMY

- ***Root pain* or *girdle pain*:** Irritation of the intercostal nerves causes severe pain which is referred to the front of the chest or abdomen, i.e. at the peripheral termination of the nerve. This is known as *root pain* or *girdle pain*.
- ***Herpes zoster*:** Herpes virus may cause infection of intercostal nerves (Fig. 14.5). If herpes infection is in 2nd thoracic nerve, there is referred pain via intercostobrachial nerve to the upper medial side of arm. the virus may spread to the skin supplied by the same cutaneous nerve and produces vesicular blisters.
- ***Thoracocentesis*:** Usually, it is done in the 8th or 9th intercostal space in the midaxillary along the upper border of the rib to prevent the injury to the intercostal nerve (that runs in costal groove) (Fig. 14.6).
- Internal thoracic artery is mobilised and its distal cut end is joined to the coronary artery distal to its narrowed segment.

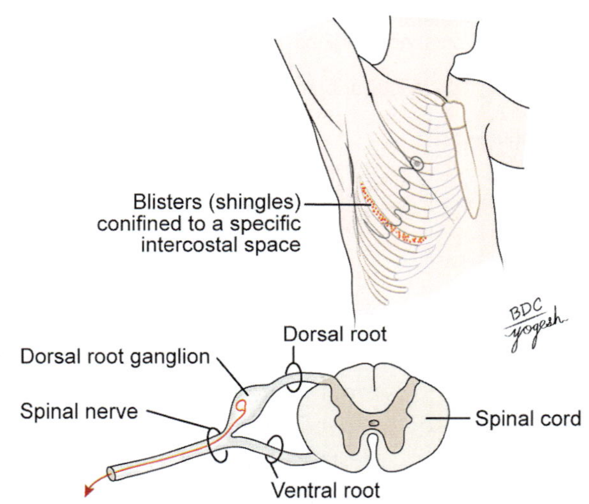

Fig. 14.5: Herpes zoster

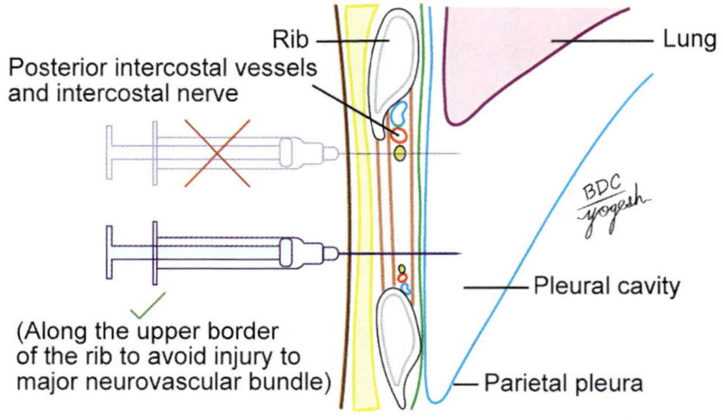

Fig. 14.6: Thoracocentesis

Section 2: Thorax

14

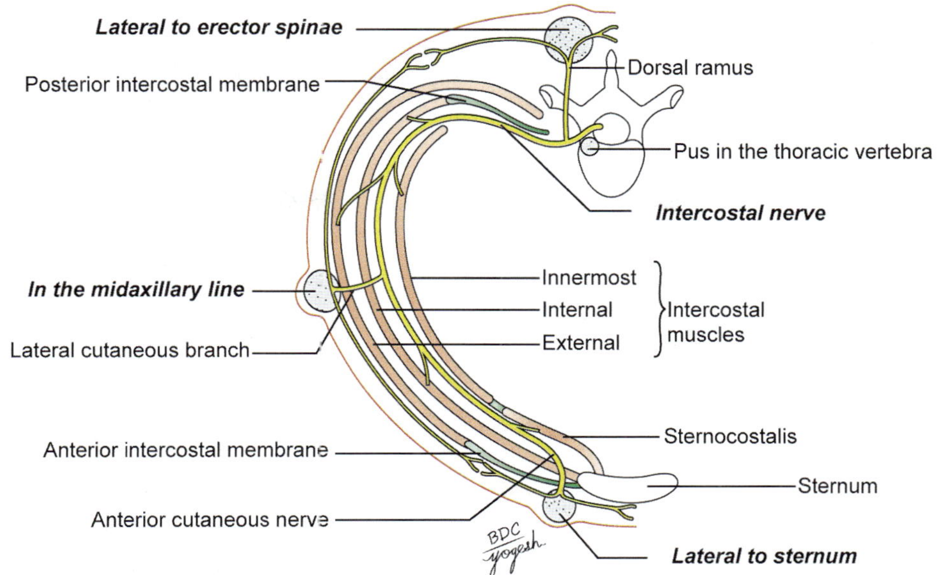

Fig. 14.7: Possible paths of cold abscess (due to TB of vertebra) along the branches of spinal nerve

- ***Sites of eruption of cold abscess on the body wall*:** Pus from the vertebral column (in cases of tuberculosis) tends to track around the thorax along the course of the neurovascular bundle, and may point at any of the three sites of exit of the branches of a thoracic nerve; one dorsal primary ramus and two cutaneous branches (Fig. 14.7).
- In ***superior vena caval obstruction*** before the entry of vena azygos, the vena azygos is the main channel which transmits the blood from the upper half of the body to distal part of superior vena cava (Flowchart 14.2). In its blockage after entry of vena azygos, flow of blood is shown in Flowchart 14.3.

DISSECTION

Detach the serratus anterior and the pectoralis major muscles from the upper ribs. Note the external intercostal muscle in the second and third intercostal spaces. Its fibres run anteroinferiorly. Follow it forwards to the external intercostal membrane which replaces it between the costal cartilages (Figs 14.1a and b and 14.2).

Cut the external intercostal membrane and muscle along the lower border of two spaces. Reflect them upwards to expose the internal intercostal muscle. The direction of its fibres is posteroinferior, at right angle to that of external oblique.

Follow the lateral cutaneous branch of one intercostal nerve to its trunk deep to internal intercostal muscle. Trace the nerve and accompanying vessels round the thoracic wall. Note their collateral branches lying along the upper margin of the rib below. Trace the muscular branches of the trunk of intercostal nerve and its collateral branch. Trace the anterior cutaneous nerve as well (Fig. 14.3).

Identify the deepest muscle in the intercostal space, the innermost intercostal muscle (Table 14.1). This muscle is deficient in the anterior and posterior ends of the intercostal spaces, where the neurovascular bundle rests directly on the parietal pleura.

Expose the internal thoracic artery 1 cm from the lateral margin of sternum by carefully removing the intercostal muscles and membranes from the upper three intercostal spaces (Fig. 14.11a).

Trace the artery through the upper six intercostal spaces and identify its two terminal branches (*see* Fig. 21.7). Trace its venae comitantes upwards till third costal cartilage where these join to form internal thoracic vein, which drains into the brachiocephalic vein.

Follow the course and branches of both anterior and posterior intercostal arteries including the course and tributaries of azygos vein.

Flowchart 14.2: Superior vena cava blockage before entry of vena azygos

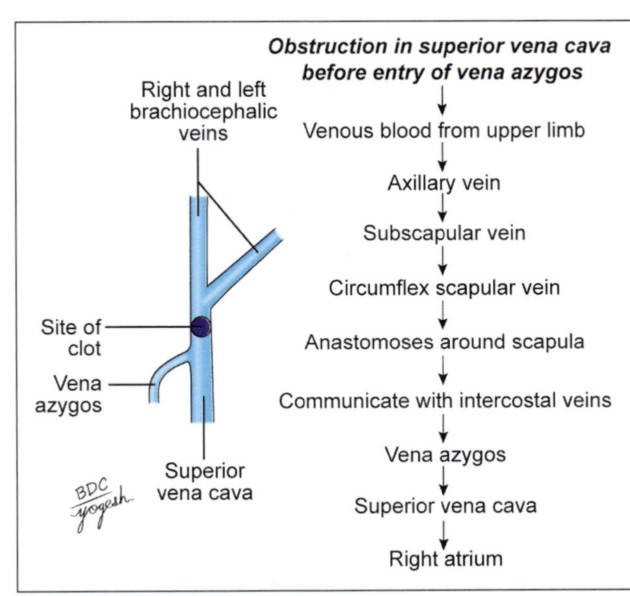

Flowchart 14.3: Superior vena cava blockage after entry of vena azygos

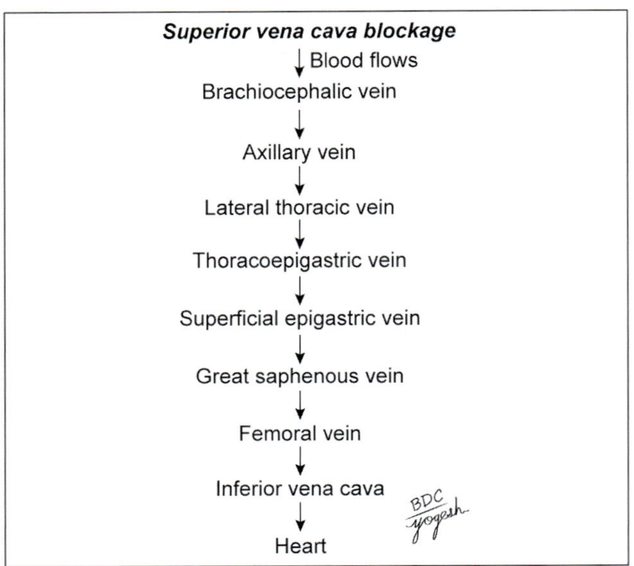

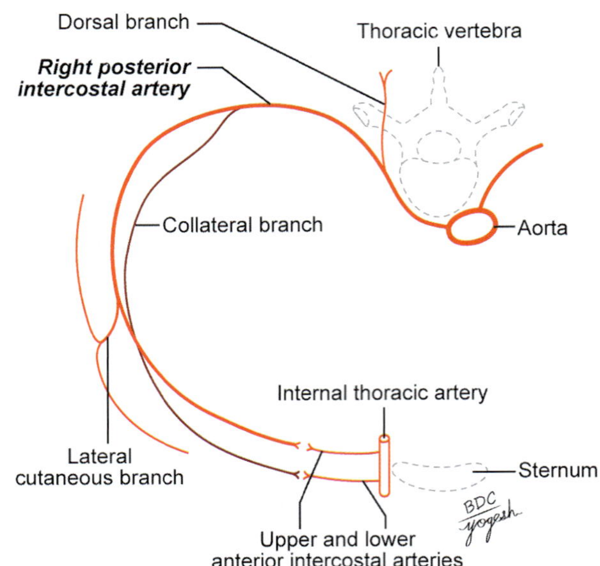

Fig. 14.8: Scheme showing the intercostal arteries. Each intercostal space contains one posterior intercostal, its collateral branch and two anterior intercostal arteries

Competencies:

AN21.6 Mention origin, course and branches/tributaries of:
1. Anterior and posterior intercostal vessels.
2. Internal thoracic vessels.

AN21.7 Mention the origin, course, relations and branches of:
1. Atypical intercostal nerve.
2. Superior intercostal artery, subcostal artery.

INTERCOSTAL ARTERIES

Each intercostal space contains (Plate 14.3, Figs 14.8 to 14.10, Flowchart 14.4)

a. One posterior intercostal artery with its collateral branch
b. Two anterior intercostal arteries.

The greater part of the space is supplied by the posterior intercostal artery.

Posterior Intercostal Arteries

These are 11 in number on each side, one in each space.

1. The 1st and 2nd posterior intercostal arteries arise from the superior intercostal artery, which is a branch of costocervical trunk of the subclavian artery.
2. The 3rd–11th arteries arise from the descending thoracic aorta (Fig. 14.10). The right-sided arteries are longer than those of the left side as aorta is to the left of median plane (Fig. 14.9).

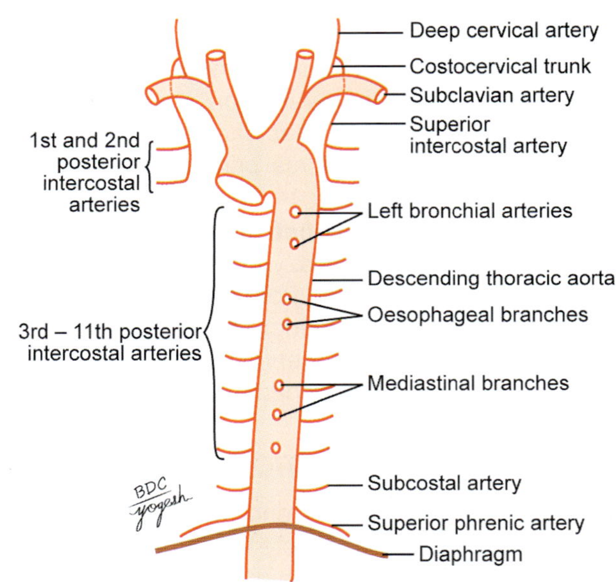

Fig. 14.9: Beginning of intercostal arteries

Course and Relations

In front of the vertebrae

- The right posterior intercostal arteries are longer than the left, and pass behind the oesophagus, the thoracic duct, the azygos vein and the sympathetic chain (Fig. 14.9).
- The left posterior intercostal arteries pass behind the hemiazygos vein and the sympathetic chain.

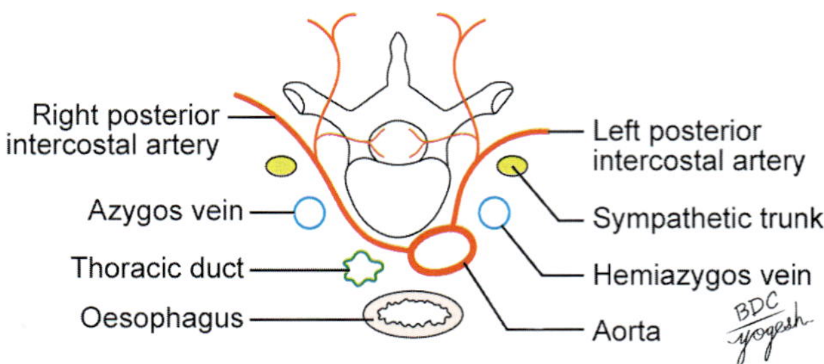

Fig. 14.10: Origin of the right and left posterior intercostal arteries

In the intercostal space

- The artery is accompanied by the intercostal vein and nerve, the relationship from above downwards being vein–artery–nerve (VAN).

Flowchart 14.4: Posterior intercostal artery

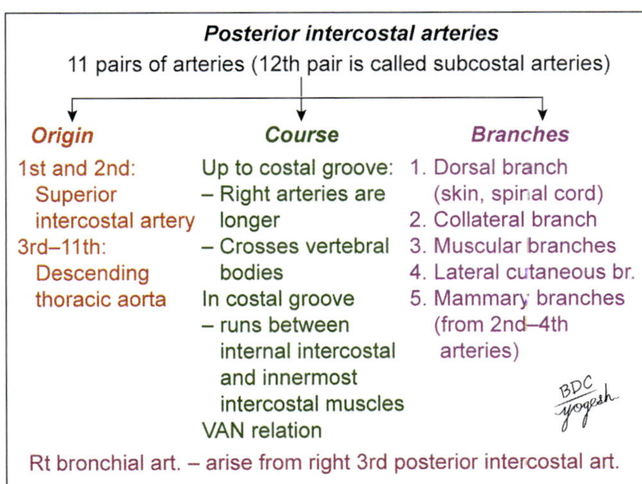

- The neurovascular bundle runs forwards in the costal groove, first between the pleura and the internal intercostal membrane and then between the internal intercostal and intercostalis intimi muscles (Plate 14.3).

Termination

Each posterior intercostal artery ends at the level of the costochondral junction by anastomosing with the upper anterior intercostal artery of the space (Fig. 14.8).

Branches

1. ***Dorsal branch*:** It supplies the muscles and skin of the back, and gives off a spinal branch to the spinal cord and vertebrae (Fig. 14.8).
2. ***Collateral branch*:** It arises near the angle of the rib, descends to the upper border of the lower rib, and ends by anastomosing with the lower anterior intercostal artery of the space.
3. ***Muscular arteries*** are given off to the intercostal muscles, the pectoral muscles and the serratus anterior.
4. ***Lateral cutaneous branch*:** It accompanies the nerve of the same name.
5. ***Mammary branches*:** They arise from the 2nd, 3rd and 4th arteries and supply the mammary gland.
6. ***Right bronchial artery*:** It arises from the right third posterior intercostal artery.

Anterior Intercostal Arteries

There are nine intercostal spaces anteriorly as only ten ribs reach front of body. There are two anterior intercostal arteries in each space.

Beginning

- In the upper six spaces, they arise from the internal thoracic artery (Fig. 14.8).
- In 7th–9th spaces, the arteries are branches of musculophrenic artery.

Termination

The two anterior intercostal arteries end at the costochondral junction by anastomosing with the respective posterior intercostal arteries and with the collateral branches of the posterior intercostal arteries.

INTERCOSTAL VEINS

Each intercostal space contains two anterior intercostal veins and one posterior intercostal vein (Plate 14.4).

Anterior Intercostal Veins

There are two ***anterior intercostal veins*** in each of the ***upper nine spaces***. They accompany the corresponding arteries.

In the upper three spaces, the veins end in the internal thoracic vein.

In 4–6 spaces, the veins end in venae comitantes accompanying internal thoracic artery.

In the succeeding spaces, they end in the venae comitantes accompanying musculophrenic artery.

Termination: In upper six spaces, they end in the internal thoracic vein. In 7th–9th spaces, they end in the musculophrenic vein.

Posterior Intercostal Veins

There is one ***posterior intercostal vein*** and one collateral vein in each intercostal space. Each vein accompanies the corresponding artery and lies superior to the artery.

***Tributaries*:** The tributaries of these veins correspond to the branches of the arteries. They include veins from the vertebral canal, the vertebral venous plexus, and the muscles and skin of the back. Vein accompanying the collateral branch of the artery drains into the posterior intercostal vein.

***Termination*:** The mode of termination of the posterior intercostal veins is different on the right and left sides as given in Table 14.2. and shown in Fig. 14.11. The azygos and hemiazygos veins are described later.

TABLE 14.2: Termination of posterior intercostal veins

Veins	*On right side they drain into*	*On left side they drain into*
1st	Right brachiocephalic vein	Left brachiocephalic vein
2nd–4th	Join to form right superior intercostal vein which drains into the azygos vein	Join to form left superior intercostal vein which drains into the left brachiocephalic vein
5th–8th	Azygos vein	Accessory hemiazygos vein
9th–11th and subcostal	Azygos vein	Hemiazygos vein

Plate 14.4: Posterior intercostal vein

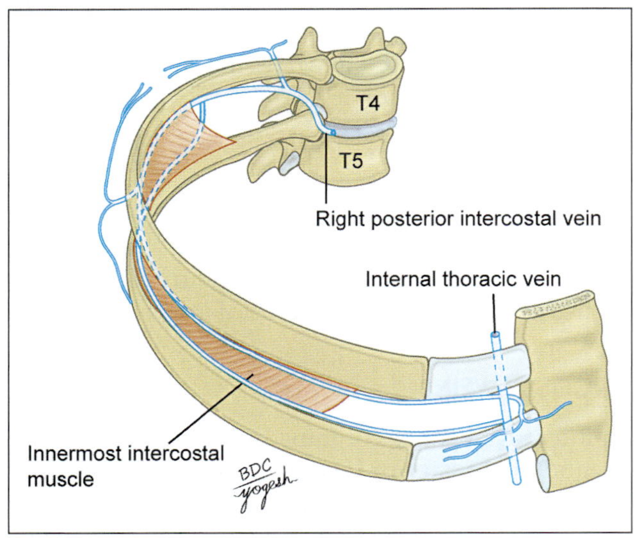

Competency:

AN23.3 Describe and demonstrate origin, course, relations, tributaries, and termination of superior vena cava, azygos, hemiazygos, and accessory hemiazygos veins. For superior vena cava, *see* Chapter 19.

AZYGOS VEIN

The azygos vein drains the thoracic wall and the upper lumbar region (Fig. 14.11, Flowchart 14.5). It forms an important channel connecting the superior and inferior venae cavae. The term 'azygos' means unpaired. The vein occupies the upper part of the posterior abdominal wall and the posterior mediastinum. It also connects portal venous system, caval venous system and vertebral venous system.

Formation

The azygos vein is formed by union of the lumbar azygos, right subcostal and right ascending lumbar veins (Fig. 14.12).

1. The ***lumbar azygos vein*** may be regarded as the abdominal part of the azygos vein. It lies to the right of the lumbar vertebrae. Its lower end communicates with the inferior vena cava.
2. The ***right subcostal vein*** accompanies the corresponding artery.
3. The ***ascending lumbar vein*** is formed by vertical anastomoses that connect the lumbar veins. The azygos vein may be formed by union of the right subcostal and ascending lumbar veins (Fig. 14.10).

Course

1. The azygos vein enters the thorax by passing through the ***aortic opening*** of the diaphragm.
2. The azygos vein then ascends up to ***T4 vertebra*** where it arches forwards over the root of the right lung and ends by joining the posterior aspect of the superior vena cava before it pierces the pericardium.

Relations

Anteriorly: Oesophagus.
Posteriorly: Lower eight thoracic vertebrae
Right posterior intercostal arteries

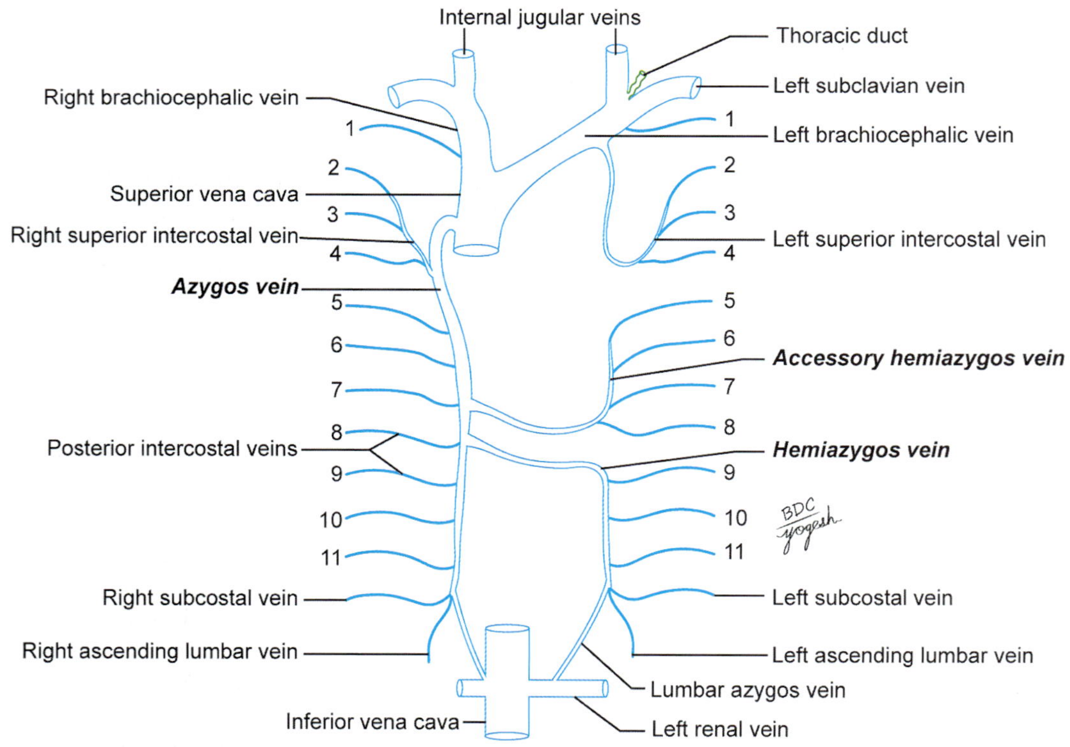

Fig. 14.11: Drainage of posterior intercostal veins

Flowchart 14.5: Azygos vein

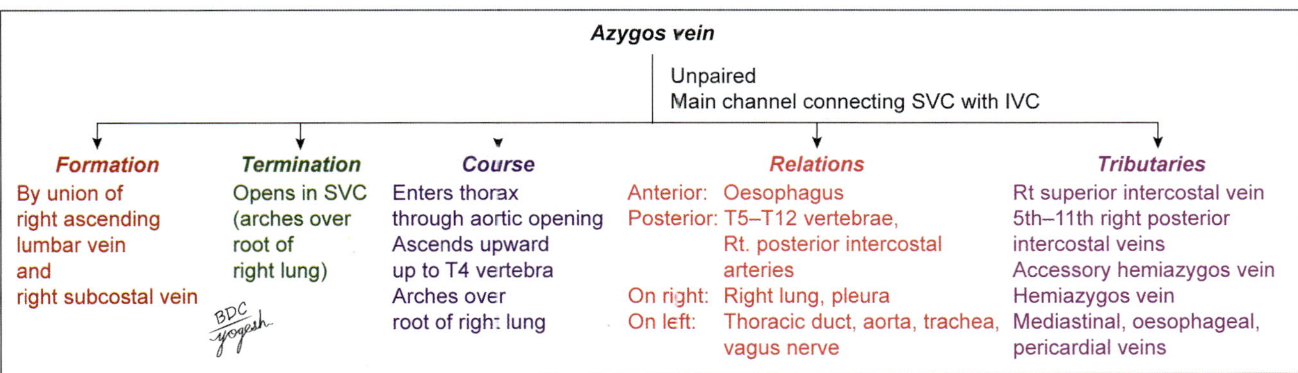

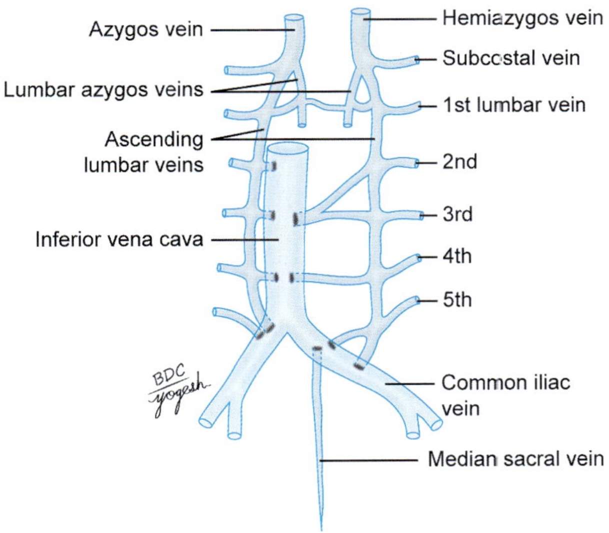

Fig. 14.12: Formation of azygos vein

To the right: Right lung and pleura
Greater splanchnic nerve

To the left: Thoracic duct and aorta in lower part
Oesophagus, trachea and vagus in the upper part.

Tributaries

1. Right superior intercostal vein formed by union of the 2nd–4th posterior intercostal veins.
2. 5th–11th right posterior intercostal veins (Fig. 14.11).
3. Hemiazygos vein at the level of lower border of T8 vertebra.
4. Accessory hemiazygos vein at the level of upper border of T8 vertebra.
5. Right bronchial vein, near the terminal end of the azygos vein.
6. Several oesophageal, mediastinal and pericardial veins.

HEMIAZYGOS VEINS

Hemiazygos vein is also called the ***inferior hemiazygos vein***. It is the mirror image of the lower part of the azygos vein. The *hemiazygos* is formed by the union of the left lumbar azygos, left ascending lumbar, and left subcostal veins (Fig. 14.10).

Course

Hemiazygos vein pierces the left crus of the diaphragm, ascends on the left side of the vertebra overlapped by the aorta. At the level of eighth thoracic vertebra, it turns to the right, passes behind the oesophagus and the thoracic duct, and joins the azygos vein (Fig. 14.10).

Tributaries

9th–11th left posterior intercostal veins and oesophageal veins.

ACCESSORY HEMIAZYGOS VEIN

Accessory hemiazygos vein is also called the ***superior hemiazygos vein***. It is the mirror image of the upper part of the azygos vein (Fig. 14.10).

Course

Accessory hemiazygos vein begins at the medial end of the 4th or 5th intercostal space, and descends on the left side of the vertebral column.

At the level of T8 vertebra, it turns to the right, passes behind the aorta and the thoracic duct, and joins the azygos vein.

Tributaries

1. 5th–8th left posterior intercostal veins
2. Sometimes the left bronchial veins.

LYMPHATICS OF AN INTERCOSTAL SPACE

- Lymphatics from the anterior part of the spaces pass to the anterior intercostal or *internal mammary nodes* which lie along the internal thoracic artery. Their efferents unite with those of the tracheobronchial and brachiocephalic nodes to form the *bronchomediastinal trunk*, which joins the *right lymphatic trunk on the right side* and the *thoracic duct on the left side.*
- Lymphatics from the posterior part of the space pass to the posterior intercostal nodes which lie on the heads and necks of the ribs. Their efferents in the lower four spaces unite to form a trunk which descends and opens into the *cisterna chyli*. The efferents from the upper spaces drain into *left bronchomediastinal lymph trunk* on the left side and into *right bronchomediastinal lymph trunk* on the right side.

INTERNAL THORACIC ARTERY

Origin

Internal thoracic artery arises from the inferior aspect of the 1st part of the subclavian artery opposite the thyrocervical trunk. The origin lies 2 cm above the sternal end of the clavicle (Plate 14.5, Fig. 14.13, and Flowchart 14.6).

Beginning, Course and Termination

Internal thoracic artery arises from lower border of 1st part of subclavian artery. It descends medially and downwards behind sternal end of clavicle, and 1st costal cartilage. Runs vertically downwards 2 cm from lateral border of sternum till 6th intercostal space.

The artery terminates in the 6th intercostal space by dividing into the superior epigastric and musculophrenic arteries.

The artery is accompanied by two venae comitantes which unite at the level of the 4th costal cartilage to form the internal thoracic or internal mammary vein. The vein runs upwards along the medial side of the artery to end in the brachiocephalic vein at the inlet of the thorax.

A chain of lymph nodes lies along the artery.

Relations

Anteriorly

Above the first costal cartilage

Here, The artery runs downwards, forwards and medially, behind:

1. Sternal end of the clavicle
2. Internal jugular vein
3. Brachiocephalic vein
4. First costal cartilage
5. Phrenic nerve. It descends in front of the cervical pleura.

Below the first costal cartilage

Here, the artery runs vertically downwards up to its termination in the 6th intercostal space. Its relations are as follows:

1. Pectoralis major
2. Upper six costal cartilages
3. External intercostal membranes
4. Internal intercostal muscles
5. The first six intercostal nerves (Fig. 14.13).

Posteriorly

The endothoracic fascia and pleura up to the 2nd or 3rd costal cartilage. Below this level, the sternocostalis muscle separates the artery from the pleura (Plate 14.5).

Branches

1. ***Pericardiophrenic artery***: It arises in the root of the neck and accompanies the phrenic nerve to reach the diaphragm. It supplies the pericardium and the pleura.
2. ***Mediastinal arteries***: They are small irregular branches that supply the thymus, in front of the pericardium, and the fat in the mediastinum.

Plate 14.5: Internal thoracic artery and its branches

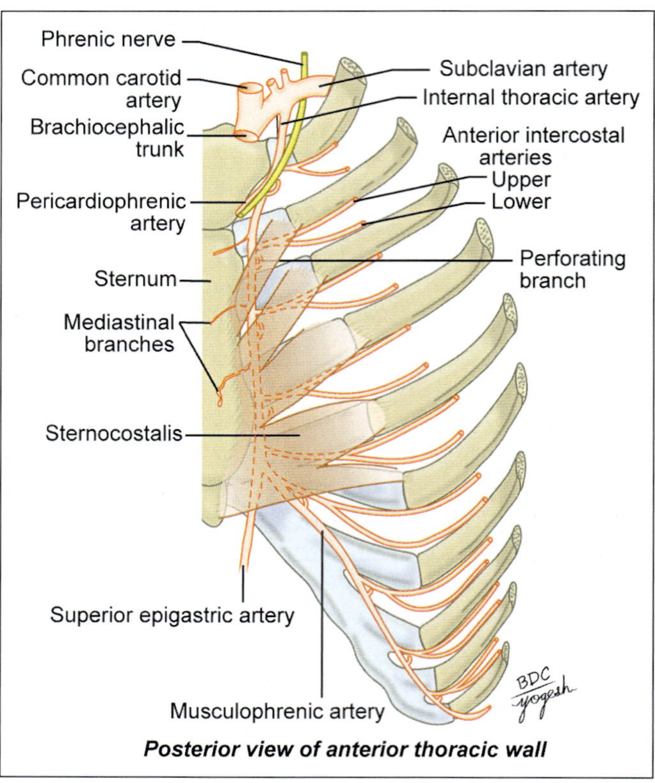

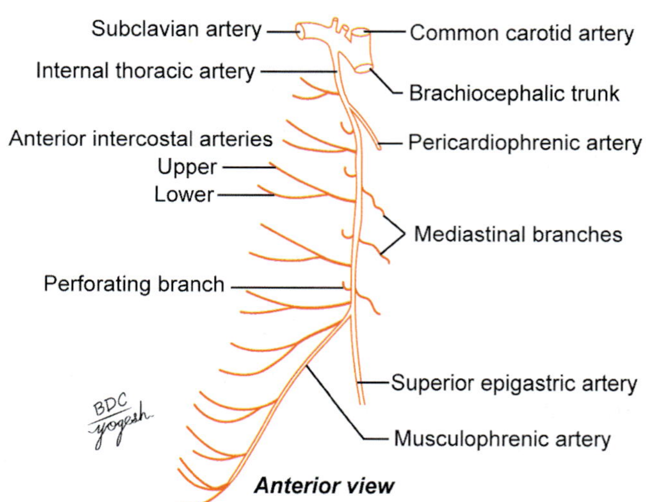

Fig. 14.13: Internal thoracic artery and its branches

Flowchart 14.6: Internal thoracic artery

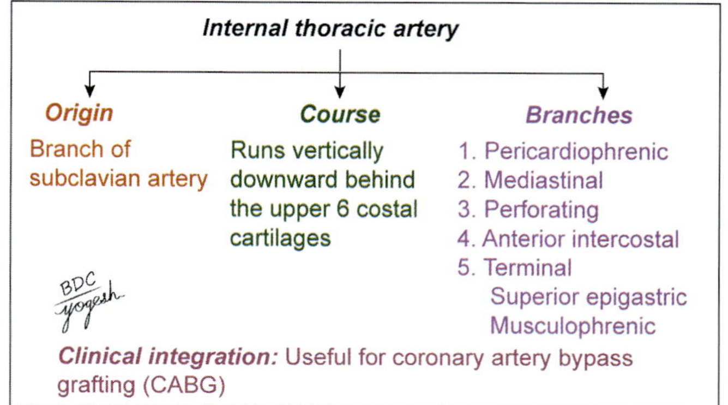

3. ***Two anterior intercostal arteries***: They are given to each of the upper six intercostal spaces.
4. ***Perforating branches*** accompany the anterior cutaneous nerves. In the female, the perforating branches in the second, third, and fourth spaces are large and supply the breast.
5. ***Superior epigastric artery***: It runs downwards behind the seventh costal cartilage and enters the rectus sheath by passing between the sternal and costal slips of the diaphragm.
6. ***Musculophrenic artery***: It runs downwards and laterally behind the 7th–9th costal cartilages. It gives two anterior intercostal branches to each of these three spaces. It perforates the diaphragm near the 9th costal cartilage and terminates by anastomosing with other arteries on the undersurface of the diaphragm. Note that through its various branches, the internal thoracic artery supplies the anterior thoracic and abdominal walls from the clavicle to the umbilicus.

Competencies:

AN23.5 Identify and mention the location and extent of thoracic sympathetic chain.

AN23.6 Describe the splanchnic nerves.

THORACIC SYMPATHETIC TRUNK

The thoracic sympathetic trunk is a ganglionated chain situated one on each side of the thoracic vertebral column. Superiorly, it is continuous with the cervical part of the chain and inferiorly with the lumbar part (Figs 14.14 and 14.15, Flowchart 14.7).

Number of Ganglions

Theoretically, the chain bears 12 ***ganglia*** corresponding to the 12 thoracic nerves. The first thoracic ganglion is commonly fused with the inferior cervical ganglion to form the cervicothoracic, or ***stellate ganglion***. The remaining thoracic ganglia generally lie at the levels of the corresponding intervertebral discs and the intercostal nerves.

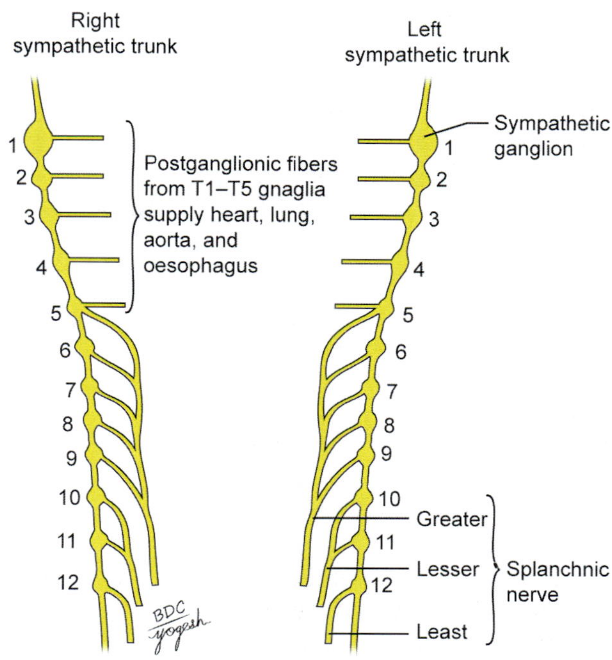

Fig. 14.14: The thoracic part of the sympathetic trunk and its splanchnic branches

Course and Relations

The chain crosses the neck of the 1st rib, the heads of the 2nd–10th ribs, and bodies of the 11th and 12th thoracic vertebrae.

The whole chain descends in front of the posterior intercostal vessels and the intercostal nerves, and passes deep to the medial arcuate ligament to become continuous with the lumbar part of the sympathetic chain.

Branches

Medial Branches for the Viscera

1. Medial branches from the upper 5 ganglia: These are ***postganglionic fibres*** and get distributed to the heart, the great vessels, the lungs and the oesophagus, through the following:
   a. Pulmonary plexuses
   b. Deep cardiac plexus
   c. Thoracic aortic plexus
   d. Oesophageal plexus (Fig. 14.14).

Flowchart 14.7: Thoracic sympathetic chain

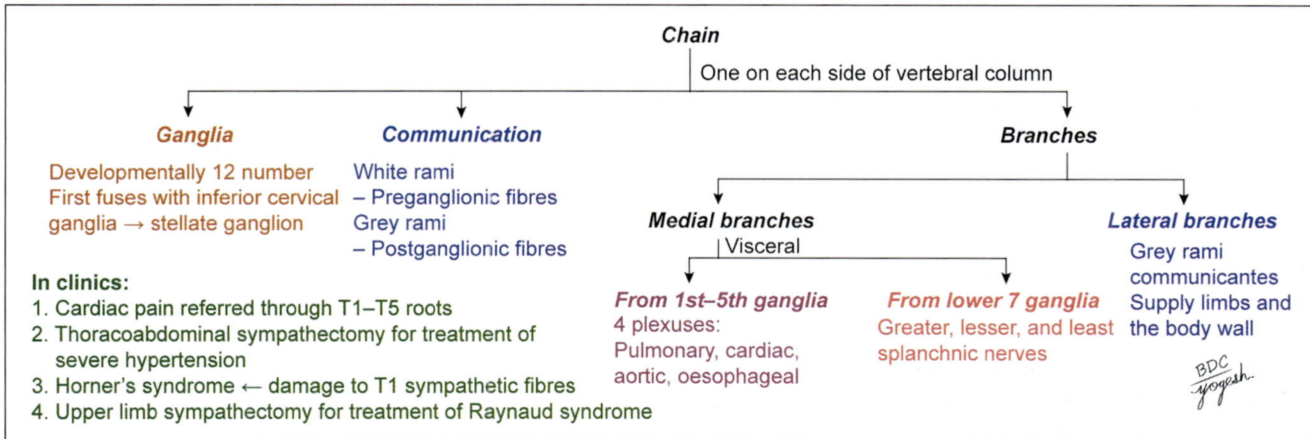

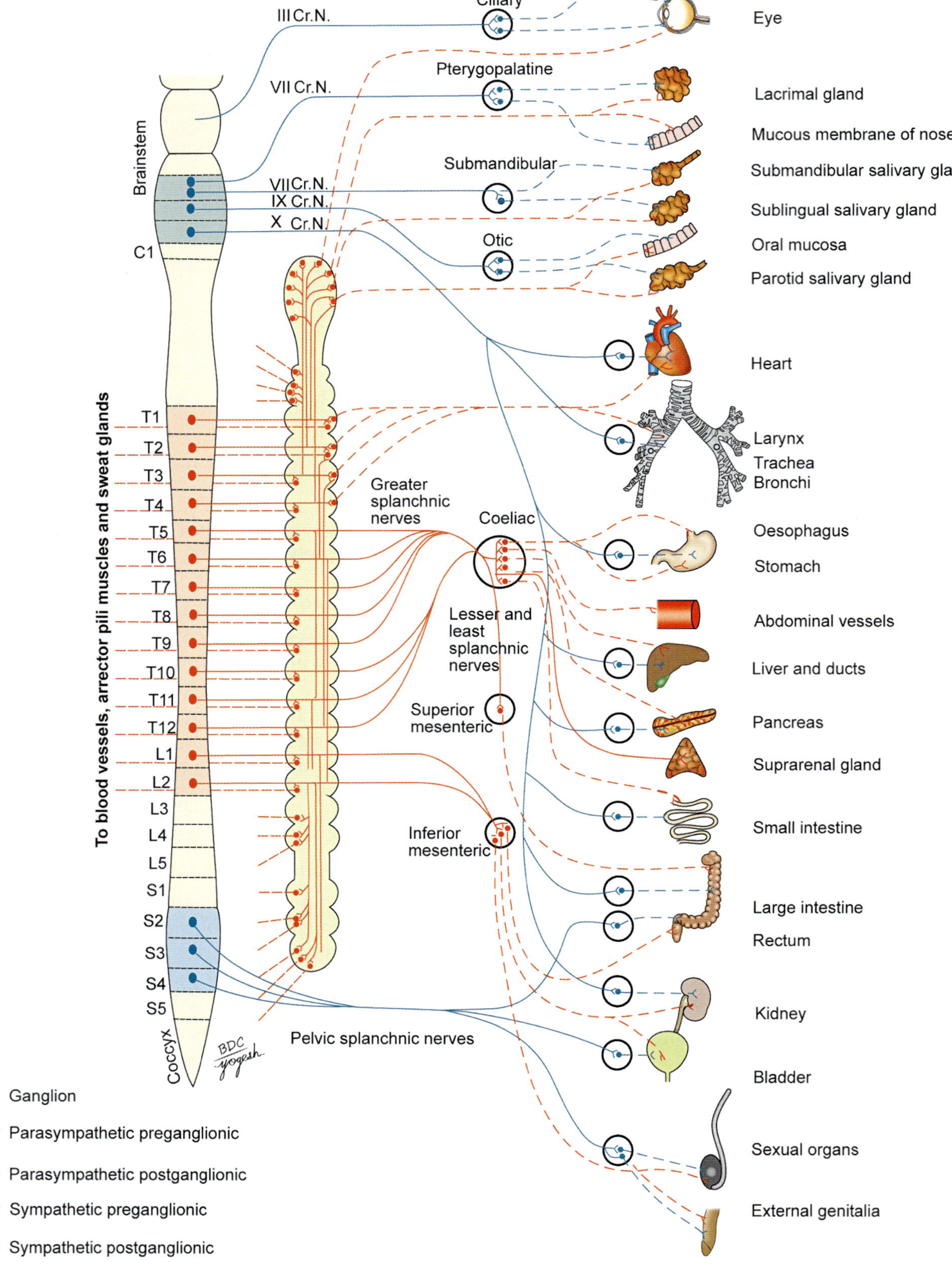

Fig. 14.15: Autonomic nervous system and its divisions: Sympathetic and parasympathetic nervous systems

2. Medial branches from the lower 7 ganglia: These are ***preganglionic fibers*** and form three splanchnic nerves.
   a. ***Greater splanchnic nerve*** is formed by 5 roots from ganglia 5–9. It descends obliquely on the vertebral bodies, pierces the crus of the diaphragm, and ends (in the abdomen) mainly in the coeliac ganglion, and partly in the aorticorenal ganglion and the *suprarenal gland*.
   b. ***Lesser splanchnic nerve*** is formed by two roots from ganglia 10 and 11. Its course is similar to that of the greater splanchnic nerve. It pierces the crus of the diaphragm, and ends in the coeliac ganglion (Fig. 14.14).

c. ***Least (lowest) splanchnic nerve (renal nerve)*** is tiny. It arises by one root from ganglion 12. It pierces the corresponding crus of the diaphragm (For details, *see* Chapter 7 of *BD Chaurasia's Handbook of General Anatomy*).

Lateral Branches for the Limbs and Body Wall

Each ganglion is connected with its corresponding spinal nerve by two rami, the *white* (preganglionic) and *grey* (postganglionic) rami communicantes.

The ***white ramus*** is distal to the grey ramus (Plate 14.6). The ***grey rami communicantes*** along with spinal nerves supply structures in the skin and blood vessels of skeletal muscles of the whole body (Fig. 14.14).

CLINICAL ANATOMY

- ***Cardiac pain***: Sympathetic fibers from T1 to T5 spinal segments carry pain sensation from the heart through the dorsal root ganglia on the left side. Hence, cardiac pain is referred along the medial side of left arm, forearm, and upper part of front of chest.
- ***Thoracoabdominal sympathectomy***: In case of severe hypertension, thoracoabdominal sympathectomy is performed. It involves surgical removal of T5–T12 ganglia and excision of splanchnic nerves.
- ***Horner's syndrome***: Injury to the stellate ganglion (T1 sympathetic fibers) causes Horner's syndrome. It is also called occulosympathetic paresis. It includes ipsilateral symptoms: Miosis (constricted pupil paralysis of dilator pupillae muscle), ptosis (weakness of superior tarsus muscle), anhidrosis (decreased sweating), and enophthalmos (posterior displacement of eyeball).
- ***Raynaud's syndrome***: It is a condition in which spasm of arteries cause episodes of reduced blood flow to fingers, toes, lips, nose, and ears. Affected part turns pale and on the return of blood flow, it causes burning sensation. To treat Raynaud syndrome, the upper limb sympathectomy (excision of ganglion chain above the level of stellate ganglion) may be useful.

Competency:

AN21.9 Describe and demonstrate mechanics and types of respiration.

RESPIRATORY MOVEMENTS

Respiration involves cyclic series of two phases: Inspiration and expiration. The ***inspiration*** is an active process that involves inhalation of air. The ***expiration*** is mostly a passive process that involves exhalation of air.

The lungs expand during inspiration and retract during expiration. These movements are governed by the following two factors.

1. Alterations in the capacity of the thorax: Increase in volume of the thoracic cavity creates a negative intrathoracic pressure which sucks air into the lungs.
2. Elastic recoil of the pulmonary alveoli and of the thoracic wall expels air from the lungs during expiration.

Plate 14.6: Grey and white rami communicantes

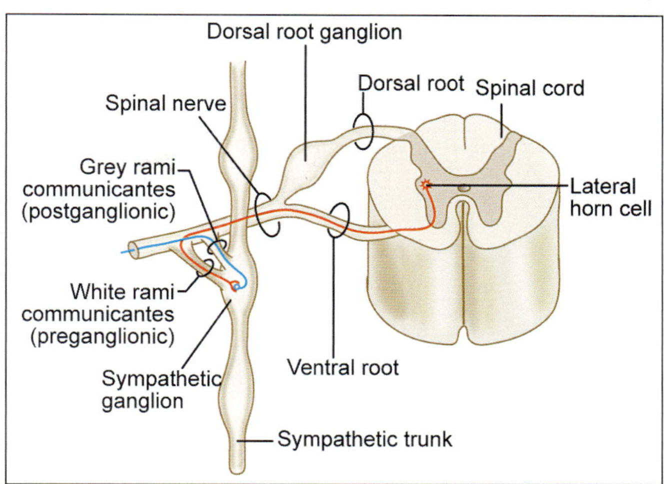

Rate of Respiration

- Rate of respiration varies according to the individual age.
  - *In infants*: 30–40 per minute
  - *In children*: 25–30 per minute
  - *In adults*: 16–20 per minute
- Respiration occurs in two phases:
  Inspiration—active phase of 1 second
  Expiration—passive phase of 3 seconds.

Diameters of Thoracic Cavity

In movements of respiration, all three diameters of thoracic cavity change. These are as follows (Fig. 14.16, Flowchart 14.8):

1. Anteroposterior diameter
2. Transverse diameter
3. Vertical diameter.

Flowchart 14.8: Movements of inspiration

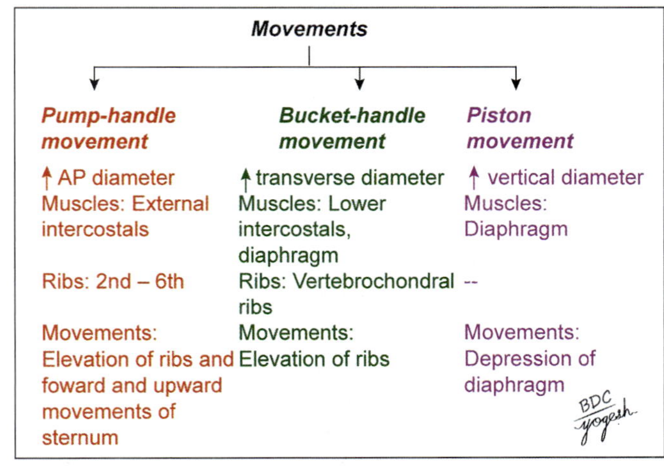

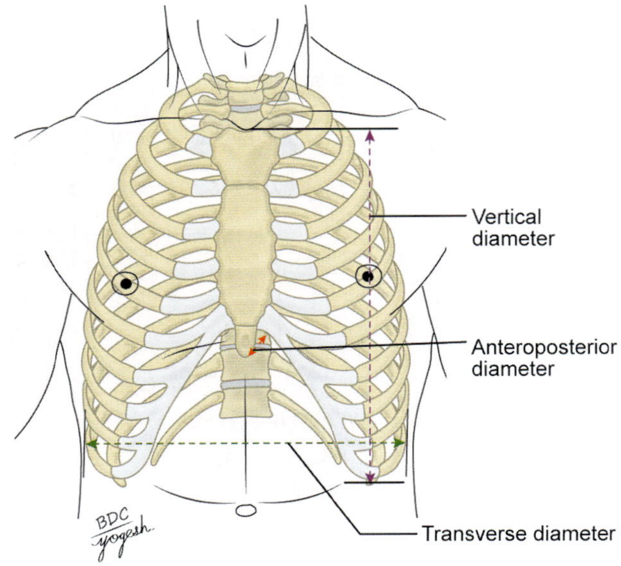

Fig. 14.16: Diameters of thoracic cage

In inspiration, these diameters increase, contributing to the increased volume of the thoracic cavity, while in expiration, these diameters decrease, leading to a reduction in the volume of the thoracic cavity.

PRINCIPLES OF MOVEMENTS

1. Each rib may be regarded as a lever, the fulcrum of which lies just lateral to the tubercle. Because of the disproportion in the length of the two arms of the lever, the slight movements at the vertebral end of the rib are greatly magnified at the anterior end (Fig. 14.17).
2. The anterior end of the rib is lower than the posterior end. Therefore, during elevation of the rib, the anterior end also moves forwards. This occurs mostly in the vertebrosternal ribs. Along with the up and down movements of the second to sixth ribs, the body of the sternum also moves up and down called ***pump-handle movements*** (Fig. 14.18). In this way, the anteroposterior diameter of the thorax is increased.
3. The middle of the shaft of the rib lies at a lower level than the plane passing through the two ends. Therefore, during elevation of the rib, the shaft also moves outwards. This causes increase in the transverse diameter of the thorax. Such movements occur in the vertebrochondral ribs and are called ***bucket-handle movements*** (Fig. 14.19).
4. The thorax resembles a cone, tapering upwards. As a result, each rib is longer than the next higher rib. On elevation, the larger lower rib comes to occupy the position of the smaller upper rib which pushes sternum forwards. This also increases the transverse diameter of the thorax.
5. Vertical diameter is increased by the '***piston movements***' of the thoracoabdominal diaphragm (Fig. 14.20).

Inspiration

In inspiration, the air is taken in (inhaled). Inspiration involves increase in the following thoracic diameters:

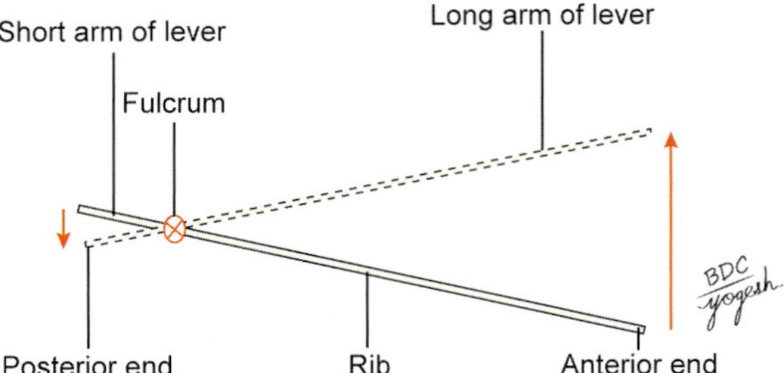

Fig. 14.17: Diagram comparing a rib to a lever

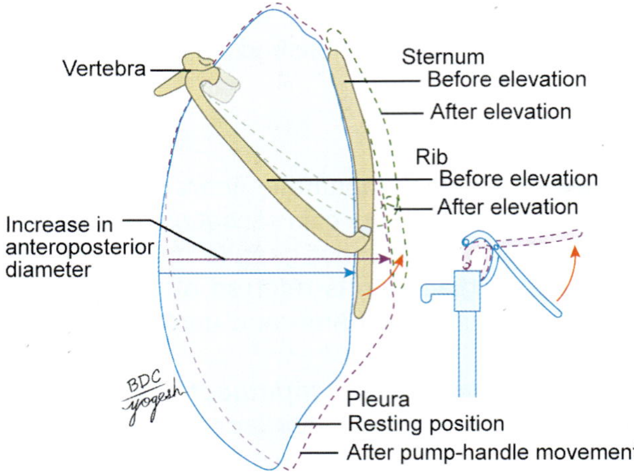

Fig. 14.18: Diagram showing how 'pump-handle' movements of the sternum bring about an increase in the anteroposterior diameter of the thorax

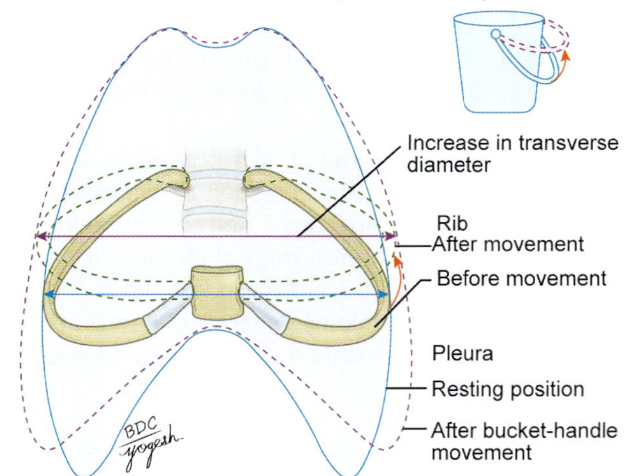

Fig. 14.19: Scheme showing how 'bucket-handle' movements of the vertebrochondral ribs bring about an increase in the transverse diameter of the thorax

Anteroposterior Diameter

- In inspiration, anteroposterior diameter increases.
- It takes place due to *pump-handle movement* that involves elevation of ribs and forward and upward movement of sternum.
- *Muscles*: External intercostal muscles.
- *Joints*: Costovertebral, costotransverse, costochondral, and sternomanubrial joints.
- ***Pump-handle movement.***

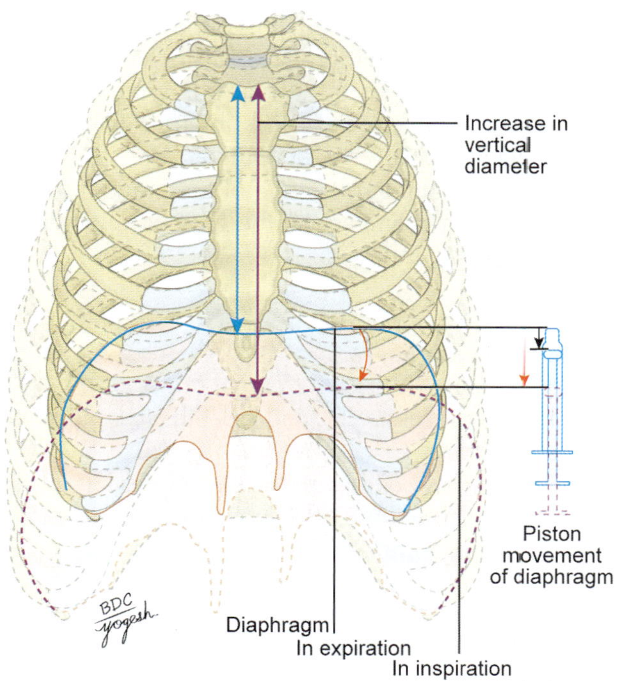

Fig. 14.20: Scheme showing how piston movements of thoraco-abdominal diaphragm bring about an increase in the vertical diameter of the thorax

***Components*:** Rib acts lever and fulcrum lies just lateral to the tubercle of the rib. Thus, rib is divided into two unequal arms: Posterior short arm (between head of the rib and tubercle) and anterior long arm (between tubercle and anterior end of the rib).

Anterior end of the rib lies at lower level than posterior end. Hence, slight depression of posterior end produces significant elevation of anterior end (pump-handle movement).

In pump-handle movement, along with anterior end of ribs, sternum moves forward and upward. Thus, anteroposterior diameter increases.

Transverse Diameter

- The transverse diameter increases in inspiration.
- Movements: Bucket-handle movement that involves outward movement of rib.
- Muscles: Lower intercostal muscles and diaphragm.
- Joints: Costovertebral, costotransverse, and costochondral joints of vertebrochondral ribs.
- Axis: It passes anteroposteriorly from costovertebral to costosternal joint.
- ***Bucket-handle movement:*** The middle portion of the shaft of rib, lies at the lower level than its anterior and posterior ends. In the elevation of rib, its shaft moves outward (similar to bucket-handle). It increases transverse diameter of thoracic cavity.

Vertical Diameter

- The vertical diameter increases in inspiration.
- Movements: Piston-movement that involves descent of diaphragm.
- Muscle: Diaphragm.
- ***Piston movement:*** Diaphragm forms the floor of thoracic cavity. During inspiration, the diaphragm contracts and causes descent of central tendon of diaphragm and flattening of its domes. It increases vertical diameter of the thoracic cavity and displaces abdominal viscera downward.

Expiration

- Expiration is a passive process that involves
  1. Relaxation of muscles of inspiration and
  2. Elastic recoil of lung alveoli.

RESPIRATORY MUSCLES

1. For inspiration—diaphragm, external intercostal muscle and interchondral part of internal intercostal of contralateral side.
2. Deep inspiration—erector spinae, scalene muscles, pectoral muscles.
3. For expiration—passive process.
4. Forced expiration—muscles of anterior abdominal wall.

DIFFERENT TYPES OF BREATHING

1. ***Quiet respiration or breathing:*** It occurs in normal individuals during resting phase at normal depth and rate as per the age of the individual.
   It involves the following muscles:
   - *For inspiration*: External intercostal, diaphragm
   - *For expiration*: It is passive and does not require any muscle.
2. ***Deep respiration:*** It is usually done during breathing exercises such as yoga. In deep respiration, depth of the respiration increases and the rate of the respiration decreases.
   In addition to the muscles of quiet respiration, the deep respiration requires the following muscles:
   - *For inspiration*: Scalene muscles, sternocleidomastoid, levator costarum, serratus posterior superior
   - *For expiration*: It is passive.
3. ***Forced respiration:*** It usually takes place during physical exercise or some diseases.
   In addition to the muscle of quiet and deep breathing, the forced breathing requires the following muscles:
   - *For inspiration*: Levator scapulae, trapezius, rhomboids, pectorals, serratus anterior.
   - *For expiration*: Quadratus lumborum, internal intercostal, transverse thoracis, serratus posterior inferior.

CLINICAL ANATOMY

- ***Dyspnoea and position of patient*:**
  In dyspnoea or difficulty in breathing, the patients are most comfortable on sitting up, leaning forwards and fixing the arms. In the sitting posture, the position of diaphragm is at the lowest allowing maximum

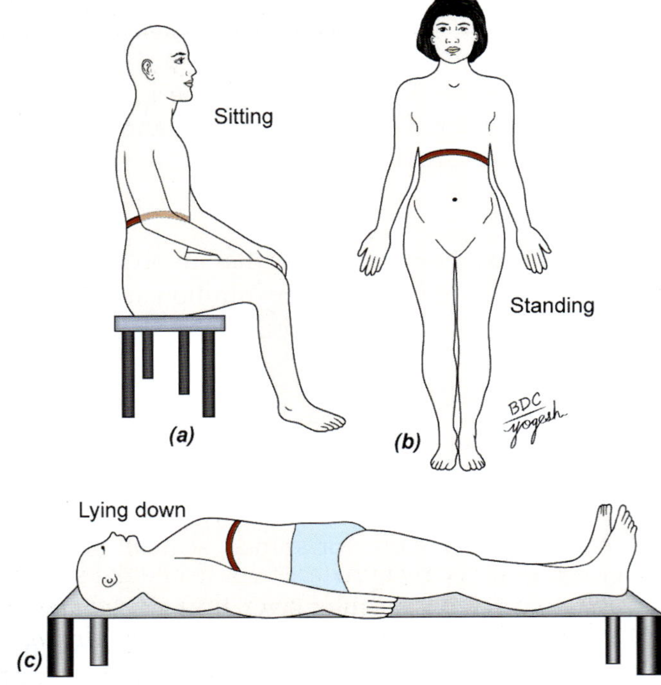

Figs 14.21a to c: Position of diaphragm: (a) Sitting, (b) standing and (c) lying down

ventilation. Fixation of the arms fixes the scapulae so that the serratus anterior and pectoralis minor may act on the ribs to good advantage.

The height of the diaphragm in the thorax is variable according to the position of the body and tone of the abdominal muscles. It is the highest on lying supine, so the patient is extremely uncomfortable, as he/she needs to exert immensely for inspiration. The diaphragm is lowest while sitting. The patient is quite comfortable as the effort required for inspiration is the least.

The diaphragm is midway in position while standing, but the patient is too ill or exhausted to stand. So dyspnoeic patients feel comfortable while sitting (Figs 14.21a to c).

- ***Respiration in children***: In young children (up to 2 years of age), the thoracic cavity is almost circular in cross-section so the scope for anteroposterior or side-to-side expansion is limited. The type of respiration in children is abdominal.
- In women of advanced stage of pregnancy, descent of diaphragm is limited, so the type of respiration in them is mainly thoracic.

Facts to Remember

- Intercostal spaces are 11, and 3rd–6th are typical intercostal spaces.
- Intercostal muscles are in 3 layers—external, internal and transversus. These correspond to the muscle layers of anterior abdominal wall.
- Neurovascular bundle lies in the upper part of the intercostal space (in subcostal groove) in between internal and innermost intercostal muscles.
- Posterior intercostal artery and its collateral branch supplies two-thirds of the intercostal space.
- Right posterior intercostal arteries are longer than the left ones.
- Subcostal nerves and vessels run below the 12th rib.
- Accessory hemiazygos vein drains 5–8 left intercostal spaces and hemiazygos vein drains 9–11 left intercostal spaces. Corresponding veins on right side drain into vena azygos.
- Most prominent role in respiration is played by diaphragm.

BDC's Anatomy *e*-book

1. Intercostal space and its contents
2. Relations of the internal thoracic vessels
3. Raynaud syndrome
4. Thoracoabdominal sympathectomy
5. Further reading
6. Viva voce questions

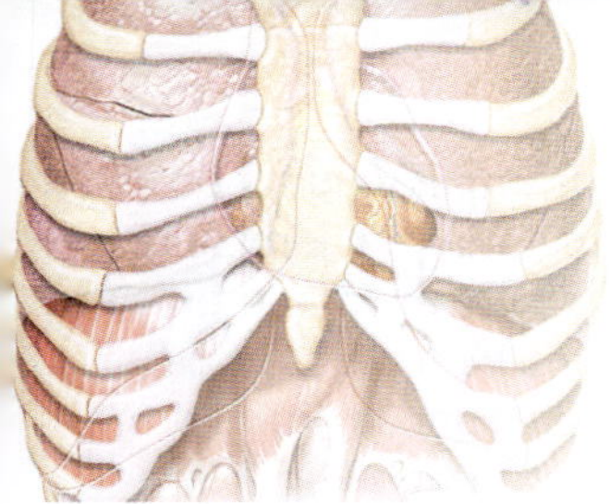

Chapter

15

Thoracic Cavity and Pleurae

THORACIC CAVITY

The spongy lungs occupying a major portion of thoracic cavity are enveloped in a serous cavity—the ***pleural cavity***. There is always slight negative pressure in this cavity. During inspiration, the pressure becomes more negative, and air is drawn into the lungs. Pleural cavity limits the expansion of the lungs (Figs 15.1a and b).

The ***mediastinum*** is the middle space in the thoracic cavity between the right and left pleural sacs. It contains major vessels and viscera of thoracic region.

PLEURAE

Like the peritoneum, the pleura is a ***serous membrane*** which is lined by ***mesothelium*** (flattened epithelium). There are two pleural sacs, one on either side of the mediastinum (Figs 15.1a and b).

Layers of The Pleura

Each pleural sac is invaginated from its medial side by the lung, so that it has an outer layer, the ***parietal pleura***, and an inner layer, the ***visceral*** or ***pulmonary pleura***.

The two layers are continuous with each other around the hilum of the lung, and enclose between them a potential space, the ***pleural cavity***.

Table 15.1 shows comparison between visceral pleura and parietal pleura.

Embryological Aspects of Pleural Cavities

- During embryonic life, foetus has two pleural sacs (initially called pericardioperitoneal canals) (*see* Fig. 7.2). Each developing lung bud invaginates one pleural sac and gets covered by two layers of pleural sac. Later, lung bud expands to form the lung and start occupying the pleural sac.

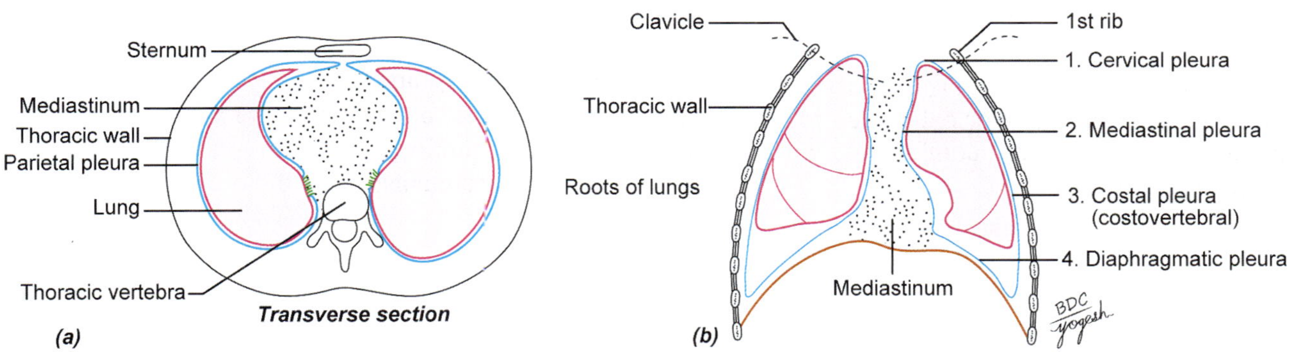

Figs 15.1a and b: (a) Schematic transverse section of the thorax showing parts of the thoracic cavity; (b) Vertical reflections of the pleura

TABLE 15.1: Comparison of visceral and parietal pleurae

	Visceral	*Parietal*
Development	Splanchnopleuric mesoderm	Somatopleuric mesoderm
Position	Lines surface of lung including the fissures	Lines thoracic wall, mediastinum, and diaphragm
Nerve supply	Sympathetic nerves from T2 to T5 ganglia Parasympathetic from vagus nerve	Thoracic nerves and phrenic nerves
Sensitivity	Insensitive to pain	Sensitive to pain which may be referred.
Blood supply	Bronchial vessels	Intercostal and pericardiacophrenic vessels
Lymph drainage	Tracheobronchial lymph nodes	Intercostal lymph nodes

Plate 15.1: Parts of parietal pleura

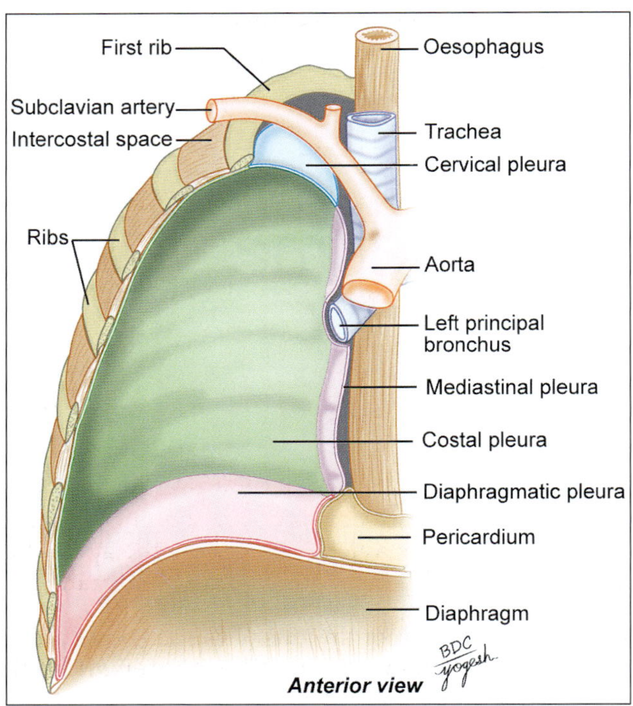

- Layer of the pleural sac covering the lung forms visceral pleura, whereas outer layer forms the parietal pleura. A thin persistent space between two layers of pleura forms pleural cavity.

DISSECTION

Divide the manubrium sterni transversely immediately inferior to its junction with the 1st costal cartilage. Cut through the parietal pleura in the 1st intercostal space on both sides as far back as possible. Cut sternum at the level of xiphisternal joint. Use a bone cutter to cut 2nd–7th ribs in midaxillary line on each side of thorax. Separate intercostal muscles in 1–6 spaces from underlying pleura.

Lift the inferior part of manubrium and body of sternum with ribs and costal cartilages and reflect it towards abdomen. Identify the pleura extending from the back of sternum onto the mediastinum to the level of lower border of heart. Trace the surface marking of parietal pleura on the skeleton.

Remove the pleura and the endothoracic fascia from the back of sternum and costal cartilages which is reflected towards abdomen. Identify the transversus thoracis muscle and internal thoracic vessels.

Note the origin of diaphragm from the xiphoid process and divide it. Identify the course and branches of intercostal nerve again. Trace the nerve medially superficial to the internal thoracic vessels.

Pull the lung laterally from the mediastinum and find its root with the pulmonary ligament extending downwards from it. Cut through the structures, i.e. bronchus/bronchi, pulmonary vessels, nerves, comprising its root from above downwards close to the lung. Remove the lung on each side.

Identify the phrenic nerve with accompanying blood vessels anterior to the root of the lung. Make a longitudinal incision through the pleura only parallel to and on each side of the phrenic nerve. Strip the pleura posterior to the nerve backwards to the intercostal spaces. Pull the anterior flap forwards to reveal part of the pericardium with the heart. Identify the following structures seen through the pleura.

Right Side

1. Bulge of the heart and pericardium anteroinferior to the root of the lung.
2. A longitudinal ridge formed by right brachiocephalic vein down to first costal cartilage and by superior vena cava up to the bulge of the heart.
3. A smaller longitudinal ridge formed by inferior vena cava between the heart and the diaphragm.
4. Phrenic nerve with accompanying vessels forming a vertical ridge on these two venae cavae passing anterior to root of the lung.
5. Vena azygos arching over root of the lung to enter the superior vena cava.
6. Trachea and oesophagus posterior to the phrenic nerve and superior vena cava.
7. Right vagus nerve descending posteroinferiorly across the trachea, behind the root of the lung.
8. Bodies of the thoracic vertebrae behind oesophagus with posterior intercostal vessels and azygos vein lying over them.
9. Sympathetic trunk on the heads of the upper ribs and on the sides of the vertebral bodies below this, anterior to the posterior intercostal vessels and intercostal nerves.

Left Side

1. Bulge of the heart.
2. Root of lung posterosuperior to it.
3. Descending aorta between (1) and (2) in front and vertebral column behind.
4. Arch of aorta over the root of the lung.
5. Left common carotid and left subclavian arteries passing superiorly from the arch of aorta.
6. Phrenic and vagus nerves descending between these vessels and the lateral surface of the aortic arch.
7. Sympathetic trunk same as on right side.

Identify longitudinally running sympathetic trunk on the posterior part of thoracic cavity. Find delicate greater and lesser splanchnic nerves arising from the trunk on the medial side. Trace the intercostal vessels above the intercostal nerve.

On the right side, identify and follow one of the divisions of trachea to the lung root and the superior and inferior venae cavae till the pericardium.

On the left side of thoracic cavity, dissect the arch of aorta. Identify the superior cervical cardiac branch of the left sympathetic trunk and the inferior cervical cardiac branch of the left vagus on the arch of the aorta between the vagus nerve posteriorly and phrenic nerve anteriorly (cardiac nerves).

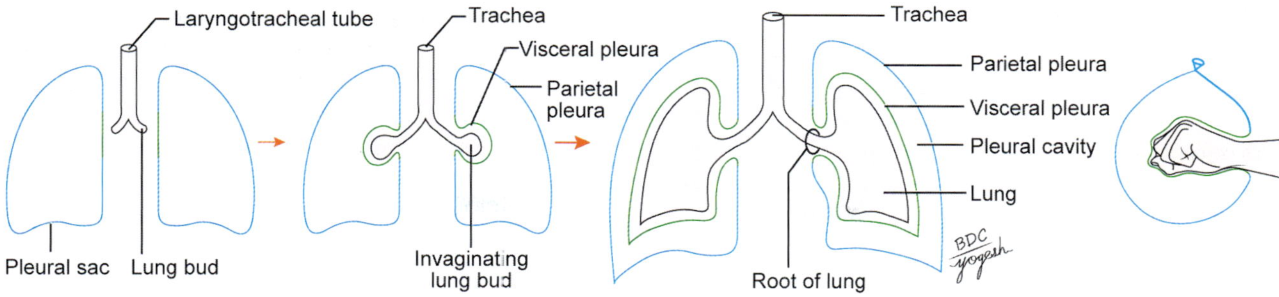

Fig. 15.2: Development of visceral and parietal pleurae (Invagination of lung in the pleural sac equates the invagination of fist in balloon)

Competency:
AN24.1 Mention the blood supply, lymphatic drainage and nerve supply of pleura, extent of pleura and describe the pleural recesses and their applied anatomy.

Pulmonary/Visceral Pleura

The serous layer of pulmonary pleura covers the surfaces and fissures of the lung, except at the hilum and along the attachment of the ***pulmonary ligament*** where it is continuous with the parietal pleura. It also extends into the depths of the fissures of the lungs. It is firmly adherent to the lung and cannot be separated from it.

Parietal Pleura

The parietal pleura is thicker than the pulmonary pleura, and is subdivided into the following four parts:

1. Costal
2. Diaphragmatic
3. Mediastinal
4. Cervical (Fig. 15.3).

Costal pleura: It lines the thoracic wall which comprises ribs and intercostal spaces to which it is loosely attached by a layer of areolar tissue called the endothoracic fascia.

Mediastinal pleura: It lines the corresponding surface of the mediastinum. It is reflected over the root of the lung and becomes continuous with the pulmonary pleura around the hilum.

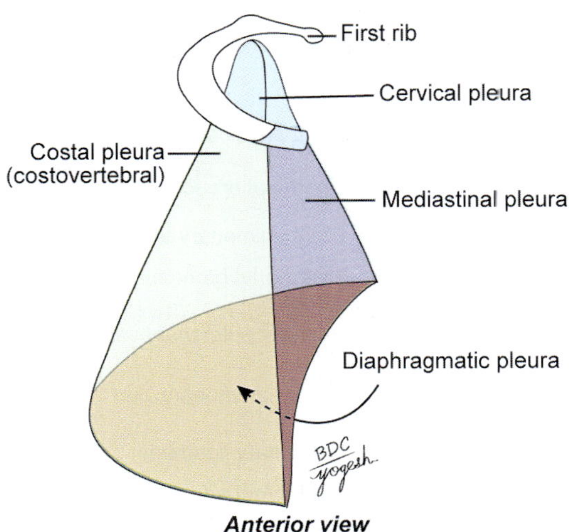

Fig. 15.3: Parts of parietal pleura (parietal pleura as a half cone)

Cervical pleura: It extends into the neck, nearly 5 cm above the first costal cartilage and 2.5 cm above the medial 1/3rd of the clavicle, and covers the apex of the lung. It is covered by the suprapleural membrane.

Relations of cervical pleura

Anterior: Subclavian artery, inner border of the first rib, scalenus anterior muscle
Posterior: Neck of the first rib
Lateral: Inner border of the first rib, scalenus medius muscle
Medial: Major vessels of the neck
Superior: Suprapleural membrane, supraclavicular part of brachial plexus
Inferior: Apex of lung.

Diaphragmatic pleura: It lines the superior aspect of diaphragm. It covers the base of the lung and gets continuous with mediastinal pleura medially and costal pleura laterally.

SURFACE MARKINGS OF PARIETAL PLEURA

Cervical Pleura or Cupola

It is marked by a curved line extending from sternoclavicular joint (C) to the junction of medial 1/3rd and middle 1/3rd of the clavicle (A). It extends about 2.5 cm (1 inch) above the medial 1/3rd of the clavicle (B) (Fig. 15.4).

Anterior Margin

It is also called costomediastinal line of pleural reflection. It can be marked as follows:

On the right: It extends vertically downward from the right sternoclavicular joint (C) to the midpoint of the sternal angle (D). Further, it extends up to midpoint of the xiphisternal joint (E).

On the left: It extends downward from the left sternoclavicular joint to the midpoint of the sternal angle. Further, it descents vertically up to the level of the 4th costal cartilage (D1) and then it arches toward left to reach left margin of sternum. Further, it descends downward to reach the 6th costal cartilage (E1). This deviation is due to the location of the heart (bare area of the heart).

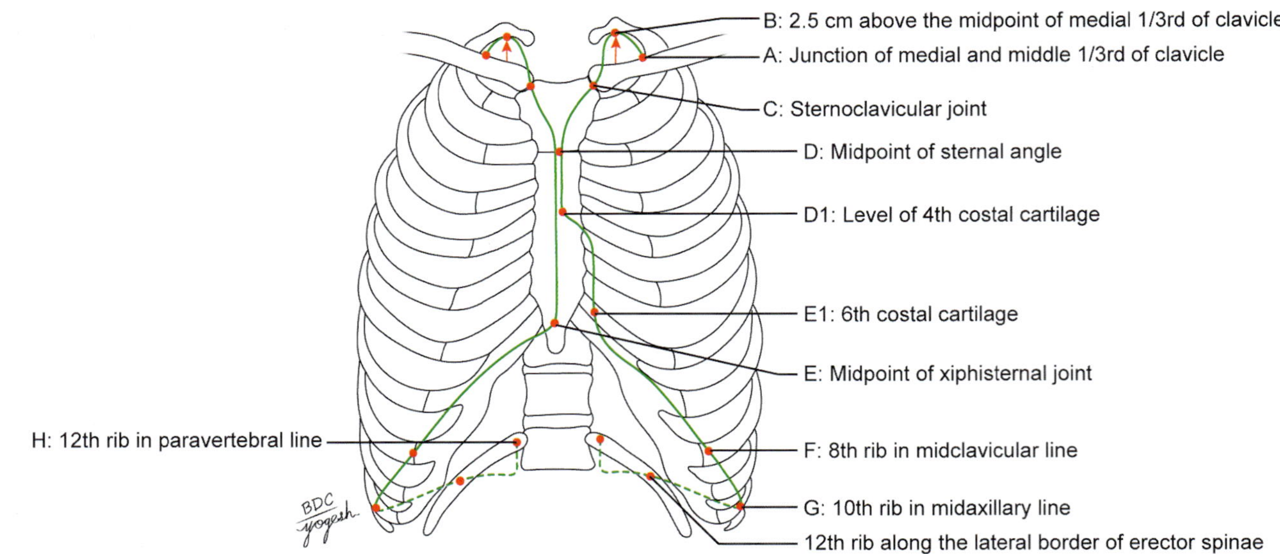

Fig. 15.4: Surface marking of pleura

Inferior Margin

It is also called costodiaphragmatic line of the pleural reflection. It can be marked as follows:

On the right: It extends laterally from the xiphisternal joint (E) and crosses the 8th rib in the midclavicular line (F), 10th rib in the midaxillary line (G), and 12th rib in paravertebral line (along the lateral border of the erector spinae muscle) (H).

On the left: It extends laterally from the left 6th costal cartilage (E1) and follows the same course as on the right (F to H).

Posterior Margins

- It is also called costovertebral line of reflection. It extends as a vertical line 2 cm lateral to the spinous processes of vertebrae from C7 to T12 vertebrae (I to H). Along this line, costovertebral pleura continues with mediastinal pleura.

Note: The surface marking of the lung and visceral pleura coincides as visceral pleura is adhered to the outer surface of lungs (*see* Fig. 16.6 for surface marking of visceral pleura or lungs).

The parietal pleurae descend below the costal margin at three places:

a. At the right xiphicostal angle
b. At the right and left costovertebral angles
c. Below the 12th rib behind the upper poles of the kidneys.

The latter fact is of surgical importance in exposure of the kidney. The pleura may be damaged at this site (Fig. 15.4).

[***Mnemonic for* surface markings of pleura:** '*All the even ribs, in order:* ***2, 4, 6, 8, 10, 12*** *show its route*': *Rib 2:* Both sides parietal pleura come close
Rib 4: The left pleura does a lateral shift to accommodate heart
Rib 6: Both diverge laterally
Rib 8: Midclavicular line
Rib 10: Midaxillary line
Rib12: The back]

PULMONARY LIGAMENT

The parietal pleura surrounding the root of the lung extends downwards beyond the root as a fold called the *pulmonary ligament* (Fig. 15.5).

Contents

1. Space of the pulmonary ligament is filled with loose areolar tissue
2. Few lymphatics
3. Sometimes accessory bronchial artery.

Functions

1. *Potential space*: Pulmonary ligament provides a potential (dead) space for the expansion of pulmonary veins.
2. *Permit descent of root of lungs*: During inspiration, pulmonary ligament provides space for the descent of root of lungs (descent of diaphragm pulls the lung downward).

RECESSES OF PLEURA

There are two recesses of parietal pleura, which act as *'reserve spaces'* for the lung to expand during deep inspiration (Plate 15.2, Fig. 15.6, Flowchart 15.1).

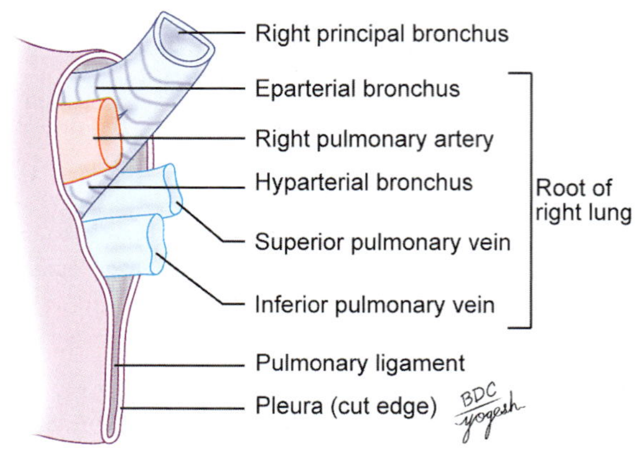

Fig. 15.5: Pulmonary ligament and pleura at root of lung

Plate 15.2: Costodiaphragmatic recess

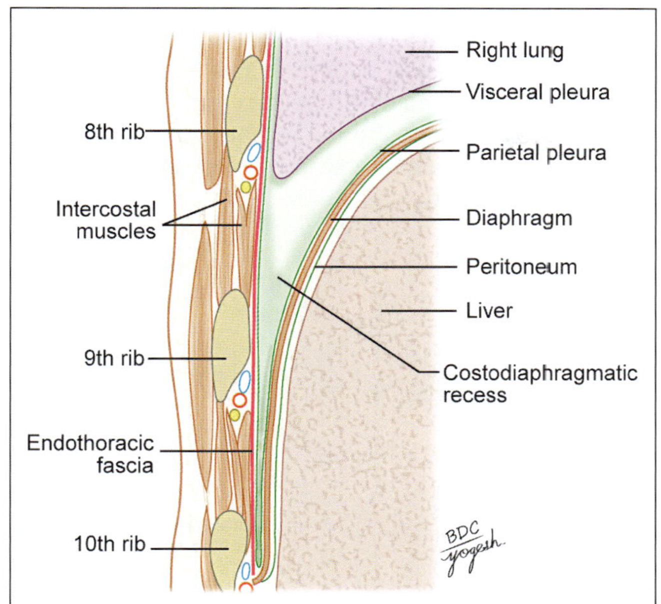

1. ***Costomediastinal recess:*** It (Fig. 15.6) lies anteriorly, behind the sternum and costal cartilages, between the costal and mediastinal pleurae, particularly in relation to the cardiac notch of the left lung. This recess is filled up by the anterior margin of the lungs even during quiet breathing. It is only obvious in the region of the cardiac notch of the lung.
2. ***Costodiaphragmatic/costovertebral recess:*** It lies inferiorly between the costal and diaphragmatic pleurae. Vertically, it measures about 5 cm, and extends from the eighth to tenth ribs along the midaxillary line (Fig. 15.6). During inspiration, the lungs expand into these recesses. So these recesses are obvious only in expiration and not in deep inspiration.

NERVE SUPPLY OF THE PLEURA

1. The ***parietal pleura*** develops from the somatopleuric layer of the lateral plate mesoderm, and is supplied by the somatic nerves. These are the intercostal and phrenic nerves (Fig. 15.7).

   The parietal pleura is ***pain sensitive***. The costal and peripheral parts of the diaphragmatic pleurae are supplied by the intercostal nerves, and the mediastinal pleura and central part of the diaphragmatic pleurae are supplied by the phrenic nerves (C4).
2. The ***pulmonary/visceral pleura*** develops from the splanchnopleuric layer of the lateral plate mesoderm, and is supplied by autonomic nerves. The sympathetic nerves are derived from 2nd to 5th sympathetic ganglia while parasympathetic nerves are drawn from the vagus nerve. The nerves accompany the bronchial vessels (Fig. 15.7).

This part of the pleura is ***not sensitive to pain***. Sympathetic system dilates the bronchi. The parasympathetic system narrows the bronchial tree and is also secretory to the glands.

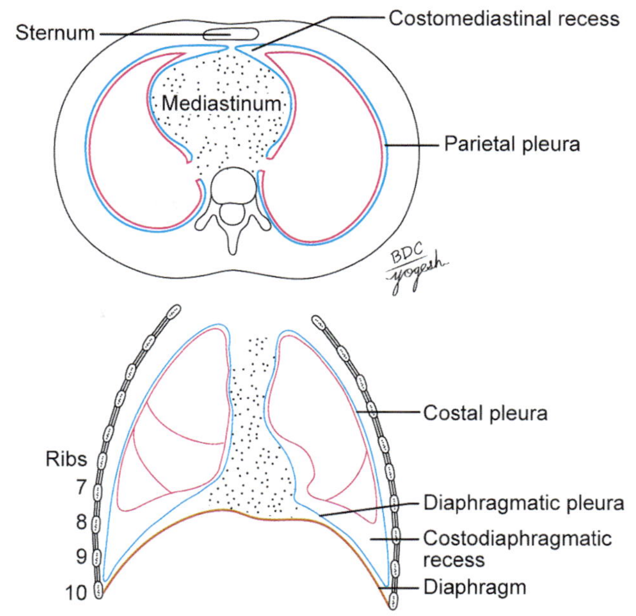

Fig. 15.6: Reflections of the pleura to show costodiaphragmatic and costomediastinal recesses

Flowchart 15.1: Pleural recesses

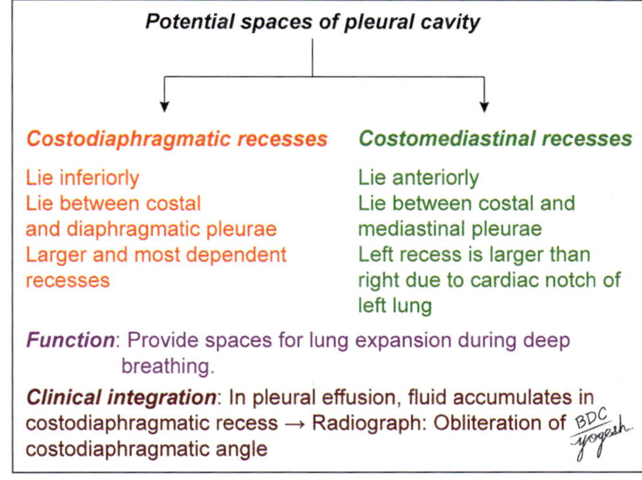

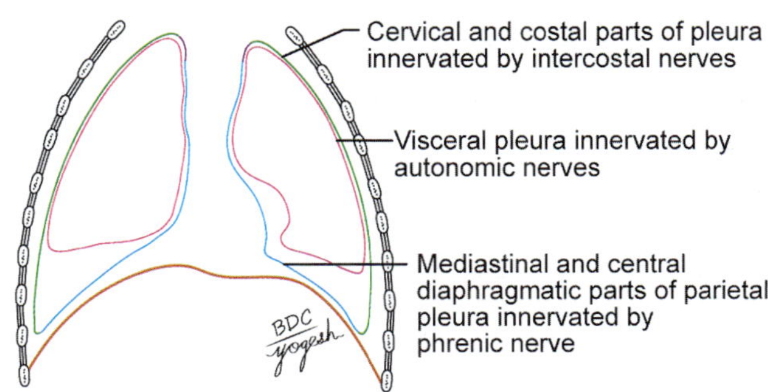

Fig. 15.7: Nerve supply of pleura

Blood Supply and Lymphatic Drainage of Pleura

1. The ***parietal pleura*** is a part and parcel of the thoracic wall. Its blood supply and lymphatic drainage are, therefore, the same as that of the body wall. It is thus supplied by intercostal, internal thoracic, and musculophrenic arteries.

2. The veins drain mostly into the azygos and internal thoracic veins. The lymphatics drain into the intercostal, internal mammary, posterior mediastinal and diaphragmatic nodes.
3. The *pulmonary pleura,* like the lung, is supplied by the bronchial arteries while the veins drain into bronchial veins. It is drained by the bronchopulmonary lymph nodes.

CLINICAL ANATOMY

- ***Paracentesis thoracis:*** Aspiration of any fluid from the pleural cavity is called *paracentesis thoracis.* It is usually done in the 8th intercostal space in the midaxillary line (Fig. 15.8). The needle is passed through the lower part of the space to avoid injury to the principal neurovascular bundle, i.e. vein, artery, and nerve (VAN).
- ***Pleurisy:*** This is inflammation of the pleura. It may be dry, but often it is accompanied by collection of fluid in the pleural cavity. The condition is called the pleural effusion. ***Dry pleurisy*** is more painful because during inspiration both layers come in contact and there is friction.
- ***Pneumothorax:*** Presence of air in the pleural cavity (Fig. 15.9).
- ***Tension pneumothorax*** is a surgical emergency. It occurs when air can enter into the pleural space but cannot escape. It occurs due to valvular air passage (one-way entry of air). It causes collapse of lungs and impairment of respiration hyperexpansion of chest, deviation of trachea to the opposite side. It requires emergency thoracostomy (insertion of needle in the 2nd intercostal space in the midclavicular line).
- ***Haemothorax:*** Presence of blood in the pleural cavity.
- ***Hydropneumothorax:*** Presence of both fluid and air in the pleural cavity.
- ***Empyema:*** Presence of pus in pleural cavity.
- ***Referred pain***: Costal and peripheral parts of diaphragmatic pleurae are innervated by intercostal nerves (Fig. 15.11). Hence, irritation of these regions causes referred pain along intercostal nerves to thoracic or abdominal wall. Mediastinal and central parts of diaphragmatic pleurae are innervated by phrenic nerve (C4). Hence, irritation here causes referred pain on tip of shoulders. Pain on right shoulder occurs due to inflammation of gallbladder, while on left shoulder is due to splenic rupture.
- Pleural effusion causes obliteration of costodiaphragmatic angle (Fig. 15.10).
- Pleura extends beyond the thoracic cage at following areas:
  - Right xiphicostal angle (Fig. 15.4)
  - Right and left costovertebral angles (Fig. 15.4)
  - Right and left sides of root of neck as cervical dome of pleura (Fig. 15.4).
- The pleura may be injured at these sites during surgical procedures. These sites have to be remembered.
- During inspiration, pure air is withdrawn in the lungs. At the same time, deoxygenated blood is received through the pulmonary arteries. Thus, an exchange of gases occurs at the level of alveoli. The deoxygenated blood gets oxygenated and sent via pulmonary veins to the left atrium of heart. The impure air containing carbon dioxide gets expelled during expiration.

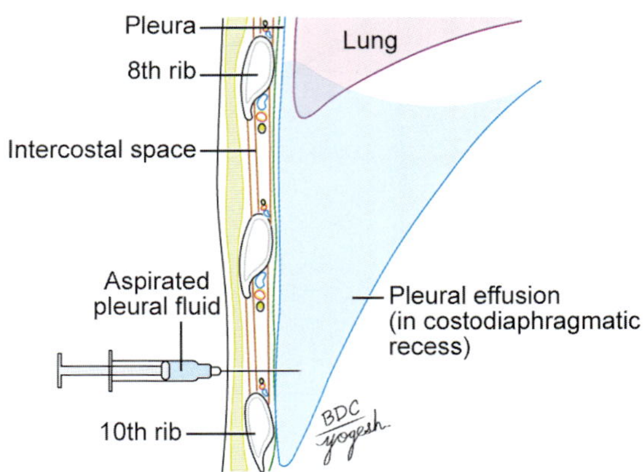

Fig. 15.8: Pleural effusion and paracentesis thoracis

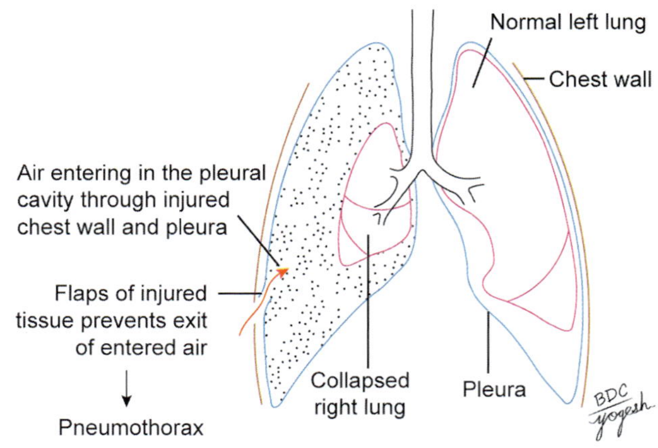

Fig. 15.9: Pneumothorax and collapsed lung

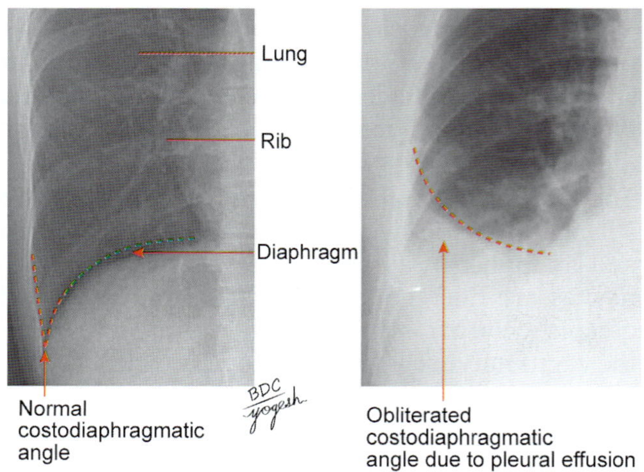

Fig. 15.10: Radiograph: Normal and obliterated costodiphragmatic angle (right, PA view)

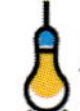

Facts to Remember

- Parietal pleura limits the expansion of the lungs.
- Visceral pleura behaves in same way as the lung.
- Parietal pleura has same nerve supply and blood supply as the thoracic wall and it is pain sensitive.
- Pleural cavity normally contains a minimal serous fluid for lubrication during movements of thoracic cage.
- Pleura lies beyond the thoracic cage at 5 places: These are right and left cervical pleurae above the 1st rib and the clavicle; right and left costovertebral angles and only right xiphicostal angle. Pleura is likely to be injured at these places.
- Costodiaphragmatic recess is the most dependent part of pleural cavity.
- *Paracentesis thoracis* is done in the lower part of the intercostal space to avoid injury to the main intercostal vessels and nerve. Its most preferred site is the 6th intercostal space in the midaxillary line.
- Pleural effusion is one of the signs of tuberculosis of the lung.

BDC's Anatomy *e*-book

1. Mediastinum as seen from the right and left sides
2. Surface marking of pleura
3. Intrapleural pressure
4. Referred pain of pleura
5. Pleurisy (pleuritis) and pleural rub
6. Atelectasis (lung collapse)
7. Further reading
8. Viva voce questions

Chapter

16

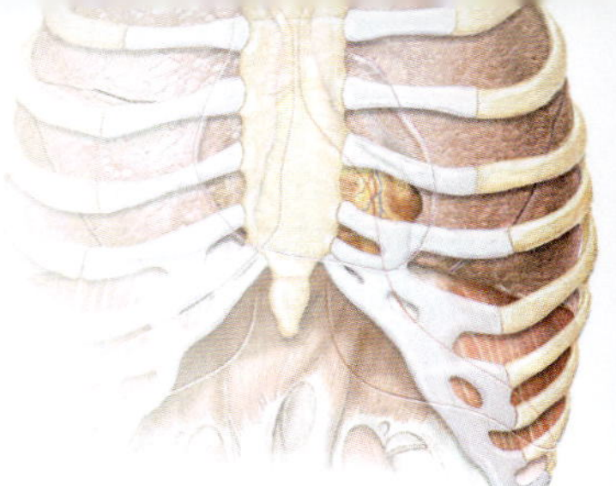

Lungs

The lungs are a pair of respiratory organs situated in the thoracic cavity. They occupy the major portions of the thoracic cavity. Each lung invaginates the corresponding pleural cavity. The right and left lungs are separated by the mediastinum.

LUNGS

Texture: The lungs are spongy in texture.

Colour: In the young, the lungs are brown or grey in colour. Gradually, they become mottled black because of the deposition of inhaled carbon particles.

Weight: The right lung weighs about 700 g; it is about 50–100 g heavier than the left lung.

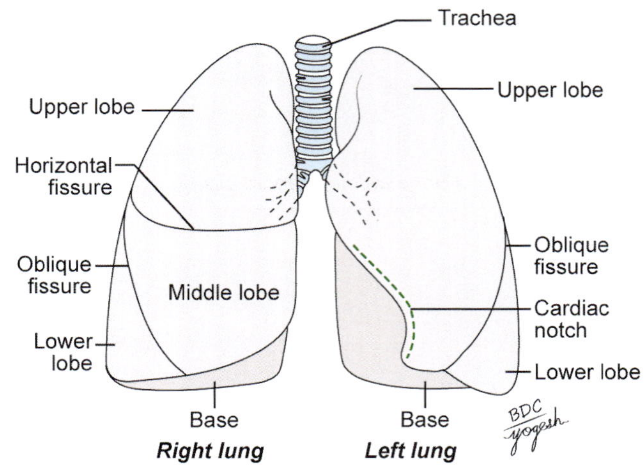

Fig. 16.1: Trachea and lungs as seen from the front

EXTERNAL FEATURES OF LUNG

Each lung is conical in shape (Plate 16.1, Figs 16.1 and 16.2, Flowchart 16.1). It has:

1. Apex (upper end)
2. Base (resting on the diaphragm)
3. Three borders: Anterior, posterior, and inferior.
4. Two surfaces: Costal and medial. The medial surface is divided into vertebral and mediastinal parts.
5. Fissures: Horizontal and oblique on the right and only oblique on the left.
6. Lobes: On the right: Superior, middle, and inferior, and on the left: Superior and inferior.

Anatomical Position and Side Determination

For anatomical position and side determination, hold the lung in such a way so that:

1. Its pointed apex is directed upward and broad base is directed downward.
2. Its thin anterior border should face anteriorly, and thick rounded posterior border should face posteriorly.
3. Its convex costal surface is directed laterally (toward the side of the lung — for right lung on the right side and for left lung on the left side) and mediastinal surface with hilum is directed medially.

Note: As number of lobes and fissures are not constant, do not determine the side of the lung using lobes and fissures.

Apex

The *apex* is blunt and lies above the level of the anterior end of the 1st rib. It reaches nearly 2.5 cm above the medial 1/3rd of the clavicle, just medial to the supraclavicular fossa. It is covered by the cervical pleura, the suprapleural membrane, and is grooved by the subclavian artery on the medial side and anteriorly (*see* Fig. 12.6).

Base

The *base/diaphragmatic surface* is semilunar and concave. It rests on the diaphragm which separates the right lung from the right lobe of the liver, and the left lung from the left lobe of the liver, the fundus of the stomach, and the spleen.

Border

The ***anterior border*** is very thin (Figs 16.2 and 16.3). It is shorter than the posterior border. On the right side, it is vertical and corresponds to the anterior or costomediastinal line of pleural reflection. The anterior border of the left lung shows a wide ***cardiac notch*** below the level of the 4th costal cartilage.

Plate 16.1: Lungs: External features

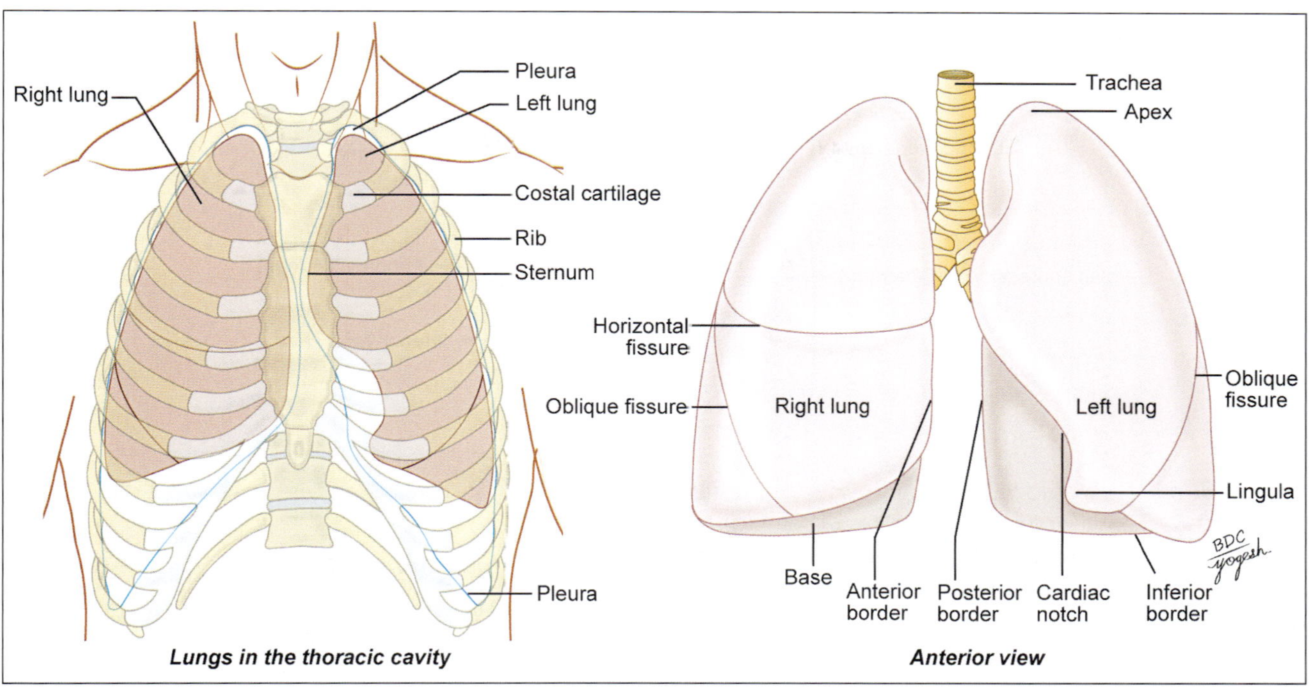

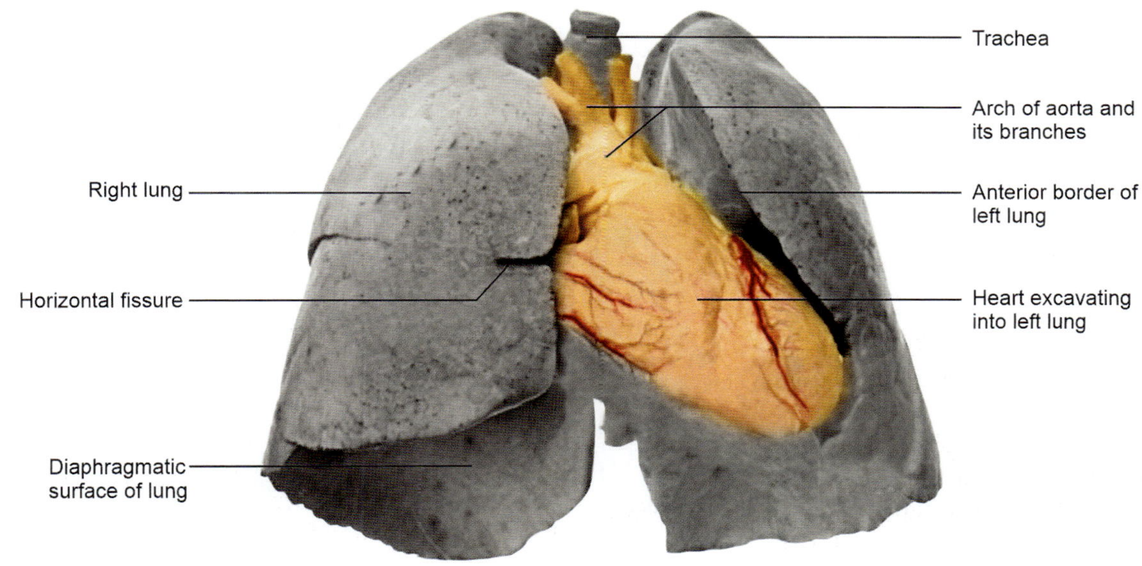

Fig. 16.2: Trachea, lungs, and heart as seen from the front

Flowchart 16.1: Features of lungs

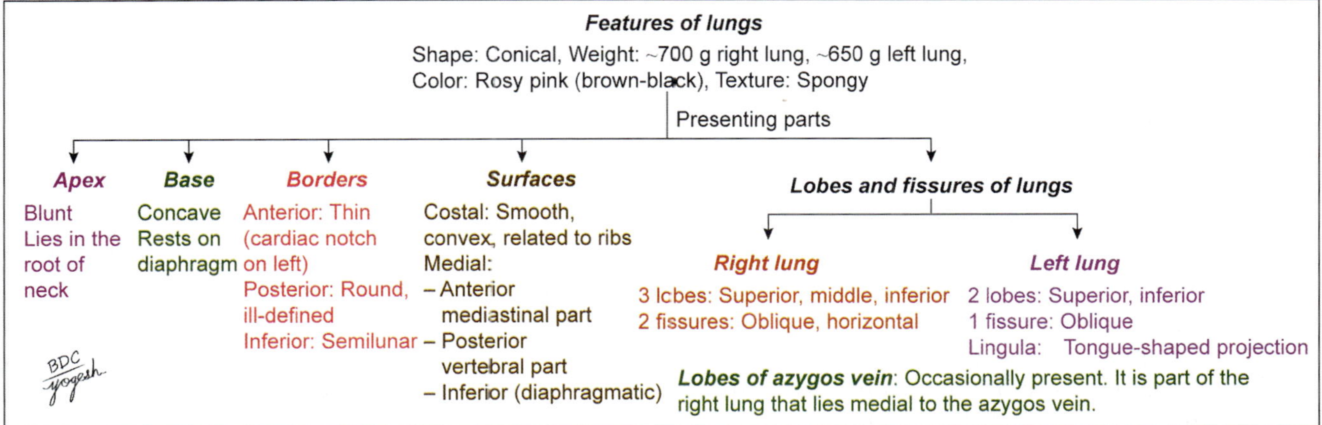

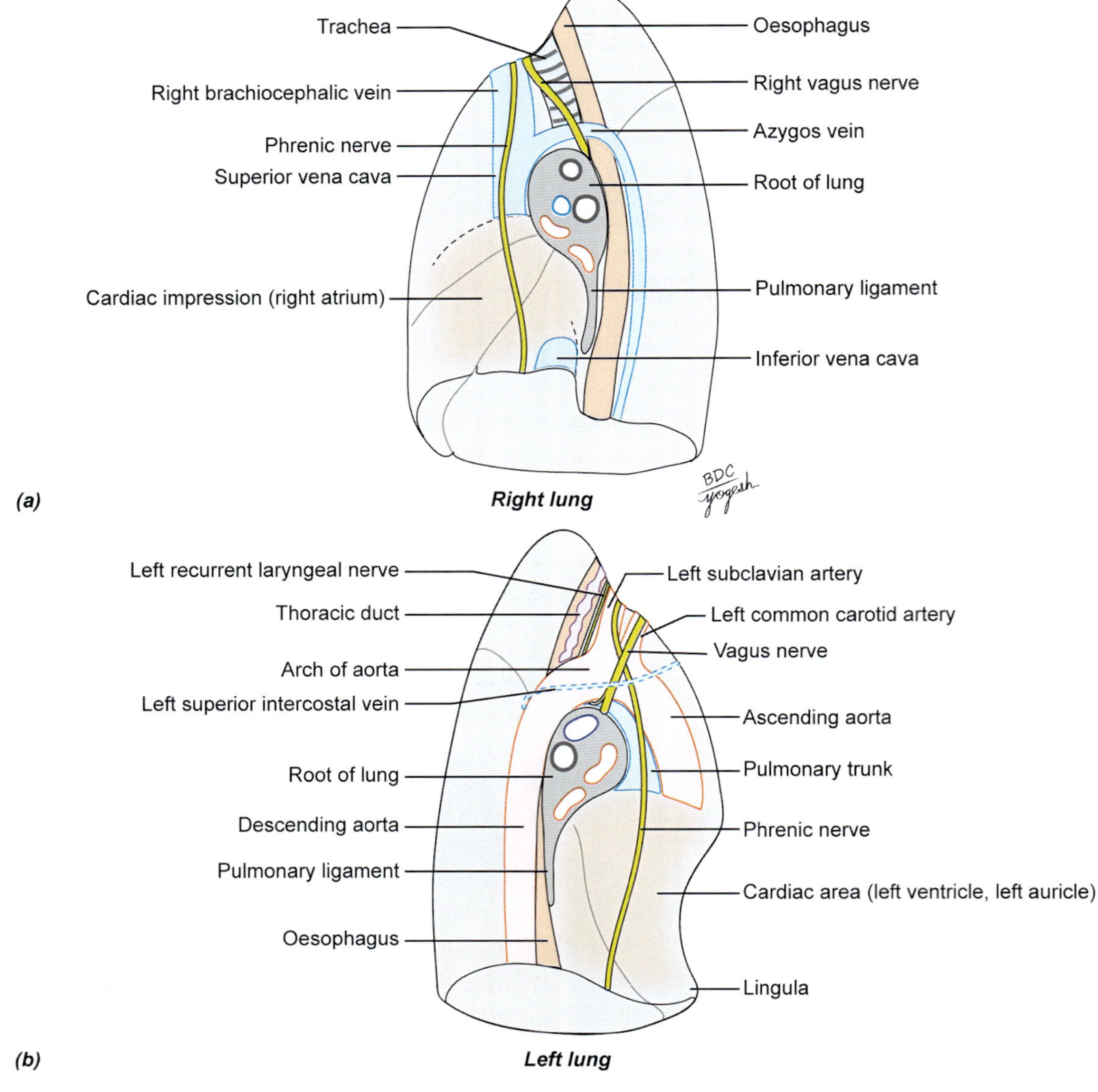

Figs 16.3a and b: Mediastinal surface of right (a) and left (b) lungs

The **posterior border** is thick and ill defined. It corresponds to the medial margins of the heads of the ribs. It extends from the level of the 7th cervical spine to the 10th thoracic spine.

The **inferior border** separates the base from the costal and medial surfaces.

Surfaces

The ***costal surface*** is large and convex. It is in contact with the costal pleura and the overlying thoracic wall.

The ***medial surface*** is divided into a posterior or *vertebral part*, and an anterior or *mediastinal part*.

a. The ***vertebral part*** is related to the vertebral bodies, intervertebral discs, the posterior intercostal vessels, and the splanchnic nerves.
b. The ***mediastinal part*** is related to the mediastinal septum and shows a cardiac impression, the hilum and a number of other impressions which differ on the two sides. Various relations of the mediastinal surfaces of the two lungs are listed in Table 16.1.

TABLE 16.1: Structures related to the mediastinal surfaces of the right and left lungs

Right side (Fig.16.2)	***Left side*** (Fig.16.3)
1. Right atrium and auricle	1. Left ventricle, left auricle, infundibulum and adjoining part of the right ventricle
2. A small part of the right ventricle	2. Pulmonary trunk
3. Superior vena cava	3. Arch of aorta
4. Lower part of the right brachiocephalic vein	4. Descending thoracic aorta
5. Azygos vein	5. Left subclavian artery
6. Oesophagus	6. Thoracic duct
7. Inferior vena cava	7. Oesophagus, trachea
8. Trachea	8. Left brachiocephalic vein
9. Right vagus nerve	9. Left vagus nerve
10. Right phrenic nerve	10. Left phrenic nerve
	11. Left recurrent laryngeal nerve

Fissures and Lobes of the Lungs

The right lung is divided into three lobes (upper, middle, and lower) by two fissures (oblique and horizontal). The left lung is divided into two lobes by the oblique fissure (Plate 16.1, Fig. 16.1).

Oblique fissure: It cuts into the whole thickness of the lung, except at the hilum. It passes obliquely downwards and forwards, crossing the posterior border about 6 cm below the apex and the inferior border about 5 cm from the median plane. Due to the oblique plane of the fissure, the lower lobe is more posterior and the upper and middle lobes are more anterior.

Horizontal fissure: In the right lung, the *horizontal fissure* passes from the anterior border up to the oblique fissure and separates a wedge-shaped middle lobe from the upper lobe. The fissure runs horizontally at the level of the 4th costal cartilage and meets the oblique fissure in the midaxillary line.

Lingula: The tongue-shaped projection of the left lung below the cardiac notch is called the *lingula*. It corresponds to the middle lobe of the right lung.

Note: The lungs expand maximally in the inferior direction because movements of the thoracic wall and diaphragm are maximal towards the base of the lung. The presence of the oblique fissure of each lung allows a more uniform expansion of the whole lung (Fig. 16.1).

DISSECTION

Identify the lungs by the thin anterior border, thick posterior border, conical apex, wider base, medial surface with hilum, and costal surface with impressions of the ribs and intercostal spaces. In addition, the right lung is distinguished by the presence of three lobes, whereas left lung comprises two lobes only (*refer to BDC App*).

On the mediastinal part of the medial surface of right lung identify two bronchi—the eparterial and hyparterial bronchi, with bronchial vessels and posterior pulmonary plexus, the pulmonary artery between the two bronchi on an anterior plane. The upper pulmonary vein is situated still on an anterior plane while the lower pulmonary vein is identified below the bronchi.

The impressions on the right lung in front of root of lung are of superior vena cava, inferior vena cava, and right atrium. The impressions behind the root of lung are those of vena azygos and oesophagus (Table 16.1).

Hilum of the left lung shows the single bronchus situated posteriorly, with bronchial vessels and posterior pulmonary plexus. The pulmonary artery lies above the bronchus. Anterior to the bronchus is the upper pulmonary vein, while the lower vein lies below the bronchus.

The mediastinal surface of left lung has the impression of left ventricle, ascending aorta. Behind the root of the left lung are the impressions of descending thoracic aorta while oesophagus leaves an impression in the lower part only.

Competency:

AN24.2 Identify side, external features, and relations of structures which form root of lung and bronchial tree and their clinical correlate.

Root of the Lung

Root of the lung is a short, broad pedicle which connects the medial surface of the lung to the mediastinum. It is formed by structures which either enter or come out of the lung at the hilum (Latin *depression*). The roots of the lungs lie opposite the bodies of the 5th–7th thoracic vertebrae.

Contents

The root is made up of the following structures.

1. Bronchus: Principal bronchus on the left side, and eparterial and hyparterial bronchi on the right
2. Pulmonary artery
3. Two pulmonary veins: Superior and inferior (Figs 16.4 and 16.5).
4. Bronchial arteries: One on the right side and two on the left
5. Bronchial veins
6. Anterior and posterior pulmonary plexuses of nerves
7. Lymphatics of the lung
8. Bronchopulmonary lymph nodes
9. Areolar tissue.

Arrangement of Structures in the Root

Right side: From posterior to anterior side:

1. Eparterial bronchus, hyparterial bronchus with bronchial vessels and posterior pulmonary plexus along their posterior walls (Figs 16.4 and 16.5, Flowchart 16.2).
2. Pulmonary artery in midplane between the two bronchi.
3. Superior and inferior pulmonary veins in anterior part.
4. Anterior pulmonary plexus, lymph nodes, and lymph vessels in the anterior and inferior parts.

Left side: From posterior to anterior side:

1. Single bronchus with bronchial vessels and posterior pulmonary plexus along its posterior wall.
2. Pulmonary artery in middle area placed above the bronchus (Figs 16.4 and 16.5).
3. Superior and inferior pulmonary veins in anterior part.
4. Anterior pulmonary plexus, lymph nodes, and lymph vessels in the anterior and inferior parts.

Relations of the Root

Anterior

1. *Common on the two sides:*
   a. Phrenic nerve
   b. Pericardiacophrenic vessels
   c. Anterior pulmonary plexus

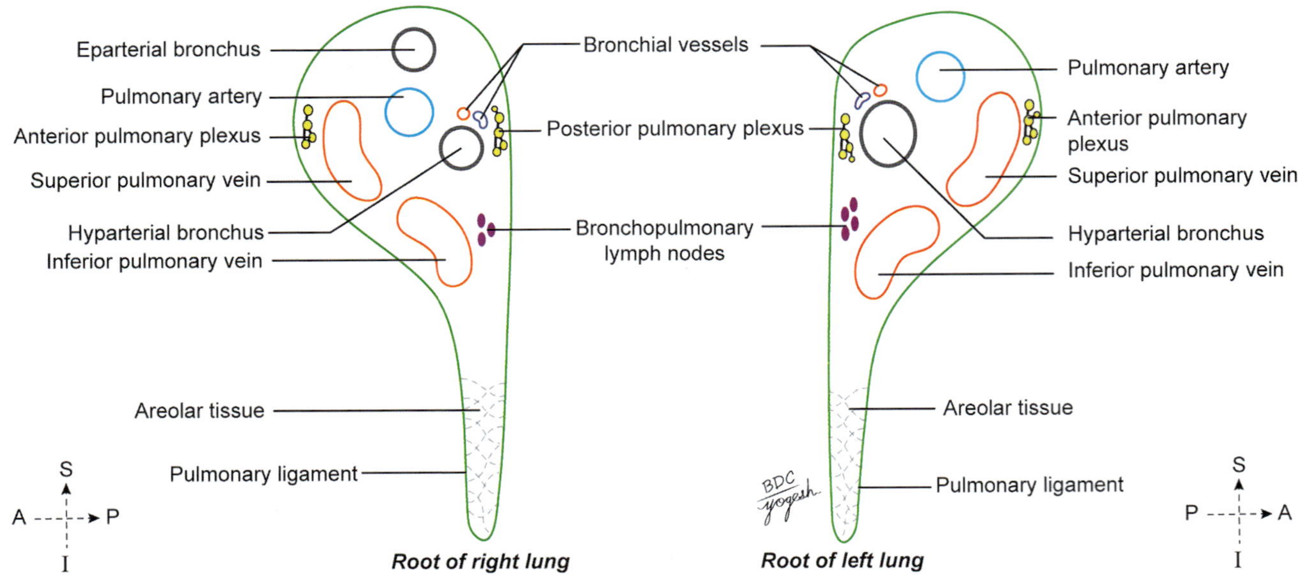

Fig. 16.4: Roots of the right and left lungs

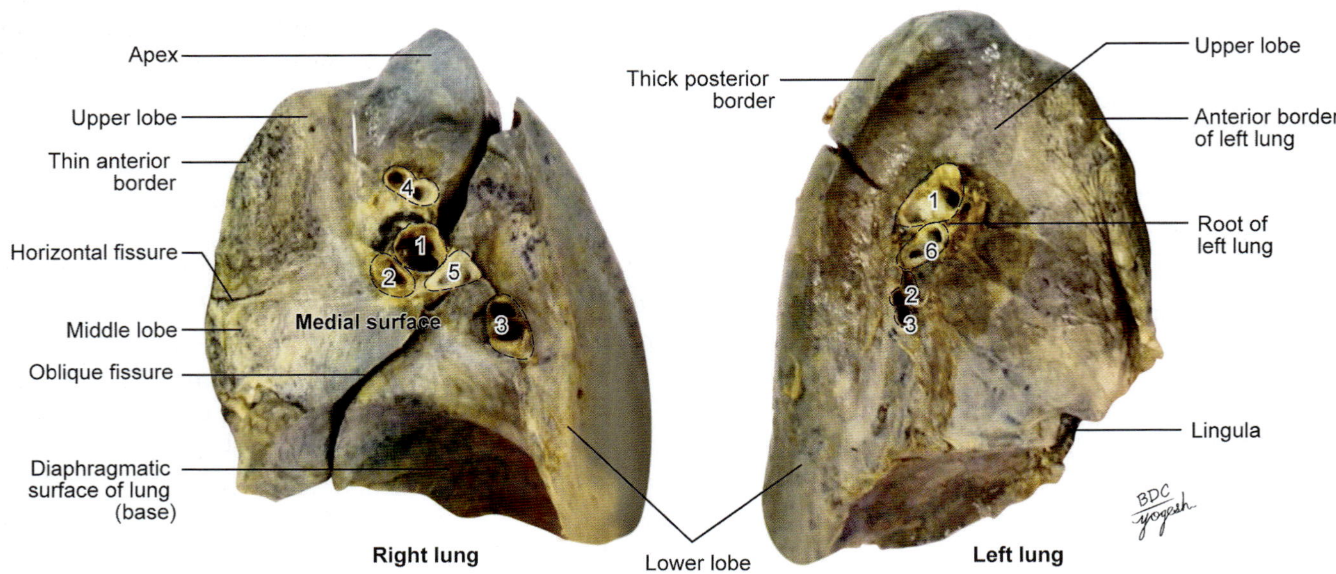

Fig. 16.5: Gross anatomy of lungs including their roots: (1) Pulmonary artery; (2) Superior pulmonary vein; (3) Inferior pulmonary vein; (4) Eparterial bronchus; (5) Hyparterial bronchus; (6) Left principal bronchus

2. *On the right side:*
   a. Superior vena cava (Fig. 16.3a)
   b. A part of the right atrium.

Posterior

1. *Common on the two sides:*
   a. Vagus nerve
   b. Posterior pulmonary plexus
2. *On left side:* Descending thoracic aorta.

Superior

1. *On right side:* Terminal part of azygos vein
2. *On left side:* Arch of the aorta.

Inferior

1. Pulmonary ligament.

Flowchart 16.2: Contents of the roots of lungs

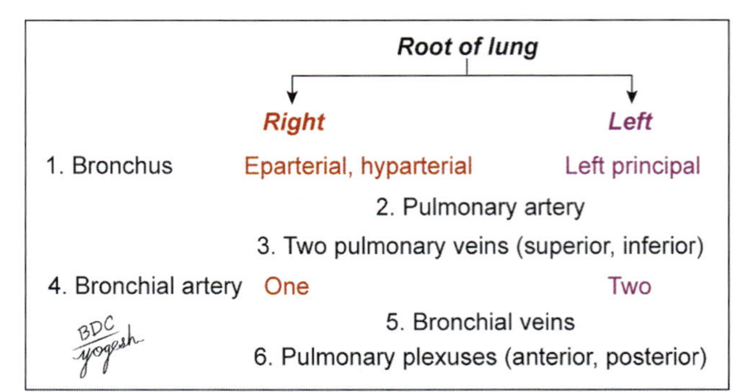

Differences between the Right and Left Lungs

Differences between right and left lungs are given in Table 16.2.

TABLE 16.2: Differences between the right and left lungs

Feature	*Right lung*	*Left lung*
Size and shape	Shorter and broader	Longer and narrower
Weight	Larger and heavier, weighs about 700 g	Smaller and lighter, weighs about 600 g
Anterior border	Straight	Interrupted by the cardiac notch
Cardiac impression	Shallow/absent	Deep
Lingula	Absent	Present
Fissures and lobes	2 fissures and 3 lobes	One fissure and 2 lobes
Hilum	2 bronchi: Eparterial, hyparterial	1 bronchus: Left principal bronchus
Bronchial artery	One	Two

SURFACE MARKING OF THE LUNG

Surface marking of lung is same as that of visceral pleura.

Apex (Fig. 16.6): It coincides with cervical pleura. It can be represented by convex line joining the following points:

A: Junction of middle and medial one-third of clavicle
B: Point 2.5 cm above medial end of clavicle
C: Midpoint of sternoclavicular joint.

Anterior border

On right: It runs vertically downward and marked by joining the following points:

C: Midpoint of sternoclavicular joint
D: Median plane of sternal angle
E: Median point of xiphisternal joint.

On left: It has cardiac notch. It is marked by joining

C: Midpoint of sternoclavicular joint
D: Median plane of sternal angle
D1: Median plane at the level of 4th costal cartilage and then forms convex lateral notch.
E-1: At 6th costal cartilage (4 cm from median plane).

Lower border: It crosses:

F: 6th rib in midclavicular line
G: 8th rib in midaxillary line
H: 10th rib in paravertebral line (2 cm lateral to 10th thoracic spine).

Posterior border: It extends from

H: 10th rib in paravertebral line to
I: 7th cervical spine level in paravertebral line.

Oblique fissure: It can be marked joining

J: Point 2 cm lateral to third thoracic spine
K: Point on 5th rib in midaxillary line
L: 6th costal cartilage 7.5 cm lateral to median plane.

Horizontal fissure: It is present only in the right lung. It can be marked by a horizontal line along the 4th costal cartilage. This line extends from anterior border (4th costal cartilage level) to the oblique fissure (at 5th rib in midaxillary line).

Competency:

AN24.5 Mention the blood supply, lymphatic drainage and nerve supply of lungs.

Arterial Supply

Bronchial arteries: The bronchial arteries supply nutrition to the bronchial tree and to the pulmonary tissue. These are small arteries that vary in number, size, and origin, but usually they are as follows (Flowchart 16.3):

1. *On the right side*, there is ***one bronchial artery*** which arises from the third right posterior intercostal artery.
2. *On the left side*, there are ***two bronchial arteries***, both of which arise from the descending thoracic aorta the upper opposite fifth thoracic vertebra and the lower just below the left bronchus.

Pulmonary arteries: Deoxygenated blood is brought to the lungs by the ***two pulmonary arteries***. There are precapillary anastomoses between bronchial and pulmonary arteries. These connections enlarge when any one of them is obstructed in disease.

Venous Drainage of the Lungs

Bronchial veins: The venous blood from the first and second divisions of the bronchi is carried by bronchial veins. Usually there are ***two bronchial veins*** on each side. The right bronchial vein drain into the azygos vein. The left bronchial veins drain into the accessory hemiazygos vein.

Pulmonary veins: Oxygenated blood from each lung is drained by two pulmonary veins (superior and inferior) that open into the left atrium.

Lymphatic Drainage

There are two sets of lymphatics, both of which drain into the bronchopulmonary nodes (Flowchart 16.3).

1. ***Superficial vessels*** drain the peripheral lung tissue lying beneath the pulmonary pleura. The vessels pass round the borders of the lung and margins of the fissures to reach the hilum.
2. ***Deep lymphatics*** drain the bronchial tree, the pulmonary vessels and the connective tissue septa. They run towards the hilum where they drain into the bronchopulmonary nodes (Fig. 16.7).

Note: The alveoli do not have lymph vessels. The superficial vessels have numerous valves and the deep vessels have only a few valves or no valves at all. Though there is no free anastomosis between the superficial and deep vessels, some connections exist which can open up, so that lymph can flow from the deep to the superficial lymphatics when the deep vessels are obstructed in disease of the lungs or of the lymph nodes.

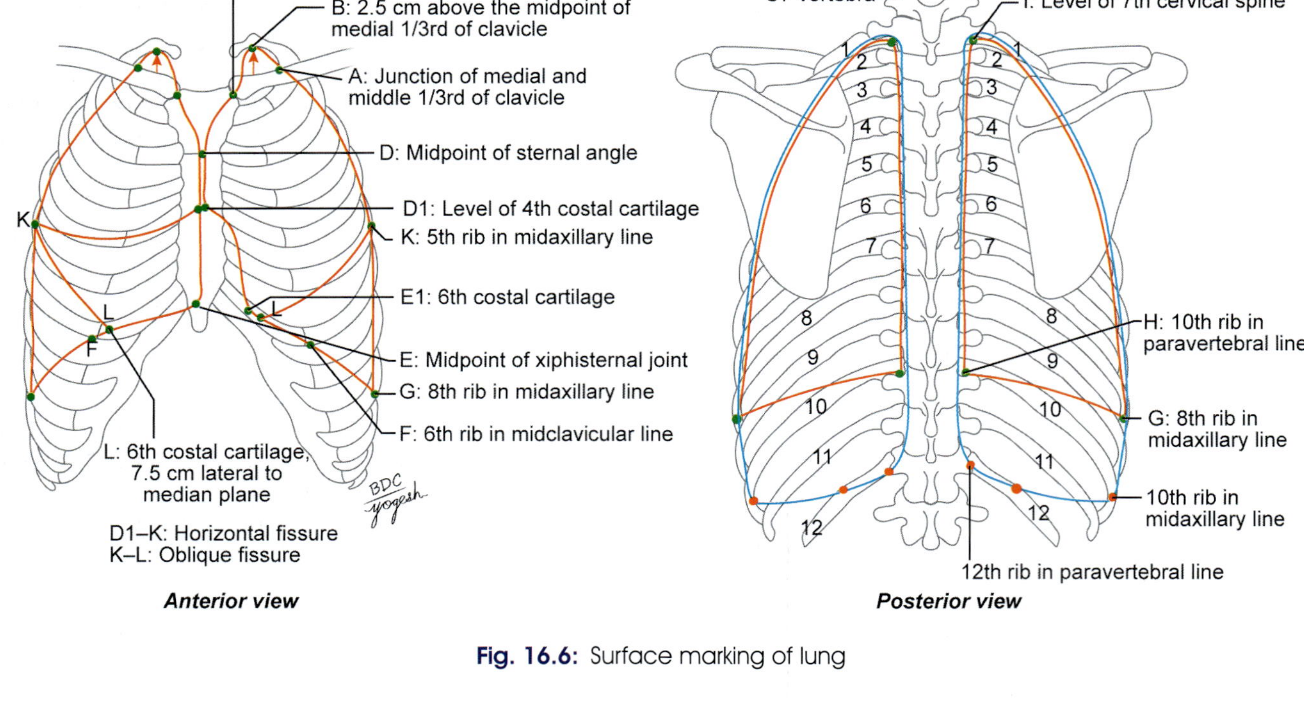

Fig. 16.6: Surface marking of lung

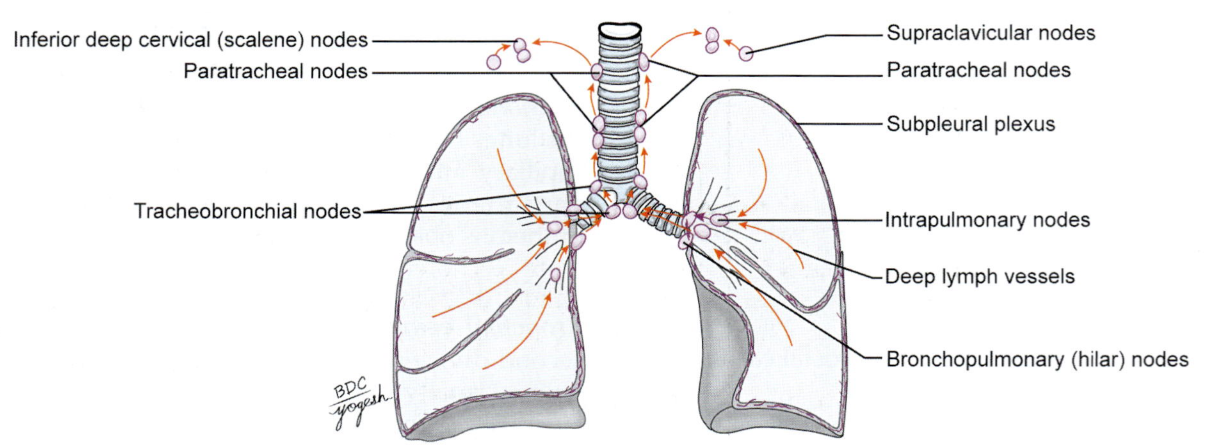

Fig. 16.7: Lymphatic drainage of lungs

Flowchart 16.3: Blood supply, lymphatic drainage, and nerve supply of lungs

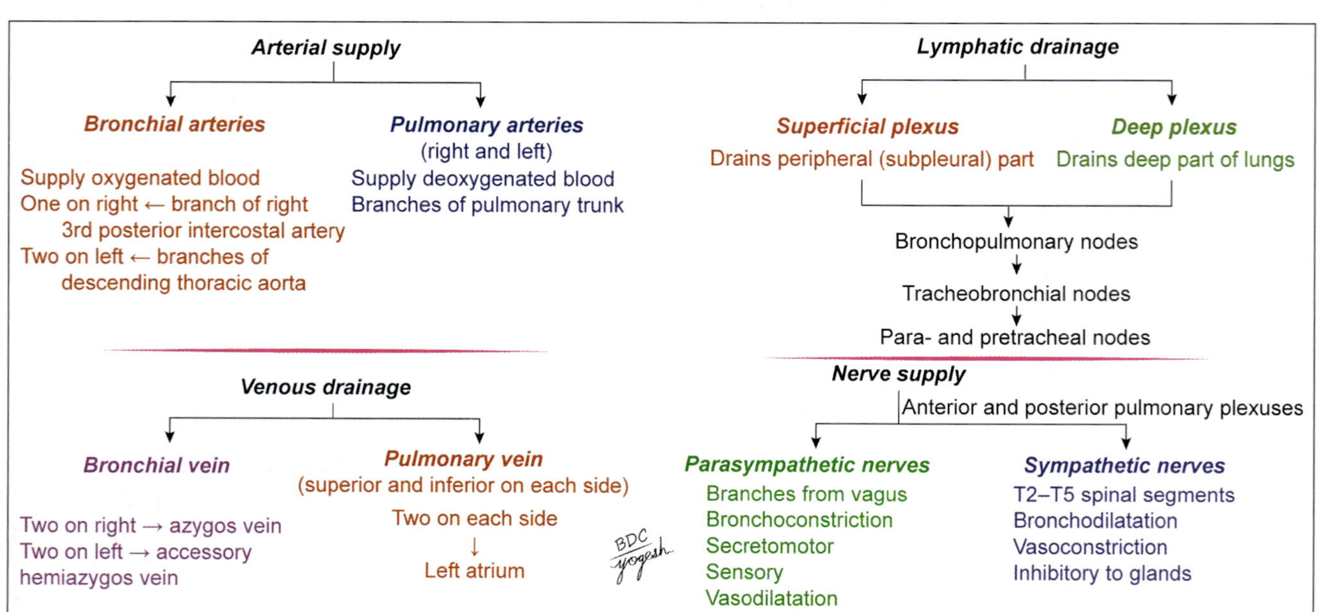

Nerve Supply

1. Parasympathetic nerves are derived from the vagus. These fibres are (Flowchart 16.3):
   a. Motor to the bronchial muscles, and on stimulation cause bronchospasm.
   b. Secretomotor to the mucous glands of the bronchial tree.
   c. Sensory fibres are responsible for the stretch reflex of the lungs, and for the cough reflex.
2. Sympathetic nerves are derived from second to fifth sympathetic ganglia. These are inhibitory to the smooth muscle and glands of the bronchial tree. That is how sympathomimetic drugs, like adrenaline, cause bronchodilatation and relieve symptoms of bronchial asthma.

Both parasympathetic and sympathetic nerves first form anterior and posterior pulmonary plexuses situated in front of and behind the lung roots: From the plexuses, nerves are distributed to the lungs along the blood vessels and bronchi (Fig. 16.4).

BRONCHIAL TREE

It consists of principal bronchi, lobar bronchi, tertiary bronchi, terminal bronchioles, and respiratory bronchioles.

Principal Bronchi

The *trachea* divides at the level of the upper half of the 4th thoracic vertebra into two primary principal bronchi, one for each lung.

1. The ***right principal bronchus*** is 2.5 cm long. It is shorter, wider and more in line with the trachea than the left principal bronchus (Plate 16.2, Fig. 16.8).
2. The ***left principal bronchus*** is 5 cm long. It is longer, narrower and more oblique than the right bronchus.

Note: Right bronchus makes an angle of 25° with tracheal bifurcation, while left bronchus makes an angle of 45° with the trachea. Inhaled particles or foreign bodies, therefore, tend to pass more frequently to the right lung, with the result that infections are more common on the right side than on the left.

Plate 16.2: Structures in conducting part of respiratory tract

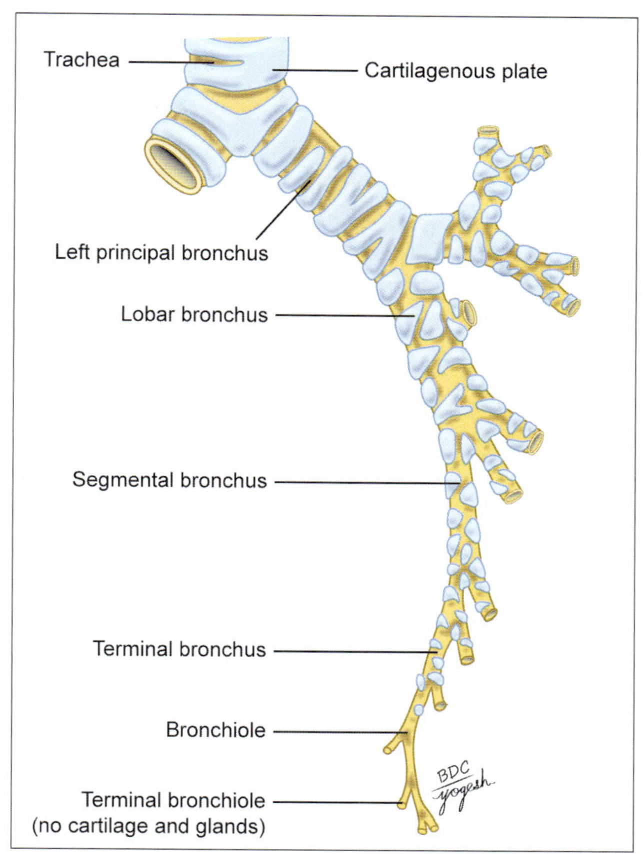

Lobar Bronchi

Each principal bronchus enters the lung through the hilum, and divides into ***secondary lobar bronchi***, one for each lobe of the lungs. Thus, there are three lobar bronchi on the right side, and only two on the left side.

Tertiary Bronchi and Bronchioles

Each lobar bronchus divides into *tertiary or segmental bronchi*, one for each bronchopulmonary segment; which are 10 on the right side and 10 on the left side. The segmental bronchi divide repeatedly to form very small branches called ***terminal bronchioles***. Still smaller branches are called ***respiratory bronchioles*** (Plates 16.2 and 16.3).

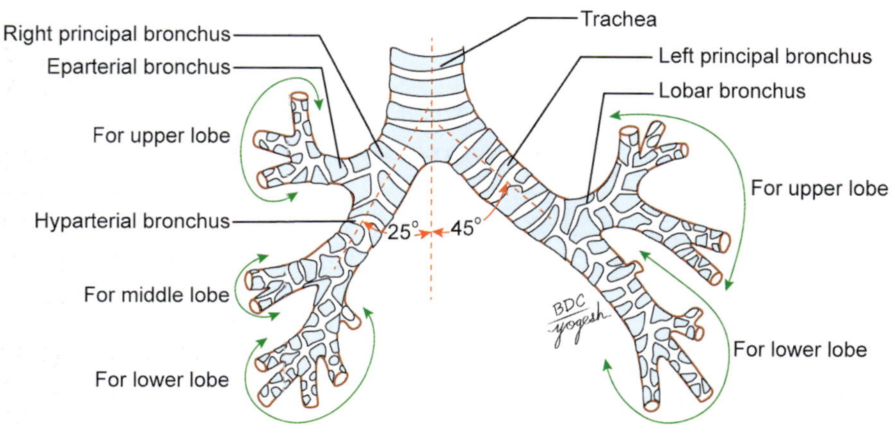

Fig. 16.8: Trachea and principal bronchi

Plate 16.3: Respiratory/pulmonary part

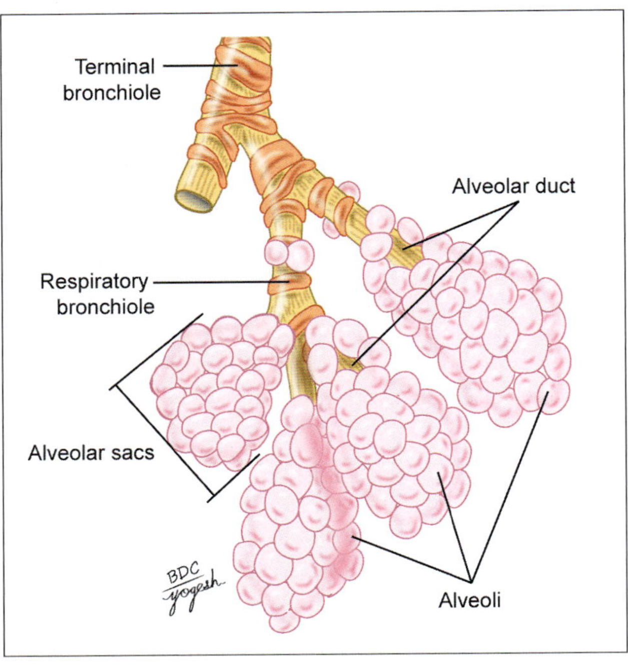

Pulmonary Unit

Each respiratory bronchiole aerates a small part of the lung known as a *pulmonary unit* which consists of the following components:

1. Alveolar ducts (Plate 16.3, Fig. 16.9)
2. Atria
3. Air saccules
4. Pulmonary alveoli (Latin *small cavity*). Gaseous exchanges take place in the alveoli.

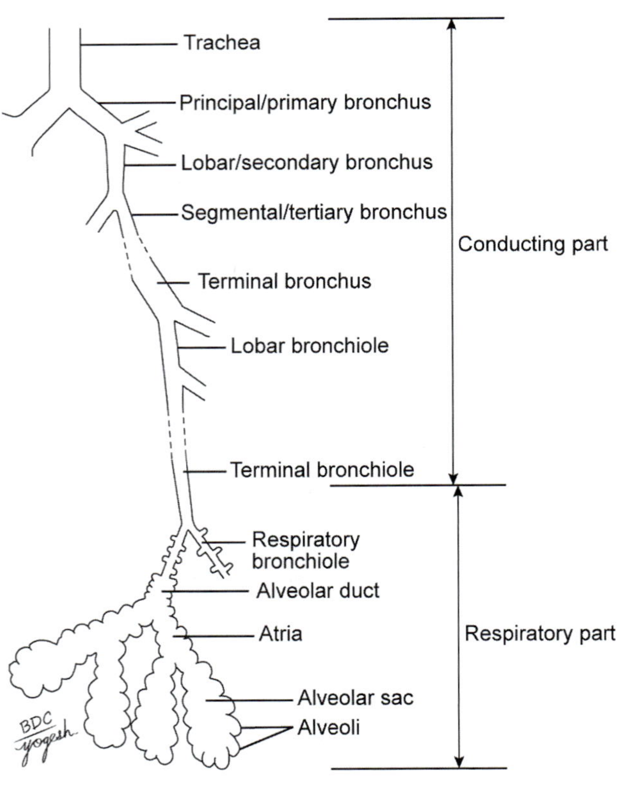

Fig. 16.9: Bronchial tree

DISSECTION

Dissect the principal bronchus into the left lung. Remove the pulmonary tissue and follow the main bronchus till it is seen to divide into two lobar bronchi. Try to dissect till these divide into the segmental bronchi (Figs 16.10 and 16.11).

Dissect the principal bronchus into the right lung. Remove the pulmonary tissue and follow the main bronchus till it is seen to divide into three lobar bronchi. Try to dissect till these divide into segmental bronchi.

Competency:
AN24.3 Describe a bronchopulmonary segment with its clinical anatomy.

BRONCHOPULMONARY SEGMENTS

Definition

Bronchopulmonary segments are well-defined, pyramidal-shaped anatomical segments aerated by tertiary/segmental bronchus.

There are 10 segments on the right side and 10 on the left side (Table 16.3, Figs 16.10 and 16.11).

Features

1. Each one is aerated by a tertiary or segmental bronchus.
2. These are well-defined anatomic, functional, and surgical sectors of the lung.

TABLE 16.3: The bronchopulmonary segments
[*Mnemonic*: '**A**ll **P**ilots **A**re **L**ike **M**ighty **S**uperheroes **M**aking **A**mazing **L**andings **P**recisely']

Lobes	*Segments*
Right lung	
A. Upper	1. **A**pical
	2. **P**osterior
	3. **A**nterior
B. Middle	4. **L**ateral
	5. **M**edial
C. Lower	6. **S**uperior (apical)
	7. **M**edial basal
	8. **A**nterior basal
	9. **L**ateral basal
	10. **P**osterior basal
Left lung	
A. Upper	
• Upper division	1. Apical
	2. Posterior
	3. Anterior
• Lower division	4. Superior lingular
	5. Inferior lingular
B. Lower	6. Superior (apical)
	7. Medial basal
	8. Anterior basal
	9. Lateral basal
	10. Posterior basal

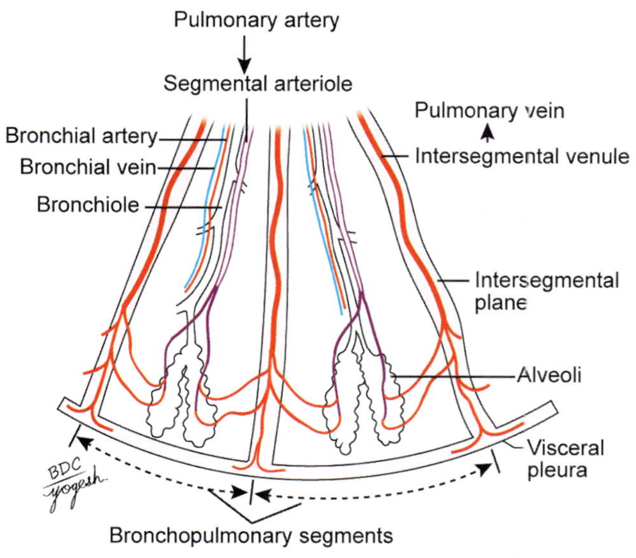

Fig. 16.10: Distal portions of adjacent bronchopulmonary segments

3. Each segment is pyramidal in shape with its apex directed towards the root of the lung and base directed towards periphery (Fig. 16.11).
4. Each segment has a segmental bronchus, segmental artery, autonomic nerves, and lymph vessels.
5. The segmental venules lie in the connective tissue between adjacent pulmonary units of bronchopulmonary segments (Fig. 16.10).
6. During segmental resection, the surgeon works along the segmental veins to isolate a particular segment.

Relation to Pulmonary Artery

The branches of the pulmonary artery accompany the bronchi. The artery lies dorsolateral to the bronchus. Thus each segment has its own separate artery (Fig. 16.10).

Relation to Pulmonary Vein

The pulmonary veins do not accompany the bronchi or pulmonary arteries. They run in the intersegmental planes. Thus, each segment has more than one vein and each vein drains more than one segment. Near the hilum, the veins are ventromedial to the bronchus.

Note: Bronchopulmonary segment have their own arterial supply; but venous drainage is shared by adjacent bronchopulmonary segment. It should be noted that the bronchopulmonary segment is not a ***bronchovascular segment*** because it does not have its own vein.

Competency:

AN25.2 Describe development of pleura, lung, and heart.

DEVELOPMENT OF RESPIRATORY SYSTEM

The lower respiratory tract primordium appears in the 3rd week of intrauterine life in the form of an outgrowth (endodermal ***respiratory diverticulum***) from the ventral

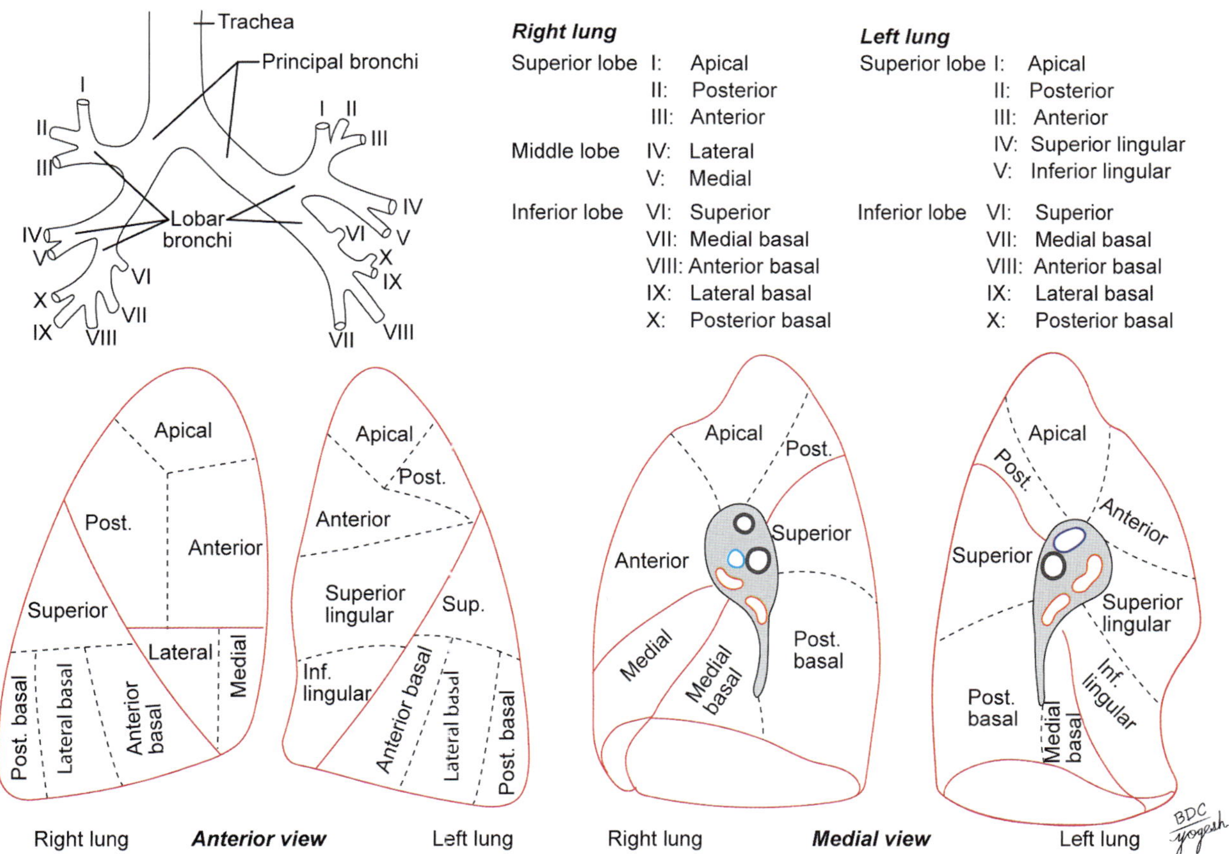

Fig. 16.11: Bronchopulmonary segments (*Reviewer*: Dr Hitant Vohra, Professor and Head, Department of Anatomy, DMC&H, Ludhiana)

Flowchart 16.4: Development of respiratory system

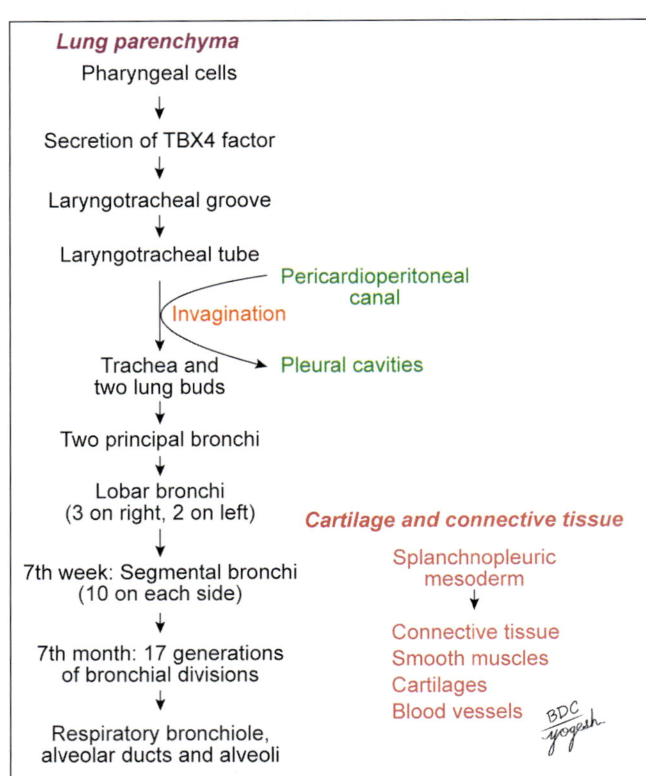

wall of the endodermal primitive pharynx. It forms the lining of the larynx, the trachea, the bronchi till the pulmonary alveoli (Flowchart 16.4).

The connective tissue, cartilage, and smooth muscles of these structures develop from splanchnic mesenchyme surrounding the foregut. As development progresses, the diverticulum separates from the foregut by the ***tracheo-oesophageal septum*** (except at the entrance to the larynx).

The respiratory diverticulum below the larynx grows caudally and forms the trachea in the midline. This bifurcates into two ***lung buds***. In the 5th week of intrauterine life, the proximal parts of each lung bud forms the principal bronchi. Each of these grows laterally and invaginates the pericardioperitoneal canals (primitive pleural cavities). Following this, the primary bronchi divide into secondary bronchi (3 on the right side and 2 on the left side). These divide dichotomously into tertiary bronchi. Each tertiary bronchus with its surrounding mesenchyme forms a bronchopulmonary segment.

By 24th week, about 17 orders of branches are formed and the lung parenchyma develops in four stages, as follows:

1. *Pseudoglandular stage* (between 5 and 17 weeks). In this stage, developing lung resembles a gland.
2. *Canalicular stage* (between 16 and 25 weeks), the lumina of bronchi and bronchioles become larger and tissue becomes more vascular.
3. *Terminal sac stage* (between 24 weeks to birth). Many saccules appear at the ends of terminal bronchioles (terminal sacs). Capillaries bulge into these sacs.

TABLE 16.4: Development of components of respiratory system

S. no.	*Component*	*Developed from*
1.	Epithelium of larynx, trachea, bronchi and alveoli	Endoderm of foregut
2.	Muscles of larynx	Branchial mesoderm of IVth and VIth arche
3.	Cartilages of larynx	All cartilages – fourth and sixth arches *except* epiglottis – hypobranchial eminence
4.	Glands of respiratory tract	Endoderm
5.	Muscles, cartilages and connective tissue of trachea and bronchi	Splanchnic mesoderm

4. *Alveolar stage* (late foetal period to 8 years after birth). The epithelial lining of the sacs becomes an extremely thin squamous layer and the alveolocapillary membrane allows exchange of gases.

By 28–32 weeks, some of the alveolar epithelial cells secrete a substance which is capable of lowering the surface tension at the air–alveolar interface and thus helps maintaining the patency of the alveoli; this is known as pulmonary surfactant. Table 16.4 and Flowchart 16.4 show the development of respiratory system.

HISTOLOGY OF LUNGS

Lung is covered by mesothelium of visceral pleura and connective tissue layer. Lung consists of intrapulmonary bronchi, bronchioles, and alveoli (Fig. 16.12).

Intrapulmonary Bronchi

These include lobar bronchus, segmental bronchus, and terminal bronchus. Intrapulmonary bronchi are lined by pseudostratified ciliated columnar epithelium with goblet cells and lamina propria (contains seromucous glands). There is a complete circumferential smooth muscle layer. Submucosa is supported by discontinuous cartilaginous plates.

Bronchioles

Bronchioles are <1 mm in diameter and do not have cartilage plates. Bronchioles show transition from ciliated pseudostratified columnar epithelium to ciliated columnar and finally simple cuboidal epithelium. In terminal bronchioles, Clara cells replace goblet cells. Bronchioles show smooth muscle layer covered by a connective tissue layer. *Respiratory bronchiole* is lined by simple cuboidal epithelium and is surrounded by smooth muscles.

Alveoli

These are thin-walled polyhedral sacs lined by simple squamous epithelium (type I pneumocytes) with few type II pneumocytes (produces surfactant). Interalveolar spaces contain a small amount of connective tissue and non-fenestrated (continuous) capillaries.

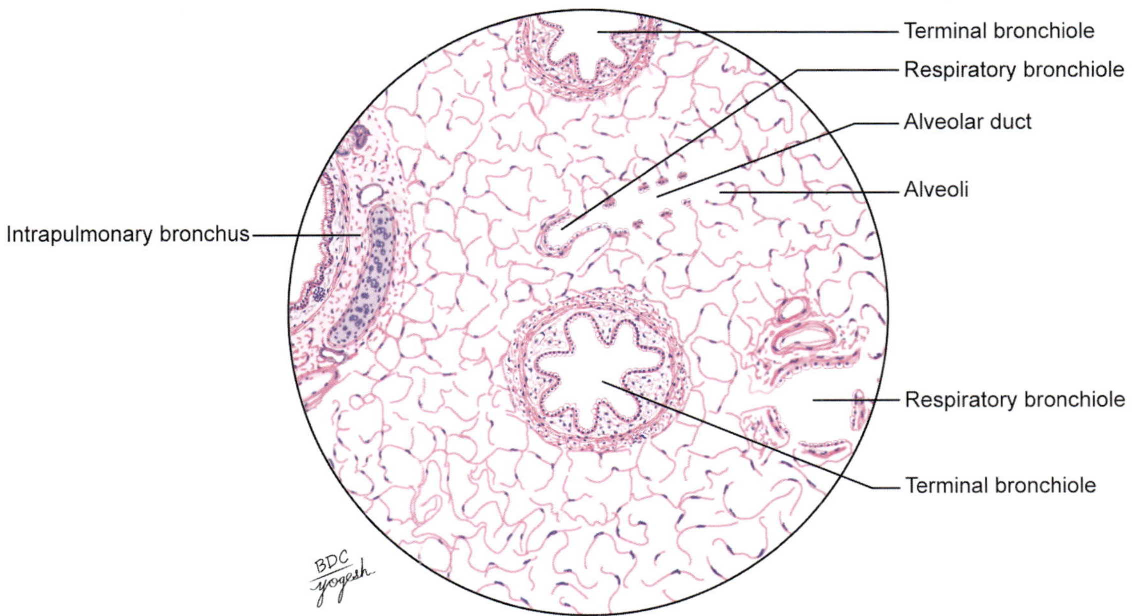

Fig. 16.12: Lung (Lung consists of intrapulmonary bronchi, bronchioles, and alveoli)

CLINICAL ANATOMY

- ***Pancoast tumour***: It is a tumour of apex of the lung. It typically spreads and compresses adjacent structures. Its signs and symptoms include:
  1. Due to involvement of T1 nerve: Horner's syndrome and pain and muscle weakness of forearm and hand
  2. Due to involvement of recurrent laryngeal nerve: hoarseness of voice.
  3. Compression of superior vena cava: Cyanosis and dilatation of veins of head and neck.
- ***Lobe of azygos vein (azygos lobe):*** Sometimes azygos vein passes through the superior lobe of the right lung and separates a part of lobe by a fissure. This separated part is called lobe of azygos vein (azygos lobe). It is not a true lobe because it does not have separate supplying bronchus, artery, and vein.
- Bronchopulmonary segments:
  1. Usually, the infection of a bronchopulmonary segment remains restricted to it, although tuberculosis and bronchogenic carcinoma may spread from one segment to another.
  2. Knowledge of the detailed anatomy of the bronchial tree helps considerably in:
     a. Segmental resection (Fig. 16.13).
     b. Visualising the interior of the bronchi through a bronchoscope passed through the mouth and trachea. The procedure is called bronchoscopy.
  3. Superior segment of lower lobe is the most dependent bronchopulmonary segment in supine position. Foreign bodies are likely to be lodged here.
- ***Bronchoscopy:*** It is a visualisation of interior of trachea and bronchi using a flexible, fibre-optic bronchoscope.
- ***Carina*** is a hook-shaped process projecting backwards from the lower margin of lowest tracheal ring. It helps to divide trachea into two primary bronchi.
- ***Foreign body aspiration:*** Foreign bodies mostly descend into right bronchus (Fig. 16.14) as it is wider and more vertical than the left bronchus. Enlarged lymph nodes present in this area may distort the carina. Right bronchus makes an angle of 25°, while left one makes an angle of 45°.
- ***Postural drainage:*** Carina (Latin *keel*) of the trachea is a sensitive area. When patient is made to lie on her/his left side, secretions from right bronchial tree flow towards the carina due to effect of gravity. This stimulates the cough reflex, and sputum is brought out. This is called *postural drainage* (Fig. 16.15).
- ***Paradoxical respiration***: During inspiration, the flail (abnormally mobile) segments of ribs are pulled inside the chest wall while during expiration the ribs are pushed out (Fig. 16.16).
- Tuberculosis of lung is one of the commonest diseases. A complete course of treatment must be taken under the guidance of a physician.
- ***Auscultation of lung***: Upper lobe is auscultated above 4th rib on both sides; lower lobes are best heard on the back. Middle lobe is auscultated between 4th and 6th ribs on right side.
- ***Bronchiectasis***: Bronchiectasis is a lung disorder caused by permanent widening of airway passage due to progressive loss of elastic fibers and smooth muscles (Fig. 16.17).
- ***Bronchial asthma*** is a common disease of respiratory system. It occurs due to bronchospasm of smooth muscles in the wall of bronchioles. Patient has difficulty especially during expiration. It is accompanied by wheezing. Epinephrine, a sympathomimetic drug, relieves the symptoms (Fig. 16.18).

- ***Emphysema*:** It is an abnormal permanent dilatation of airway distal to terminal bronchiole. Cigarette smoking and air pollution are common causative agents (Fig. 16.19).
- ***Bronchogenic carcinoma*** (type of lung cancer)**:** It is the most common cancer in men. It is mainly caused by cigarette smoking. It spreads to bronchopulmonary lymph nodes and supraclavicular nodes. It also spreads (metastasize) via blood (hematogenous root) to brain, bone, suprarenal glands, and another lung (Fig. 16.20).

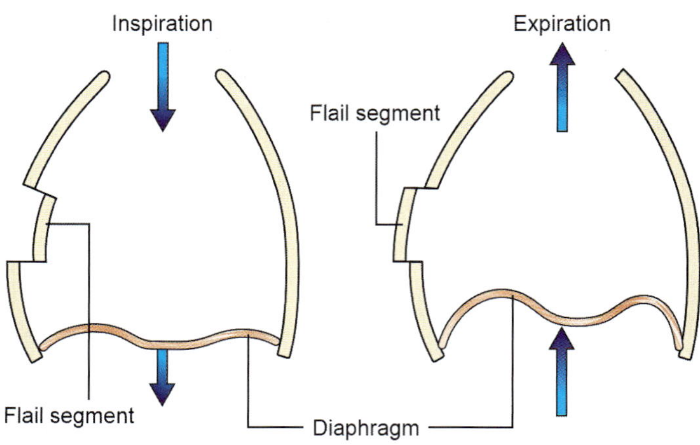

Fig. 16.16: Paradoxical respiration

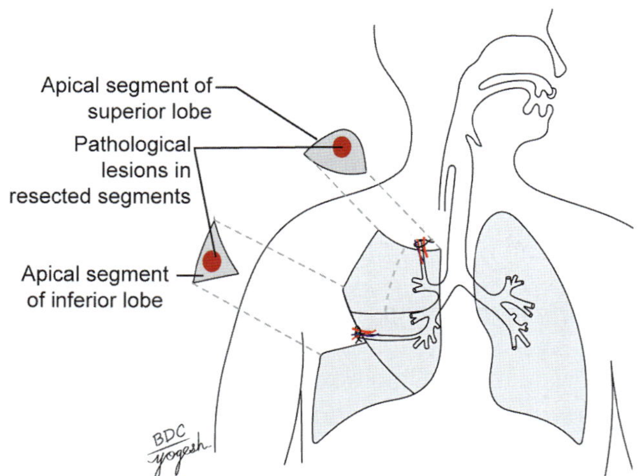

Fig. 16.13: Segmental resection of lung

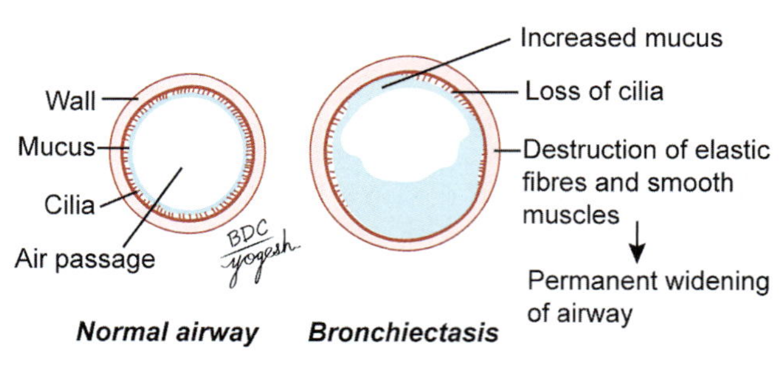

Fig. 16.17: Bronchiectasis

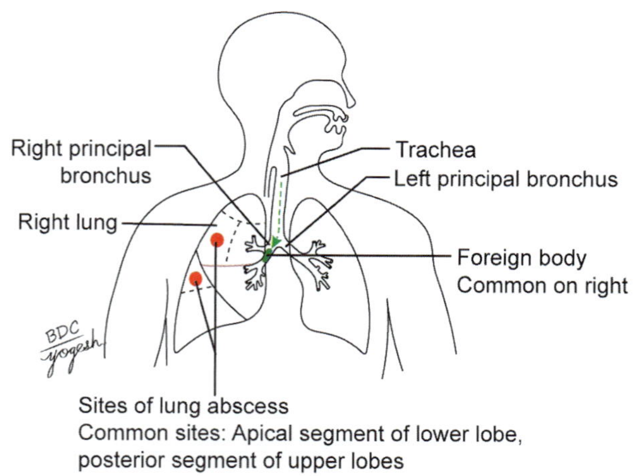

Fig. 16.14: Foreign body aspiration and lung abscess

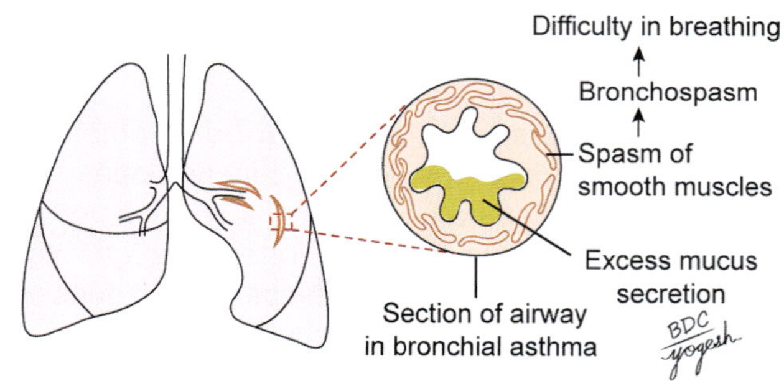

Fig. 16.18: Bronchial asthma

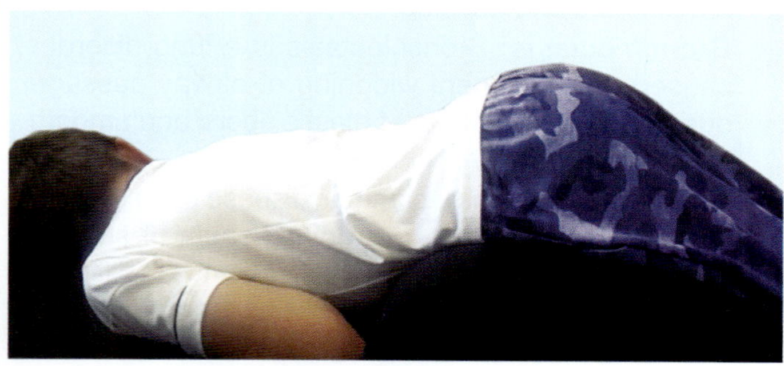

Fig. 16.15: Postural drainage from right lung

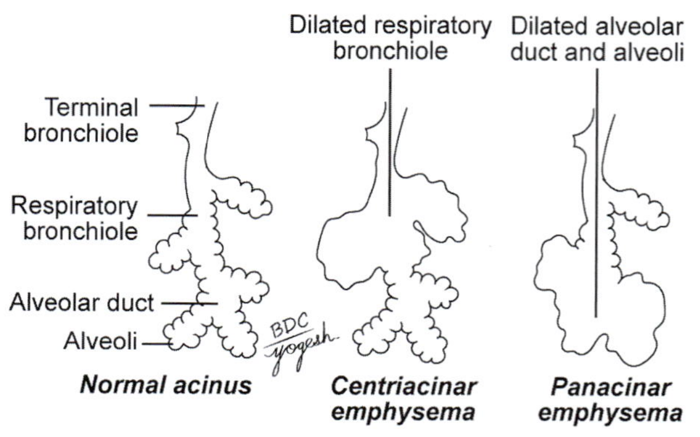

Fig. 16.19: Emphysema

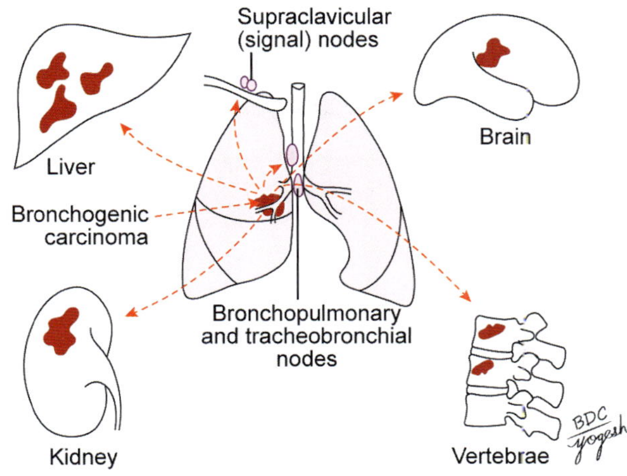

Fig. 16.20: Sites of spread of bronchogenic carcinoma

Facts to Remember

- Left lung has cardiac notch and lingula.
- Bronchopulmonary segments are independent functional units of lung.
- Lungs are subjected to lot of insult by the smoke of cigarette/bidis/pollution.
- Tuberculosis of lung is one of the commonest killers in an underdeveloped or a developing country. It most commonly affects the apical region of lungs.
- Inhaled foreign particles mostly enter the right principal bronchus.
- Right lower lobe is the commonest site for lung abscess.
- Bronchogenic carcinoma is the commonest cancer of the lungs.

BDC's Anatomy *e*-book

1. Molecular regulation of lung development
2. Congenital anomalies of respiratory system
3. Hering-Breuer and cough reflexes
4. Pancoast tumour
5. Lobe of azygos vein (azygos lobe)
6. Area of superficial cardiac dullness
7. Mendelson's syndrome
8. Further reading
9. Viva voce questions

Chapter

17

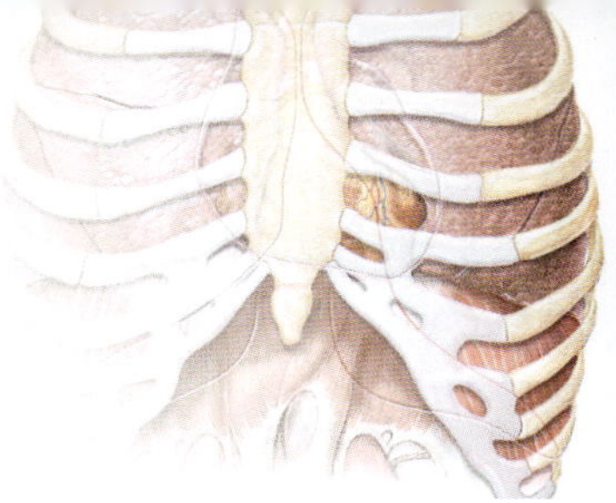

Mediastinum

Competency:

AN21.11 Mention boundaries and contents of the superior, anterior, middle, and posterior mediastinum.

Definition: Mediastinum (plural—mediastina) (Latin *intermediate*) is the middle space left in the thoracic cavity in-between the lungs.

Boundaries of Mediastinum (Fig. 17.1)

Anterior:	Sternum
Posterior:	Vertebral column
Superior:	Thoracic inlet
Inferior:	Diaphragm
On each side (lateral):	Mediastinal pleurae.

Contents of Mediastinum

The contents of the mediastinum are as follows (Plate 17.1):

1. *Viscera*: Thymus, heart enclosed in pericardial sac, trachea, oesophagus
2. *Vessels*: Thoracic aorta, pulmonary trunk, superior and inferior vena cava
3. *Lymphatics*: Lymph nodes, thoracic duct
4. *Nerves*: Vagus nerves, sympathetic trunks, and phrenic nerves.
5. Mediastinal pleurae.

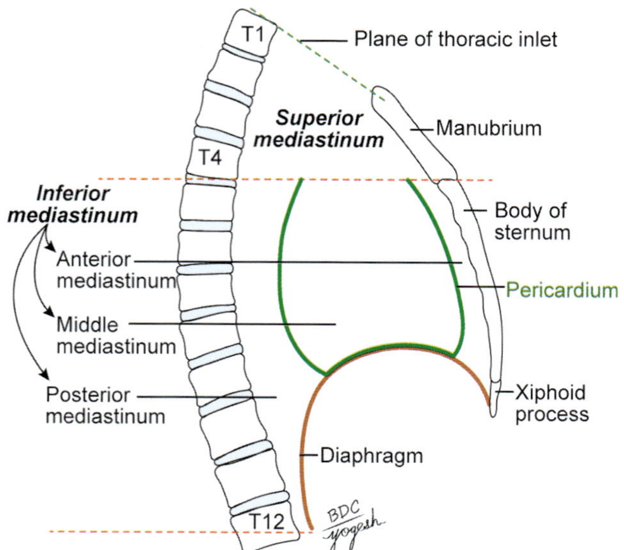

Fig. 17.1: Subdivisions of the mediastinum

DIVISIONS OF MEDIASTINUM

Divisions

For descriptive purposes, the mediastinum is divided into the *superior mediastinum* and the *inferior mediastinum* by an imaginary plane passing through the sternal angle anteriorly and the lower border of the body of the 4th thoracic vertebra posteriorly.

The inferior mediastinum is further divided into the *anterior, middle,* and *posterior* mediastina by the pericardium (Fig. 17.1, Flowchart 17.1). The area in front of the pericardium is the anterior mediastinum. The area behind the pericardium is the posterior mediastinum. The pericardium and its contents form the middle mediastinum.

DISSECTION

Reflect the upper half of manubrium sterni upwards and study the boundaries and contents of superior and three divisions of the inferior mediastinum.

SUPERIOR MEDIASTINUM

Boundaries

Anteriorly:	Manubrium sterni (Fig. 17.1)
Posteriorly:	Upper four thoracic vertebrae
Superiorly:	Plane of the thoracic inlet
Inferiorly:	An imaginary plane passing through the sternal angle in front, and the lower border of the body of the 4th thoracic vertebra behind.
On each side:	Mediastinal pleura.

Contents (Fig. 17.2, Plate 17.1)

1. ***Trachea and oesophagus***
2. ***Arteries:***
   i. Arch of aorta
   ii. Brachiocephalic artery
   iii. Left common carotid artery
   iv. Left subclavian artery.

Plate 17.1: Contents of mediastinum

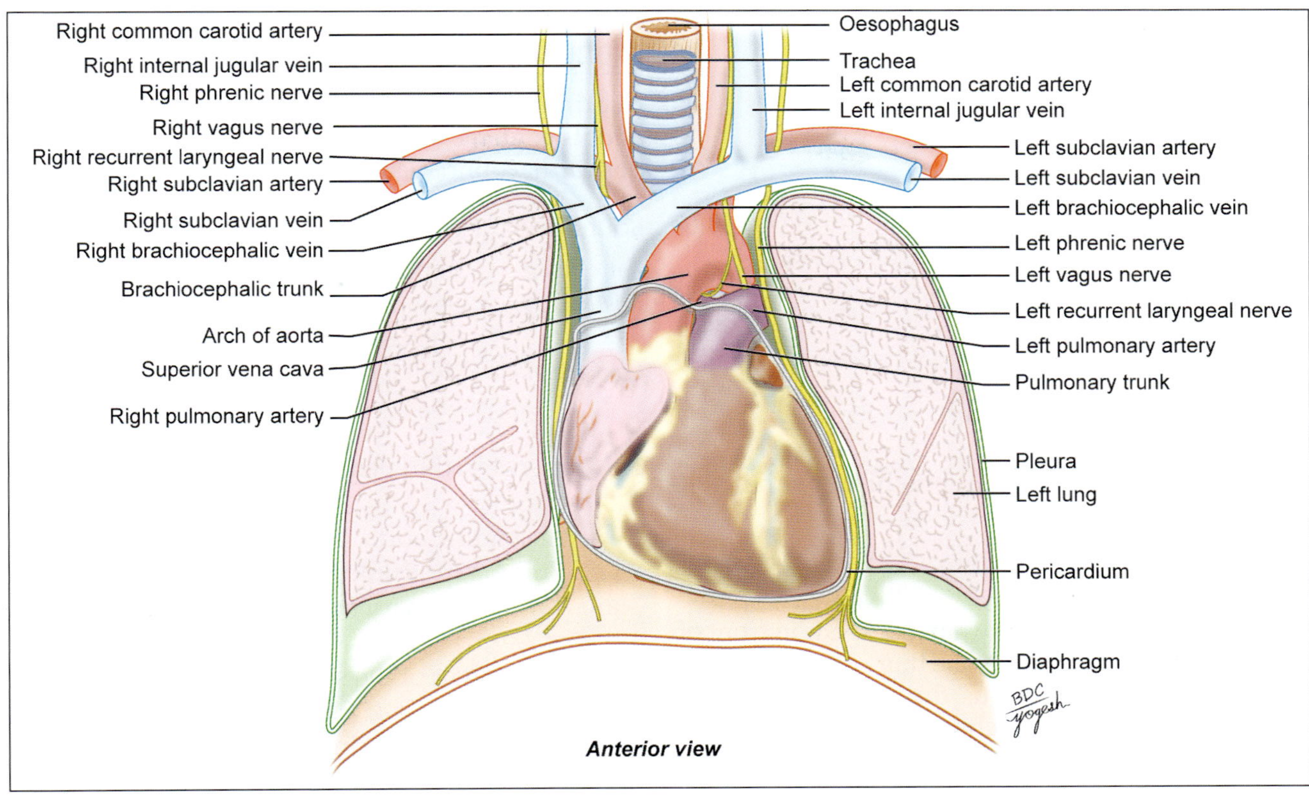

Flowchart 17.1: Divisions and contents of mediastinum

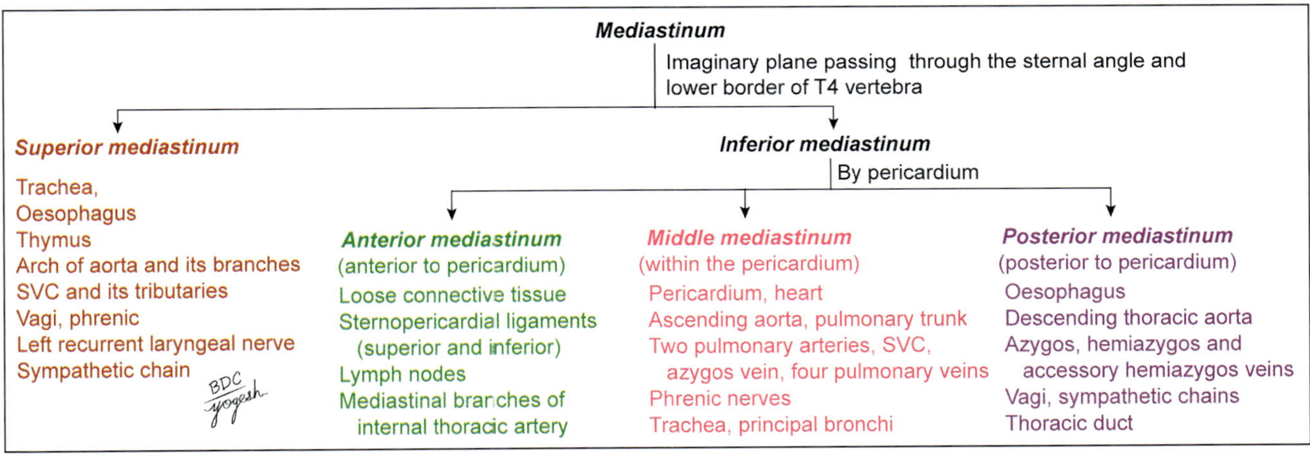

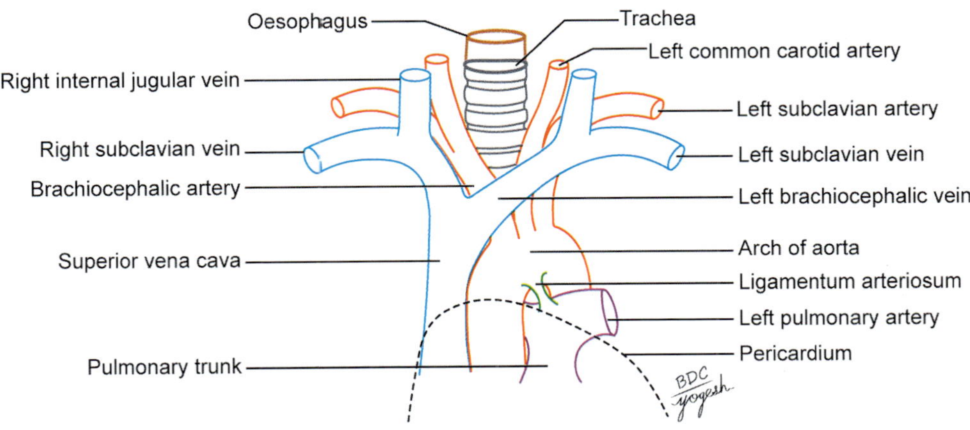

Fig. 17.2: Arrangement of the large structures in the superior mediastinum. Note the relationship of superior vena cava, ascending aorta and pulmonary trunk to each other in the middle mediastinum, i.e. within the pericardium. The bronchi are not shown

3. ***Veins:***
   i. Right and left brachiocephalic veins
   ii. Upper half of the superior vena cava
   iii. Left superior intercostal vein.
4. ***Nerves:***
   i. Vagus
   ii. Phrenic
   iii. Cardiac nerves of both sides
   iv. Left recurrent laryngeal nerve.
5. ***Thymus***
6. ***Muscles:***
   i. Sternohyoid
   ii. Sternothyroid
   iii. Lower ends of longus colli.
7. ***Thoracic duct***
8. ***Lymph nodes:*** Paratracheal, brachiocephalic, and tracheobronchial.

ANTERIOR MEDIASTINUM

Anterior mediastinum is a very narrow space in front of the pericardium, overlapped by the thin anterior borders of both lungs. It is continuous through the superior mediastinum with the pretracheal space of the neck. It contains areolar tissue and part of thymus gland.

Boundaries (Fig. 17.1)

Anteriorly: Body of sternum
Posteriorly: Pericardium
Superiorly: Imaginary plane separating the superior mediastinum from the inferior mediastinum.
Inferiorly: Superior surface of diaphragm
On each side: Mediastinal pleura.

Contents

1. Sternopericardial ligaments (Fig. 17.3)
2. Lymph nodes with lymphatics
3. Small mediastinal branches of the internal thoracic artery
4. The lowest part of the thymus
5. Areolar tissue.

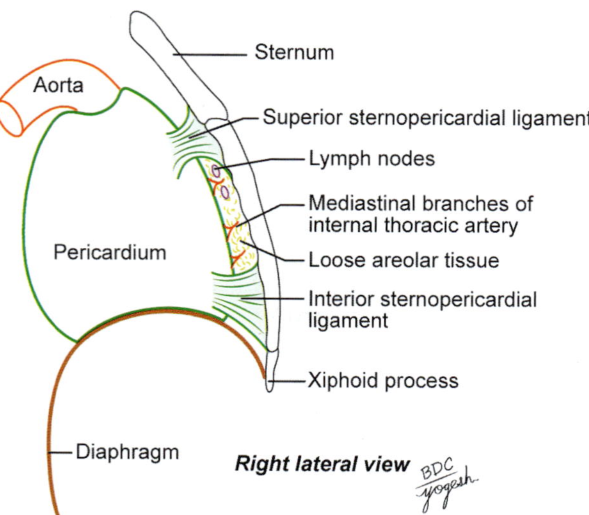

Fig. 17.3: Contents of anterior mediastinum

MIDDLE MEDIASTINUM

Middle mediastinum is occupied by the pericardium and its contents, along with the phrenic nerves and the pericardiacophrenic vessels.

Boundaries (Fig. 17.1)

Anteriorly: Sternopericardial ligaments
Posteriorly: Oesophagus, descending thoracic aorta, azygos vein
On each side: Mediastinal pleura.

Contents

1. *Heart* enclosed in pericardium (Plate 17.1)
2. ***Arteries:***
   i. Ascending aorta
   ii. Pulmonary trunk
   iii. Two pulmonary arteries.
3. ***Veins:***
   i. Lower half of the superior vena cava
   ii. Terminal part of the azygos vein
   iii. Right and left pulmonary veins.
4. ***Nerves:***
   i. Phrenic
   ii. Deep cardiac plexus.
5. ***Lymph nodes:*** Tracheobronchial nodes.

POSTERIOR MEDIASTINUM

Boundaries (Fig. 17.1)

Anteriorly:
   i. Pericardium
   ii. Bifurcation of trachea
   iii. Pulmonary vessels
   iv. Posterior part of the upper surface of the diaphragm.

Posteriorly: Lower eight thoracic vertebrae and intervening discs.
On each side: Mediastinal pleura.

Contents

1. ***Oesophagus*** (Fig. 17.4).
2. ***Arteries:*** Descending thoracic aorta and its branches.
3. ***Veins:***
   i. Azygos vein
   ii. Hemiazygos vein
   iii. Accessory hemiazygos vein.
4. ***Nerves:***
   i. Vagi
   ii. Splanchnic nerves: Greater, lesser and least, arising from the lower eight thoracic ganglia of the sympathetic chain.
5. ***Lymph nodes and lymphatics:***
   i. Posterior mediastinal lymph nodes lying alongside the aorta.
   ii. The thoracic duct (Fig. 17.4).

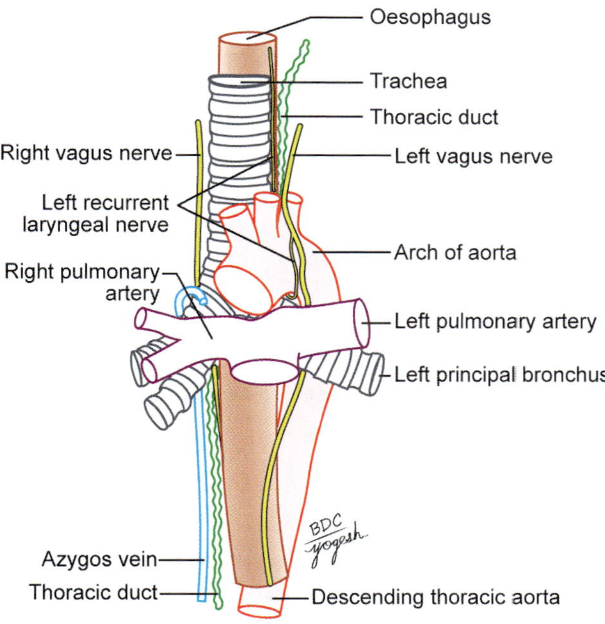

Fig. 17.4: Contents of superior and posterior mediastinum

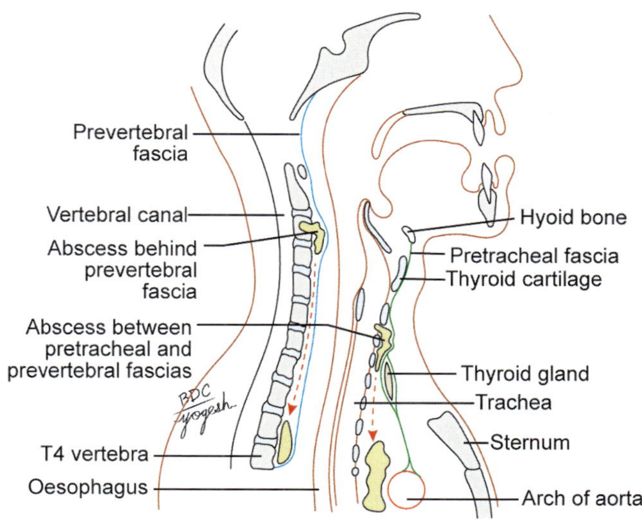

Fig. 17.5: Spread of infection to mediastinum

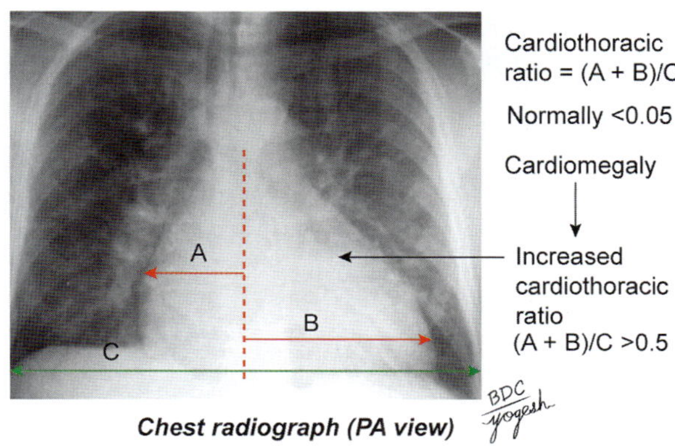

Fig. 17.6: Widening of mediastinum. Here, cardiothoracic ratio [(A + B)/C] is more than 0.5 and indicative of cardiomegaly and widening of mediastinum

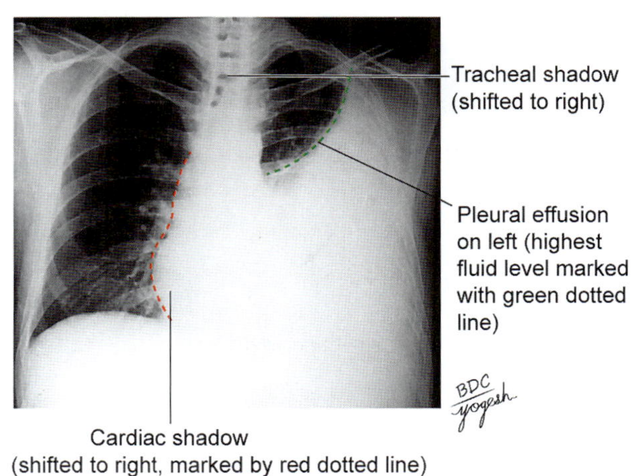

Fig. 17.7: Mediastinal shift. The mediastinal structures are deviated to the right due to left pleural effusion

CLINICAL ANATOMY

- The ***prevertebral layer*** of the deep cervical fascia extends to the superior mediastinum, and is attached to the fourth thoracic vertebra. An infection present in the neck behind this fascia can pass down into the superior mediastinum but not lower down (Fig. 17.5).
- The ***pretracheal fascia*** of the neck also extends to the superior mediastinum, where it blends with the arch of the aorta. Neck infections between the pretracheal and prevertebral fasciae can spread into the superior mediastinum, and through it into the posterior mediastinum. Thus mediastinitis can result from infections in the neck (Fig. 17.5).
- There is very little loose connective tissue between the mobile organs of the mediastinum. Therefore, the space can be readily dilated by inflammatory fluids, neoplasms, etc.
- ***Mediastinum — as a potential dead space***: In the superior mediastinum, all large veins are on the right side and the arteries on the left side. During increased blood flow, veins expand enormously, while the large arteries do not expand at all. Thus there is much 'dead space' on the right side and it is into this space that tumour or fluids of the mediastinum tend to project (Fig. 17.5).
- ***Widening of mediastinum***: Widening of mediastinum can be observed in chest radiographs. Causes of mediastinal widening: Haemorrhage from lacerated blood vessels, enlarged lymph nodes, enlarged heart (hypertrophy), and so on (Fig. 17.6).
- ***Mediastinal shift*** (Fig. 17.7): In some cases, mediastinum shifts on one side instead of its usual position. In case of lung collapse (atelectasis), mediastinum shifts toward the side of the collapsed lung. In case of pleural effusion, mediastinum may shift to the opposite side. Normally, on palpation, the trachea is felt as a central structure in the suprasternal notch. In mediastinal shift, trachea also shifts towards the side of mediastinal shift.
- ***Mediastinal syndrome***: Compression of mediastinal structures by any tumour gives rise to a group of

symptoms known as *mediastinal syndrome*. The common symptoms are as follows:

a. Obstruction of superior vena cava gives rise to engorgement of veins in the upper half of the body.
b. Pressure over the trachea causes dyspnoea and cough.
c. Pressure on oesophagus causes dysphagia.
d. Pressure or the left recurrent laryngeal nerve gives rise to hoarseness of voice (dysphonia).
e. Pressure on the phrenic nerve causes paralysis of the diaphragm on that side.
f. Pressure on the intercostal nerves gives rise to pain in the area supplied by them. It is called *intercostal neuralgia*.
g. Pressure on the vertebral column may cause erosion of the vertebral bodies.
h. The common causes of mediastinal syndrome are bronchogenic carcinoma, Hodgkin's disease causing enlargement of the mediastinal lymph nodes, aneurysm or dilatation of the aorta, etc.

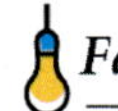

Facts to Remember

- Mediastinum is the middle space between the lungs.
- It is chiefly occupied by the heart enclosed in pericardium with blood vessels and nerves.
- Unit structures in the superior mediastinum are trachea, oesophagus, left recurrent laryngeal nerve between the two tubes and thoracic duct on the left of the oesophagus.
- The commonest cause of the mediastinal shift on the side of the disease is collapse of lung, whereas to the opposite side of the disease is pneumothorax or hydrothorax.

BDC's Anatomy *e*-book

1. Extension of infection from neck to the mediastinum
2. Anterior mediastinitis
3. Position of the thoracic viscera
4. Viva voce questions

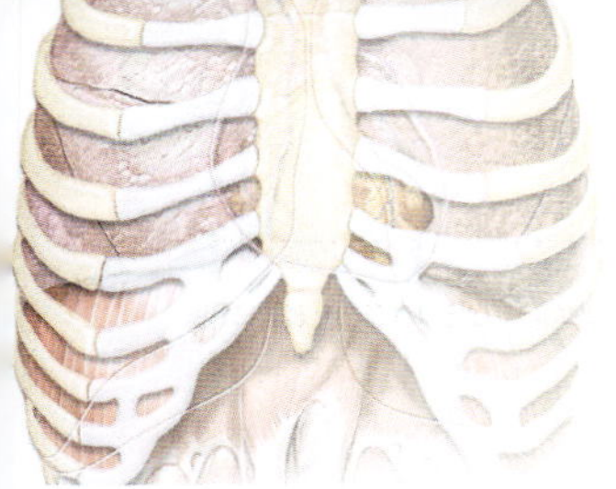

Chapter

18

Pericardium and Heart

Competency:

AN22.1 Describe and demonstrate subdivisions, sinuses in pericardium, blood supply, and nerve supply of pericardium.

PERICARDIUM

The pericardium (Greek *around heart*) is a fibroserous sac which encloses the heart and the roots of the great vessels. It is situated in the middle mediastinum. It consists of the *fibrous pericardium* and the *serous pericardium* (Fig. 18.1).

Functions of Pericardium

The functions of pericardium are:
1. Protection of heart (shock absorption).
2. Restriction of excessive movements of the heart.
3. Prevention of overexpansion of the heart when blood volume increases.
4. Prevents kinking of the great blood vessels.
5. Minimizes friction between the heart and the surrounding structures.
6. Mechanical barrier for the spread of infection and other pathologies to the heart.

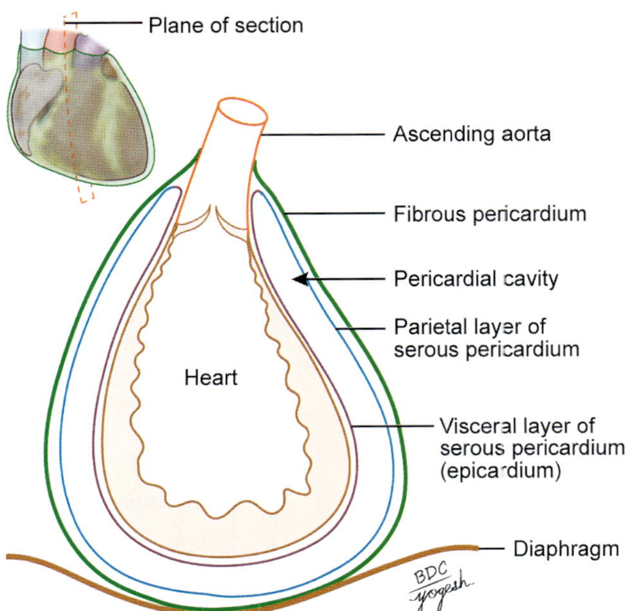

Fig. 18.1: Layers of the pericardium

Subdivisions

The pericardium has two components (Plate 18.1, Fig. 18.1, Flowchart 18.1):
1. ***Fibrous pericardium*:** It is the outer layer of pericardium. It forms a single-layered, thick, and cone-shaped sac that encloses heart and fuses with roots of the major vessels.
2. ***Serous pericardium*:** It is an inner double-layered blind sac of the pericardium. It has two layers:
   a. ***Parietal layer*:** It lines the inner surface of the fibrous pericardium.
   b. ***Visceral layer*** or ***epicardium*:** It lines the outer surface of the heart and the great blood vessels.

Development

The subdivisions of pericardium can be better explained with the help of development of the pericardium (Plate 18.2, Fig. 18.2). When head fold of the embryo is formed, the pericardial sac comes to lie in front of the developing heart tube. This heart tube undergoes folding and projects into the posterior wall of the sac. Arterial and venous ends of the heart tube are connected by a fold of pericardium called dorsal mesocardium. Later, the dorsal mesocardium degenerates and a gap called transverse sinus develops.

Flowchart 18.1: Subdivisions of pericardium

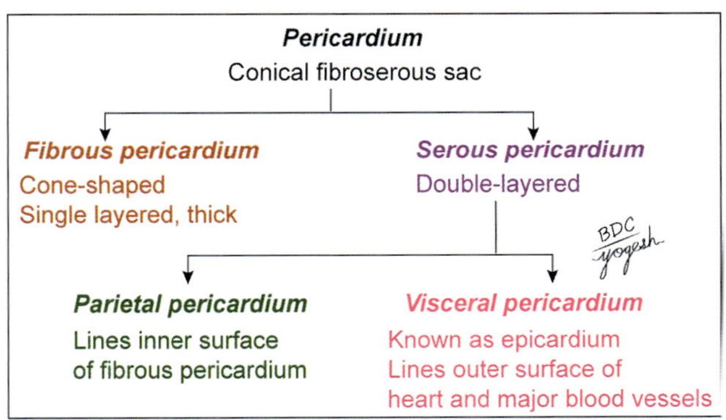

Plate 18.1: Layers of pericardium

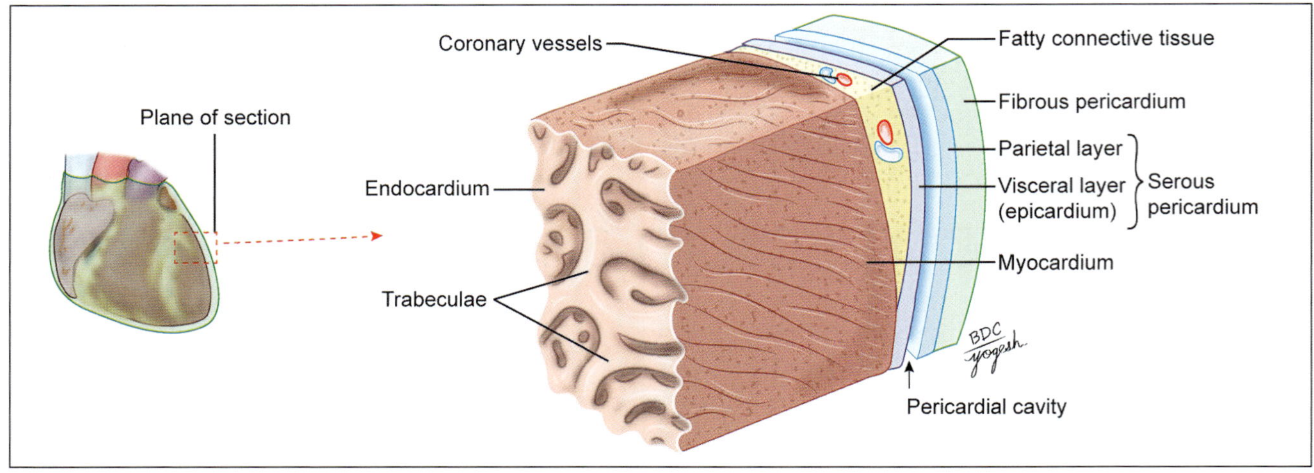

Plate 18.2: Development of pericardium

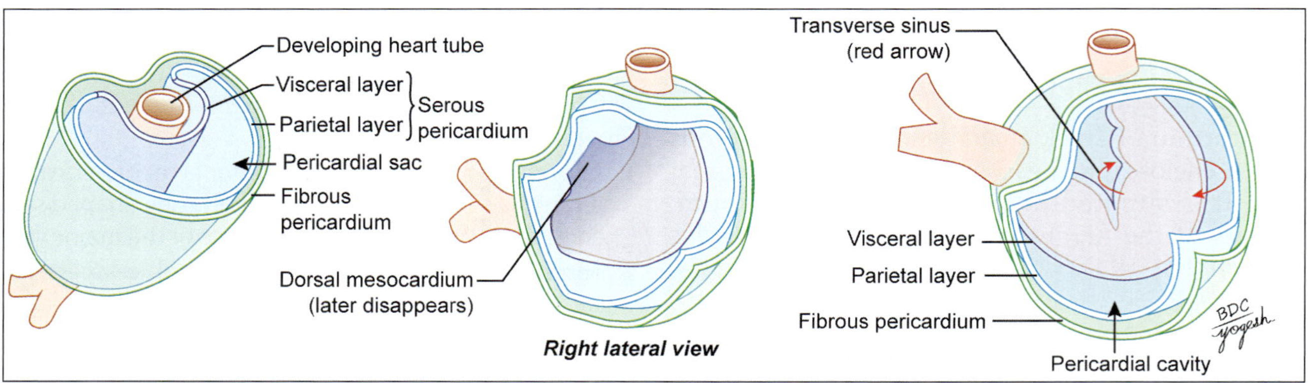

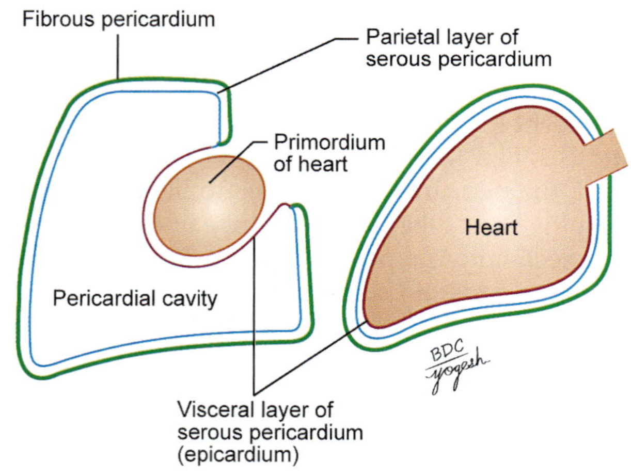

Fig. 18.2: Development of the layers of serous pericardium

Fibrous pericardium and parietal layer of the serous pericardium develop from the somatopleuric layer of the pericardial sac. Visceral layer of serous pericardium develops from splanchnopleuric layer of the pericardial sac.

Fibrous Pericardium

Fibrous pericardium is a conical sac made up of fibrous tissue. The parietal layer of serous pericardium is attached to its deep surface. The following features of the fibrous pericardium are noteworthy (Fig. 18.3).

1. ***Apex*** is blunt and lies at the level of the sternal angle. It is fused with the roots of the great vessels and with the pretracheal fascia.
2. Its ***base*** is broad and inseparably blended with the central tendon of the diaphragm.
3. Anteriorly, it is connected to the upper and lower ends of body of the sternum by weak superior and inferior *sternopericardial ligaments* (Fig. 18.3).

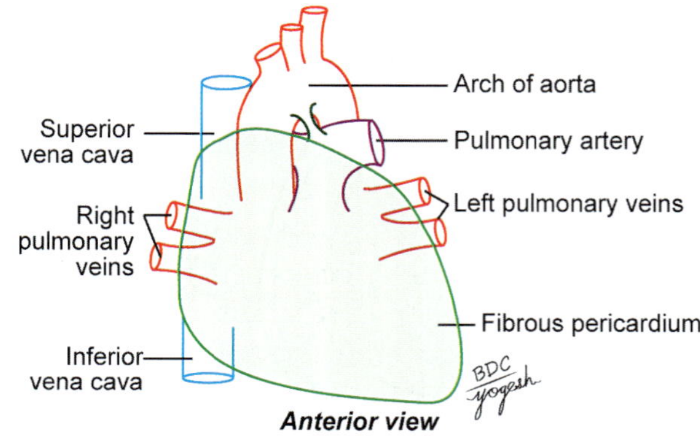

Fig. 18.3: Relations of the fibrous pericardium to the roots of the great vessels

4. Posteriorly, it is related to the principal bronchi, the oesophagus with the nerve plexus around it and the descending thoracic aorta.
5. On each side, it is related to the mediastinal pleura, the mediastinal surface of the lung, the phrenic nerve, and the pericardiacophrenic vessels.
6. It protects the heart against sudden overfilling and prevents overexpansion of the heart.

Serous Pericardium

Serous pericardium is thin, double-layered serous membrane lined by mesothelium (Fig. 18.1).

a. The outer layer or ***parietal pericardium*** is fused with the fibrous pericardium.
b. The inner layer or the ***visceral pericardium***, or ***epicardium*** is fused to the heart, except along the cardiac grooves, where it is separated from the heart by blood vessels.

The two layers are continuous with each other at the roots of the great vessels, i.e. ascending aorta, pulmonary trunk, two venae cavae, and four pulmonary veins.

PERICARDIAL CAVITY

The ***pericardial cavity*** is a potential space between the parietal pericardium and the visceral pericardium (Fig. 18.1).

Normally, it contains a thin film of serous fluid (15–20 ml) which lubricates the apposed surfaces and allows the heart to beat smoothly.

Differences between parietal and visceral pericardia are listed in Table 18.1.

CONTENTS OF PERICARDIUM

1. Heart with cardiac veins, coronary arteries and nerves
2. Ascending aorta
3. Pulmonary trunk
4. Lower half of the superior vena cava
5. Terminal part of the inferior vena cava
6. The terminal parts of the pulmonary veins.

BLOOD SUPPLY

The fibrous and parietal pericardia are supplied by branches from:

1. Internal thoracic arteries
2. Musculophrenic arteries
3. The descending thoracic aorta
4. Veins drain into corresponding veins.

NERVE SUPPLY

1. The fibrous and parietal pericardia are supplied by the phrenic nerves. They are sensitive to pain.
2. The epicardium is supplied by autonomic nerves of the heart and is not sensitive to pain.

Note: Pain of pericarditis originates in the parietal pericardium alone. On the other hand, cardiac pain or angina originates in the cardiac muscle or in the vessels of the heart.

TABLE 18.1: Differences between parietal and visceral pericardia

Parietal pericardium	*Visceral pericardium (epicardium)*
Outer layer of serous pericardium	Inner layer of serous pericardium
Lines the inner surface of fibrous pericardium	Lines the external surface of the heart
Firmly adherent to fibrous pericardium	Separated from myocardium by subserous areolar tissue and blood vessels
Develops from somatopleuric mesoderm	Develops from splanchnopleuric mesoderm
Innervated by somatic nerves	Innervated by autonomic nerves
Pain sensitive	Pain insensitive

SINUSES OF PERICARDIUM

The sinuses of pericardium are the communicating zones that are developed by the reflection of serous pericardium. There are two sinuses of pericardium (Plate 18.3, Flowchart 18.2):

1. Transverse sinus
2. Oblique sinus.

The epicardium at the roots of the great vessels is arranged in form of two tubes. The arterial tube encloses the ascending aorta and the pulmonary trunk at the arterial end of the heart tube, and the venous tube encloses the venae cavae and pulmonary veins at the venous end of the heart tube. The passage between the two tubes is known as the *transverse sinus* of pericardium.

During development, to begin with, the veins of the heart are crowded together. As the heart increases in size and these veins separate out, a pericardial reflection surrounds all of them and forms the *oblique pericardial sinus*. This cul-de-sac is posterior to the left atrium (Fig. 18.4).

Flowchart 18.2: Sinuses of pericardium

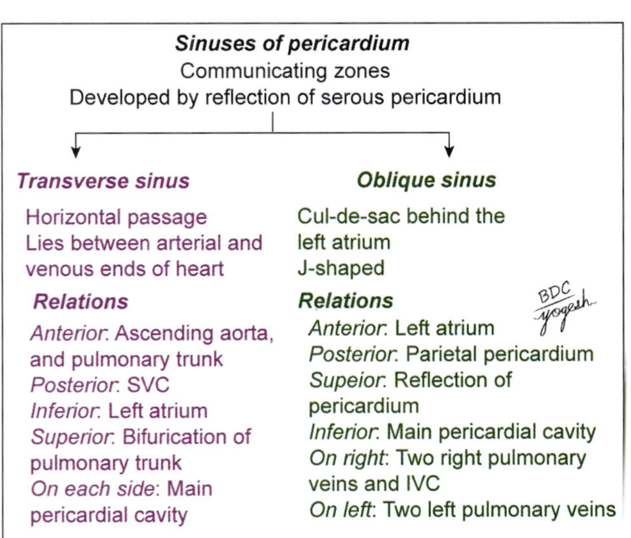

Plate 18.3: Sinuses of pericardium

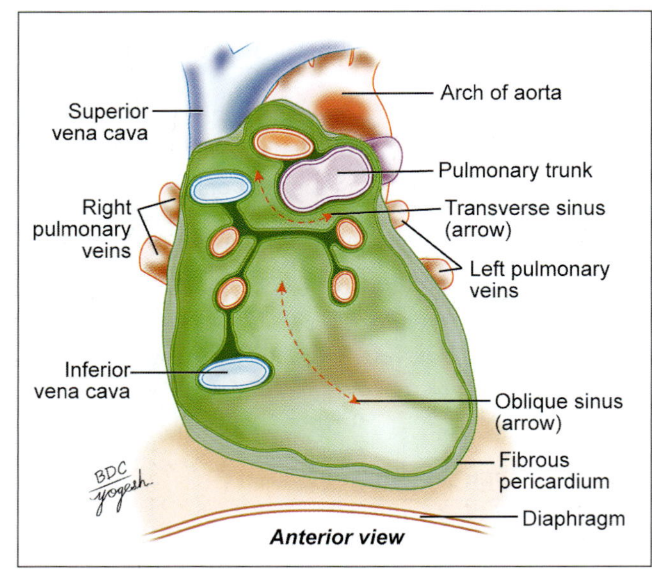

Transverse Sinus

The *transverse sinus* is a horizontal gap between the arterial and venous ends of the heart tube (Fig. 18.4). It develops from degeneration of the central part of dorsal mesocardium.

Boundaries

Anterior:	Ascending aorta, pulmonary trunk
Posterior:	Superior vena cava
Inferior:	Left atrium
Superior:	Bifurcation of pulmonary trunk
On each side:	Opens into the main pericardial cavity.

Oblique Sinus

The *oblique sinus* is a narrow gap behind the heart. The oblique sinus permits pulsations of the left atrium to take place freely (Figs 18.4 and 18.5). It develops due to rearrangement of veins at the venous end.

Boundaries

Anterior:	Left atrium
Posterior:	Parietal pericardium
On the right:	Two right pulmonary veins and inferior vena cava
On the left:	Two left pulmonary veins
Superior:	Reflection of visceral pericardium along the right and left superior pulmonary veins (along the upper margin of left atrium)
Inferior:	Communicates with the main pericardial cavity.

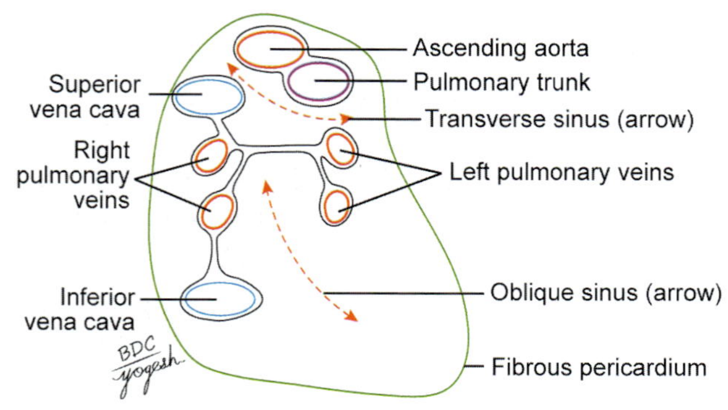

Fig. 18.4: Pericardial cavity seen after removal of the heart. Note the reflections of pericardium, and the mode of formation of the transverse and oblique sinuses

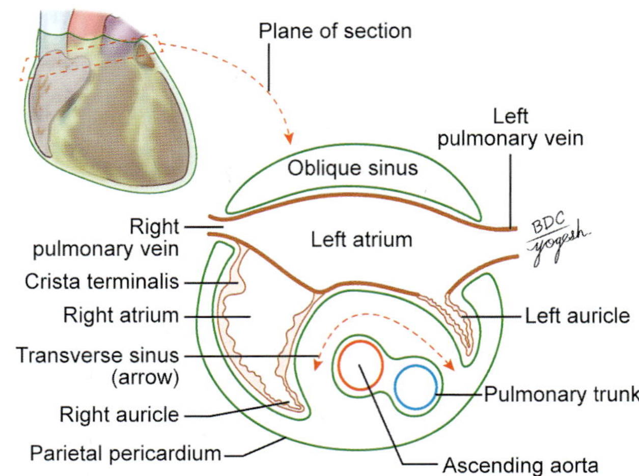

Fig. 18.5: Transverse section through the upper part of the heart. Note that oblique sinus forms posterior boundary of left atrium

CLINICAL ANATOMY

- ***Significance of transverse pericardial sinus*:** During heart surgery, the ligature is passed through the transverse sinus around aorta and the pulmonary trunk (Fig. 18.6).
- ***Pericarditis*:** It is an inflammation of the pericardium. As fibrous and parietal pericardia are pain sensitive, pericarditis induces pain (Fig. 18.7).
- ***Pericardial friction rub*:** In pericarditis, smooth opposing surfaces of serous pericardium become rough. It results in pericardial friction rub. It can be heard as the rustle of silk with the use of stethoscope (Fig. 18.7).
- ***Pericardial effusion*:** Collection of fluid in the pericardial cavity is referred to as *pericardial effusion* (Fig. 18.8). The fluid compresses the heart and restricts venous filling during diastole. It also reduces cardiac output. Radiologically, it shows ***water-bottle heart*** on chest radiograph. It has enlarged cardiac shadow in the form of a shape of a flask or water bottle (Fig. 18.9).
- ***Pericardiocentesis*:** Pericardial effusion can be drained by puncturing the left 5th or 6th intercostal space just lateral to the sternum, or in the angle between the xiphoid process and left costal margin, with the needle directed upwards, backwards and to the left (Fig. 18.8).
- ***Cardiac tamponade*:** It is a type of pericardial effusion that results in compression of the heart (Fig. 18.10). It occurs due to inelastic nature of tough fibrous pericardium. Cardiac tamponade reduces filling of

cardiac chambers during diastole and thus reduces cardiac output.
- In mitral stenosis, left atrium enlarges and compresses the oesophagus causing dysphagia.

DISSECTION

Make a vertical cut through each side of the pericardium immediately anterior to the line of the phrenic nerve. Join the lower ends of these two incisions by a transverse cut approximately 1 cm above the diaphragm. Turn the flap of pericardium upwards and sideways to examine the pericardial cavity. See that the turned flap comprises fibrous and parietal layer of visceral pericardium. The pericardium enclosing the heart is its visceral layer (Fig. 18.1).

Pass a probe from the right side behind the ascending aorta and pulmonary trunk till it appears on the left just to the right of left atrium. This probe is in the *transverse sinus of the pericardium* (Fig. 18.4).

Lift the apex of the heart upwards. Put a finger behind the left atrium into a cul-de-sac, bounded to the right and below by inferior vena cava and above and to left by lower left pulmonary vein. This is the *oblique sinus of pericardium*.

Define the borders, surfaces, grooves, apex, and base of the heart.

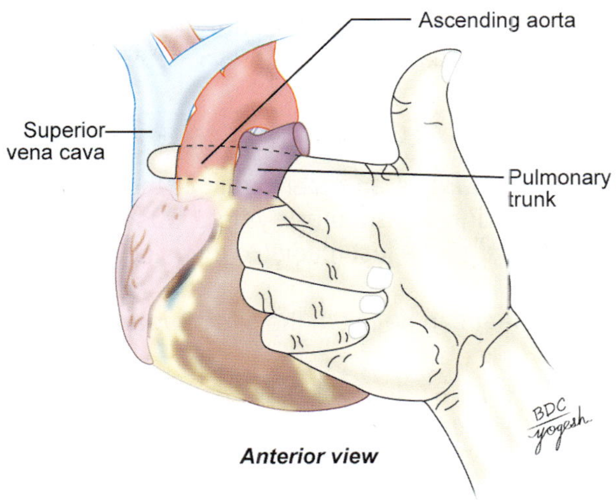

Fig. 18.6: Transverse sinus of pericardium (passage for ligature around ascending aorta and pulmonary trunk through the transverse sinus is shown with index finger)

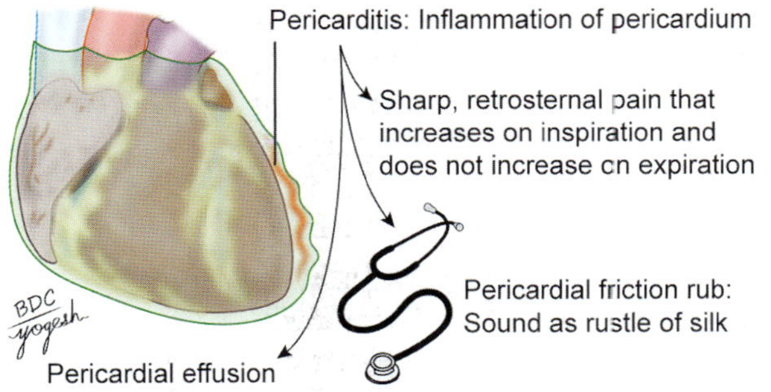

Fig. 18.7: Pericarditis: Clinical presentation and examination

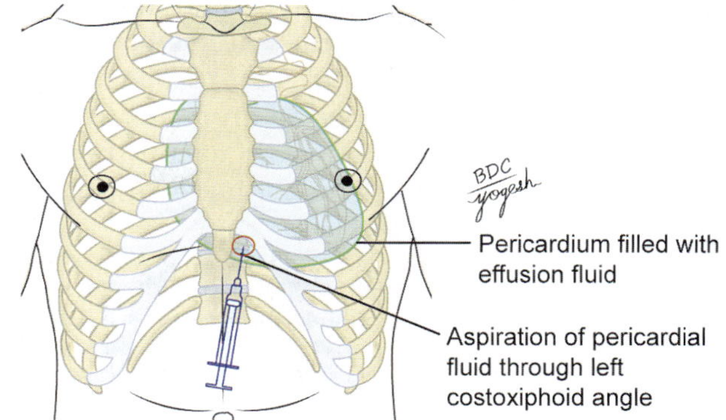

Fig. 18.8: Drainage of pericardial effusion

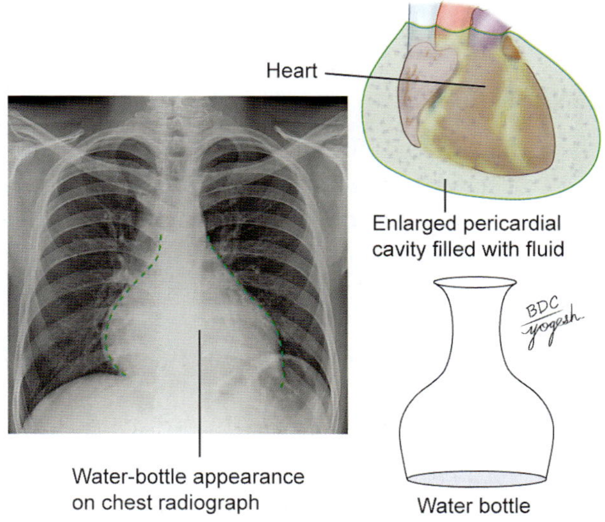

Fig. 18.9: Radiological finding in pericardial effusion (chest radiograph, PA view)

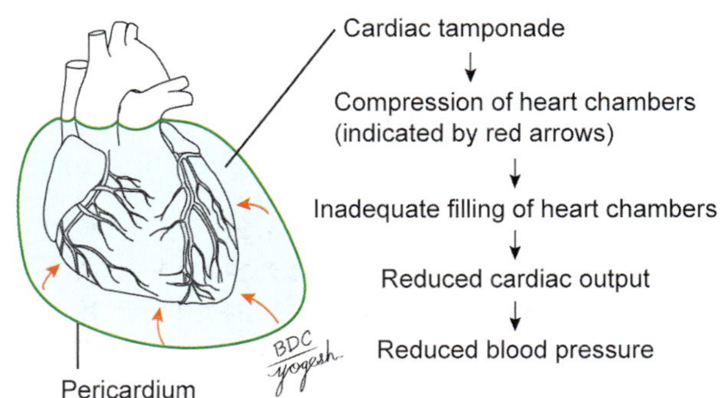

Fig. 18.10: Cardiac tamponade

HEART

The heart is a conical hollow muscular organ situated in the middle mediastinum. It is enclosed within the pericardium. The Greek name for the heart is *cardia* from which we have the adjective *cardiac*. The Latin name for the heart is *cor* from which we have the adjective *coronary*.

The heart is placed obliquely behind the body of the sternum and adjoining parts of the costal cartilages, so that 1/3rd of it lies to the right and 2/3rd to the left of the median plane.

The human heart has four chambers. These are the right and left atria and the right and left ventricles. The atria (Latin *chamber*) lie above and behind the ventricles. On the surface of the heart, they are separated from the ventricles by an *atrioventricular groove*. The atria are separated from each other by an *interatrial groove*. The ventricles are separated from each other by an *interventricular groove*, which is subdivided into anterior and posterior parts (Fig. 18.11).

Note: The names given to the heart chamber as right and left does not fully correspond to their location in the heart.

Measurements

- *Shape*: Conical or pyramidal
- *Length*: 12 cm (from base to apex)
- *Width*: 8–9 cm (broadest transverse diameter)
- *Weight*: 300 g in adult males, 250 g in adult female

EXTERNAL FEATURES

The heart has (Plates 18.4 and 18.5, Flowchart 18.3):

- Apex directed downwards, forwards and to the left.
- Base (posterior surface) directed backwards
- Surfaces: Anterior/sternocostal, inferior, right pulmonary and left pulmonary [*Reference*: 42nd edn. Gray's Anatomy]
- *Borders:* The surfaces are demarcated by upper, inferior, right and left borders.

Note: *Previous concept: Heart has three surfaces: Anterior, inferior, and left.*

Grooves or Sulci

The heart shows the following sulci (Fig. 18.11):

1. ***Atrioventricular*** or ***coronary sulcus:*** The atria are separated from the ventricles by a circular *atrioventricular* or *coronary sulcus.*
   It is divided into anterior and posterior parts.
   a. ***Anterior part*** consists of right and left halves. It is overlapped anteriorly by the ascending aorta and the pulmonary trunk.
      Right half is oblique between right auricle and right ventricle, lodging right coronary artery.
      Left part is small between left auricle and left ventricle, lodges circumflex branch of left coronary artery.
   b. ***Posterior part*** intervenes between the base and the diaphragmatic surface of the heart. It lodges coronary sinus.
2. ***Interatrial groove:*** It is faintly visible posteriorly, while anteriorly, it is hidden by the aorta and pulmonary trunk.
3. ***Anterior interventricular groove:*** It is nearer to the left margin of the heart. It runs downwards and to the left. The lower end of the groove separates the apex from the rest of the inferior border of the heart.
4. ***Posterior interventricular groove:*** It is situated on the diaphragmatic or inferior surface of the heart. It is nearer to the right margin of this surface (Plate 18.5). The two interventricular grooves meet at the inferior border near the apex.

Note: ***Crux of the Heart*** is the meeting point of interatrial, atrioventricular and posterior interventricular grooves.

Apex of the Heart

Apex of the heart is formed entirely by the left ventricle. It is directed downwards, forwards and to the left and is overlapped by the anterior border of the left lung.

Location: It is situated in the left 5th intercostal space 9 cm lateral to the midsternal line just medial to the midclavicular line (Fig. 18.11).

CLINICAL ANATOMY

- ***Apex impulse*** is an outer thrust of the apex of the heart during ventricular systole observed in 5th intercostal space just medial to the midclavicular line (Fig. 18.12).
- ***Apex beat*** can be felt at the site of apex impulse.

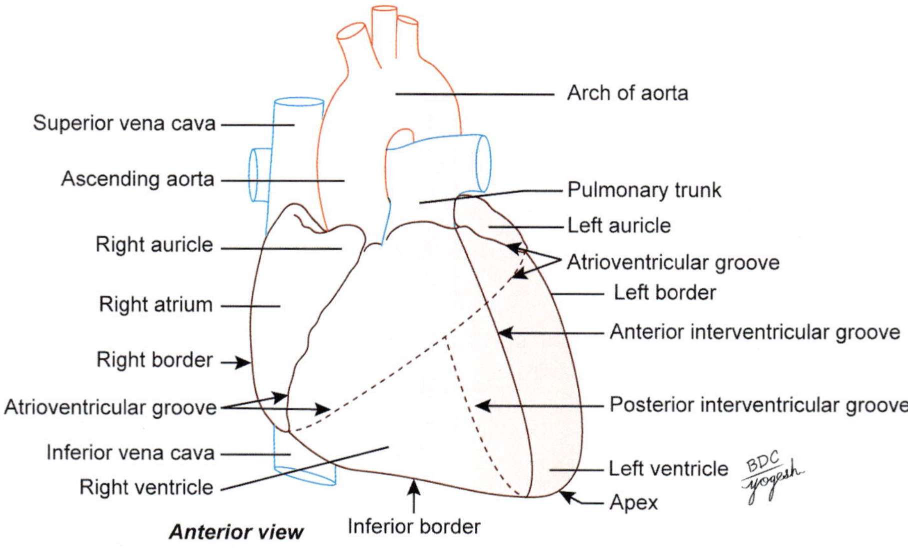

Fig. 18.11: Gross features: Sternocostal surface of heart

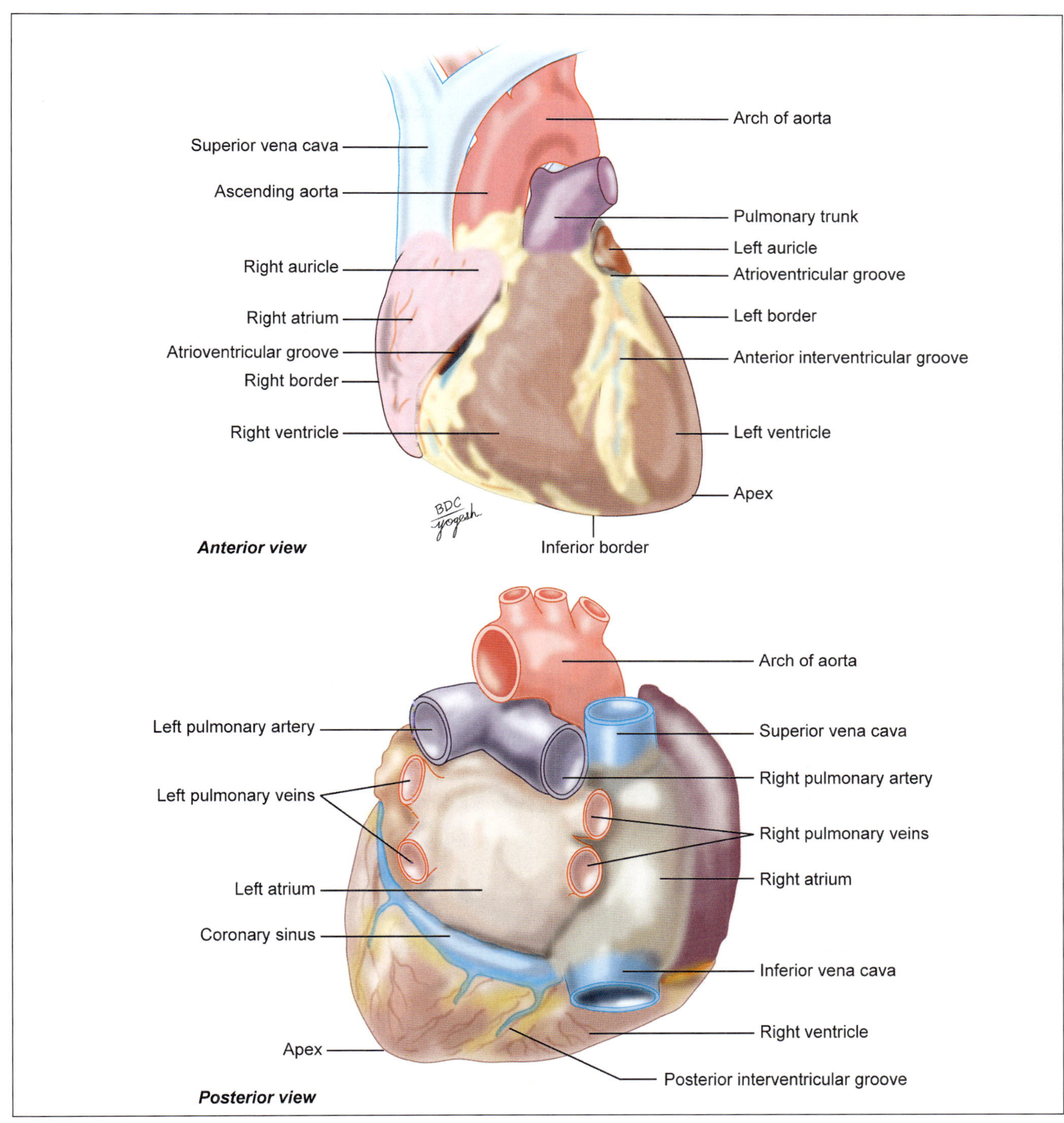

- In children below 2 years, apex is situated in the left 4th intercostal space in midclavicular line.
- Normally, the cardiac apex or apex beat is on the left side. In the condition called ***dextrocardia***, the apex is on the right side (Fig. 18.13). Dextrocardia may be part of a condition called *situs inversus* in which all thoracic and abdominal viscera are a mirror image of normal.

Base (Posterior Surface) of the Heart

The *base* of the heart is also called its ***posterior surface***. It is formed mainly by the left atrium and by a small part of the right atrium (Fig. 18.14).

Features

1. The base has the openings of
   a. four pulmonary veins which open into the left atrium
   b. superior and inferior venae cavae which open into the right atrium.
2. *Level*: It is related to T5 to T8 vertebrae in the lying posture, and descends by one vertebra in the erect posture.
3. It is separated from the vertebral column by the pericardium, the right pulmonary veins, the oesophagus, and the aorta.

Plate 18.5: Posteroinferior view of heart

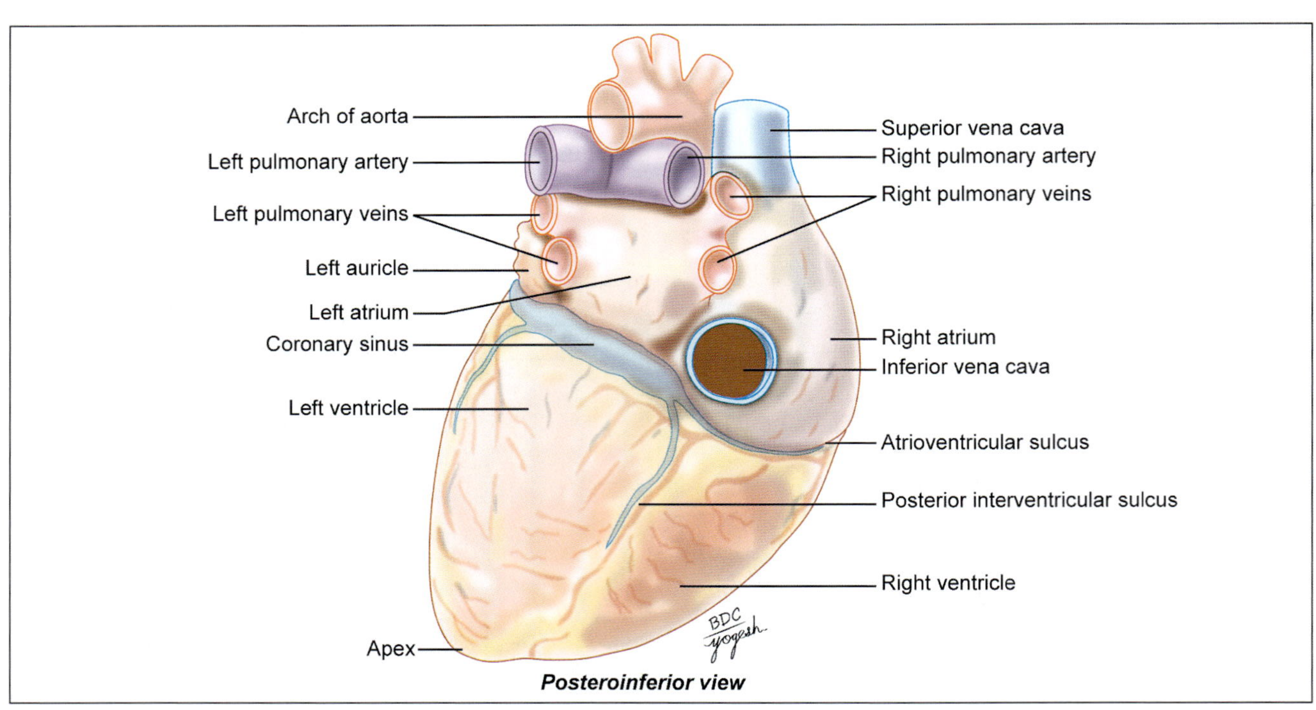

Posteroinferior view

Flowchart 18.3: External features of heart

External features of heart

- ***Apex***
  - Conical
  - Formation: Left ventricle
- ***Base***
  - Posterior surface
  - Formation: 2/3rd by left atrium, 1/3rd by right atrium
- ***Surfaces***
  1. Anterior
  2. Inferior
  3. Left
  4. Right
- ***Borders***
  1. Right
  2. Left
  3. Inferior
  4. Upper

Grooves (sulci) of the heart

- ***Coronary (AV) sulcus***
  - Separates atria from ventricles
  - Contents: Trunk and circumflex branch of LCA, coronary sinus, RCA, anterior cardiac vein
- ***Interventricular sulcus***
  - Separates ventricles
  - ***Anterior*** — Contents: Anterior interventricular branch of LCA, great cardiac vein
  - ***Posterior (inferior)*** — Contents: Posterior interventricular branch of coronary artery, middle cardiac vein
- ***Interatrial sulcus***
  - Separates atria
  - Indicates attachment of interatrial septum

Surfaces of heart

	Anterior (sternocostal) surface	***Inferior (diaphragmatic) surface***	***Left surface***	***Right surface***
Formation	Right atrium, right auricle, left auricle, left ventricle, right ventricle	Left ventricle, right ventricle	Left auricle, left atrium	Right atrium
Features	Atrioventricular groove Anterior interventricular groove	Posterior interventricular groove	Convex, rounded Left atrioventricular groove	Rounded Sulcus terminalis

Borders of heart

	Right border	***Left border***	***Inferior border***	***Upper border***
Formation	Right atrium	Mainly by left ventricle, partly by left auricle	Mainly by right ventricle, partly by left ventricle	Right and left atria
Extension	From opening of SVC to opening of IVC	From left auricle to apex of the heart	From opening of IVC to apex of the heart	From upper end of right heart border to left heart border

BDC yogesh

Borders of the Heart (Plate 18.6)

1. ***Right border***: It is more or less vertical and is formed by the right atrium. It extends from superior vena cava to inferior vena cava (IVC).
2. ***Left border***: It is oblique and curved. It is formed mainly by the left ventricle, and partly by the left auricle. It separates the anterior and left surfaces of the heart (Fig. 18.11). It extends from apex to left auricle.

Plate 18.6: **Borders of heart**

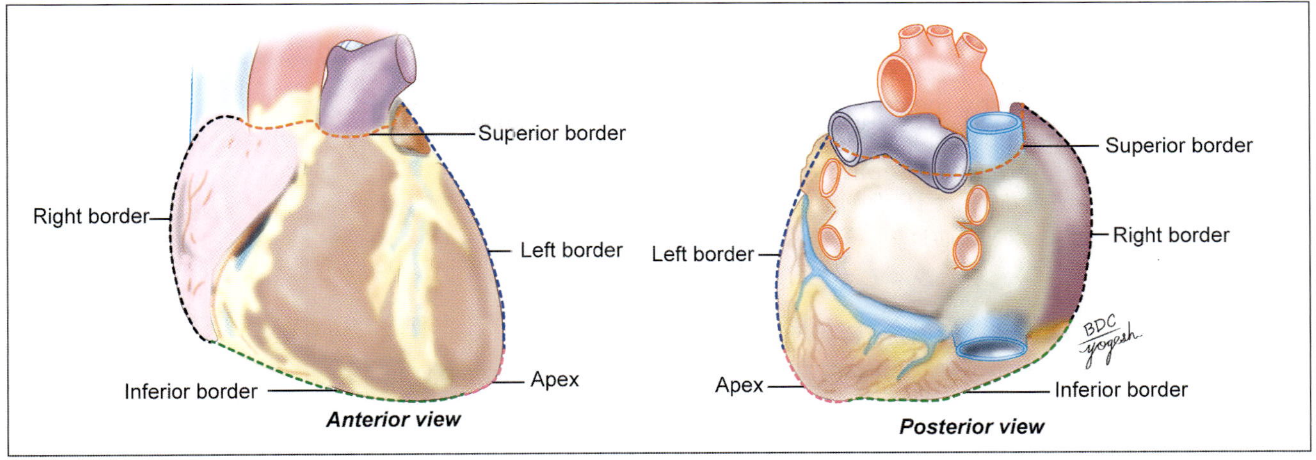

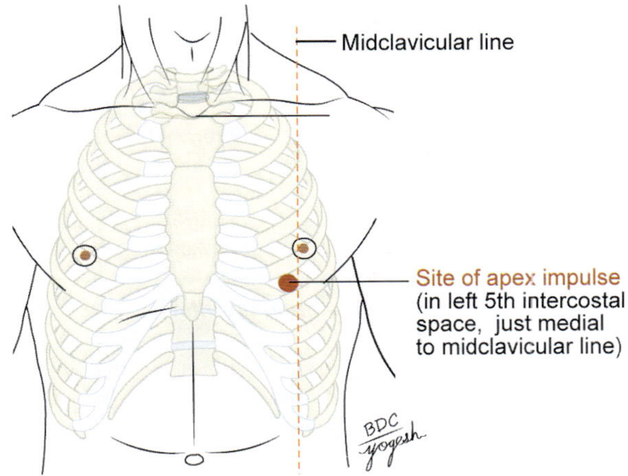

Fig. 18.12: Site of apex impulse and apex beat

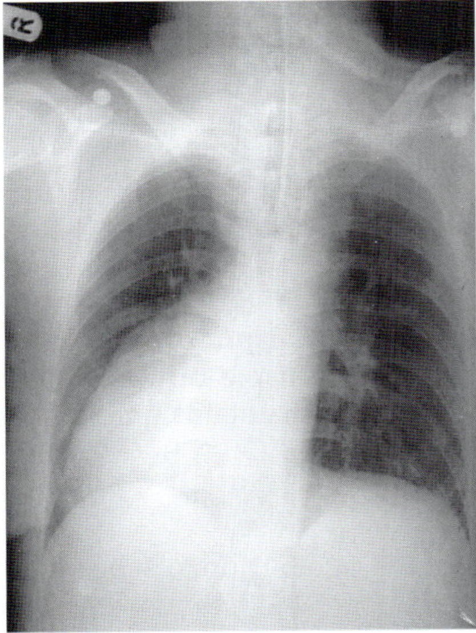

Fig. 18.13: Dextrocardia

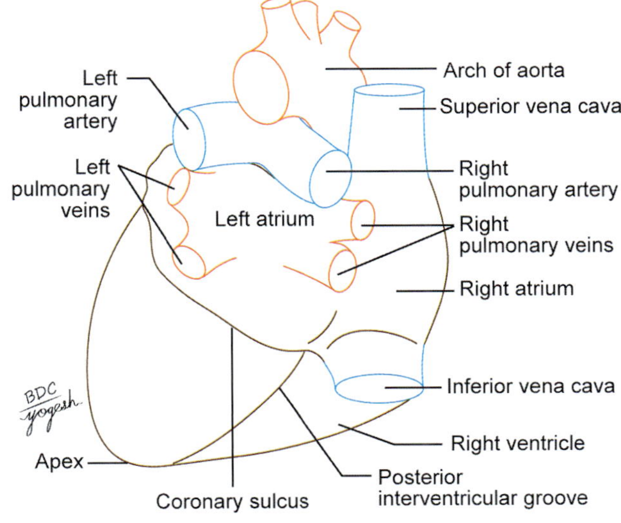

Fig. 18.14: Base or posterior surface of the heart

3. ***Inferior border***: It is nearly horizontal and is formed mainly by the right ventricle. A small part of it near the apex is formed by left ventricle. It extends from IVC to apex. *Incisura apicis cordis* is a small notch on the inferior border near the apex of the heart. It gives passage to anterior interventricular branch of left coronary artery.
4. ***Upper border***: It is slightly oblique, and is formed by the two atria, chiefly the left atrium. Anteriorly, the upper border is overlapped by pulmonary trunk and aorta.

Surfaces of the Heart

1. ***Anterior*** or ***sternocostal surface***: It is formed mainly by the right atrium and right ventricle, and partly by the left ventricle and left auricle (Fig. 18.11). The left atrium is not seen on the anterior surface as it is covered by the aorta and pulmonary trunk. Most of the sternocostal surface is covered by the lungs, but a part of it that lies behind the cardiac notch of the left lung is uncovered. The uncovered area is dull on percussion. Clinically, it is referred to as the *area of superficial cardiac dullness*.
2. ***Inferior*** or ***diaphragmatic surface***: It rests on the central tendon of the diaphragm. It is formed in its left 2/3rd by the left ventricle, and in its right 1/3rd

by the right ventricle. It is traversed by the posterior interventricular groove, and is directed downwards and slightly backwards (Fig. 18.14).

3. ***Left surface*:** It is formed mostly by the left ventricle, and at the upper end by the left auricle. In its upper part, the surface is crossed by the coronary sulcus.
4. ***Right surface*:** It is rounded and formed by the right atrial wall. The sulcus terminalis separates the right surface from the anterior surface [*Reference*: 42nd edn. Gray's Anatomy].

Types of Circulation

There are two main types of circulations—systemic and pulmonary. Flowchart 18.4 shows their comparison.

Competency:
AN22.2 Describe and demonstrate external and internal features of each chamber of heart.

RIGHT ATRIUM

Position

The right atrium is the right upper chamber of the heart. It receives venous blood from the whole body, pumps it to the right ventricle through the right atrioventricular or tricuspid opening. It forms the right border, part of the upper border, the sternocostal surface, and the base of the heart (Fig. 18.7, Flowchart 18.5).

External Features

1. The chamber is elongated vertically, receiving the superior vena cava at the upper end and the inferior vena cava at the lower end (Fig. 18.11).
2. The upper end is prolonged to the left to form the ***right auricle*** (Latin *little ear*). The auricle covers the root of the ascending aorta and partly overlaps the infundibulum of the right ventricle. Its margins are notched and the interior is sponge-like, which prevents free flow of blood.
3. Along the right border of the atrium, there is a shallow vertical groove which passes from the superior vena cava to the inferior vena cava. This groove is called the ***sulcus terminalis***. It is produced by an internal muscular ridge called the *crista terminalis* (Fig. 18.11). The upper part of the sulcus contains the *sinuatrial* or ***SA node*** which acts as the pacemaker of the heart.
4. The *right atrioventricular groove* separates the right atrium from the right ventricle. It is more or less vertical and lodges the right coronary artery and the small cardiac vein.

Tributaries or Inlets of the Right Atrium

1. Superior vena cava
2. Inferior vena cava
3. Coronary sinus
4. Anterior cardiac veins
5. Venae cordis minimae (Thebesian veins)
6. Sometimes the right marginal vein

Flowchart 18.4: Comparing the systemic circulation and pulmonary circulation

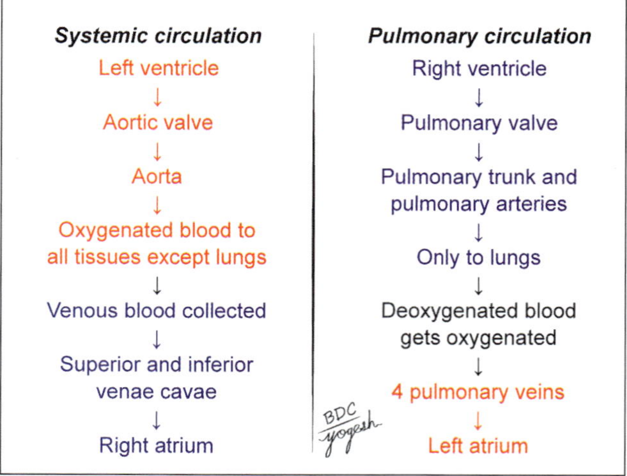

Flowchart 18.5: Right atrium

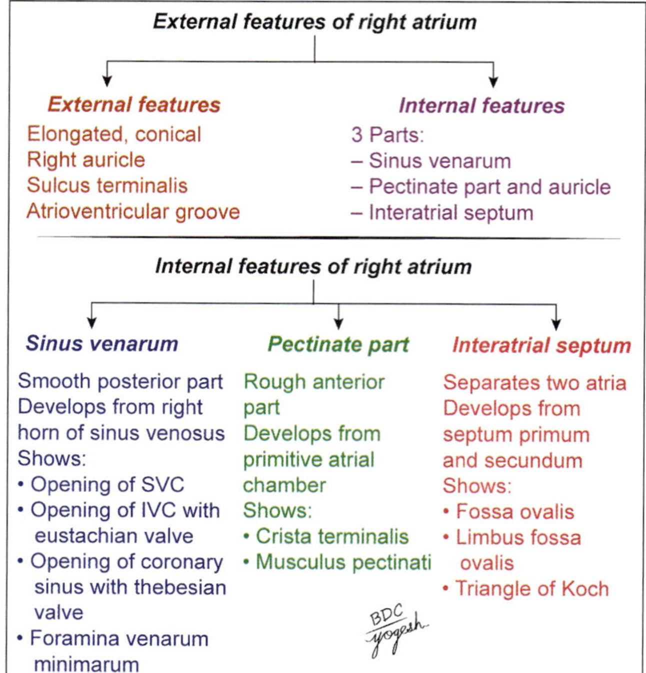

Right Atrioventricular Orifice

Blood passes out of the right atrium through the right atrioventricular or ***tricuspid orifice*** and goes to the right ventricle. The tricuspid orifice is guarded by the tricuspid valve which maintains unidirectional flow of blood (Fig. 18.15).

Internal Features

The interior of the right atrium can be broadly divided into three parts (Plate 18.7): Sinus venarum, pectinate part, and interatrial septum.

Smooth Posterior Part or Sinus Venarum

1. Developmentally, it is derived from the right horn of the sinus venosus.
2. Most of the tributaries except the anterior cardiac veins open into it.
   a. The *superior vena cava* opens at the upper end.

Plate 18.7: Interior of right atrium (cut along coronary sulcus)

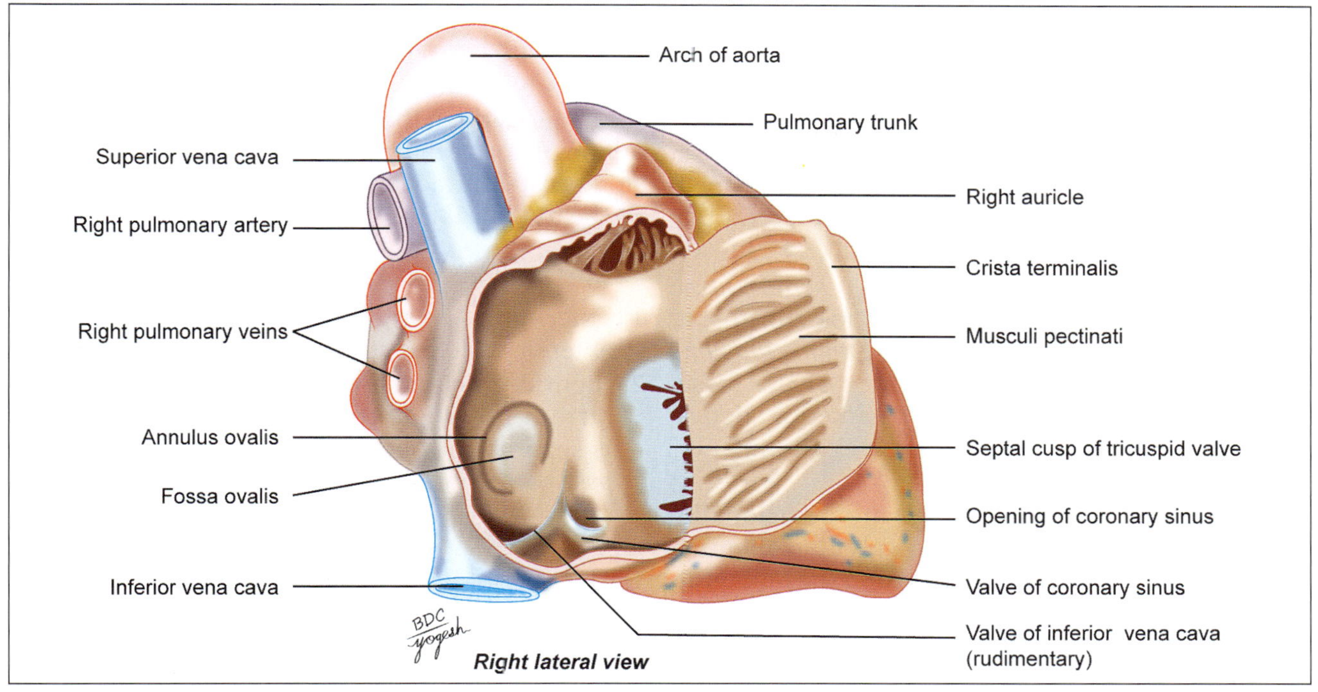

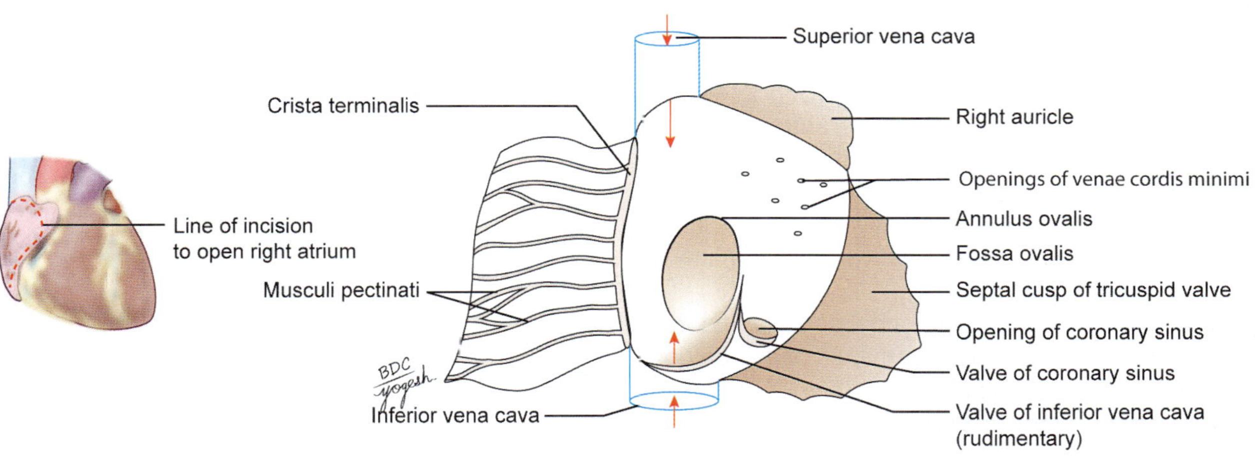

Fig. 18.15: Interior of right atrium (cut along sulcus terminalis)

b. The *inferior vena cava* opens at the lower end (Fig. 18.15).

The opening of inferior vena cava is guarded by a rudimentary valve of the inferior vena cava or ***Eustachian valve***. During embryonic life, the valve guides the inferior vena caval blood to the left atrium through the *foramen ovale*.

c. The *coronary sinus* opens between the opening of the inferior vena cava and the right atrioventricular orifice. The opening is guarded by the *valve of the coronary sinus* or *thebesian valve*.

d. The *venae cordis minimae* are numerous small veins present in the walls of all the four chambers. They open into the right atrium through small foramina.

3. The ***intervenous tubercle* of *Lower*** is a very small projection, scarcely visible, on the posterior wall of the atrium just below the opening of the superior vena cava. During embryonic life, it directs the superior caval blood to the right ventricle.

4. ***Triangle of Koch*** is bounded by ostium of coronary sinus, septal leaflet of tricuspid valve and tendon of Todaro, a subendocardial ridge. AV node lies at the apex, of this triangle.

Rough Anterior Part or Pectinate Part, including the Auricle

1. Developmentally, it is derived from the primitive atrial chamber.
2. It presents a series of transverse muscular ridges called ***musculi pectinati*** (Fig. 18.15).

They arise from the ***crista terminalis*** and run forwards and downwards towards the atrioventricular orifice, giving the appearance of the teeth of a comb. In the auricle, the muscles are interconnected to form a reticular network.

Interatrial Septum

1. Developmentally, it is derived from the *septum primum* and *septum secundum*.
2. It presents the ***fossa ovalis***, a shallow saucer-shaped depression, in the lower part. The fossa represents the site of the embryonic septum primum.
3. The ***annulus ovalis*** or *limbus* (Latin *a border) fossa ovalis* is the prominent margin of the fossa ovalis. It represents the lower free edge of the *septum secundum*. It is distinct above and at the sides of the fossa ovalis, but is deficient inferiorly. Its anterior edge is continuous with the left end of the valve of the inferior vena cava.
4. The remains of the *foramen ovale* are occasionally present. This is a small slit-like valvular opening between the upper part of the fossa and the limbus. It is normally occluded after birth, but may sometimes persist.

DISSECTION

Cut along the upper edge of the right auricle by an incision from the anterior end of the superior vena caval opening to the left side. Similarly cut along its lower edge by an incision extending from the anterior end of the inferior vena caval opening to the left side. Incise the anterior wall of the right atrium near its left margin and reflect the flap to the right (Fig. 18.16).

On its internal surface, see the vertical crista terminalis and horizontal pectinate muscles.

The fossa ovalis is on the interatrial septum and the opening of the coronary sinus is to the left of the inferior vena caval opening.

Define the three cusps of tricuspid valve.

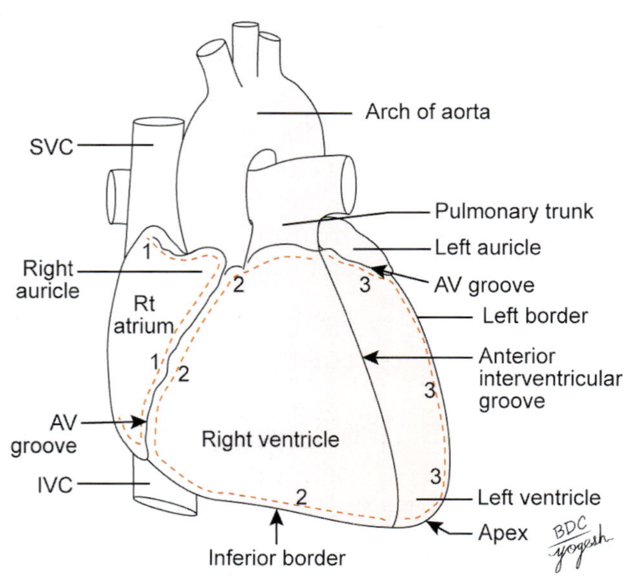

Fig. 18.16: Heart: Line of incisions

RIGHT VENTRICLE

Position

The right ventricle is a triangular chamber which receives blood from the right atrium and pumps it to the lungs through the pulmonary trunk and pulmonary arteries. It forms the inferior border and 2/3rd part of the sternocostal surface and 1/3rd part of inferior surface of the heart (Fig. 18.11, Flowchart 18.6).

External Features

1. Externally, the right ventricle has two surfaces—anterior or sternocostal and inferior or diaphragmatic.
2. Right ventricle is separated externally from the right atrium by *atrioventricular groove*. Right ventricle is separated from the left ventricle by *anterior and posterior (inferior) interventricular grooves*.

Internal Features

1. The interior has two parts (Plate 18.8):
   a. ***Inflowing part***: It is rough due to the presence of muscular ridges called ***trabeculae carneae***. It develops from the proximal part of bulbus cordis of the heart tube.
   b. ***Outflowing part*** or ***infundibulum***: It is smooth and forms the upper conical part of the right ventricle which gives rise to the pulmonary trunk. It develops from the midportion of the bulbus cordis. The two parts are separated by a muscular ridge called the ***supraventricular crest*** or infundibuloventricular crest situated between the tricuspid and pulmonary orifices.
2. The interior shows two orifices:
   a. The right atrioventricular or ***tricuspid orifice***, guarded by the tricuspid valve.
   b. The ***pulmonary orifice*** guarded by the pulmonary valve (Fig. 18.17).

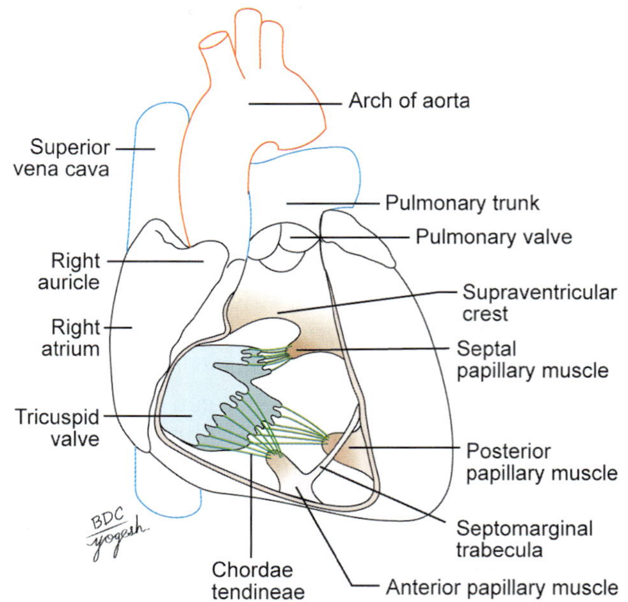

Fig. 18.17: Interior of the right ventricle. Note the moderator band and the supraventricular crest

Plate 18.8: Internal view of right ventricle

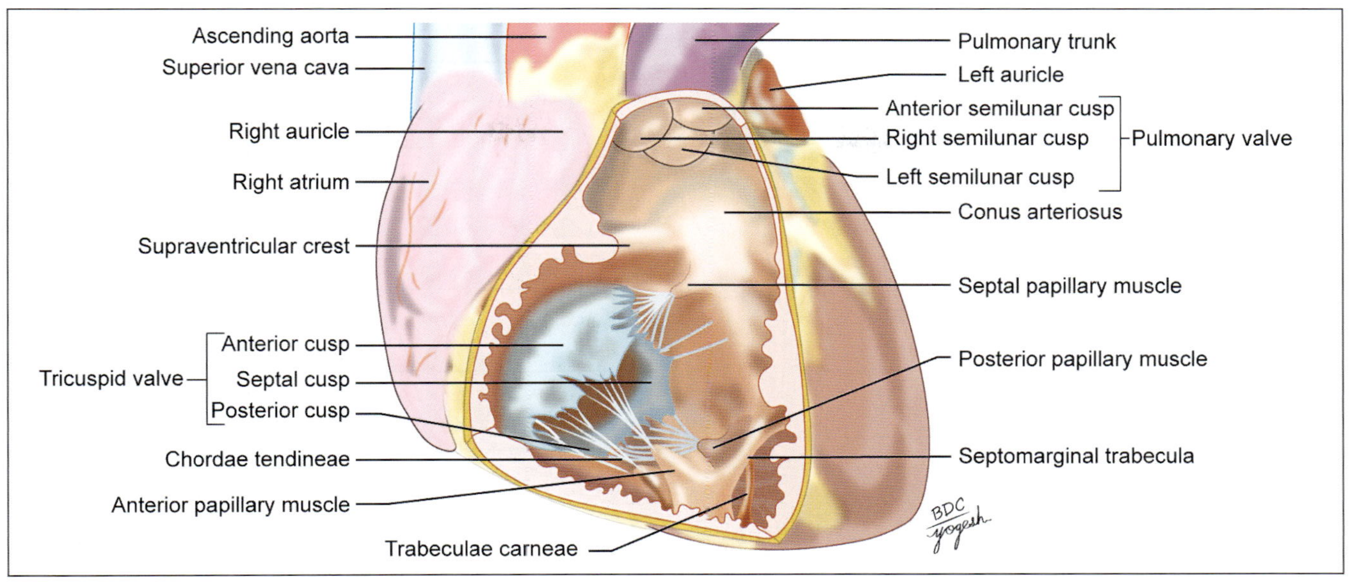

Flowchart 18.6: Features of right ventricle

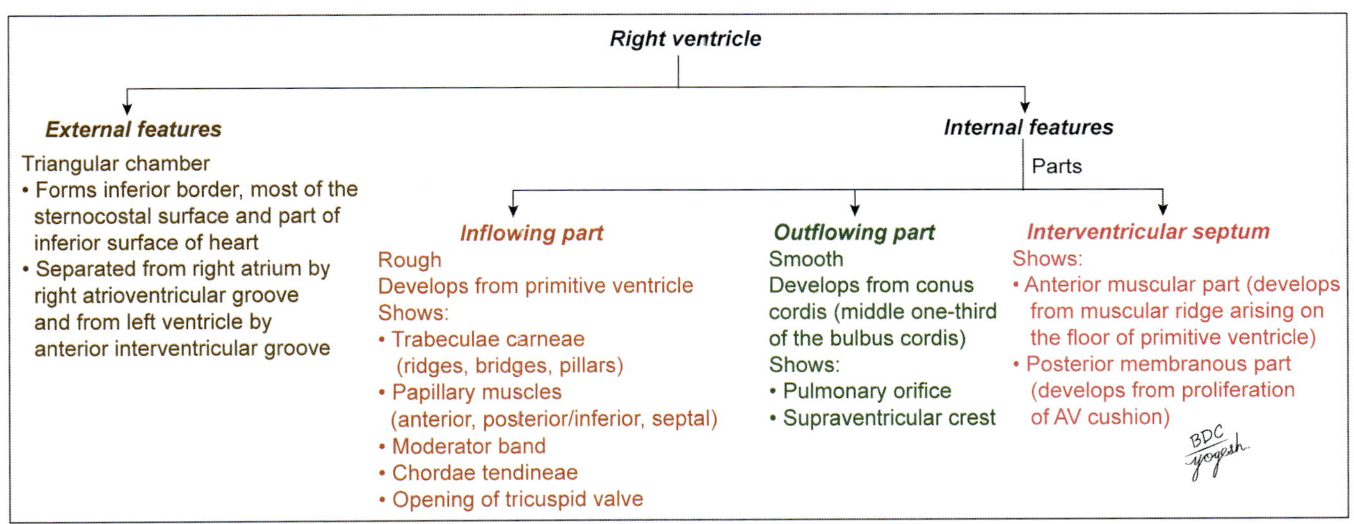

3. The interior of the inflowing part shows ***trabeculae carneae*** or muscular ridges of three types:
   a. ***Ridges*** or fixed elevations
   b. ***Bridges***
   c. ***Papillary muscles*** *(pillars)* with one end attached to the ventricular wall, and the other end connected to the cusps of the tricuspid valve by ***chordae tendineae*** (Latin *strings to stretch*). There are three papillary muscles in the right ventricle:
      i. *Anterior muscle* is the largest (Fig. 18.17).
      ii. *Posterior* or *inferior muscle* is small and irregular.
      iii. *Septal muscle* is divided into a number of little nipples. Each papillary muscle is attached by chordae tendineae to the contiguous sides of two cusps (Fig. 18.18).
4. The *septomarginal trabecula* or ***moderator band*** is a muscular ridge extending from the ventricular septum to the base of the anterior papillary muscle. It contains the right branch of the AV bundle (Fig. 18.17).
5. The cavity of the right ventricle is crescentic in section because of the forward bulge of the interventricular septum (Fig. 18.18).
6. The wall of the right ventricle is thinner than that of the left ventricle in a ratio of 1:3.

Interventricular Septum

The septum is placed obliquely. Its one surface faces forwards and to the right and the other faces backwards and to the left. It has two parts:

a. *Membranous part:* The upper part of the septum is thin and membranous and separates not only the two ventricles but **also the right atrium and left ventricle**.
b. *Muscular part:* The lower part is thick muscular and separates the two ventricles (Fig. 18.18). Its position is indicated by the anterior and posterior interventricular grooves.

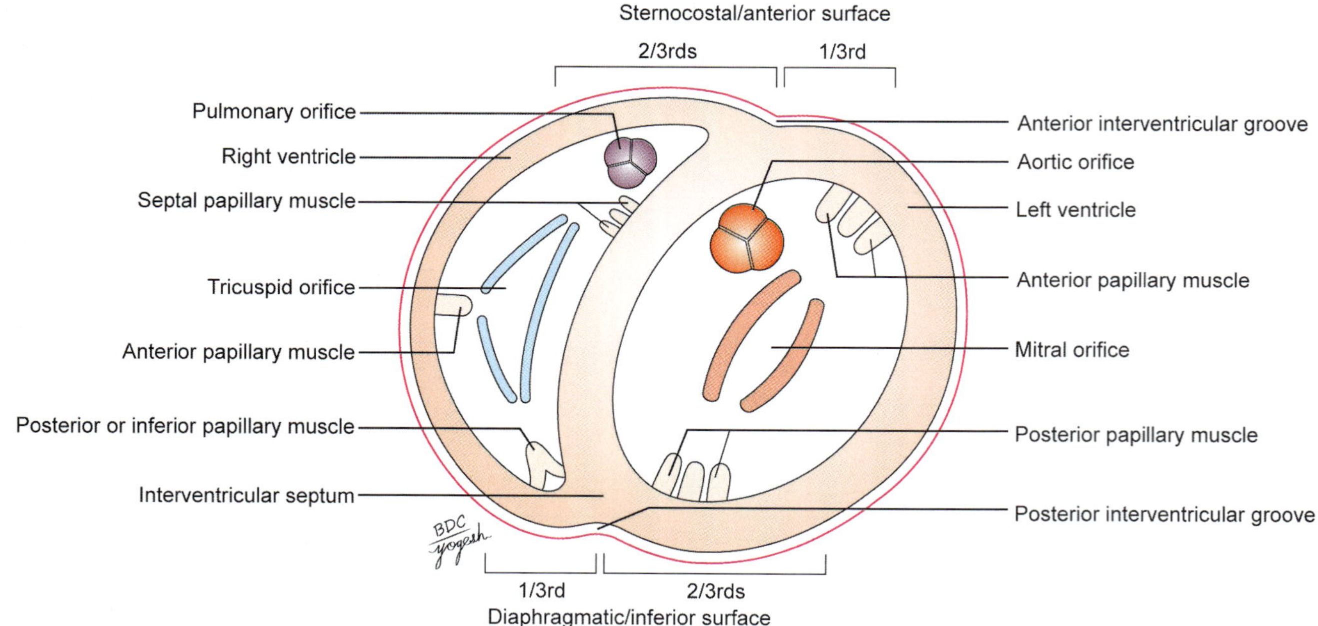

Fig. 18.18: Schematic transverse section through the ventricles of the heart showing the atrioventricular orifices, papillary muscles, and the pulmonary and aortic orifices

DISSECTION

Incise along the ventricular aspect of right AV groove, till you reach the inferior border. Continue to incise along the inferior border till the inferior end of anterior interventricular groove. Next cut along the infundibulum. Now the anterior wall of right ventricle is reflected to the left to study its interior (Fig. 18.16).

LEFT ATRIUM

Position

The left atrium is a quadrangular chamber situated posteriorly. It receives oxygenated blood from the lungs through four pulmonary veins, and pumps it to the left ventricle through the left atrioventricular or bicuspid (Latin *two tooth point*) or mitral orifice (Latin *like bishop's mitre*) which is guarded by the valve of the same name.

External Features

1. Its appendage, the ***left auricle*** projects anteriorly to overlap the infundibulum of the right ventricle.
2. The left atrium forms the left 2/3rd of the base of the heart, the greater part of the upper border, parts of the sternocostal and left surfaces and the left border.
3. The posterior surface of the atrium forms the anterior wall of the oblique sinus of pericardium (Fig. 18.5).

Internal Features (Fig. 18.19)

1. ***Anterior wall:*** The anterior wall of the atrium is formed by the ***interatrial septum***. The septal wall shows the ***fossa lunata*** corresponding to the fossa ovalis of the right atrium.

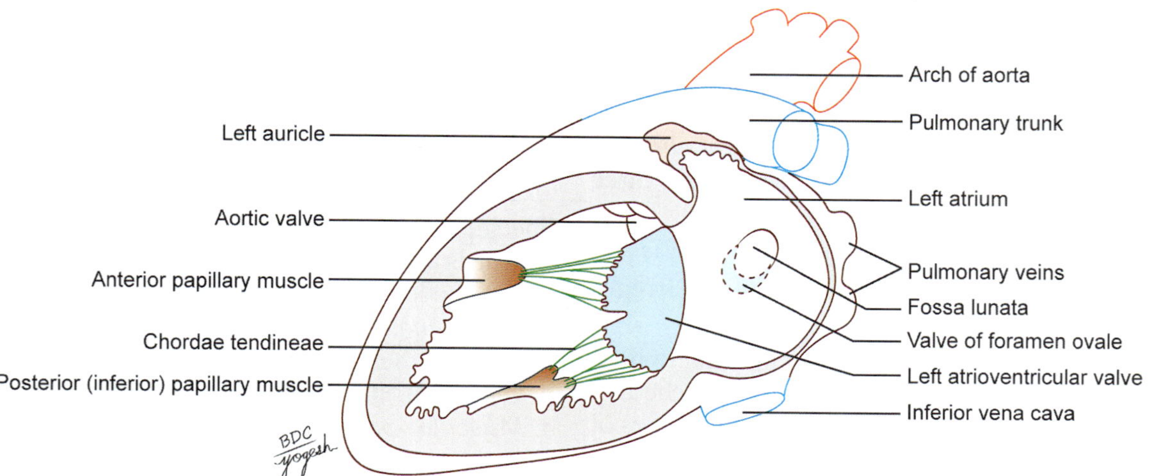

Fig. 18.19: Interior of left atrium and left ventricle

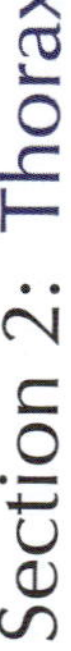

2. ***Posterior wall***: Two *pulmonary veins* open into the atrium on each side of the posterior wall.
3. The greater part of the interior of the atrium is smooth walled. It is derived embryologically from the absorbed pulmonary veins which open into it.
4. ***Musculi pectinati*** are present only in the auricle where they form a reticulum. This part develops from the original *primitive atrial chamber* of the heart tube.
5. In addition to the four pulmonary veins, the tributaries of the atrium include a few *venae cordis minimae*.

Table 18.2 compares the right atrium and the left atrium.

TABLE 18.2: Comparison of right atrium and left atrium

Right atrium	*Left atrium*
Receives venous blood of the body	Receives oxygenated blood from lungs
Pushes blood to right ventricle through tricuspid valve	Pushes blood to left ventricle through bicuspid valve
Forms right border, part of sternocostal and small part of base of the heart	Forms major part of base of the heart
Enlarged in tricuspid stenosis	Enlarged in mitral stenosis

DISSECTION

Cut off the pulmonary trunk and ascending aorta, immediately above the three cusps of the pulmonary and aortic valves. Remove the upper part of the left atrium to visualise its interior (Fig. 18.8). See the upper surface of the cusps of the mitral valve. Revise the fact that left atrium forms the anterior wall of the oblique sinus of the pericardium (Fig. 18.5).

LEFT VENTRICLE

Position

The left ventricle receives oxygenated blood from the left atrium and pumps it into the aorta (Flowchart 18.7).

External Features

1. It forms the apex of the heart, a part of the sternocostal surface, most of the left border and left surface, and the left 2/3rd of the diaphragmatic surface (Fig. 18.19).
2. Externally, the left ventricle has three surfaces—anterior or sternocostal, inferior or diaphragmatic, and left.

Internal Features

1. The interior is divisible into two parts (Plate 18.9):
   a. The lower rough part with *trabeculae carneae* develops from the primitive ventricle of the heart tube (Fig. 18.19).
   b. The upper smooth part or ***aortic vestibule*** gives origin to the ascending aorta: It develops from the midportion of the bulbus cordis. The vestibule lies between the membranous part of the interventricular septum and the anterior or aortic cusp of the mitral valve.
2. The interior of the ventricle shows two orifices:
   a. The left atrioventricular or bicuspid or ***mitral orifice***, guarded by the *bicuspid* or *mitral valve*.
   b. The ***aortic orifice***, guarded by the aortic valve (Fig. 18.18).
3. There are two well-developed ***papillary muscles***—anterior and posterior. *Chordae tendineae* from both muscles are attached to both the cusps of the mitral valve.
4. The cavity of the left ventricle is circular in cross-section (Fig. 18.18).
5. The walls of the left ventricle are three times thicker than those of the right ventricle.

Table 18.3 compares the right ventricle and the left ventricle.

TABLE 18.3: Comparison of right ventricle and left ventricle

Right ventricle	*Left ventricle*
Thinner than left, one-third thickness of left ventricle	Much thicker than right, 3 times thicker than right ventricle
Pushes blood only to the lungs	Pushes blood to top of the body and down to the toes
Contains three small papillary muscles	Contains two strong papillary muscles
Cavity is crescentic	Cavity is circular
Contains deoxygenated blood	Contains oxygenated blood
Forms two-thirds sternocostal and one-third diaphragmatic surfaces	Forms one-third sternocostal and two-thirds diaphragmatic surfaces

Flowchart 18.7: Features of left ventricle

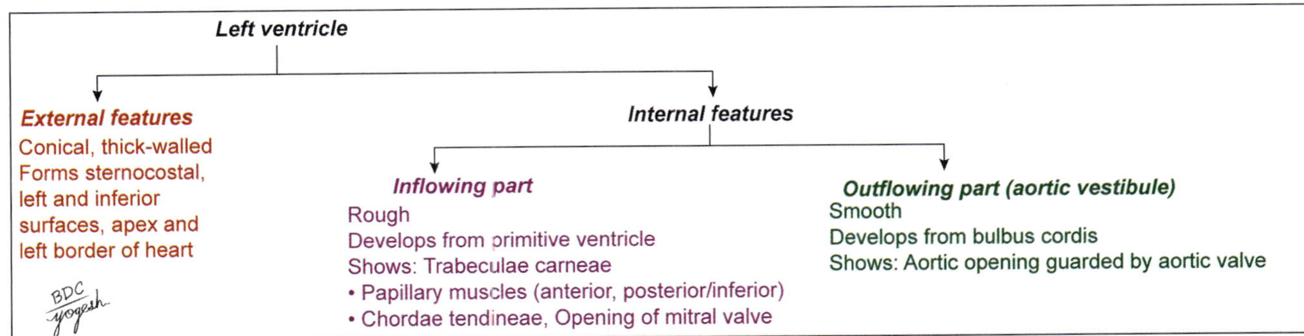

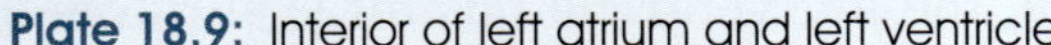

Plate 18.9: Interior of left atrium and left ventricle

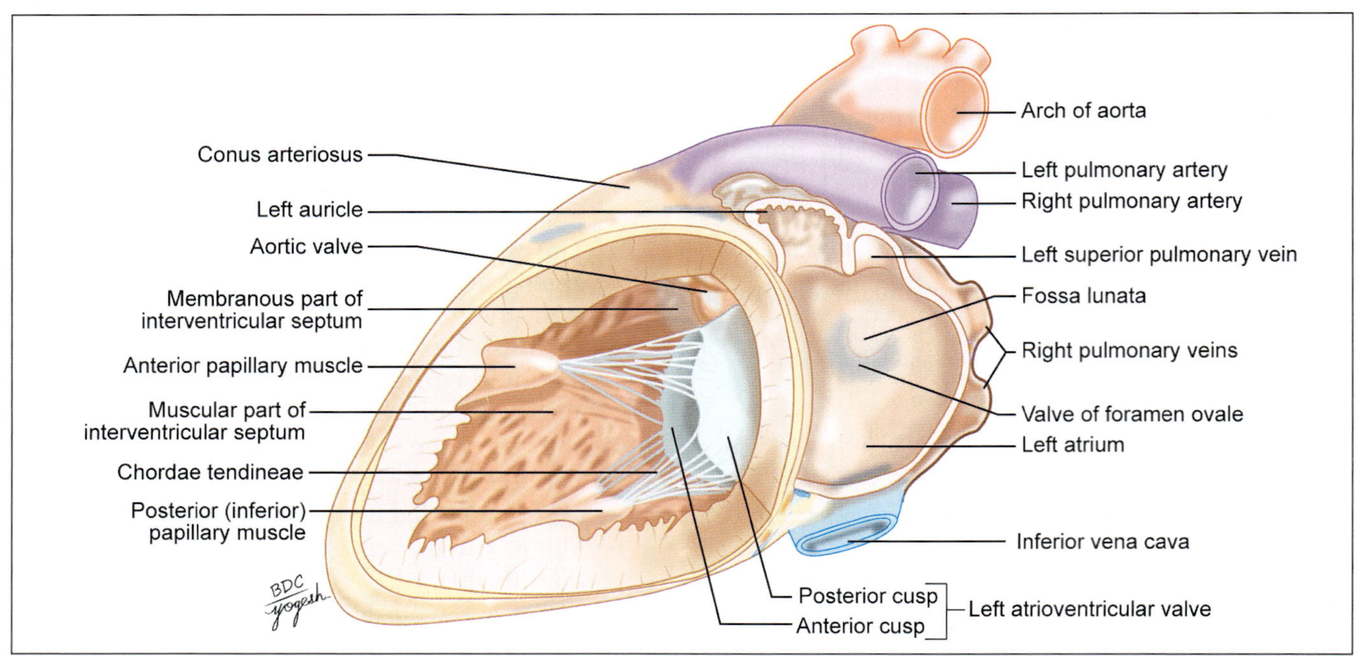

DISSECTION

Open the left ventricle by making a bold incision on the ventricular aspect of atrioventricular groove below left auricle and along whole thickness of left ventricle from above downwards till its apex. Curve the incision towards right till the inferior end of anterior interventricular groove. Reflect the flap to the right and clean the atrioventricular and aortic valves (Fig. 18.16).

Remove the surface layers of the myocardium. Note the general directions of its fibres and the depth of the coronary sulcus, the wall of the atrium passing deep to the bulging ventricular muscle. Dissect the musculature and the conducting system of the heart.

CLINICAL ANATOMY

- The area of the chest wall overlying the heart is called the ***precordium***.
- Inflammation of the heart can involve more than one layer of the heart. Inflammation of the pericardium is called ***pericarditis***; of the myocardium is ***myocarditis***; and of the endocardium is ***endocarditis***.
- Normally, the diastolic pressure in ventricles is zero. A positive diastolic pressure in the ventricle is evidence of its failure. Any one of the four chambers of the heart can fail separately, but ultimately the rising back pressure causes right sided failure (congestive cardiac failure or CCF) which is associated with increased venous pressure, oedema on feet, and breathlessness on exertion. Heart failure (right sided) due to lung disease is known as ***cor pulmonale***.

STRUCTURE OF HEART

VALVES OF HEART

The valves of the heart maintain unidirectional flow of the blood and prevent its regurgitation in the opposite direction. There are two pairs of valves in the heart (Plate 18.10):

1. Pair of atrioventricular valves
   a. Right atrioventricular valve or tricuspid valve — has three cusps
   b. Left atrioventricular valve or bicuspid or mitral valve — has two cusps.
2. Pair of semilunar valves — having three semilunar cusps
   a. Aortic valve
   b. Pulmonary valves.

   The cusps are folds of endocardium, strengthened by an intervening layer of fibrous tissue.

Atrioventricular Valves

1. Both valves are made up of the following components.
   a. A ***fibrous ring*** to which the cusps are attached (Fig. 18.20).
   b. The ***cusps*** are flat and project into the ventricular cavity. Each cusp has an attached and a free margin, and an atrial and a ventricular surface. The atrial surface is smooth (Fig. 18.19). The free margins and ventricular surfaces are rough and irregular due to the attachment of chordae tendineae.
2. The ***chordae tendineae*** connect the free margins and ventricular surfaces of the cusps to the apices of the *papillary muscles*. They prevent eversion of the free margins and limit the amount of ballooning of the cusps towards the cavity of the atrium.

Plate 18.10: Tricuspid and mitral valves

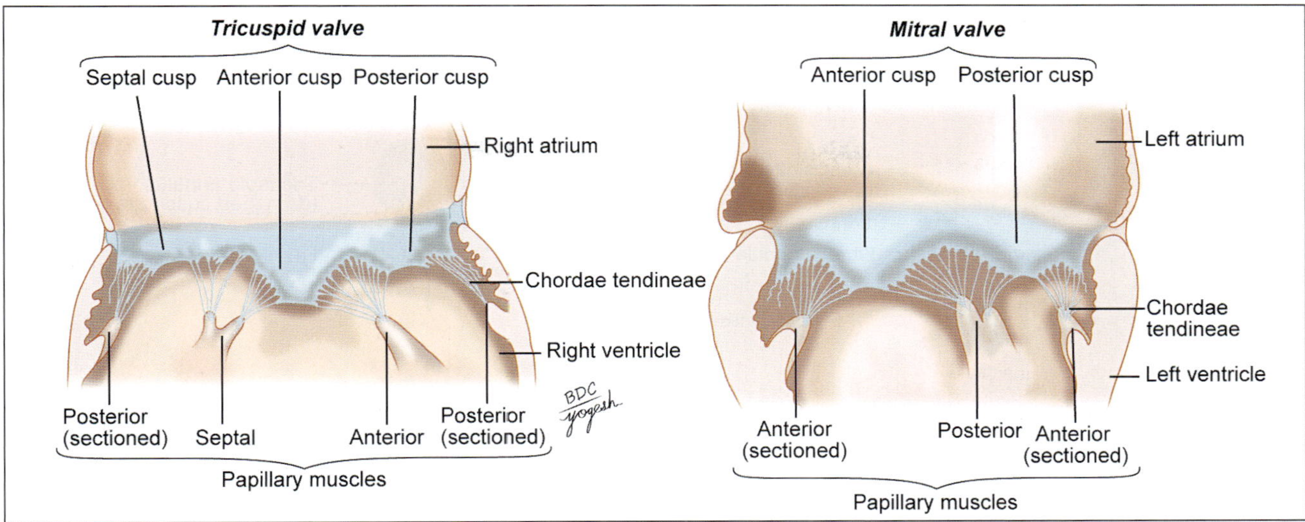

3. **Tricuspid valve:** It has three cusps. The three cusps—the anterior, posterior or inferior, and septal. Of the three papillary muscles, the anterior is the largest, the inferior is smaller and irregular, and the septal is represented by a number of small muscular elevations.
4. **Mitral or bicuspid valve:** It has two cusps—a large anterior or aortic cusp, and a small posterior cusp. The anterior cusp lies between the mitral and aortic orifices. The mitral cusps are smaller and thicker than those of the tricuspid valve (Fig. 18.21).

Note:

a. *The valves are closed during ventricular systole* (Greek *contraction*) by apposition of the atrial surfaces near the serrated margins (Fig. 18.18).
b. The atrioventricular valves are kept competent by active contraction of the *papillary muscles*, which pull on the chordae tendineae during ventricular systole. Each papillary muscle is connected to the contiguous halves of two cusps (Fig. 18.20).
c. Blood vessels are present only in the fibrous ring and in the basal 1/3rd of the cusps. Nutrition to the central 2/3rd of the cusps is derived directly from the blood in the cavity of the heart.

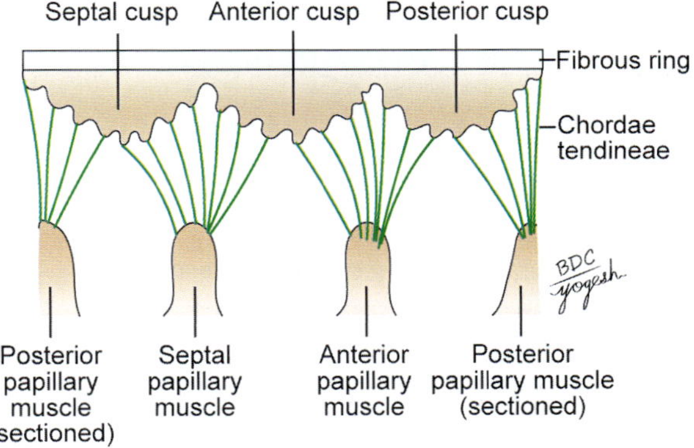

Fig. 18.20: Structure of an atrioventricular/tricuspid valve

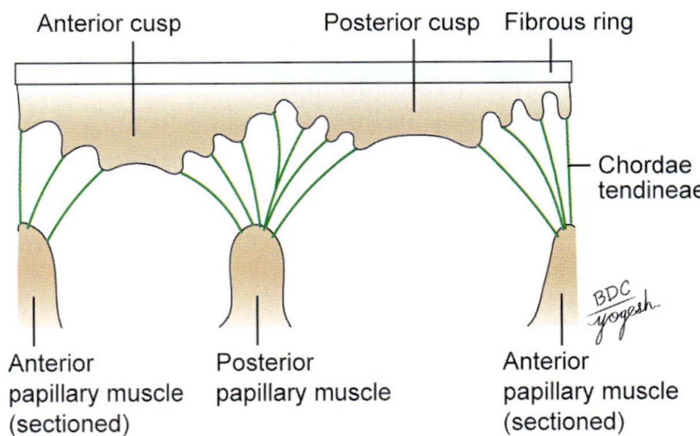

Fig. 18.21: Structure of mitral valve

Semilunar Valves

1. The aortic and pulmonary valves are called semilunar valves because their cusps are semilunar in shape. Both valves are similar to each other (Plate 18.11).
2. Each valve has **three cusps** which are attached to the vessel wall. The free margin of each cusp contains a central fibrous ***nodule*** from each side of which a thin smooth margin *the* ***lunule*** extends up to the base of the cusp.

Note:

a. These valves are closed during ventricular diastole when each cusp bulges towards the ventricular cavity.
b. Opposite the cusps, the vessel walls are slightly dilated to form the aortic and pulmonary sinuses.
c. The coronary arteries arise from the anterior and the left posterior aortic sinuses (Plate 18.11, Fig. 18.22).

CLINICAL ANATOMY

- ***Heart sounds***: The first heart sound is produced by closure of the atrioventricular valves. The second heart sound is produced by closure of the semilunar valves. The first and second heart sounds are heard as '***LUB***' and '***DUB***', respectively.
- ***Stenosis***: Narrowing of the valve orifice due to fusion of the cusps is known as 'stenosis', viz. mitral stenosis, aortic stenosis, etc.

Plate 18.11: Aortic valve

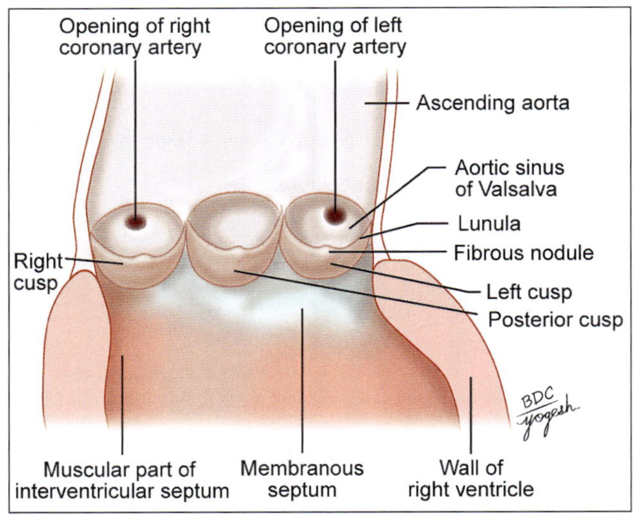

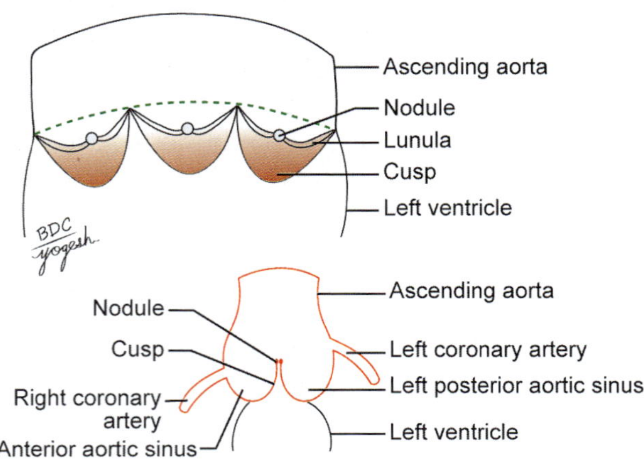

Fig. 18.22: Structure of the aortic valve

- ***Valve incompetence/regurgitation***: Dilatation of the valve orifice, or stiffening of the cusps causes imperfect closure of the valve leading to back flow of blood. This is known as incompetence or regurgitation, e.g. aortic incompetence or aortic regurgitation.
- ***Valvuloplasty***: Surgical replacement of the valve is called valvuloplasty (Fig. 18.23).

Competency:
AN22.6 Describe the fibrous skeleton of heart.

FIBROUS SKELETON OF HEART

The fibrous rings surrounding the atrioventricular and arterial orifices, along with some adjoining masses of fibrous tissue, constitute the fibrous skeleton of the heart. It provides attachment to the cardiac muscle and keeps the cardiac valves competent (Fig. 18.24).

Components

The fibrous skeleton of heart consists of the following components:

1. Four rings that surround two atrioventricular and aortic and pulmonary orifices.

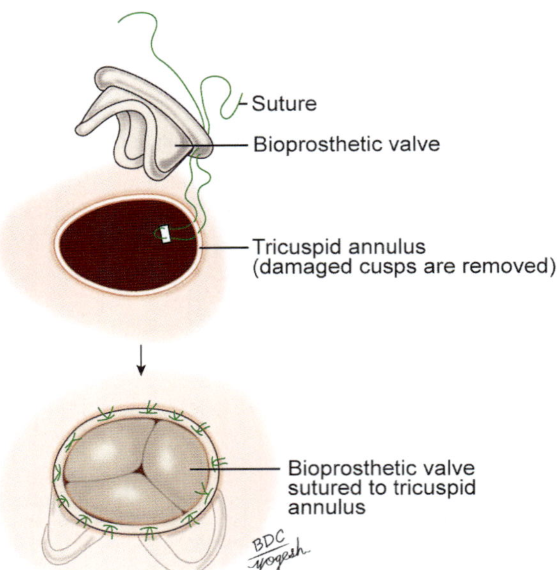

Fig. 18.23: Bioprosthetic tricuspid valve replacement

2. Tendon of infundibulum: It is a fibrous septum. It connects pulmonary ring with aortic ring.
3. Right fibrous trigone (*trigonum fibrosum dextrum*): It is a fibrous thickening where right and left atrioventricular rings fuse.
4. Left fibrous trigone (*trigonum fibrosum sinistrum*): It is a fibrous thickening where aortic and left atrioventricular rings fuse.

Note:
The *atrioventricular fibrous rings* are in the form of the *figure of 8*. The atria, the ventricles, and the membranous part of the interventricular septum are attached to them.

There is no muscular continuity between the atria and ventricles across the rings except for the atrioventricular bundle or *bundle of His*.

Functions of Skeleton of Heart

1. *Support*: Fibrous skeleton provides attachment to the musculature of the heart and supports it.
2. *Discontinuity between atria and ventricles*: Fibrous skeleton creates discontinuity between atrial and ventricular musculature. Hence, conducting system is required to transmit the atrial impulses to the ventricles.
3. *Maintain valvular function*: By supporting cusps of heart valves, fibrous skeleton helps to maintain unidirectional blood flow.

Competency:
AN22.7 Mention the parts, position and arterial supply of the conducting system of heart.

CONDUCTING SYSTEM

The conducting system is made up of myocardium that is specialised for initiation and conduction of the cardiac impulse. Its fibres are finer than other myocardial fibres, and are completely cross-striated.

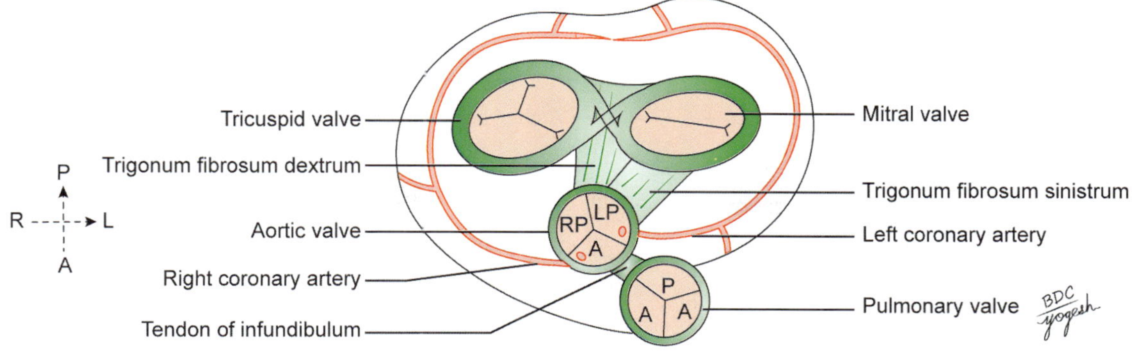

Fig. 18.24: Heart seen from above after removing the atria. The tricuspid, mitral, aortic and pulmonary orifices and their valves are seen. The fibrous skeleton of the heart is also shown (anatomical position)

The conducting system has the following parts (Plate 18.12):

1. Sinoatrial (SA) node
2. Atrioventricular (AV) node
3. Atrioventricular bundle of His (AV bundle): Right and left branches
4. Subendocardial plexus of Purkinje fibres.

1. ***Sinuatrial node or SA node of Keith–Flack:*** It is known as the ***'pacemaker'*** of the heart. It generates impulses at the rate of about 70–100 beats/min and initiates the heartbeat. It is horseshoe-shaped and is situated in the upper part of the sulcus terminals, just below the opening of superior vena cava. The impulse travels through the atrial wall to reach the AV node (Fig. 18.25).
2. ***Atrioventricular node or AV node of Tawara:*** It is smaller than the SA node and is situated in the lower part of the atrial septum just above the opening of the coronary sinus. It is capable of generating impulses at a rate of about 40–60 beats/minute.
3. ***Atrioventricular bundle or AV bundle or bundle of His:*** It is the only muscular connection between the atrial and ventricular musculatures. It begins as the atrioventricular (AV) node crosses AV ring and descends along the posteroinferior border of the membranous part of the ventricular septum. At the upper border of the muscular part of the septum, it divides into right and left branches.
   a. *The* ***right branch*** of the AV bundle passes down the right side of the interventricular septum. A large part enters the moderator band to reach the anterior wall of the right ventricle where it divides into Purkinje fibres (Fig. 18.25).
   b. *The* ***left branch*** of the AV bundle descends on the left side of the interventricular septum and is distributed to the left ventricle after dividing into Purkinje fibres.
4. *The* ***Purkinje fibres*** form a subendocardial plexus. They are large pale fibres striated only at their margins. They usually possess double nuclei. These generate impulses at the rate of 20–35 beats/minute.

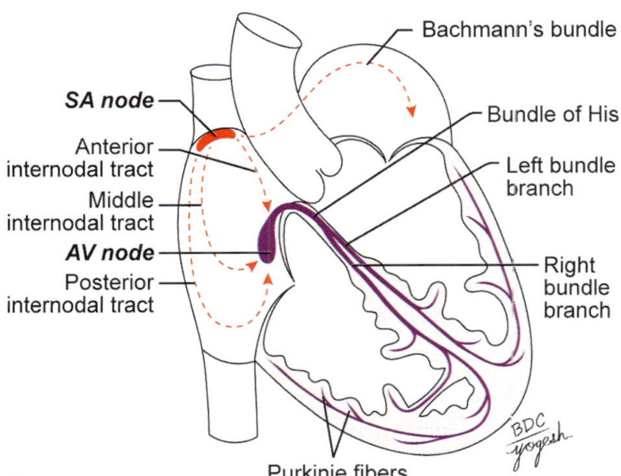

Fig. 18.25: Conducting system of the heart

Note:

Blood supply: Whole of conducting system except left branch of AV bundle is supplied by right coronary artery. In 40% cases, left coronary artery supplies SA node.

Internodal Tracts: SA node is connected with AV node by three internodal tracts (Fig. 18.25):

A. *Anterior tract of Bachmann*: It connects anterosuperior part of SA node with AV node. It passes in front of superior vena caval opening and then along the interatrial septum.
B. *Middle tract of Wenckebach*: It connects posteroinferior part of SA node with AV node. It passes behind orifice of superior vena cava and then along the interatrial septum.
C. *Posterior tract of Torel*: It connects posteroinferior part of SA node with AV node. It passes along the crista terminalis and the valve of inferior vena cava.

CLINICAL ANATOMY

Sinus rhythm: Normally, SA node acts as a pacemaker and produces heart rate of 70 beats/minute. This is called sinus rhythm.

- Rapid pulse or increased heart rate is called ***tachycardia*** (Greek *rapid heart*).
- Slow pulse or decreased heart rate is called ***bradycardia*** (Greek *slow heart*).
- Irregular pulse or irregular heart rate is called ***arrhythmia***.
- Consciousness of one's heartbeat is called ***palpitation***.

Plate 18.12: Conducting system of heart

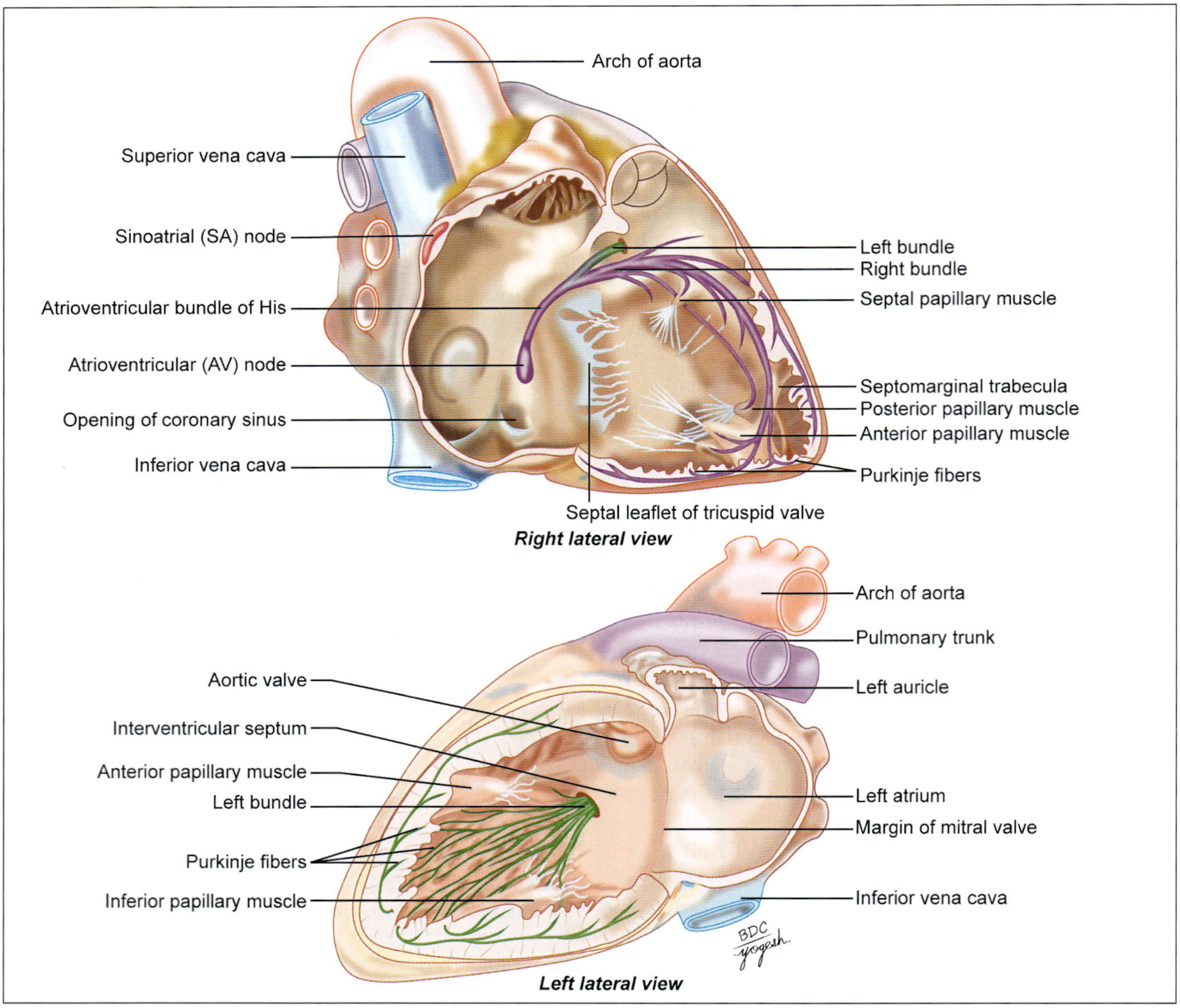

Arch of aorta
Superior vena cava
Sinoatrial (SA) node
Atrioventricular bundle of His
Atrioventricular (AV) node
Opening of coronary sinus
Inferior vena cava
Left bundle
Right bundle
Septal papillary muscle
Septomarginal trabecula
Posterior papillary muscle
Anterior papillary muscle
Purkinje fibers
Septal leaflet of tricuspid valve

Right lateral view

Arch of aorta
Pulmonary trunk
Left auricle
Aortic valve
Interventricular septum
Anterior papillary muscle
Left bundle
Purkinje fibers
Inferior papillary muscle
Left atrium
Margin of mitral valve
Inferior vena cava

Left lateral view

Cardiac arrhythmias: Defects or damage to conducting system results in cardiac arrhythmias, i.e. defects in the normal rhythm of contraction. Vascular lesions of the heart can cause a variety of arrhythmias.

Heart block: Due to loss of blood supply of AV node or bundle of His, the ventricles functionally get dissociated from SA node. This is called heart block. In this condition, atria contracts at a normal speed under SA nodal rhythm (70 times/minute), whereas ventricles contract at a slower speed (25–30 times/minute).

Artificial cardiac pacemaker (Fig. 18.26)**:** It is a small device (about the size of wristwatch) that is placed in the chest to control the heartbeat. Pacemaker has a pulse generator with battery, wire, and electrode to stimulate the ventricles. Pacemaker is useful in patients with cardiac arrhythmias and heart block.

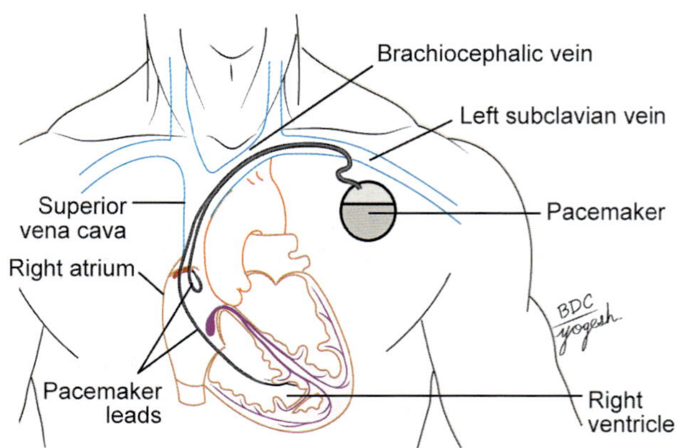

Fig. 18.26: Pacemaker with two leads

Cardiopulmonary resuscitation (CPR) (Fig. 18.27)**:** In case of cardiac arrest, CPR is useful to restart the heart and to restore cardiac output and pulmonary ventilation. It is a life-saving emergency procedure. *Procedure*: It is performed by applying pressure on sternum at the rate of 100–120 per minute, with the depth of 2 inches in adult. Increased pressure pushes the blood out of heart and great blood vessels and decreasing external pressure helps in venous return to the heart.

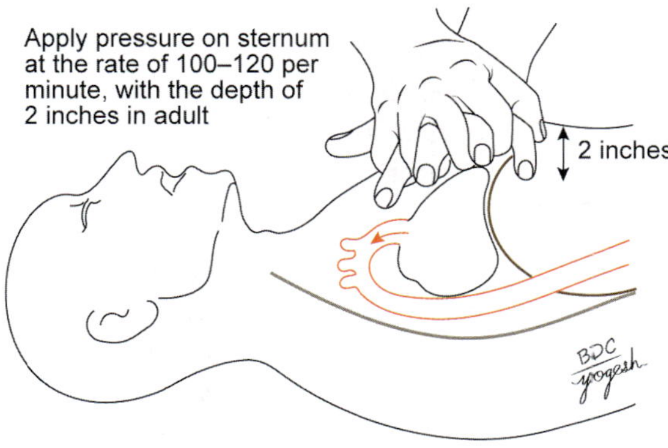

Fig. 18.27: Cardiopulmonary resuscitation (CPR)

Competency:
AN22.3 Describe and demonstrate origin, course and branches of coronary arteries.

ARTERIES SUPPLYING THE HEART

The heart is supplied by two coronary arteries, arising from the ascending aorta. Both arteries run in the coronary sulcus (Flowchart 18.8).

Features of Coronary Arteries

1. The blood flows through these arteries during diastole of heart.
2. Left coronary is larger in calibre and supplies more myocardium.
3. These arteries are *'functional end arteries'*. Though their branches anastomose with each other but one cannot compensate for the other artery in case of thrombosis.
4. The origin of posterior interventricular artery determines the dominance of the artery.
5. Sympathetic stimulation dilates the intramuscular arteries and constricts the epicardial arteries.
6. They are prone for development of atherosclerosis.

RIGHT CORONARY ARTERY

Position

Right coronary artery is smaller than the left coronary artery. It arises from the ***anterior aortic sinus*** (Fig. 18.28, Flowchart 18.8) of ascending aorta.

Course

The course of the artery can be divided into two segments as follows:

1. ***First segment:*** It first passes forwards and to the right to emerge on the surface of the heart between the root of the pulmonary trunk and the right auricle. It then runs downwards in the right anterior coronary sulcus to the junction of the right and inferior borders of the heart.
2. ***Second segment:*** It winds round the inferior border to reach the diaphragmatic surface of the heart. Here, it runs backwards and to the left in the right posterior coronary sulcus to reach crux of the heart.

It terminates by anastomosing with the circumflex branch of left coronary artery at the crux (60%).

Branches (Plate 18.13, Fig. 18.28)

1. ***Atrial branches*** are anterior, posterior, and lateral. One of the anterior atrial branches is called ***SA nodal artery***. It arises from right coronary artery in 60% cases. In 40% cases it arises from circumflex branch of left coronary artery.
2. ***Right conus artery*** forms an arterial circle around pulmonary trunk with a similar branch from the left coronary artery. The circle is called, ***'annulus of Vieussens'***.
3. ***Ventricular branches*** are as anterior and posterior groups. The anterior group lies on the sternocostal surface while posterior group traverses the diaphragmatic surface of the heart.
4. ***Right marginal artery*** arises as the right coronary artery crosses the right border of heart. It runs along its inferior border till the apex of heart.
5. ***Posterior interventricular branch*** arises close to the crux of heart and lies in the posterior interventricular groove. It gives:
    a. Septal branches for posteroinferior 1/3rd of interventricular septum.
    b. Nodal branch in 60% individuals for AV node.
    c. Ventricular branches for inferior surface of the right and left ventricles.

Area of Distribution

1. Right atrium
2. Ventricles:
    a. Greater part of the right ventricle, except the area adjoining the anterior interventricular groove.
    b. A small part of the left ventricle adjoining the posterior interventricular groove.
3. Posterior 1/3rd part of the interventricular septum.
4. Whole of the conducting system of the heart except a part of the left branch of the AV bundle. The SA node is supplied by the left coronary artery in about 40% of cases.

DISSECTION

Carefully remove the fat from the coronary sulcus. Identify the right coronary artery in the depth of the right part of the atrioventricular sulcus (Fig. 18.28). Trace the right coronary artery superiorly to its origin from the right aortic sinus and inferiorly till it turns onto the posterior surface of the heart to lie in its atrioventricular sulcus. It gives off the posterior interventricular branch which is seen in posterior interventricular groove. The right coronary artery ends by anastomosing with the circumflex branch of left coronary artery or by dipping itself deep in the myocardium there.

Plate 18.13: Branches of coronary artery

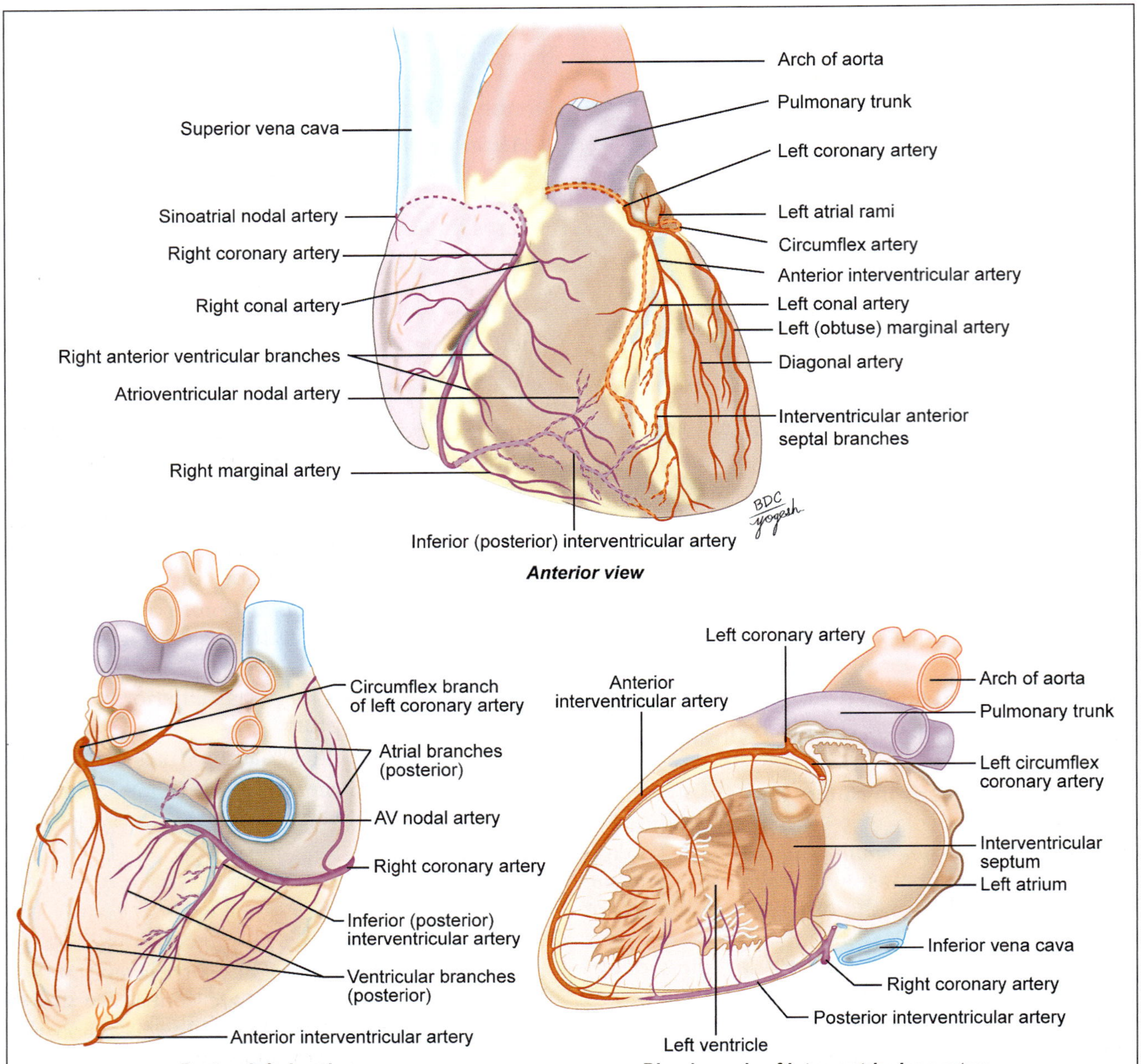

Arch of aorta
Pulmonary trunk
Superior vena cava
Left coronary artery
Sinoatrial nodal artery
Left atrial rami
Right coronary artery
Circumflex artery
Anterior interventricular artery
Right conal artery
Left conal artery
Left (obtuse) marginal artery
Right anterior ventricular branches
Diagonal artery
Atrioventricular nodal artery
Interventricular anterior septal branches
Right marginal artery
Inferior (posterior) interventricular artery
BDC yogesh

Anterior view

Circumflex branch of left coronary artery
Atrial branches (posterior)
AV nodal artery
Right coronary artery
Inferior (posterior) interventricular artery
Ventricular branches (posterior)
Anterior interventricular artery

Posteroinferior view

Left coronary artery
Anterior interventricular artery
Arch of aorta
Pulmonary trunk
Left circumflex coronary artery
Interventricular septum
Left atrium
Inferior vena cava
Right coronary artery
Posterior interventricular artery
Left ventricle

Blood supply of interventricular septum

Flowchart 18.8: Coronary arteries

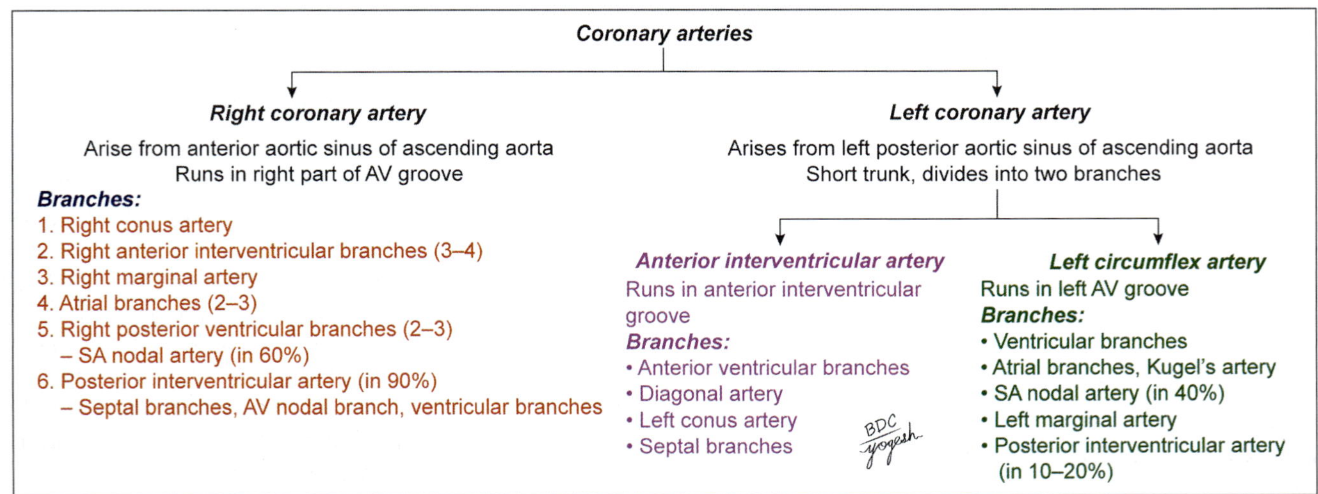

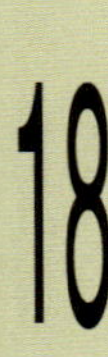

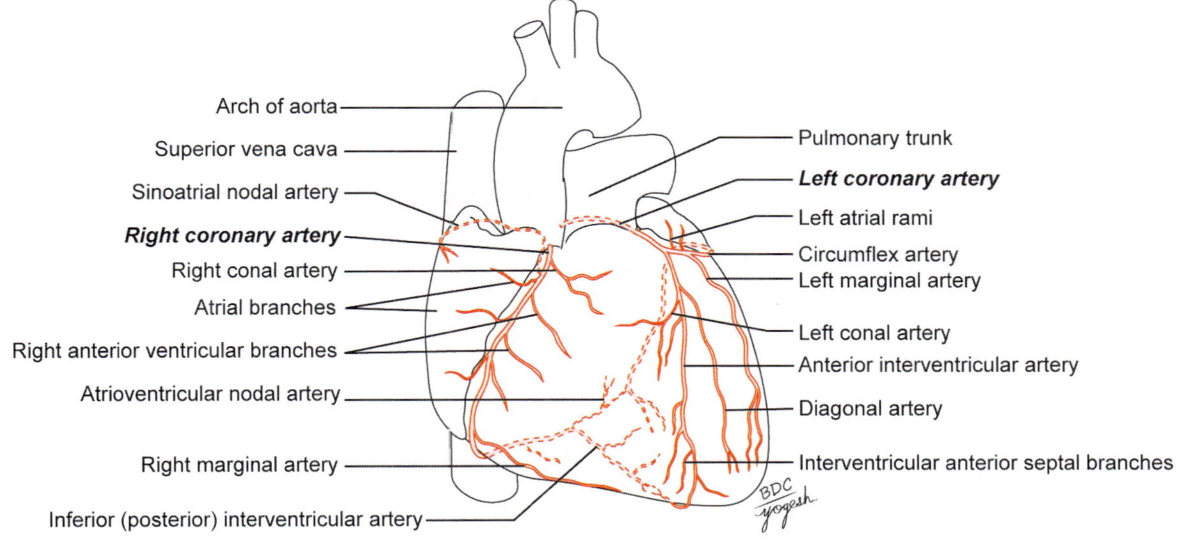

Fig. 18.28: Arterial supply of heart

LEFT CORONARY ARTERY

Position

Left coronary artery is larger than the right coronary artery. It arises from the *left posterior aortic sinus* of ascending aorta.

Course

1. The artery first runs forwards and to the left and emerges between the pulmonary trunk and the left auricle. Here it gives the *anterior interventricular branch* which runs downwards in the groove of the same name. The further continuation of the left coronary artery is called the *circumflex artery* (Figs 18.28 and 18.29).
2. *Anterior interventricular artery* descends along the anterior interventricular groove. It turns around the inferior heart border and enters the posterior interventricular groove, where it ends by anastomosing with posterior interventricular artery.
3. The *circumflex artery* runs to the left in the left anterior coronary sulcus. It winds round the left border of the heart and continues in the left posterior coronary sulcus. Near the posterior interventricular groove, it terminates by anastomosing with the right coronary artery.

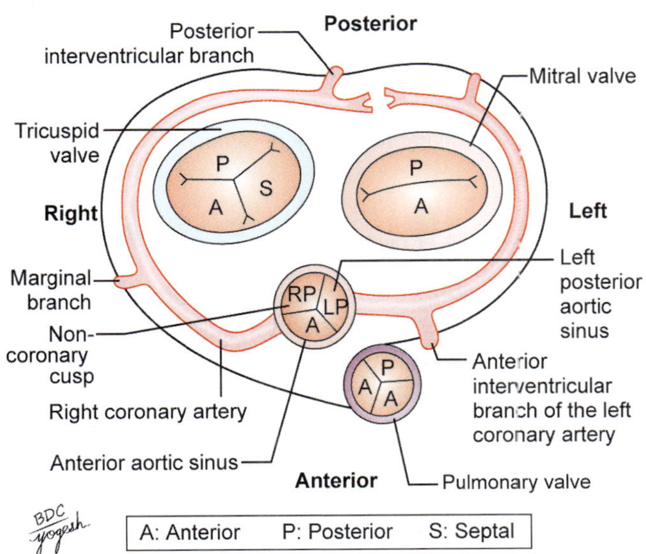

Fig. 18.29: Origin of the coronary arteries from the aortic sinuses and their course in the coronary sulcus, as seen after removal of the atria (anatomical position)

Branches (Plate 18.13)

1. *Anterior interventricular artery* or left anterior descending (LAD) artery: It gives:
   a. Anterior ventricular branches that supply sternocostal surface of right and left ventricles.
   b. *Diagonal artery*: It is the largest anterior ventricular artery. Occasionally it arises from the junction of anterior interventricular artery and left circumflex coronary artery.
   c. *Left conus artery*: It supplies pulmonary conus. Septum branches: They supply anterior 2/3rd of interventricular septum.
2. *Left circumflex coronary artery:* It gives the following branches:
   a. *Ventricular branches* to supply sternocostal, left, and inferior surfaces of the left ventricle.
   b. *Atrial branches* to supply adjacent area of left atrium.
   c. Sinoatrial nodal artery arises from left circumflex coronary artery in 40% individuals.
   d. *Left marginal artery* runs along the left heart border toward the apex.
   e. *Posterior interventricular artery*: Left circumflex coronary artery continues as posterior interventricular artery in 10–20% individuals.
   f. *Kugel's artery*: It is an atrial branch of left coronary artery that anastomoses with similar branch of right coronary artery along the anterior wall of atria.

Area of Distribution

1. Left atrium
2. *Ventricles*:
   a. Greater part of the left ventricle, except the area adjoining the posterior interventricular groove.
   b. A small part of the right ventricle adjoining the anterior interventricular groove.
3. Anterior 2/3rd of the interventricular septum (Fig. 18.30).
4. A part of the left branch of the AV bundle.

CARDIAC DOMINANCE

In about 10% of hearts, the right coronary is rather small and is not able to give the posterior interventricular branch. In these cases, the circumflex artery, the continuation of left coronary, provides the posterior interventricular branch as well as to the AV node. Such cases are called ***left dominant.*** Mostly, the right coronary gives posterior interventricular artery. Such hearts are ***right dominant***. Thus the artery giving the posterior interventricular branch is the dominant artery.

DISSECTION

Strip the visceral pericardium from the sternocostal surface of the heart. Expose the anterior interventricular branch of the left coronary artery and the great cardiac vein by carefully removing the fat from the anterior interventricular sulcus. Note the branches of the artery to both ventricles and to the interventricular septum which lies deep to it. Trace the artery inferiorly to the diaphragmatic surface and superiorly to the left of the pulmonary trunk (Fig. 18.28). Trace the circumflex branch of left coronary artery on the left border of heart into the posterior part of the sulcus, where it may end by anastomosing with the right coronary artery or by dipping into the myocardium.

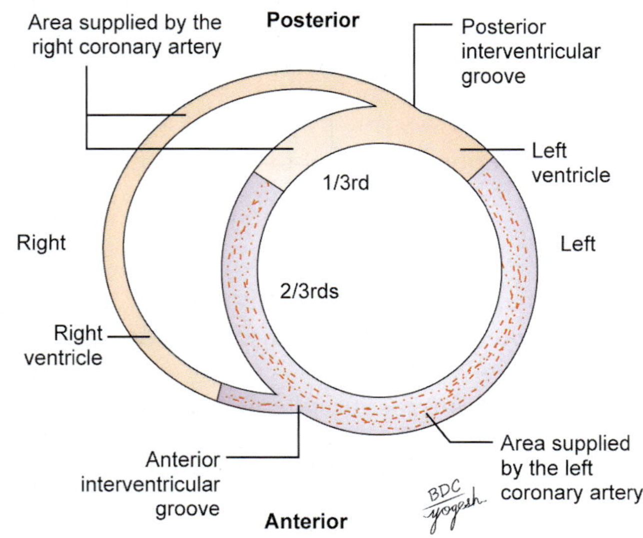

Fig. 18.30: Transverse section through the ventricles showing the areas supplied by the two coronary arteries

ANASTOMOSIS OF CORONARY ARTERIES

Interarterial Circulation

The coronary arteries though end arteries do anastomose in interventricular septum, as Kugel's arteries near crux of heart and as annulus of Vieussens around pulmonary trunk. Rate of anastomosis is better in older persons.

Arteriovenous Anastomosis

Blood from a blocked artery flows back into the veins and into coronary sinus, giving nutrition to myocardium. Branches of coronary arteries divide into number of sinusoids, which drain into coronary sinus. Some branches of coronary artery may open directly into the chambers of the heart. Venae cordis minimi open directly into the cavity of right-sided chambers. Blood in the various chambers supply some of the myocardium.

Cardiac Anastomoses

The two coronary arteries anastomose with each other in myocardium.

Extracardiac Anastomoses

The coronary arteries anastomose with the following.

1. Vasa vasorum of the aorta
2. Vasa vasorum of the pulmonary arteries
3. The internal thoracic arteries
4. The bronchial arteries
5. The pericardiacophrenic arteries.

The last three anastomose through the pericardium. These channels may open up in emergencies when both coronary arteries are obstructed.

Retrograde flow of blood in the veins may irrigate the myocardium. These anastomoses are of some practical value. They may be able to provide an alternative source of blood in case of blockage of a branch of a coronary artery.

Blockage of arteries or coronary thrombosis usually leads to death of myocardium. The condition is called ***myocardial infarction***.

Competency:
AN22.4 Describe anatomical basis of ischaemic heart disease.

CLINICAL ANATOMY

- ***Ischaemic heart disease*** is condition in which myocardium does not receive adequate supply of blood and oxygen. Coronary atherosclerosis is the major cause of ischaemic heart disease (Fig. 18.31). The ischaemic heart diseases are classified based on severity as follows:
  1. Angina pectoris (stable and unstable)
  2. Myocardial infarction
  3. Heart failure
  4. Arrhythmias
  5. Sudden cardiac death

- ***Angina pectoris*:** It is a pain which occurs in the chest due to reduced blood (oxygen) supply to the heart. Angina is paroxysmal and usually recurrent attacks of substernal or precordial chest discomfort. It is caused by transient (15 seconds to 15 minutes) myocardial ischemia that is insufficient to induce necrosis of cardiac myocytes. It is described as heavy, tight or gripping pain that is typically retrosternal. It is also referred to the left shoulder and medial side of the arm and forearm (Fig. 18.32). ***Stable angina*** is a type of angina that begins on exercise or physical activity, whereas the ***unstable angina*** occurs at rest and last for more than 20 minutes. Pain gets relieved by putting sorbitrate tablets below the tongue.
- ***Myocardial infarction (heart attack)*:** A sudden occlusion of the branch of coronary artery leads to complete loss of blood supply of a specific area of the heart. At this area, myocardium undergoes infarction (reduced blood supply) and finally into necrosis (tissue death). Myocardial infarction produces the following symptoms:
  - Angina pectoris that lasts longer than 30 minutes
  - Nausea, vomiting
  - Shortness of breath
  - Sweating
- Commonly involved vessels in coronary occlusion:
  1. Anterior interventricular artery (left anterior descending) (LAD) artery in 40–50% cases
  2. Right coronary artery in 30–40% cases
  3. Left circumflex coronary artery in 15–20% cases.
- ***Cardiac arrest*:** It is a sudden loss of blood flow to the body due to failure of pumping function of the heart. Myocardial infarction is most common cause of cardiac arrest.
- ***Coronary angiography*** determines the site(s) of narrowing or occlusion of the coronary arteries or their branches.
- ***Angioplasty*** helps in removal of small blockage. It is done using small stent or small inflated balloon (Fig. 18.33) through a catheter passed upwards through femoral artery, aorta, into the coronary artery.
- If there are large segments or multiple sites of blockage, ***coronary artery bypass grafting*** (CABG) is done using either great saphenous vein or internal thoracic artery as graft(s) (Fig. 18.34).

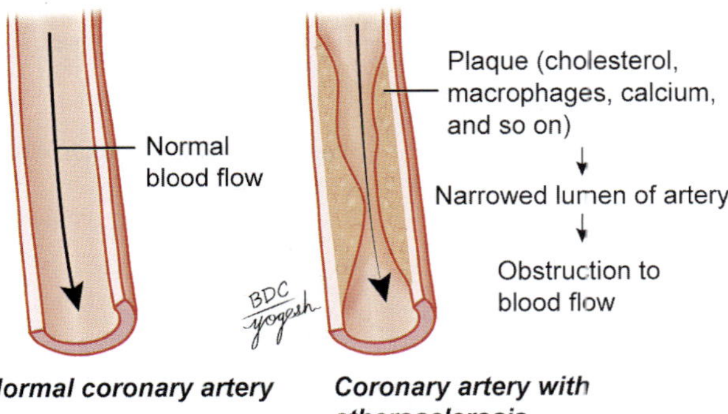

Fig. 18.31: Coronary atherosclerosis

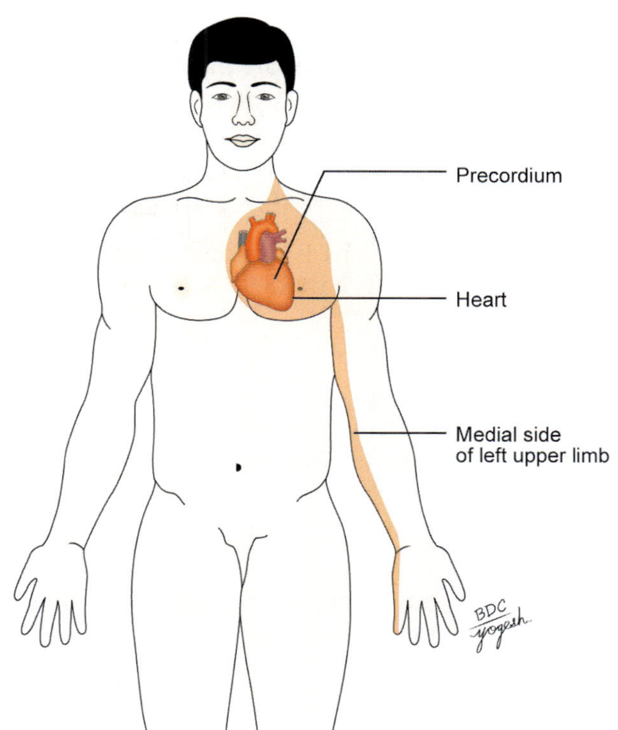

Fig. 18.32: Pain of angina pectoris felt in precordium and along medial border of left arm

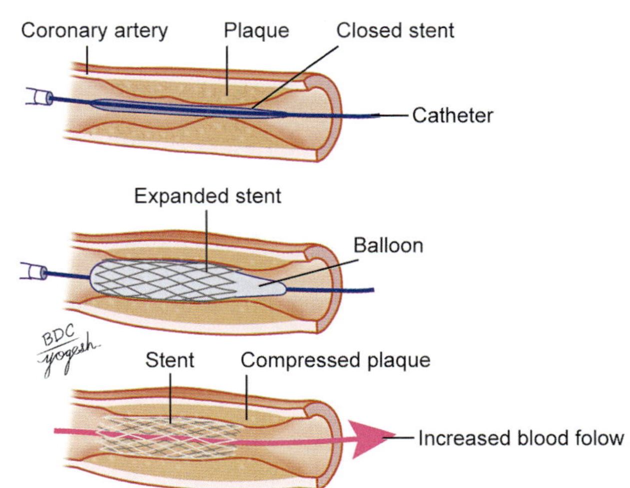

Fig. 18.33: Stent passed in the blocked coronary artery

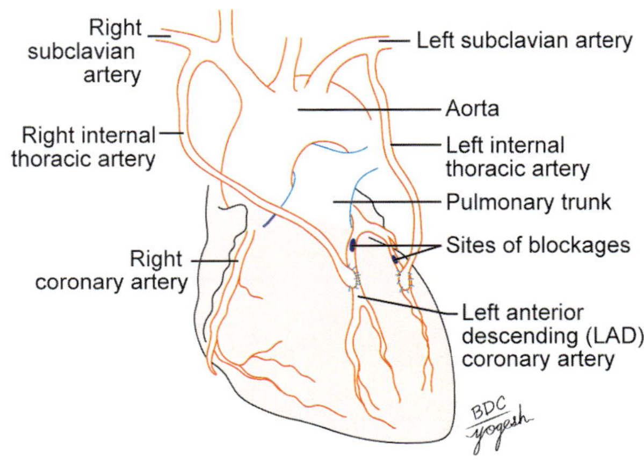

Fig. 18.34: Coronary artery bypass grafting using internal thoracic artery

Competency:

AN22.5 Describe and demonstrate the formation, course, tributaries and termination of coronary sinus.

VEINS OF THE HEART

Venous blood of the heart is drained by the following veins (Plate 18.14, Flowchart 18.9):

1. Great cardiac vein
2. Middle cardiac vein
3. Right marginal vein
4. Posterior vein of the left ventricle
5. Oblique vein of the left atrium
6. Anterior cardiac veins
7. Venae cordis minimae (Figs 18.35a and b).

All veins except the last two drain into the coronary sinus which opens into the right atrium. The anterior cardiac veins and the venae cordis minimae open directly into the right atrium.

Coronary Sinus

The coronary sinus is the largest vein of the heart. It is situated in the left posterior coronary sulcus. It is about 2–3 cm long. It ends by opening into the posterior wall of the right atrium.

Tributaries

It receives the following tributaries:

1. ***Great cardiac vein*:** It accompanies first the anterior interventricular artery and then the circumflex artery to enter the left end of the coronary sinus (Figs 18.35a to c). It receives the left marginal vein from the left ventricle.
2. ***Middle cardiac vein*:** It accompanies the posterior interventricular artery, and joins the middle part of the coronary sinus.
3. ***Small cardiac vein*:** It accompanies the right coronary artery in the right posterior coronary sulcus and joins the right end of the coronary sinus. The ***right marginal vein*** may drain into the small cardiac vein (Fig. 18.35b).
4. ***Posterior vein of the left ventricle*:** It runs on the diaphragmatic surface of the left ventricle and ends in the coronary sinus.
5. ***Oblique vein of the left atrium of Marshall*:** It is a small vein running on the posterior surface of the left atrium. It terminates in the left end of the coronary sinus. It develops from the left common cardinal vein or *duct of Cuvier* which may sometimes form a large left superior vena cava.
6. ***Right marginal vein*:** It accompanies the marginal branch of the right coronary artery. It may either drain into the small cardiac vein, or may open directly into the right atrium.

Anterior Cardiac Veins

The *anterior cardiac veins* are three or four small veins which run parallel to one another on the anterior wall of the right ventricle and usually open directly into the right atrium through its anterior wall.

Venae Cordis Minimae

The *venae cordis minimae* or *Thebesian veins* or *smallest cardiac veins* are numerous small valveless veins present in all four chambers of the heart which open directly into the cavity. These are more numerous on the right side of the heart than on the left. This may be one reason why left-sided infarcts are more common.

LYMPHATICS OF HEART

Lymphatics of the heart accompany the coronary arteries and form two trunks. The right trunk ends in the brachiocephalic nodes, and the left trunk ends in the tracheobronchial lymph nodes at the bifurcation of the trachea.

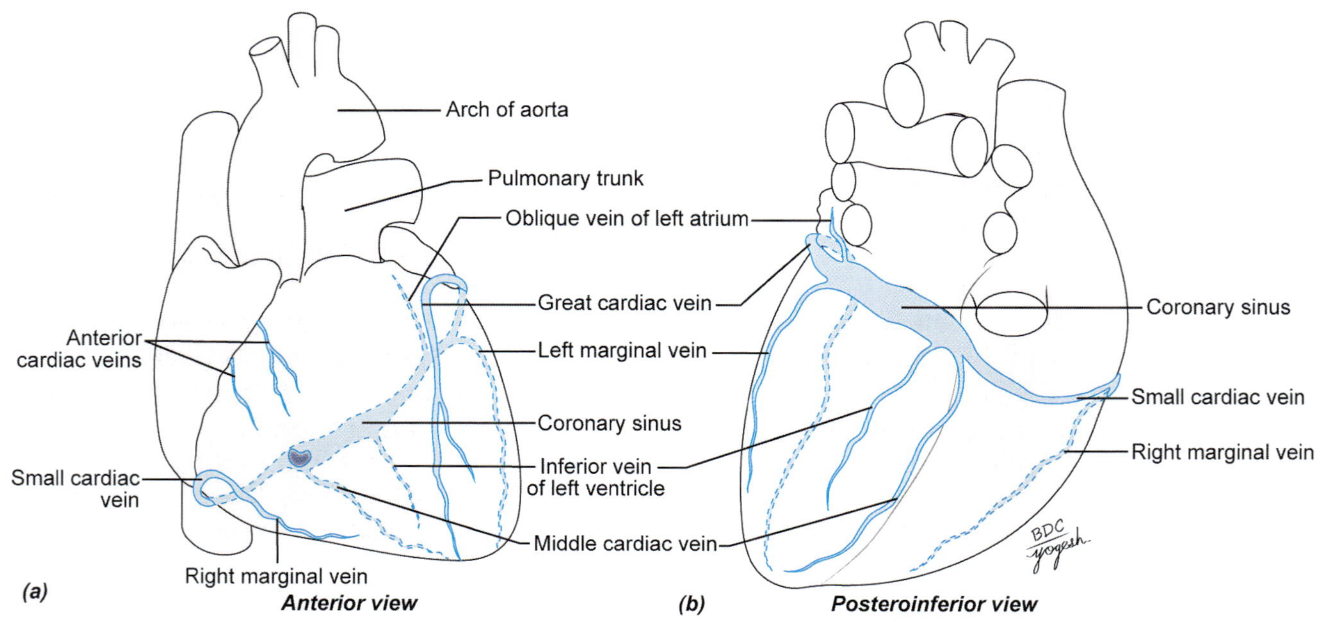

Figs 18.35a and b: Veins of the heart: (a) Sternocostal surface; (b) Posteroinferior view

Plate 18.14: Principal veins of the heart

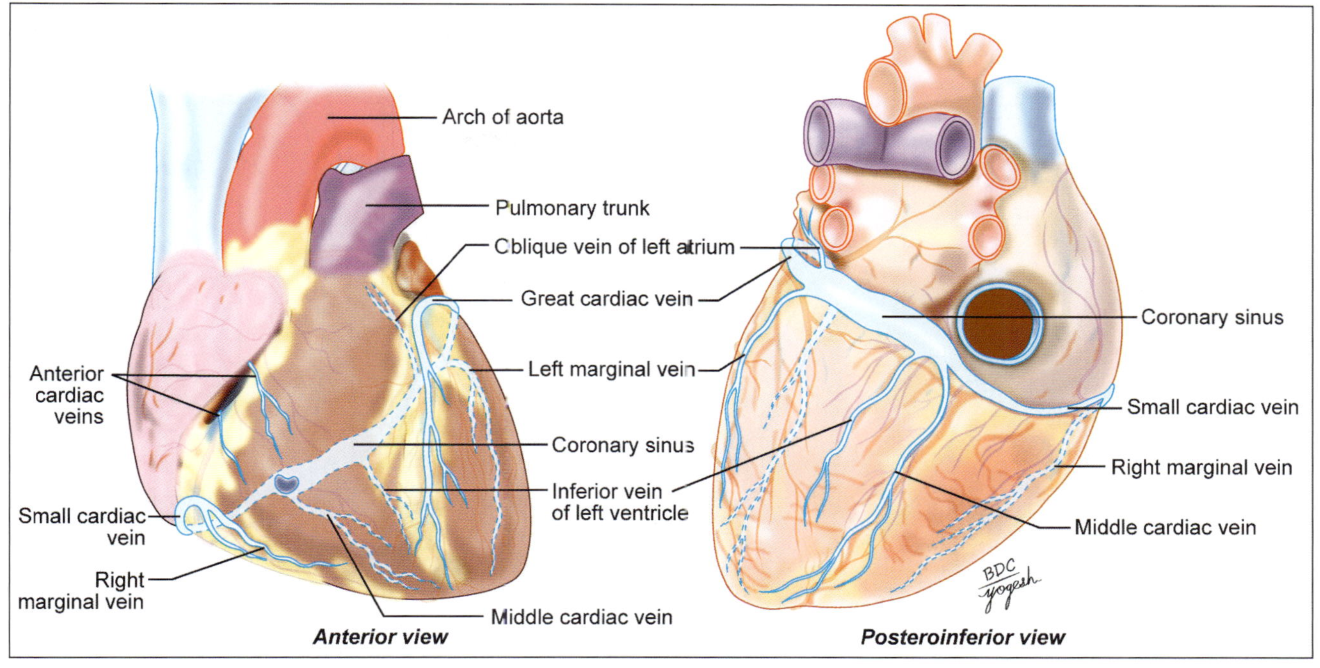

Flowchart 18.9: Venous drainage of heart

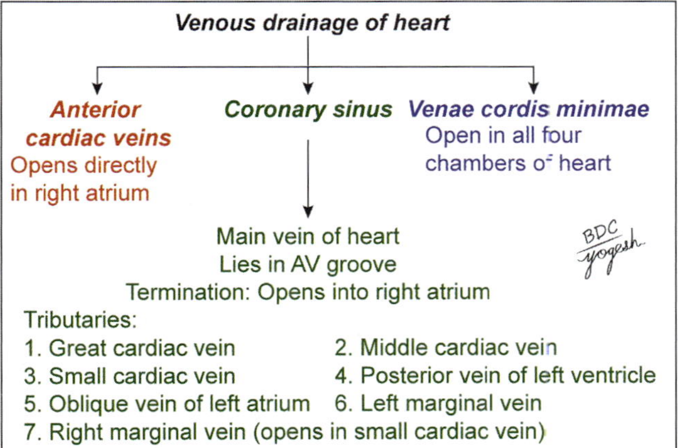

Flowchart 18.10: Nerve supply of heart

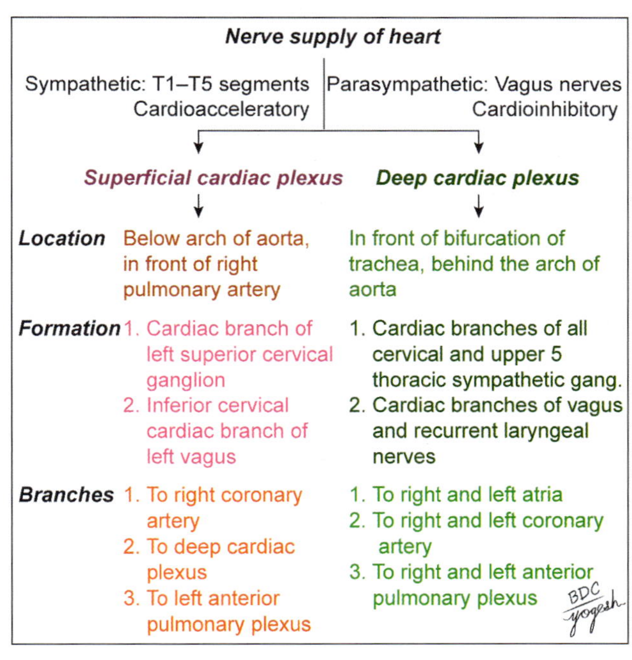

NERVE SUPPLY OF HEART

1. *Parasympathetic nerves* reach the heart via the vagus. These are cardioinhibitory; on stimulation, they slow down the heart rate (Flowchart 18.10).
2. *Sympathetic nerves* are derived from the upper 4–5 thoracic segments of the spinal cord. These are cardioacceleratory, and on stimulation, they increase the heart rate, and also dilate the coronary arteries.

Both parasympathetic and sympathetic nerves form the superficial and deep cardiac plexuses, the branches of which run along the coronary arteries to reach the myocardium.

1. ***Superficial cardiac plexus*** is situated below the arch of the aorta in front of the right pulmonary artery. It is formed by:
   a. The superior cervical cardiac branch of the left sympathetic chain.
   b. The inferior cervical cardiac branch of the left vagus nerve.

   Branches: Superficial cardiac plexus gives:
   a. Branch to the right coronary artery
   b. Communicating branch to deep cardiac plexus
   c. Communicating branch to the left anterior pulmonary plexus (Fig. 18.36).
2. ***Deep cardiac plexus*** is situated in front of the bifurcation of the trachea, and behind the arch of the aorta. It is formed by:
   a. All the cardiac branches derived from all the cervical and upper thoracic ganglia of the sympathetic chain

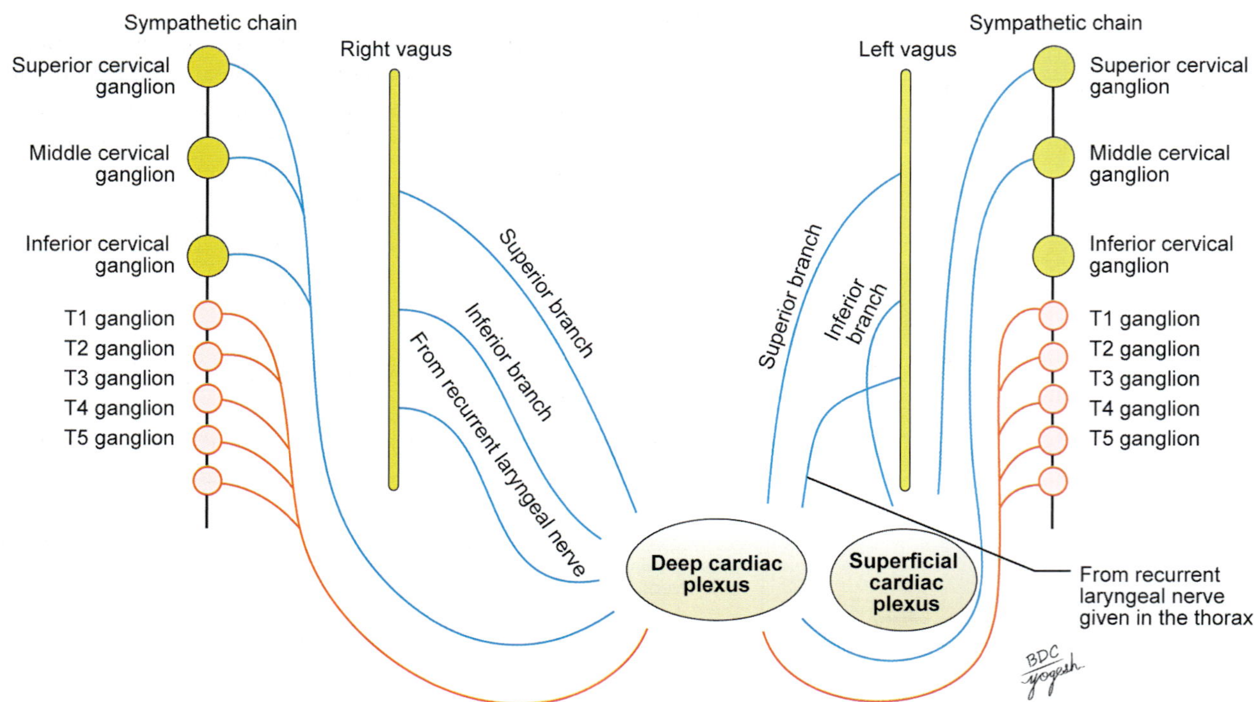

Fig. 18.36: Formation of superficial and deep cardiac plexuses

b. Cardiac branches of the vagus and recurrent laryngeal nerves, except those which form the superficial plexus.

Branches: Deep cardiac plexus comprises right and left half that gives the following branches:

a. To the right and left atria.
b. Right and left coronary artery through right and left coronary plexus.
c. Communicating branch to the right and left anterior pulmonary plexus.

Separate branches are given to the atria.

CLINICAL ANATOMY

- ***Cardiac pain*** is an ischaemic pain caused by incomplete obstruction of a coronary artery.
  Pathway: Axons of pain fibres conveyed by the sensory sympathetic cardiac nerves reach thoracic T1–T5 segments of spinal cord mostly through the dorsal root ganglia of the left side. Since these dorsal root ganglia also receive sensory impulses from the medial side of arm, forearm and upper part of front of chest, the pain gets referred to these areas.
- Viscera have low amount of sensory output, whereas skin is an area of high amount of sensory output. So pain arising from area of low sensory output area is projected as coming from high sensory output area.

Competency:

AN25.2 Describe development of respiratory system and heart. Development of respiratory system has been described in Chapter 16 and development of heart is described in this Chapter.

DEVELOPMENTAL COMPONENTS

1. Right atrium
   - Rough trabeculated part of right atrium and right auricle from right half of primitive atrium.
   - Smooth part of right atrium (sinus venarum) from sinus venosus.
   - Crista terminalis, valve of inferior vena cava, and valve of coronary sinus develop from right venous valve.
   - A small area of most ventral smooth part develops from right half of atrioventricular canal.
2. Left atrium
   - Anterior rough part of left atrium and left auricle develop from left half of primitive atrium.
   - Posterior smooth part (between openings of pulmonary veins) develops from absorption of pulmonary veins.
   - Ventral smooth part develops from left half of atrioventricular canal.
3. Right ventricle
   a. Rough part—proximal portion of bulbus cordis
   b. Smooth part—the conus cordis or middle portion of bulbus cordis.
4. Left ventricle
   a. Rough part—whole of primitive ventricular chamber.
   b. The conus cordis or the middle portion of bulbus cordis forms the smooth part.
5. Interatrial septum
   a. Septum primum—fossa ovalis.
   b. Septum secundum—limbus fossa ovalis.
6. Interventricular septum
   - Muscular part—from muscular ridge arising on the floor of bulboventricular cavity.

- Bulbar part—from right and left bulbar ridges arising from conus cordis.
- Membranous part—from proliferation of AV cushion that fills the gap between muscular and bulbar parts.

7. Truncus arteriosus or distal part of bulbus cordis forms the ascending aorta and pulmonary trunk, as separated by spiral septum.

Spiral septum is responsible for triple relation of ascending aorta and pulmonary trunk. At the beginning, pulmonary trunk is anterior to ascending aorta, then it is to the left, and finally the right pulmonary artery is posterior to ascending aorta. Heart is fully functional at the end of 2nd month of intrauterine life.

Competency:

AN25.4 Describe embryological basis of: (1) Atrial septal defect, (2) Ventricular septal defect, (3) Fallot's tetralogy.

CLINICAL ANATOMY

1. *Atrial septal defect:* Normally septum primum fuses with septum secondum to obliterate interatrial foramen. Incomplete fusion of the two septa leads to atrial septal defect.
2. *Ventricular septal defect:* Ventricular septal defect is due to defect in the formation of membranous part of interventricular septum. This septum is formed by right and left bulbar ridges and proliferating posterior endocardial cushion.

   Improper fusion of these three leads to ventricular septal defect. The membranous part of interventricular septum is of neural crest origin.
3. *Fallot's tetralogy:* The components of Fallot's tetralogy are:
   a. Patent interventricular foramen
   b. Overriding of the aorta
   c. Pulmonary stenosis
   d. Right ventricular hypertrophy.

Facts to Remember

- The pericardium consists of outer fibrous and inner serous pericardium. The serous pericardium has outer parietal inner visceral layer.
- Heart is a pump for pushing blood to the lungs and for rest of the organs of the body. Due to sympathetic stimulation, it is felt thumping against the chest wall.
- Crux of the Heart is the meeting point of interatrial, atrioventricular and posterior interventricular grooves.
- Triangle of Koch is bounded by ostium of coronary sinus, septal leaflet of tricuspid valve and tendon of Todaro, a subendocardial ridge.
- All the components of left ventricle are thicker as it has to push the blood from top of head to the toes of foot.
- Left atrium forms most of the base of the heart.
- Coronary arteries are functional end arteries.
- Right conus artery forms an arterial circle around pulmonary trunk with a similar branch from the left coronary artery. The circle is called, 'annulus of Vieussens'.
- Kugel's artery is an atrial branch of left coronary artery that anastomoses with similar branch of right coronary artery along the anterior wall of atria.
- Oblique vein of the left atrium of Marshall develops from the duct of Cuvier.
- Pain of heart due to myocardial infarction is referred to left side of chest between 3rd and 6th intercostal spaces. It also get extended to medial side of left upper limb in the area of distribution of C8 and T1 spinal segments.

BDC's Anatomy *e*-book

1. Triangle of Koch
2. Area of superficial cardiac dullness
3. Musculature of the heart
4. Molecular regulation of cardiac development
5. Foetal circulation
6. Blood circulation through right atrium in embryonic life
7. Atrial septal defects
8. Tetralogy of Fallot
9. Ligament of left vena cava
10. Coronary angiography
11. Echocardiography
12. Myocardial infarction (heart attack)
13. Heart sounds
14. Further reading
15. Viva voce questions

Chapter

19

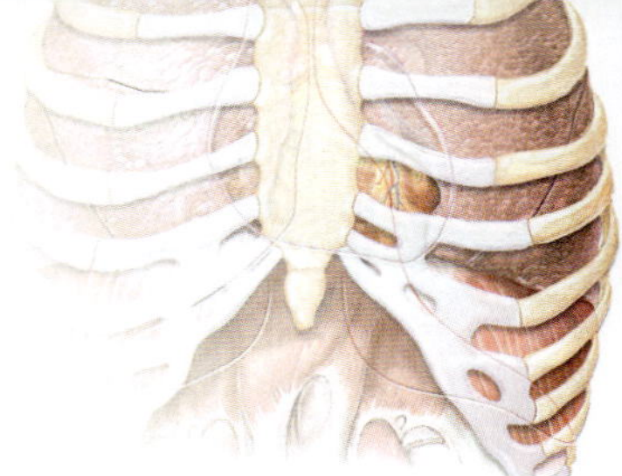

Superior Vena Cava, Aorta and Pulmonary Trunk

Superior vena cava brings deoxygenated blood from the head and neck, upper limbs, and thorax to the heart. Aorta and pulmonary trunk are the only two exit channels from the heart, developing from a single truncus arteriosus (Plate 19.1).

Competency:
AN23.3 Describe and demonstrate origin, course, relations, tributaries and termination of superior vena cava (described below), azygos, hemiazygos and accessory hemiazygos veins (described in Chapter 14).

SUPERIOR VENA CAVA

Superior vena cava (SVC) is a large venous channel which collects blood from the upper half of the body and drains it into the right atrium. It has ***no valves***.

Formation

It is formed by the union of the right and left brachiocephalic or innominate veins behind the lower border of the 1st right costal cartilage close to the sternum. Each brachiocephalic vein is formed behind the corresponding sternoclavicular joint by the union of the internal jugular and subclavian veins (Fig. 19.1).

Course

The superior vena cava is about 7 cm long. It begins behind the lower border of the sternal end of the 1st right costal cartilage, pierces the pericardium opposite the 2nd right costal cartilage.

It terminates by opening into the upper part of the right atrium behind the 3rd right costal cartilage (Fig. 19.1).

[*Mnemonic:* Relations to the important venous structures:
Behind **sternoclavicular** joints: Brachiocephalic veins begin.
Behind the **1st costal cartilage** on the right: Superior vena cava begins.
Behind the **2nd costal cartilage** on the right: Azygos vein ends.
Behind the **3rd costal cartilage** on the right: Superior vena cava ends.]

Relations

Anterior

1. Chest wall
2. Internal thoracic vessels
3. Anterior margin of the right lung and pleura
4. The vessel is covered by pericardium in its lower half (Fig. 19.2).

Posterior

1. Trachea and right vagus (posteromedial to the upper part of the vena cava)
2. Root of right lung posterior to the lower part

Medial

1. Ascending aorta
2. Brachiocephalic artery

Lateral

1. Right phrenic nerve with accompanying vessels
2. Right pleura and lung

Tributaries

1. *Formative tributaries*: Right and left brachiocephalic veins.
2. The ***azygos vein*** arches over the root of the right lung and opens into the superior vena cava at the level of the second costal cartilage, just before the latter enters the pericardium.
3. Several small mediastinal and pericardial veins drain into the vena cava.

CLINICAL ANATOMY

Obstruction of superior vena cava

a. When the superior vena cava is obstructed ***above the opening of the azygos vein***, the venous blood of the upper half of the body is returned through the azygos vein; and the superficial veins are dilated on the chest up to the costal margin (Fig. 19.3). Blood from upper limb is returned through the communicating veins joining the veins around the scapula with the intercostal veins. The latter veins of both sides drain into vena azygos.

Plate 19.1: Major vessels of thoracic region

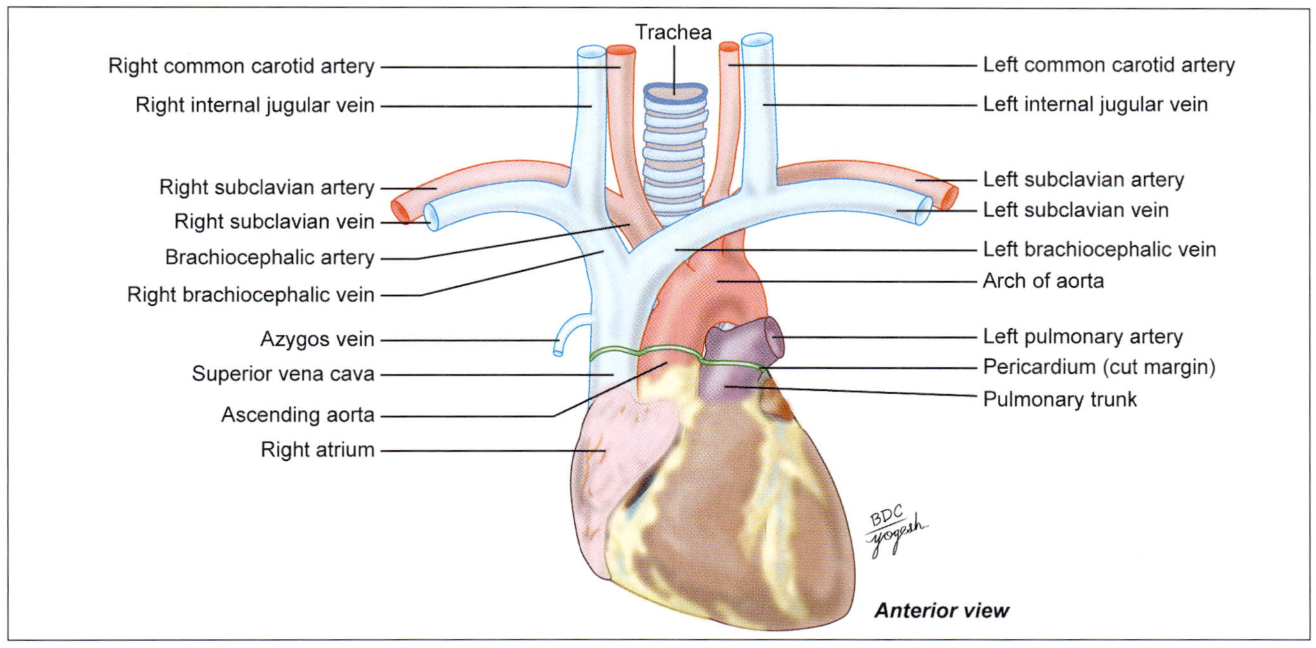

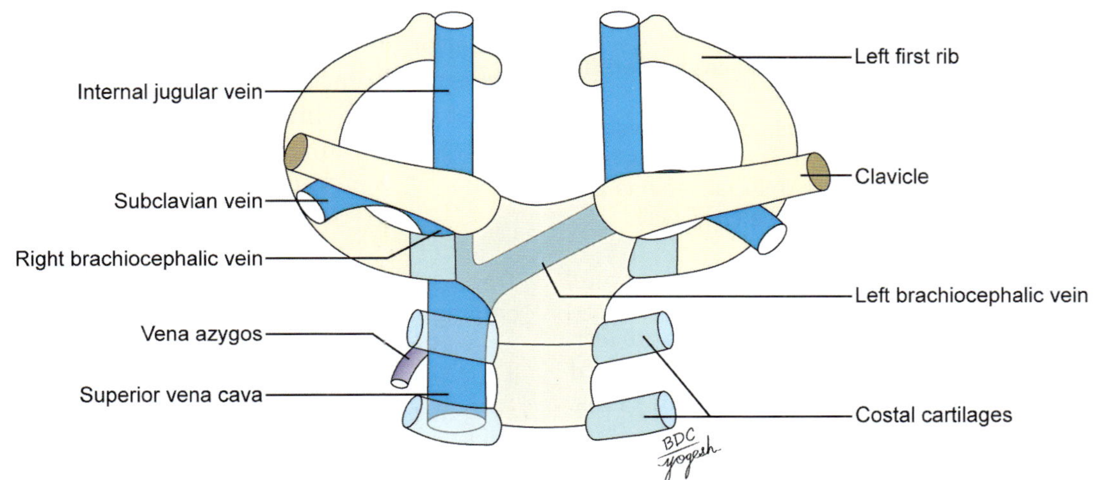

Fig. 19.1: Formation of superior vena cava

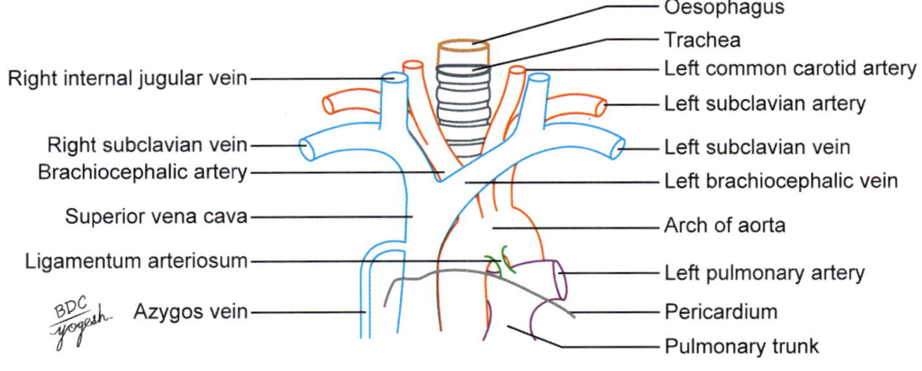

Fig. 19.2: Superior vena cava and its relations

b. When the superior vena cava is obstructed ***below the opening of the azygos veins***, the blood is returned through the inferior vena cava via the femoral vein; and the superior veins are dilated on both the chest and abdomen up to the saphenous opening in the thigh. The superficial vein connecting the lateral thoracic vein with the superficial epigastric vein is known as the ***thoracoepigastric vein*** (Fig. 19.3).

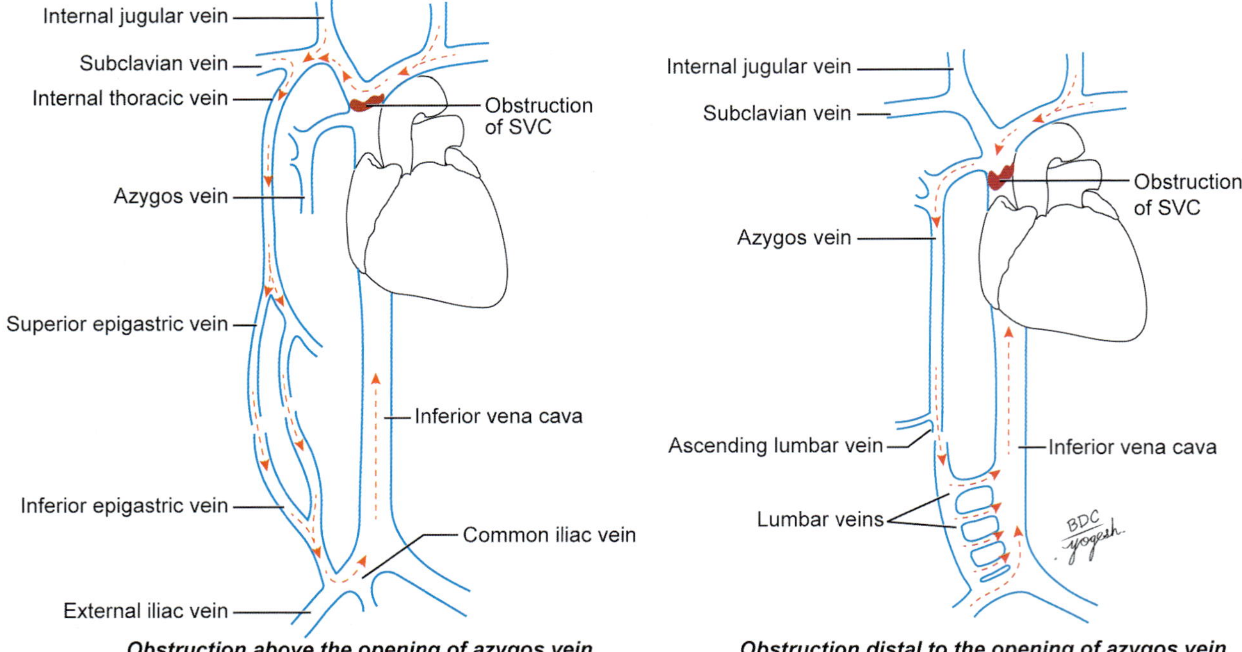

Fig. 19.3: Obstruction to superior vena cava

Note:
- Azygos vein opens in SVC just before SVC pierces the pericardium.
- Patients of SVC obstruction may complain of facial swelling, chest pain, cough, dysphagia, and so on. These patients have distention of veins of neck and chest wall, facial oedema and upper limb oedema, and dilated veins on the chest wall.

BRACHIOCEPHALIC VEINS

There are two brachiocephalic veins, right and left. Each brachiocephalic vein is formed by union of corresponding internal jugular and subclavian veins. Both (right and left) brachiocephalic veins unite to form superior vena cava. Each brachiocephalic vein extends from corresponding sternoclavicular joint to the lower border of the 1st right costal cartilage where they form SVC.

The differences between right and left brachiocephalic veins are listed in Table 19.1.

Tributaries

1. Formative tributaries:
   a. Internal jugular vein
   b. Subclavian vein.
2. Vertebral vein

TABLE 19.1: Difference between the right and left brachiocephalic veins

Feature	*Right brachiocephalic vein*	*Left brachiocephalic vein*
Length	2.5 cm (shorter)	6 cm (longer)
Course	Vertical	Oblique
Tributaries	Do not drain right superior intercostal vein	Drain left superior intercostal vein

3. Inferior thyroid vein
4. Internal thoracic vein
5. First posterior intercostal vein
6. Left superior intercostal vein.

DISSECTION

Trace superior vena cava from level of first right costal cartilage where it is formed by union of left and right brachiocephalic veins till the third costal cartilage where it opens into right atrium (Fig. 19.1).

Trace the ascending aorta from the vestibule of left ventricle upwards between superior vena cava and pulmonary trunk (Fig. 19.2).

Arch of aorta is seen above the bifurcation of pulmonary trunk.

Cut ligamentum arteriosum as it connects the left pulmonary artery to the arch of aorta.

Trace the left recurrent laryngeal nerve to the medial aspect of arch of aorta.

Lift the side of oesophagus forwards to expose the anterior surface of the descending aorta.

Lift the diaphragm forwards and expose the aorta in the inferior part of the posterior mediastinum.

AORTA

The aorta is the great arterial trunk which receives oxygenated blood from the left ventricle and distributes it to all parts of the body. It is studied in thorax in the following three parts:
1. Ascending aorta
2. Arch of the aorta
3. Descending thoracic aorta.

ASCENDING AORTA

Origin and Course

The ascending aorta arises from the upper end of the left ventricle. It is about 5 cm long and is enclosed in the pericardium (Fig. 19.4, Flowchart 19.1). It begins behind the left half of the sternum at the level of the lower border of the third costal cartilage. It runs upwards, forwards and to the right and becomes continuous with the arch of the aorta at the sternal end of the upper border of the second right costal cartilage.

At the root of the aorta, there are three dilatations of the vessel wall, called the *aortic sinuses*. The sinuses are anterior, left posterior, and right posterior.

Relations

Anterior

1. Sternum
2. Right lung and pleura
3. Infundibulum of the right ventricle
4. Root of the pulmonary trunk (Fig. 19.2)
5. Right auricle.

Posterior

1. Transverse sinus of pericardium
2. Left atrium
3. Right pulmonary artery
4. Right bronchus.

To the Right

1. Superior vena cava
2. Right atrium.

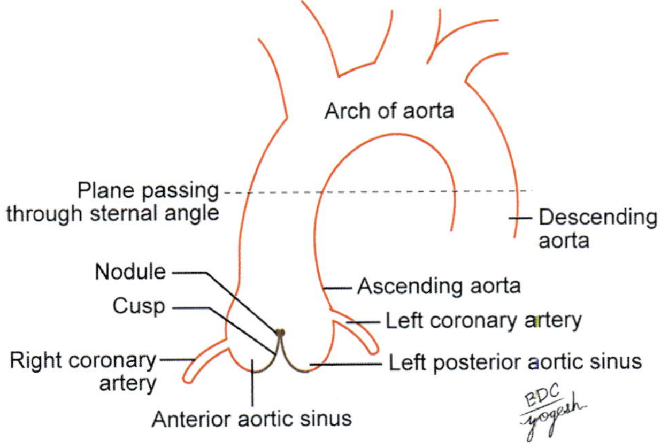

Fig. 19.4: Ascending aorta and arch of aorta

Flowchart 19.1: Ascending aorta

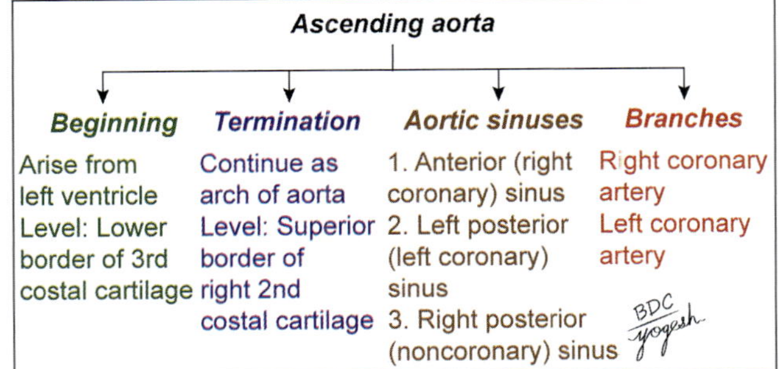

To the Left

1. Pulmonary trunk above
2. Left atrium below.

Branches

1. The right coronary artery arises from anterior aortic sinus.
2. Left coronary artery arises from the left posterior aortic sinus.

Note:

Aortic sinuses (sinuses of the Valsalva): The root of the ascending aorta shows three dilatations of vessel wall. These dilatations are called aortic sinuses of Valsalva. There are three dilatations (Fig. 19.4):

1. *Anterior aortic* or *right coronary sinus*: Anterior aortic sinus gives rise to the right coronary artery. Hence, it is also called right coronary sinus.
2. *Left posterior aortic* or *left coronary sinus*: Left posterior aortic sinus gives rise to the left coronary artery. Hence, it is also called left coronary sinus.
3. *Right posterior aortic* or *noncoronary sinus*: The right posterior aortic sinus does not give rise to any coronary artery. Hence, it is called non-coronary sinus.

Competencies:

AN23.4 Mention the extent, branches and relations of arch of aorta and descending thoracic aorta.

AN25.5 Describe developmental basis of congenital anomalies, transposition of great vessels, dextrocardia, patent ductus arteriosus and coarctation of aorta.

ARCH OF AORTA

Arch of the aorta is the continuation of the ascending aorta. It is situated in the superior mediastinum behind the lower half of the manubrium sterni.

Course

1. It begins behind the upper border of the 2nd right sternochondral joint (Fig. 19.4, Flowchart 19.2).
2. It runs upwards, backwards and to the left across the left side of the bifurcation of trachea. Then it passes downwards behind the left bronchus and on the left side of the body of the 4th thoracic vertebra. It thus arches over the root of the left lung.

Flowchart 19.2: Arch of aorta

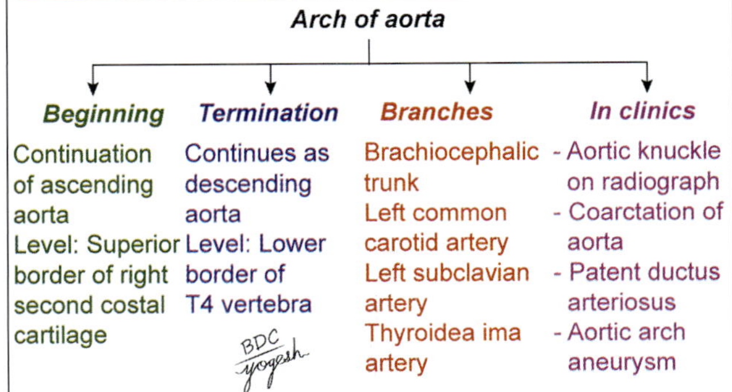

3. It ends at the lower border of the body of the fourth thoracic vertebra by becoming continuous with the descending aorta. Thus, the beginning and the end of arch of aorta are at the same level, although it begins anteriorly and ends posteriorly.

Relations

Anteriorly and to the Left

1. Four nerves from before backwards:
   a. Left phrenic
   b. Lower cervical cardiac branch of the left vagus
   c. Superior cervical cardiac branch of left sympathetic chain.
   d. Left vagus (Figs 19.5 and 19.6).
2. Left superior intercostal vein, deep to the phrenic nerve and superficial to the vagus nerve
3. Left pleura and lung
4. Remains of thymus.

Posteriorly and to the Right

1. Trachea, with the deep cardiac plexus and the tracheobronchial lymph nodes
2. Oesophagus
3. Left recurrent laryngeal nerve
4. Thoracic duct
5. Vertebral column.

Superior

1. Three branches of the arch of the aorta:
   a. Brachiocephalic
   b. Left common carotid
   c. Left subclavian artery (Figs 19.7 and 19.8)
2. All three arteries are crossed close to their origin by the left brachiocephalic vein.

Inferior

1. Bifurcation of the pulmonary trunk (Fig. 19.2).
2. Left bronchus
3. Ligamentum arteriosum with superficial cardiac plexus on it.
4. Left recurrent laryngeal nerve (Fig. 19.9).

Branches

1. Brachiocephalic artery which divides into the right common carotid and right subclavian arteries (Fig. 19.9).
2. Left common carotid artery
3. Left subclavian artery
4. Occasional branch—thyroidea ima artery.

[*Mnemonic*: "Know your **ABC'S**": **A**ortic arch gives rise to: **B**rachiocephalic trunk, Left **C**ommon Carotid, Left **S**ubclavian]

DESCENDING THORACIC AORTA

Descending thoracic aorta is the continuation of the arch of the aorta. It lies in the posterior mediastinum. It continues as abdominal aorta which ends by dividing into right and left common iliac arteries.

Course

1. It begins on the left side of the lower border of the body of the 4th thoracic vertebra (Fig. 19.4).
2. It descends with an inclination to the right and terminates at the lower border of the 12th thoracic vertebra.

Relations (Fig. 19.10)

Anterior

1. Root of left lung
2. Pericardium and heart
3. Oesophagus in the lower part
4. Diaphragm

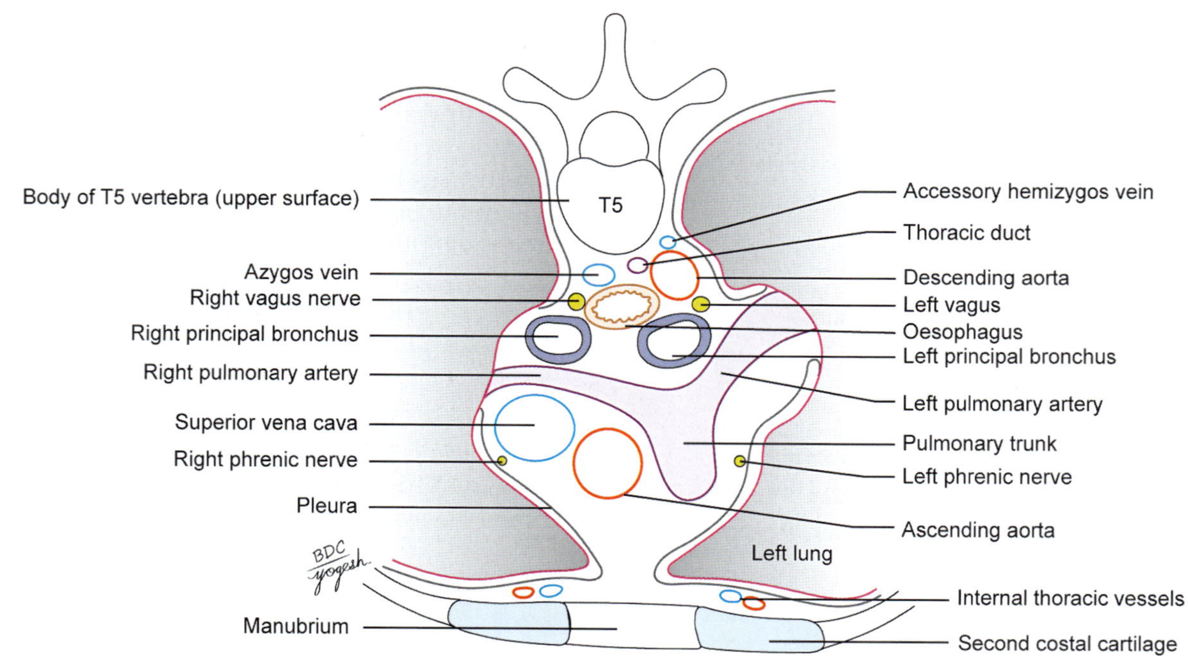

Fig. 19.5: Transverse section of the thorax passing through the T5 vertebra

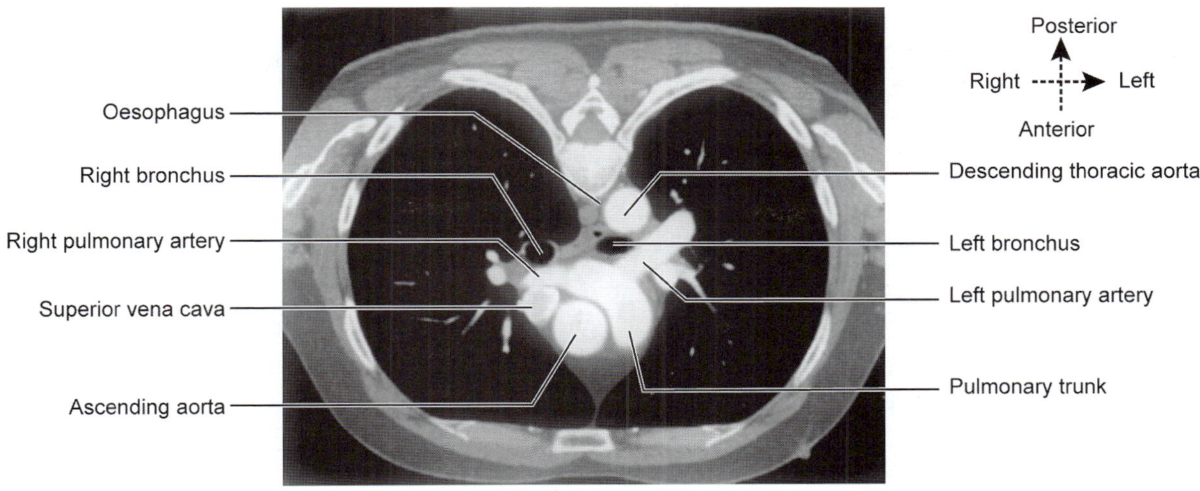

Fig. 19.6: CT scan section of the thorax passing through the T5 vertebra

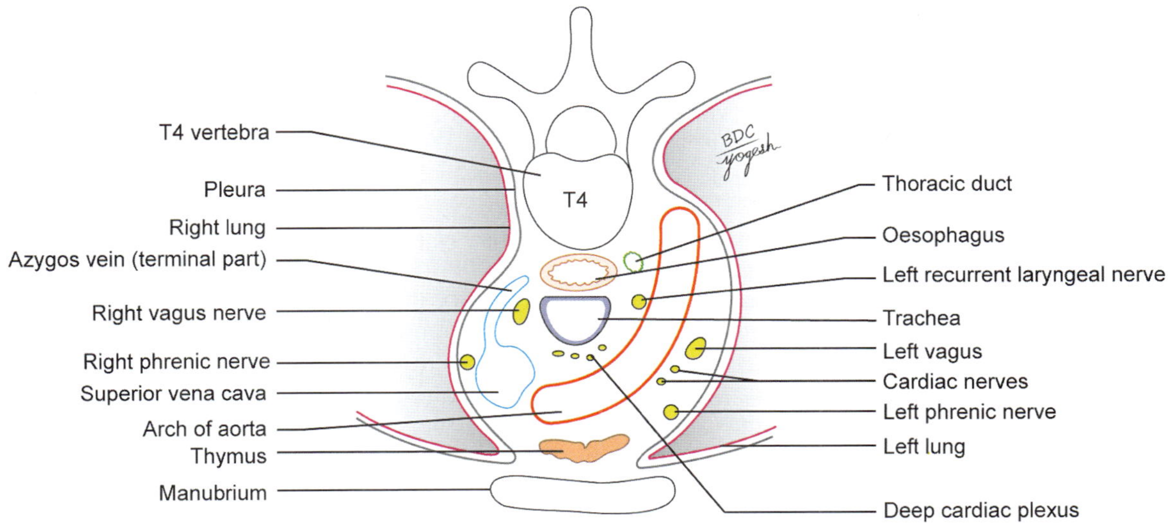

Fig. 19.7: Transverse section of the thorax passing through the T4 vertebra

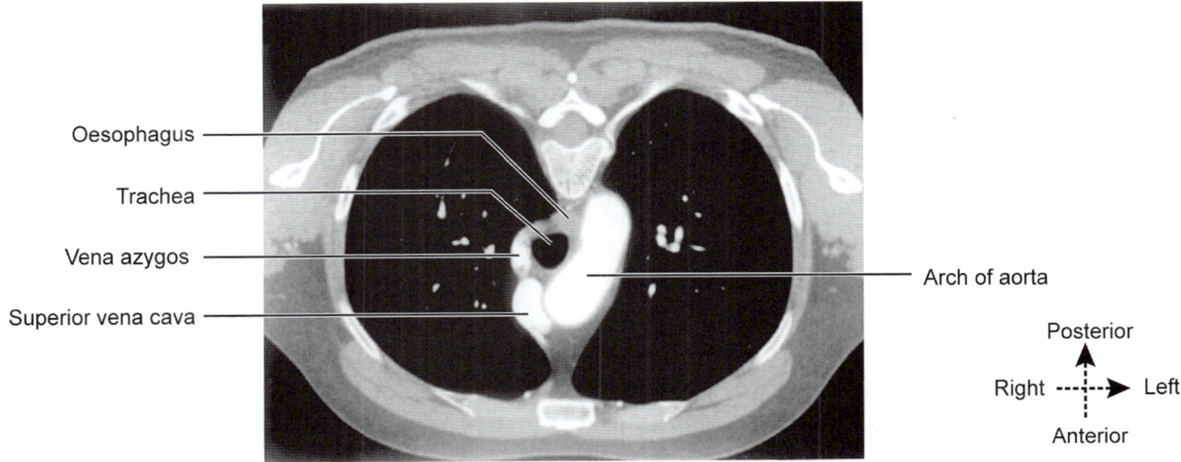

Fig. 19.8: CT scan section of the thorax passing through the T4 vertebra

Posterior

1. Vertebral column
2. Hemiazygos veins

To the Right Side

1. Oesophagus in the upper part
2. Azygos vein

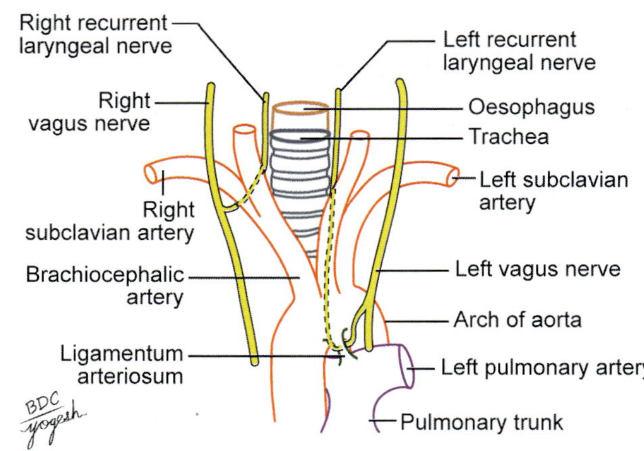

Fig. 19.9: Relations of aorta with vagus and recurrent laryngeal nerve

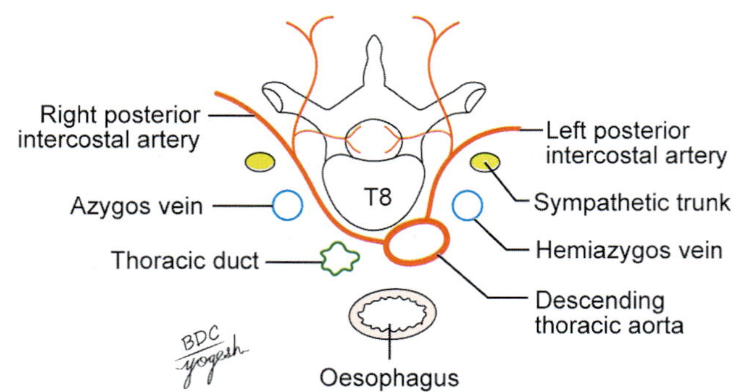

Fig. 19.10: Origin of posterior intercostal arteries from descending thoracic aorta

3. Thoracic duct
4. Right lung and pleura.

To the Left Side

Left lung and pleura.

Branches

1. Nine posterior intercostal arteries on each side for the 3rd to 11th intercostal spaces (Fig. 19.11).
2. The subcostal artery on each side.
3. Two left bronchial arteries. The right bronchial artery arises from the 3rd right posterior intercostal artery.
4. Oesophageal branches, supplying the middle 1/3rd of the oesophagus.
5. Pericardial branches, to the posterior surface of the pericardium.
6. Mediastinal branches, to lymph nodes and areolar tissue of the posterior mediastinum.
7. Superior phrenic arteries to the posterior part of the superior surface of the diaphragm. Branches of these arteries anastomose with those of the musculophrenic and pericardiacophrenic arteries.

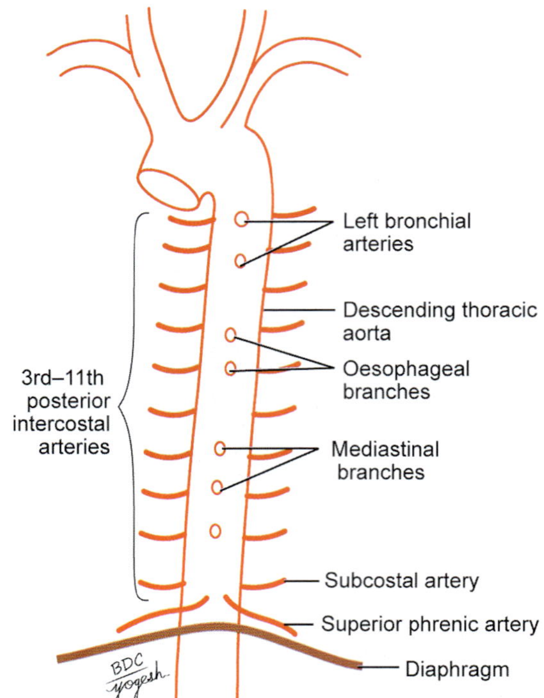

Fig. 19.11: Branches of descending thoracic aorta

CLINICAL ANATOMY

- ***Aortic knuckle:*** In posteroanterior view of radiographs of the chest, the arch of the aorta is seen as a projection beyond the left margin of the mediastinal shadow. The projection is called the aortic knuckle. It becomes prominent in old age (Fig. 19.12).
- ***Coarctation of the aorta*** is a localised narrowing of the aorta opposite to or just beyond the attachment of the ductus arteriosus. An extensive collateral circulation develops between the branches of the subclavian arteries and those of the descending aorta. These include the anastomoses between the anterior and posterior intercostal arteries. These arteries enlarge greatly and produce a characteristic ***notching on the ribs*** (Figs 19.13 and 19.14).
- ***Ductus arteriosus, ligamentum arteriosum** and **patent ductus arteriosus:*** During foetal life, the *ductus arteriosus* is a short wide channel connecting the beginning of the left pulmonary artery with the arch of the aorta immediately distal to the origin of the left subclavian artery. It conducts most of the blood from the right ventricle into the aorta, thus short circuiting the lungs. After birth, it is closed functionally within about a week and anatomically within about 8 weeks. The remnants of the ductus form a fibrous band called the *ligamentum arteriosum.* The left recurrent laryngeal nerve hooks around the ligamentum arteriosum. The ductus may remain patent after birth. This condition is called ***patent ductus arteriosus*** (*patent = open*) and may cause serious problems. The condition can be surgically treated.
- ***Aortic arch aneurysm*** is a localised dilatation of the aorta which may press upon the left recurrent laryngeal nerve leading to paralysis of left vocal cord and hoarseness. It may also press upon the surrounding structures and cause the mediastinal syndrome (Fig. 19.15), i.e. dyspnoea, dysphagia, dysphonia, etc.

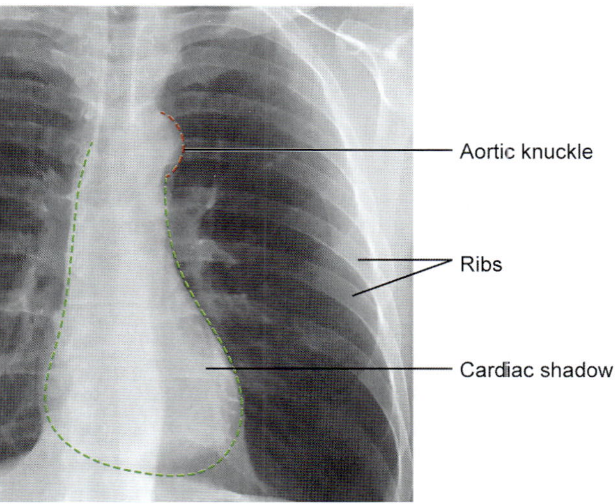

Fig. 19.12: Aortic knuckle (chest radiograph, PA view)

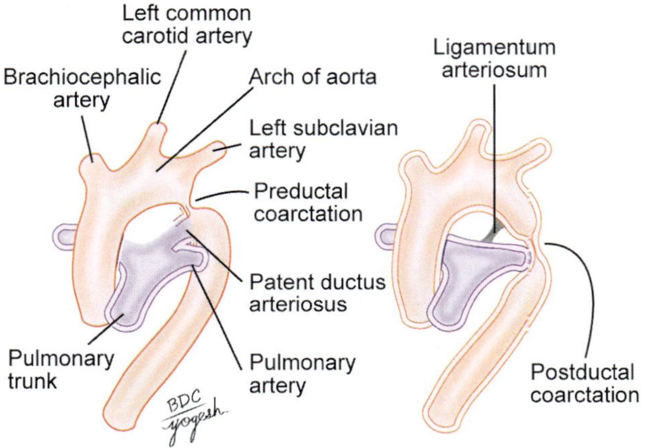

Fig. 19.13: Coarctation of aorta and patent ductus arteriosus. Coarctation of aorta is a congenital narrowing of arch of aorta distal to the origin of left subclavian artery. Preductal coarctation is narrowing proximal to the ductus arteriosus, whereas postductal coarctation is a narrowing distal to the ductus arteriosus (*Source*: Textbook of Human Embryology, Yogesh Sontakke, 2e, CBS Publisher).

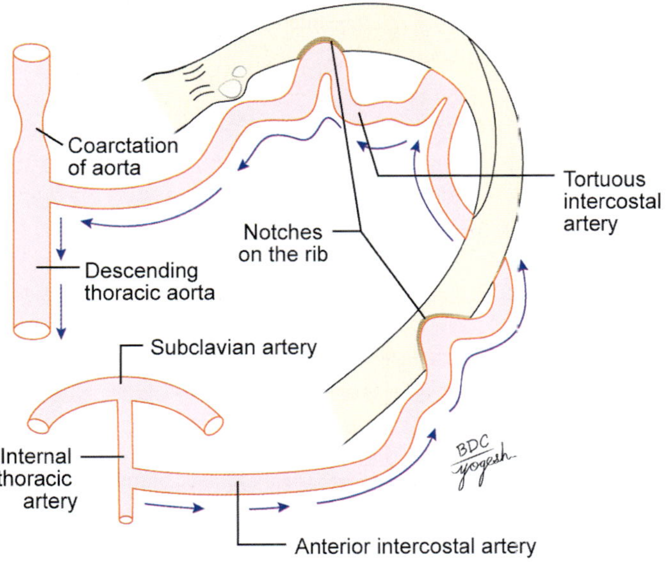

Fig. 19.14: Notching of ribs in coarctation of aorta

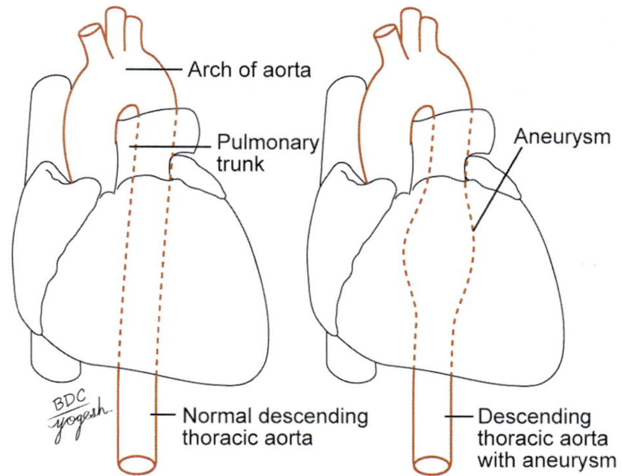

Fig. 19.15: Aneurysm of aorta

PULMONARY TRUNK

The wide pulmonary trunk starts from the summit of infundibulum of right ventricle. Both the ascending aorta and pulmonary trunk are enclosed in a common sleeve of serous pericardium, in front of transverse sinus of pericardium.

Pulmonary trunk carrying deoxygenated blood overlies the beginning of ascending aorta. It courses to the left and divides into right and left pulmonary arteries under the concavity of aortic arch at the level of sternal angle (Plate 19.1, Fig. 19.2).

The right pulmonary artery courses to the right behind ascending aorta, and superior vena cava and anterior to oesophagus to become part of the root of the lung. It gives off its 1st branch to the upper lobe before entering the hilum. Within the lung, the artery descends posterolateral to the main bronchus and divides like the bronchi into lobar and segmental arteries.

The left pulmonary artery passes to the left anterior to descending thoracic aorta to become part of the root of the left lung. At its beginning, it is connected to the inferior aspect of arch of aorta by ligamentum arteriosus, a remnant of ductus arteriosus. Rest of the course is same as of the right branch.

Branches

1. Right pulmonary artery: It carries deoxygenated blood to the right lung.
2. Left pulmonary artery: It carries deoxygenated blood to the left lung.

CLINICAL ANATOMY

Sudden occlusion of pulmonary trunk: Thrombus from right ventricle or large veins may cause sudden occlusion of pulmonary trunk.

Pulmonary artery catheterization (right heart catheterization): It involves insertion of catheter into pulmonary artery through internal jugular vein or subclavian vein (→ SVC → right atrium → right ventricle → pulmonary

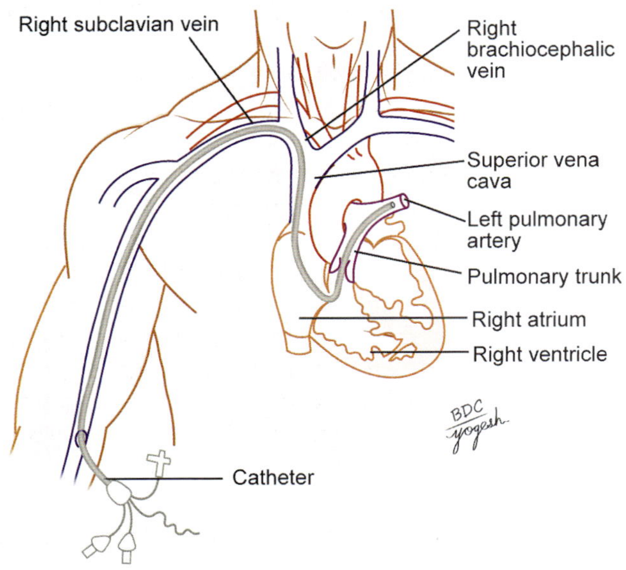

Fig. 19.16: Pulmonary artery characterization

trunk) (Fig. 19.16). It is useful for assessment of respiratory distress, assessment of right-sided cardiac functions, and so on.

Competency:
AN24.4 Identify phrenic nerve and describe its formation and distribution.

PHRENIC NERVE

Phrenic nerve arising from (C3–C5) cervical nerves is a mixed nerve carrying motor fibres to the diaphragm and sensory fibres from mediastinal pleura, pericardium and part of peritoneum (Fig. 19.17, Flowchart 19.3).

Course

Right phrenic nerve: Right phrenic nerve is shorter, vertical and deeply placed. It crosses 2nd part of right subclavian artery. It runs along right side of venous system and passes through vena caval opening of the diaphragm.

Left phrenic nerve: Left phrenic nerve is longer, oblique and not deeply placed. It crosses 1st part of left subclavian artery. It runs along left side of arterial system and pierces the left cupola of the diaphragm.

Flowchart 19.3: Phrenic nerve

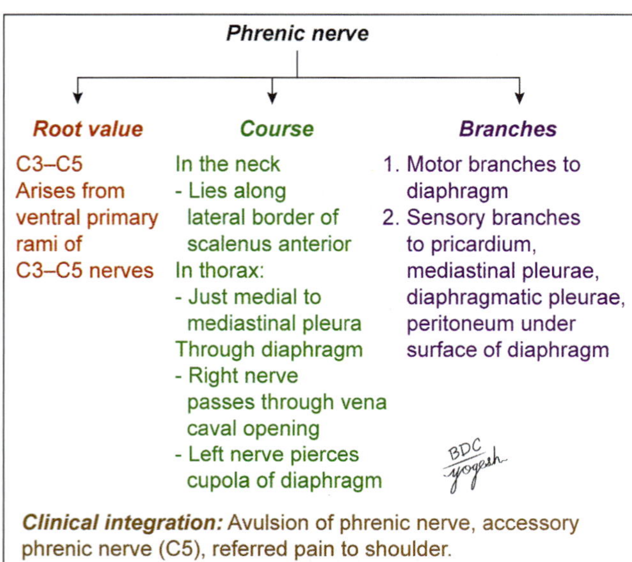

Branches (Fig. 19.17)

1. It supplies diaphragm from its under surface through four sets of branches on each side — anteromedial, anterolateral, posteromedial, and posterolateral.
2. Right phrenic nerve — right half of the diaphragm, part of right crus.
3. Left phrenic nerve — left half of the diaphragm, left crus, and part of right crus.
4. Also supplies pleura and peritoneum.

CLINICAL ANATOMY

- ***Avulsion of phrenic nerve*** (old surgical method): Crushing or avulsion of phrenic nerve was done to paralyze half part of the diaphragm. It was useful in the treatment of severe lung disease.
- ***Accessory phrenic nerve*** (root value C5) (Fig. 19.18): It is the branch of nerve to subclavius (C5). It may descend in front of subclavian vein and then join phrenic nerve in the thorax. Accessory phrenic nerve, if present, may damage the subclavian vein during avulsion of phrenic nerve → severe bleeding.
- ***Referred pain of diaphragm:*** Pain from the diaphragm get referred from phrenic nerve (C3–C5) to the shoulder region through supraclavicular nerves (C3–C4).

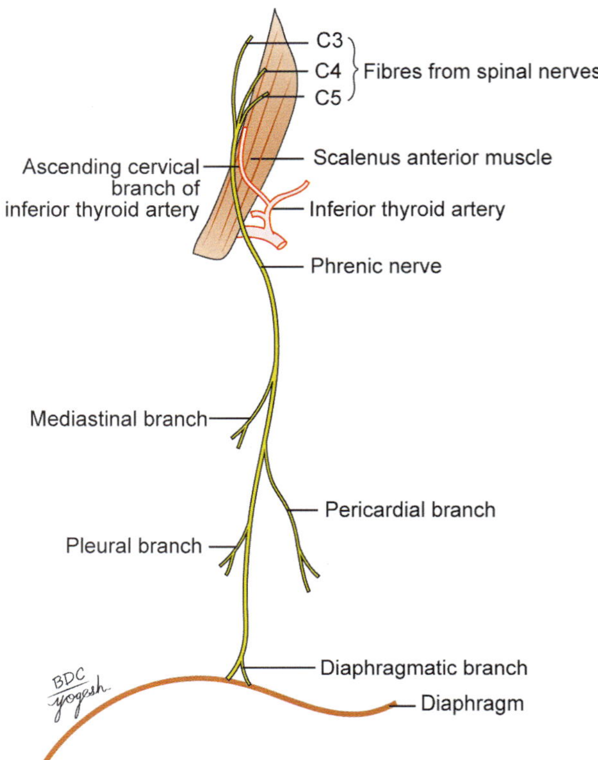

Fig. 19.17: Phrenic nerve (right)

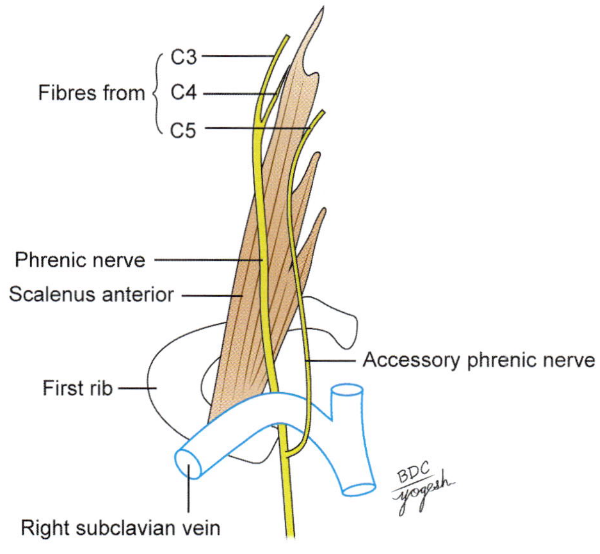

Fig. 19.18: Accessory phrenic nerve

Competency:

AN25.6 Mention development of aortic arch arteries, SVC, IVC and coronary sinus.

DEVELOPMENT OF MAJOR VESSELS (Fig. 19.19)

- *Brachiocephalic artery:* Right aortic sac
- *Right subclavian artery:* Proximal part from the right 4th aortic arch artery and remaining part from right 7th cervical intersegmental artery.
- *Left subclavian artery:* Only left 7th cervical intersegmental artery.
- *Common carotid:* Third aortic arch, distal to the external carotid bud and original dorsal aorta cranial to the attachment of third aortic arch.
- *External carotid artery:* Develop as sprout from the third aortic arch.
- *Pulmonary trunk:* Part of truncus arteriosus.
- *Arch of aorta:* Left aortic sac. Left 4th aortic arch. Left dorsal aorta.
- Relation to recurrent laryngeal nerve. Recurrent laryngeal is given off from vagi in relation to distal part of 6th arch artery. Since this distal part forms ligamentum arteriosum on left side only, the recurrent laryngeal nerve hooks around this ligamentum in thorax to reach tracheo-oesophageal groove. On the right side, there is no ligamentum arteriosum. The recurrent laryngeal nerve slips upwards in the neck and hooks around the right subclavian artery to reach the tracheo-oesophageal groove.
- Development of superior vena cava
  - Upper half of superior vena cava (extrapericardial) develops from caudal part of right anterior cardinal vein.
  - Lower half of superior vena cava (intrapericardial) develops from right common cardinal vein.
- Coronary sinus is a remnant of left horn of sinus venosus. Great, middle, and anterior cardiac veins drain into this sinus.

Facts to Remember

- Superior vena cava is the second largest vein of the body.
- Vena azygos brings the venous blood from the posterior parts of thoracic and abdominal wall.
- Aorta is the largest elastic artery of the body. It takes oxygenated blood to all parts of the body except the lungs.
- There is a gradual transition from its elastic nature to muscular nature of its branches.

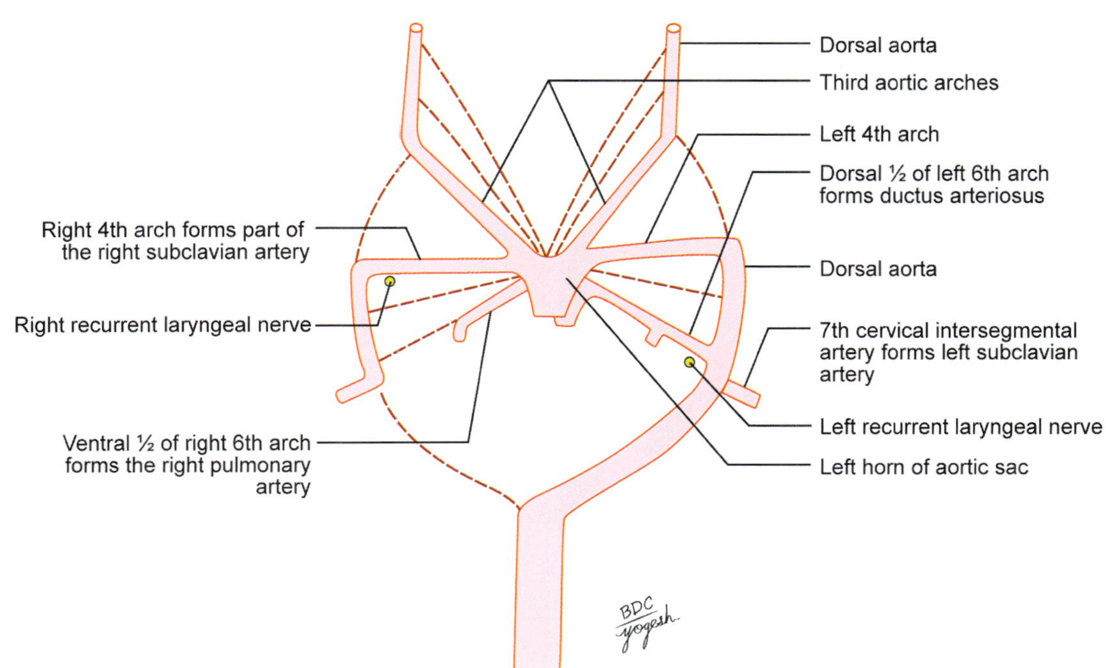

Fig. 19.19: Foetal aortic arches showing development of arch arteries

- Pulmonary trunk arises from the right ventricle. It soon divides into right and left pulmonary arteries which carry deoxygenated blood from right ventricle to the lungs for oxygenation.
- Pulmonary trunk and ascending aorta develop from a common source, the truncus arteriosus.
- There is triple relationship between these two vessels:
  - Close to heart, pulmonary trunk lies anterior to ascending aorta.
  - At upper border of heart, pulmonary trunk lies to the left of ascending aorta (Fig. 19.2).
  - A little above this, the right pulmonary artery lies posterior to the ascending aorta.

BDC's Anatomy *e*-book

1. Major vessels of thoracic region
2. Viva voce questions

HEART

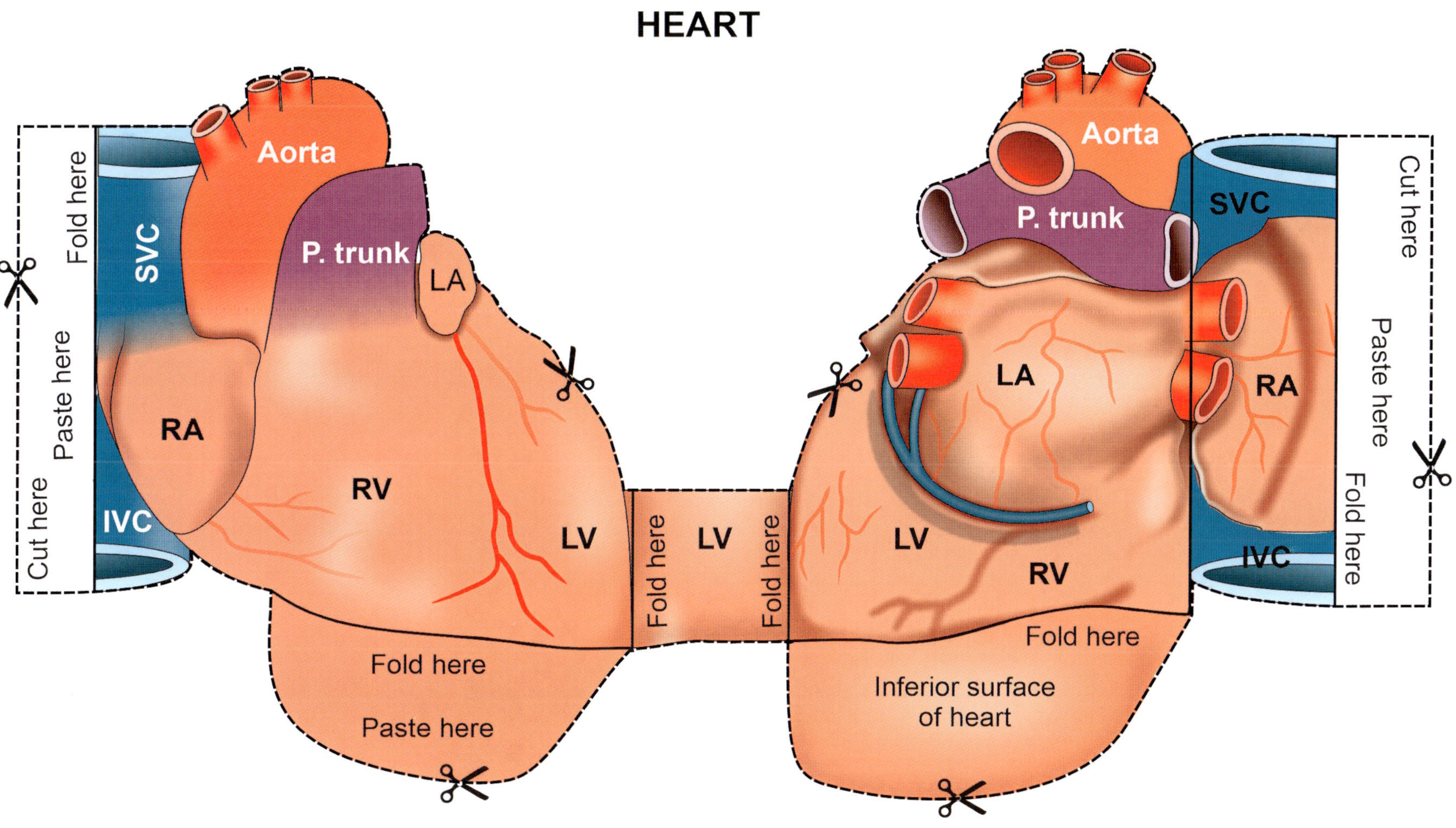

- Cut, fold and paste at the appropriate sites
- Fill it with cotton carefully

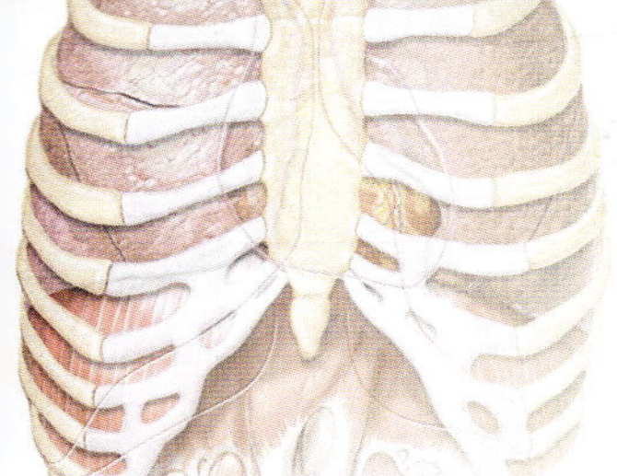

Chapter

20

Trachea, Oesophagus and Thoracic Duct

Competency:

AN24.6 Describe the extent, length, relations, blood supply, lymphatic drainage, and nerve supply of trachea.

TRACHEA

The trachea or *windpipe* (Latin *air vessel*) is a wide tube lying more or less in the midline, in the lower part of the neck, and in the superior mediastinum. Its upper end is continuous with the lower end of the larynx.

Note: The trachea has a fibroelastic wall supported by a cartilaginous skeleton formed by C-shaped rings. The rings are about 16 – 20 in number and make the tube convex anterolaterally. Posteriorly, there is a gap that is closed by a fibroelastic membrane and contains transversely arranged smooth muscle known as the ***trachealis***.

As the tracheal rings are incomplete posteriorly, the oesophagus can dilate during swallowing. This also allows the diameter of the trachea to be controlled by the trachealis muscle. This muscle narrows the calibre of the tube, compressing the contained air, if the vocal cords are closed. This increases the explosive force of the blast of compressed air, as occurs in coughing and sneezing.

Location

1. The trachea in the neck is covered by the isthmus of the thyroid gland and acts as a shield for trachea. At its lower end, the trachea ends by dividing into the right and left principal bronchi (Fig. 20.1).
2. The upper end of the trachea lies at the lower border of the cricoid cartilage, opposite the 6th cervical vertebra.
3. It bifurcates at the level of the body of the 5th or 6th thoracic vertebra or the T5–T6 intervertebral disc (*Reference*: 42nd Gray's Anatomy). [*Previous concept*: Trachea bifurcates at the lower border of T4 vertebra.]
4. Thus, the upper part of the trachea is located in the neck (***cervical part***) and lower part in the superior mediastinum (***thoracic part***).

Dimensions

The trachea is 10 – 11 cm in length.

Its external diameter measures about 2 cm in males and about 1.5 cm in females.

Lumen of the trachea:

1. The lumen is smaller in the living than in the cadaver.
2. It is about 3 mm at one year of age.
3. During childhood, it corresponds to the age in years, with a maximum of about 12 mm in adults, i.e. it increases 1 mm per year up to 12 years.

Course

Over most of its length, the trachea lies in the median plane, but near the lower end, it deviates slightly to the right. As it runs downwards, the trachea passes slightly backwards following the curvature of the spine.

Relations of the Thoracic Part

(Plate 20.1, Figs 20.1 and 20.2)

Anteriorly

1. Manubrium sterni
2. Sternothyroid muscles
3. Remains of the thymus
4. Left brachiocephalic and inferior thyroid veins
5. Aortic arch, brachiocephalic and left common carotid arteries
6. Deep cardiac plexus
7. Some lymph nodes.

Posteriorly

1. Oesophagus
2. Vertebral column.

On the Right Side

1. Right lung and pleura
2. Right vagus
3. Azygos vein (Plate 20.1).

On the Left Side

1. Arch of aorta, left common carotid and left subclavian arteries.
2. Left recurrent laryngeal nerve (Plate 20.1).

Arterial supply: Inferior thyroid arteries.

Venous drainage: Into the left brachiocephalic vein.

Lymphatic drainage: To the pretracheal and paratracheal nodes.

Plate 20.1: Relations of trachea and oesophagus

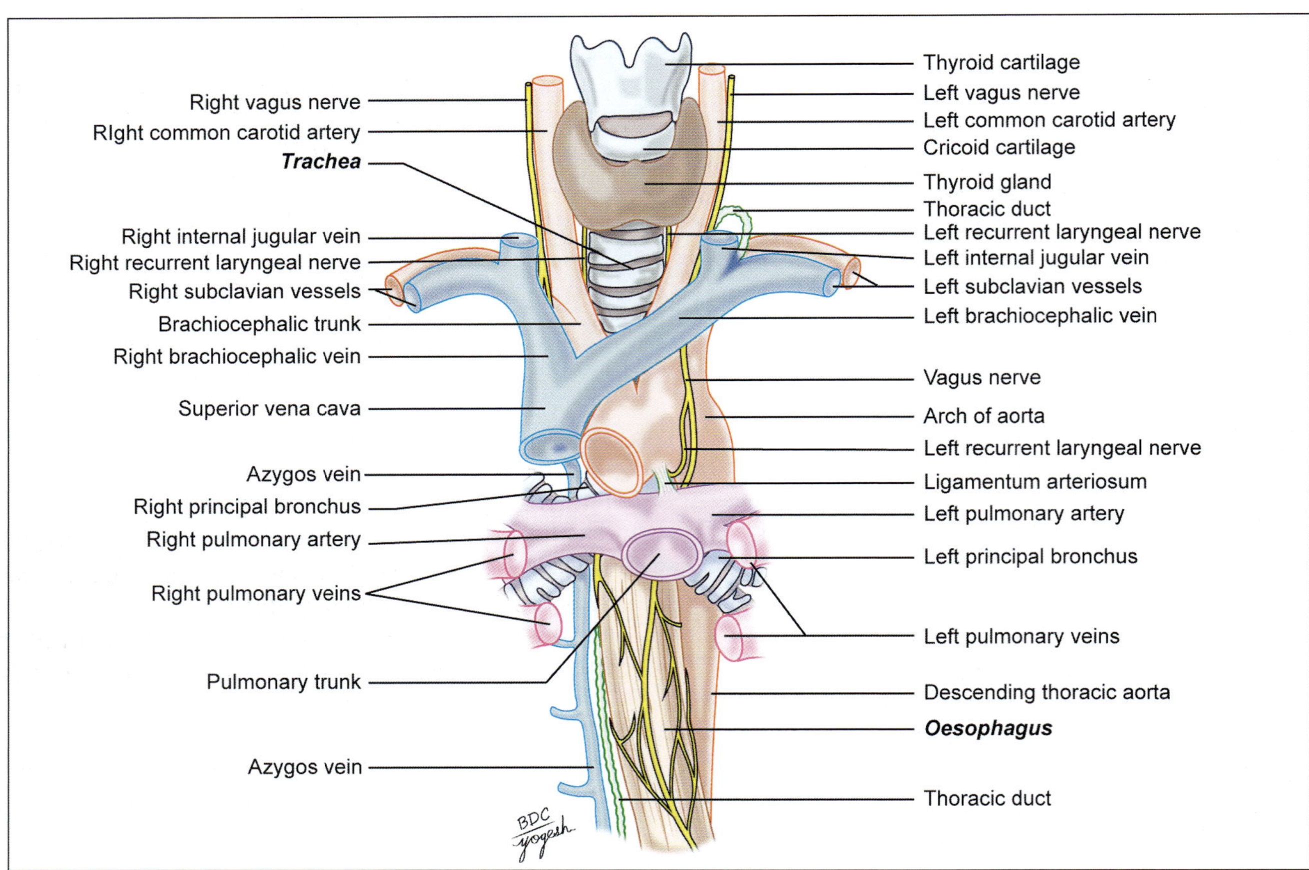

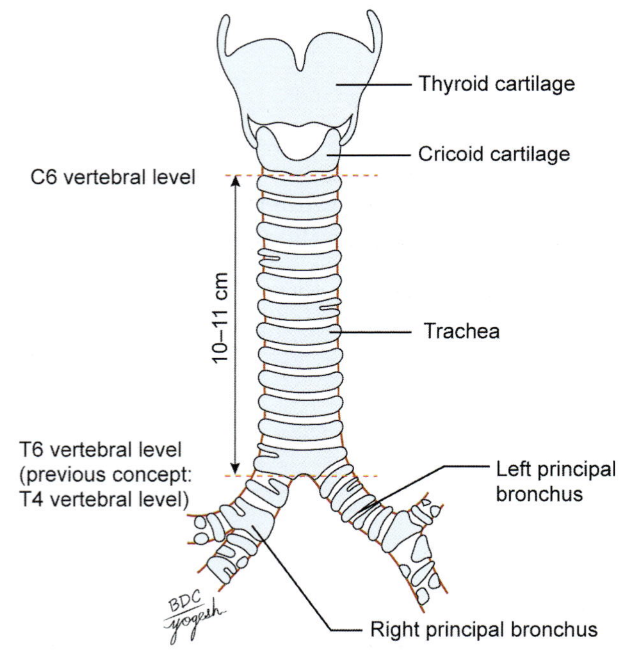

Fig. 20.1: Trachea

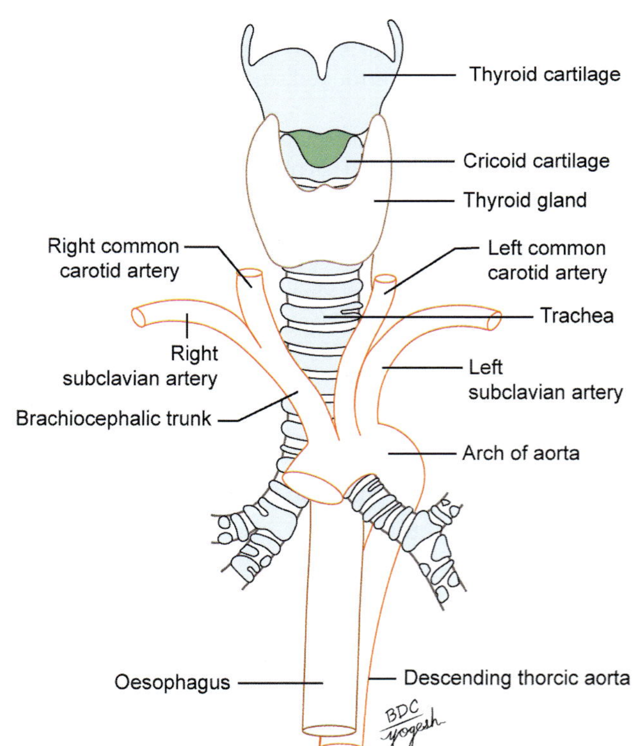

Fig. 20.2: Relations of the trachea with arch of aorta and thyroid gland

Nerve Supply

1. *Parasympathetic:* Nerves through vagi and recurrent laryngeal nerves. It is:
   a. Sensory and secretomotor to the mucous membrane.
   b. Motor to the trachealis muscle.
2. *Sympathetic:* Fibres from the middle cervical ganglion reach it along the inferior thyroid arteries and are vasomotor.

Competency:
AN25.1 Identify, draw, and label a slide of trachea and lung.

STRUCTURE (HISTOLOGY) OF TRACHEA

Trachea has four layers: Mucosa, submucosa, cartilage – muscle layer, and adventitia (Fig. 20.3, Flowchart 20.1).

1. Mucosa has ***pseudostratified ciliated columnar epithelium*** that has ciliated columnar cells, goblet cells (mucous secreting), brush cells (sensory), small granule cells (enteroendocrine-like), and basal cell (germinal cells).
2. The epithelium rests on thick basement membrane and lamina propria that has bronchus-associated lymphatic tissue (BALT).
3. Trachea has 16–20 C-shaped hyaline cartilages. Gaps of tracheal rings are filled by fibroelastic tissue and trachealis (smooth) muscle.
4. Trachea is externally covered by fibroelastic tissue of adventitia.

CLINICAL ANATOMY

- ***Tracheal shadow in radiograph:*** In radiographs, the trachea is seen as a vertical translucent shadow due to the contained air in front of the cervicothoracic spine (Fig. 20.4).
- ***Palpation of trachea:*** Clinically, the trachea is palpated in the suprasternal notch. Normally, it is median in position. Shift of the trachea to any side indicates a mediastinal shift.
- During swallowing when the larynx is elevated, the trachea elongates by stretching because the tracheal bifurcation is not permitted to move by the aortic arch. Any downward pull due to sudden and forced inspiration or aortic aneurysm will produce a physical sign known as '***tracheal tug***'.
- ***Tracheostomy:*** It is a surgical procedure which allows air to enter directly into trachea. It is done in cases of blockage of air pathway in nose or larynx (Fig. 20.5).
- ***Importance of mucous secretion in trachea:*** *Mucus secretions* help in trapping inhaled foreign particles, and the soiled mucus is then expelled by coughing. The cilia of the mucous membrane beat upwards, pushing the mucus towards the pharynx.
- The trachea may get compressed by pathological enlargements of the thyroid, the thymus, lymph nodes and the aortic arch. This causes dyspnoea, irritative cough, and often a husky voice.
- ***Carina***: It is a median ridge in the trachea at the bifurcation of the trachea. It is richly supplied by sensory nerves that can induce cough reflex (Fig. 20.6).
- Endotracheal tube should be selected according to the age of individual up to the age of 12 years (Fig. 20.7) because luminal diameter increases by 1 mm per year up to the age of 12 years.

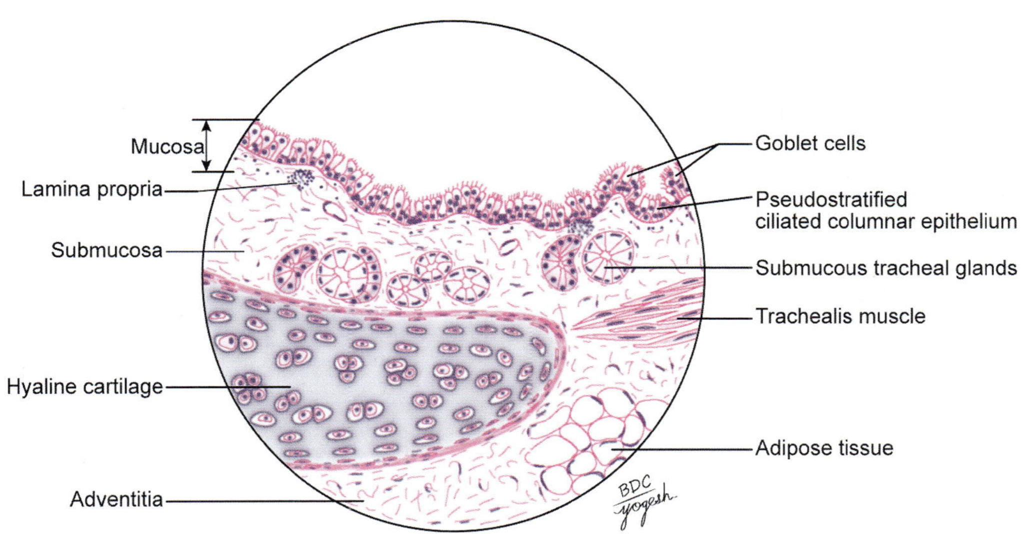

Fig. 20.3: Histology of the trachea

Flowchart 20.1: Histology of trachea

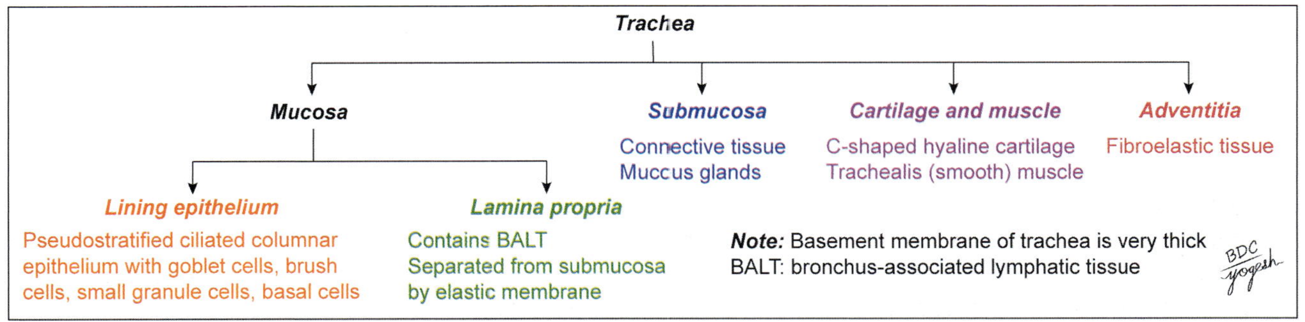

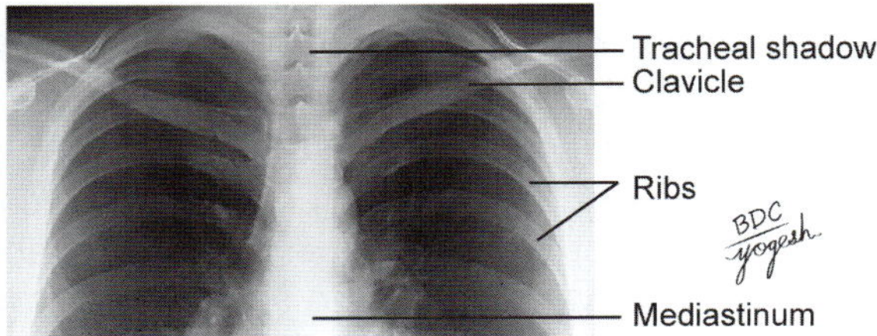

Fig. 20.4: Tracheal shadow

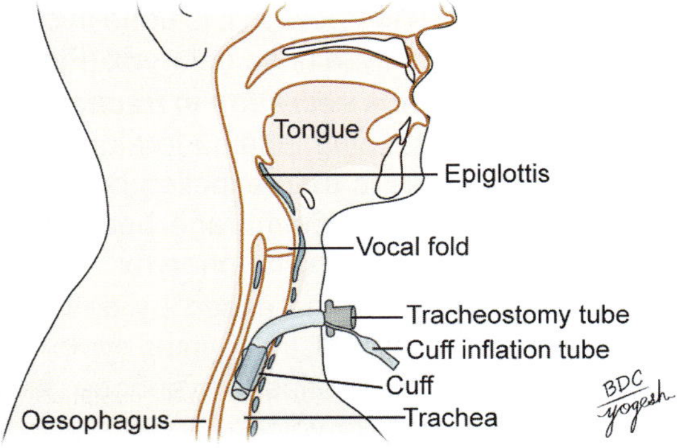

Fig. 20.5: Tracheostomy

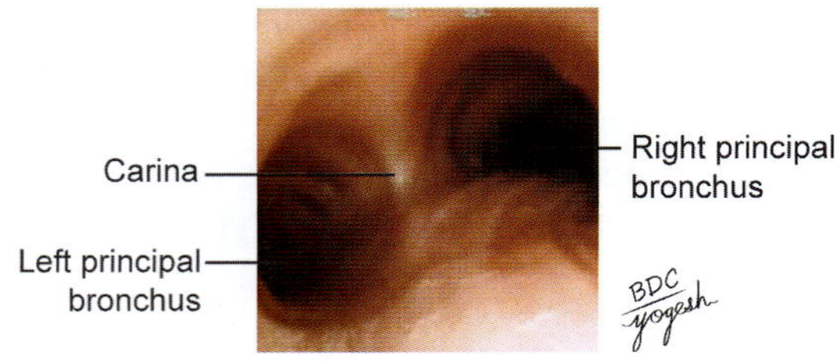

Fig. 20.6: Carina of trachea

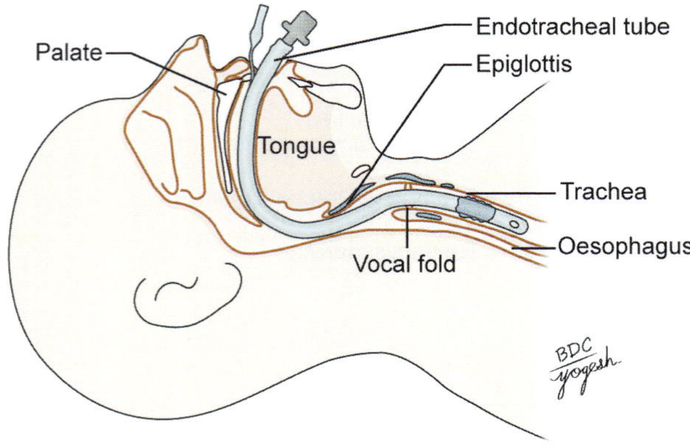

Fig. 20.7: Endotracheal tube intubation

DISSECTION

Remove the posterior surface of the parietal pericardium between the right and left pulmonary veins. This uncovers the anterior surface of the oesophagus in the posterior mediastinum. Find the azygos vein and its tributaries on the vertebral column to the right of the oesophagus. Find and follow the thoracic duct on the left of azygos vein.

Identify the sternal, sternocostal, interchondral, and costochondral joints on the anterior aspect of chest wall which was reflected downwards. Expose the ligaments which unite the heads of the ribs to the vertebral bodies and intervertebral discs.

Competency:

AN23.1 Describe and demonstrate the external appearance, relations, blood supply, nerve supply, lymphatic drainage and applied anatomy of oesophagus.

OESOPHAGUS

Features

The oesophagus is a narrow muscular tube, forming the food passage between the pharynx and stomach. It extends from the lower part of the neck to the upper part of the abdomen (Plate 20.1, Fig. 20.8, Flowchart 20.2).

Dimensions

The oesophagus is about 25 cm long and 2 cm wide.

The tube is flattened antero-posteriorly and the lumen is kept collapsed; it dilates only during the passage of the food bolus.

Note: The pharyngo-oesophageal junction is the narrowest part of the alimentary canal except for the vermiform appendix.

Course

The oesophagus begins in the neck at the lower border of the cricoid cartilage, where it is continuous with the lower end of the pharynx (Fig. 20.8). It descends in front of the vertebral column through the superior and posterior parts of the mediastinum, and pierces the diaphragm at the level of 10th thoracic vertebra. It ends by opening into the stomach at its cardiac end at the level of eleventh thoracic vertebra.

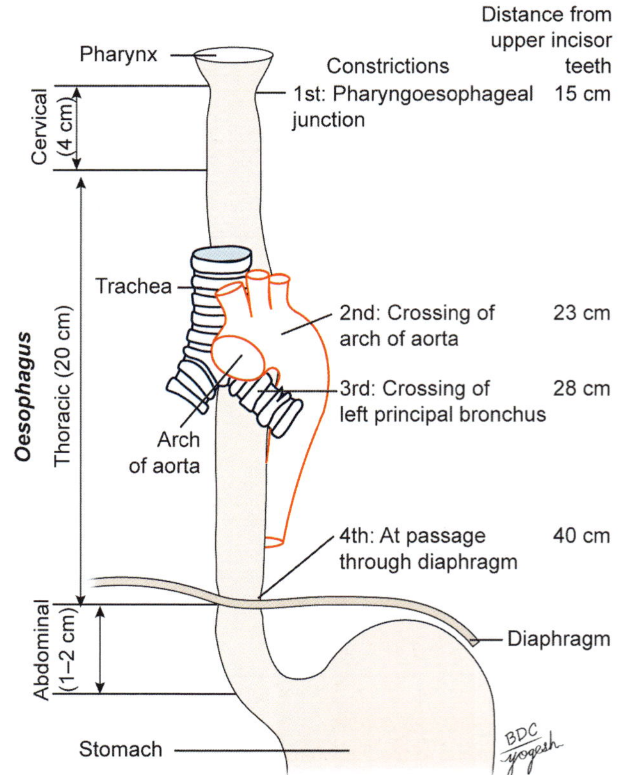

Fig. 20.8: Constrictions and parts of oesophagus

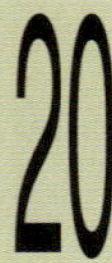

Flowchart 20.2: Morphology of oesophagus

Oesophagus
Mucomuscular tube

- ***Measurements***
  - Length: 25 cm
  - Width: 2 cm
  - Lumen: Normally closed, opens for passage of food
- ***Course***
  - Continuation of pharynx
  - Level: Lower border of cricoid cartilage
  - Pierces diaphragm at T10
  - Opens in stomach at T11
- ***Curvatures***
  - 2 anteroposterior
  - 2 left curvatures
- ***4 constrictions***
  - At
  - Pharyngoesophageal junction
  - Crossing of arch of aorta
  - Crossing of left bronchus
  - Passage through diaphragm
- ***Blood supply***
  - ***Arteries***
    - Inferior thyroid artery
    - Oesophageal branches of aorta
    - Left gastric and phrenic arteries
  - ***Veins***
    - Inferior thyroid vein
    - Azygos, hemiazygos veins
    - Left gastric veins

In clinics
- Oesophageal varices – dilated tortuous veins ← portal hypertension
- Referred pain of oesophagus
- Oesophagoscopy
- Dysphagia
- Achalasia cardia
- Tracheo-oesophageal fistula

BDC yogesh

Curvatures

Oesophagus has the following curvatures

1. ***Anteroposterior curvatures*:** First corresponds to the curvature of cervical vertebrae, whereas second corresponds to the curvature of thoracic vertebrae.
2. ***Lateral curvatures*** (side by side)**:** Oesophagus deviates two times toward left
   a. First at the root of neck
   b. Second at the level of T7 vertebra.

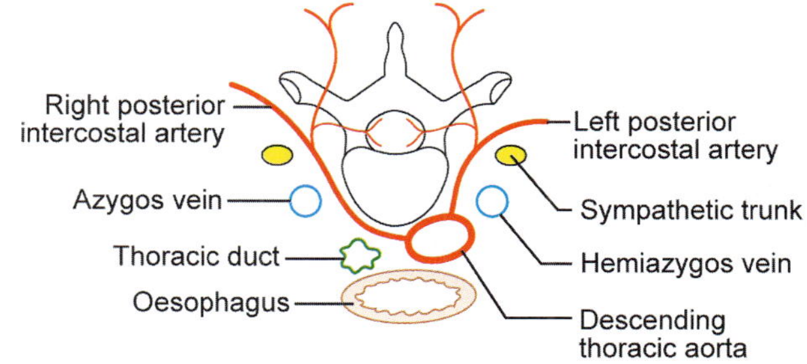

Fig. 20.9: Posterior relations of oesophagus

Constrictions

Normally, the oesophagus shows ***four constrictions*** as follows (Fig. 20.8):

1. At its beginning, 15 cm (6 inches) from the incisor teeth, where it is crossed by cricopharyngeus, part of inferior constrictor muscle.
2. Where it is crossed by the aortic arch, 22.5 cm (9 inches) from the incisor teeth.
3. Where it is crossed by the left bronchus, 27.5 cm (11 inches) from the incisor teeth (Fig. 20.8).
4. Where it pierces the diaphragm 37.5 cm (15 inches) from the incisor teeth.

Note: The distances from the incisor teeth are important in passing instruments like endoscope into the oesophagus.

For the sake of convenience, the relations of the oesophagus may be studied in three parts—cervical, thoracic and abdominal. The relations of the cervical part are described in *BD Chaurasia's Human Anatomy*, Volume 3, and those of the abdominal part in Volume 2.

Relations of the Thoracic Part of the Oesophagus

Anteriorly

1. Trachea
2. Right pulmonary artery
3. Left bronchus
4. Pericardium with left atrium
5. The diaphragm.

Posteriorly (Figs 20.9 and 20.10a to c)

1. Vertebral column
2. Right posterior intercostal arteries
3. Thoracic duct
4. Azygos vein with the terminal parts of the hemiazygos veins
5. Thoracic aorta
6. Right pleural recess
7. Diaphragm.

To the Right

1. Right lung and pleura
2. Azygos vein
3. The right vagus (Figs 20.10a to c).

To the Left

In the superior mediastinum

1. Aortic arch
2. Left subclavian artery
3. Thoracic duct
4. Left lung and pleura
5. Left recurrent laryngeal nerve.

In the posterior mediastinum

1. The descending thoracic aorta
2. The left lung and mediastinal pleura.

Arterial Supply

1. The ***cervical part*** including the segment up to the arch of aorta is supplied by the inferior thyroid arteries.
2. The ***thoracic part*** is supplied by the oesophageal branches of the aorta.
3. The ***abdominal part*** is supplied by the oesophageal branches of the left gastric artery.

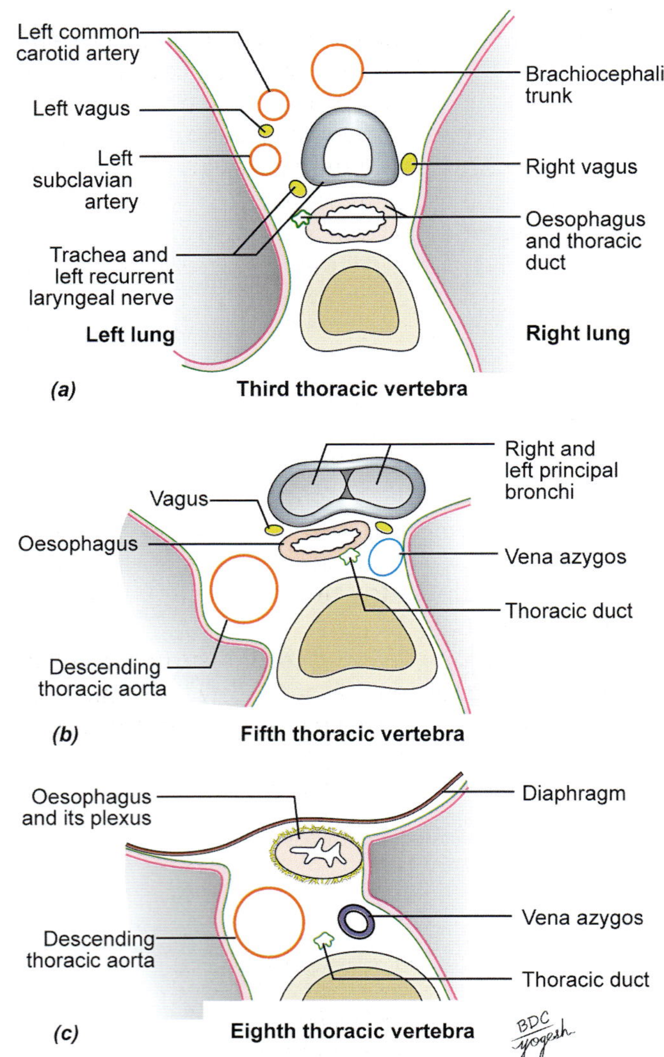

Figs 20.10a to c: Outline drawings of three sections through the oesophagus at different levels of thoracic vertebrae

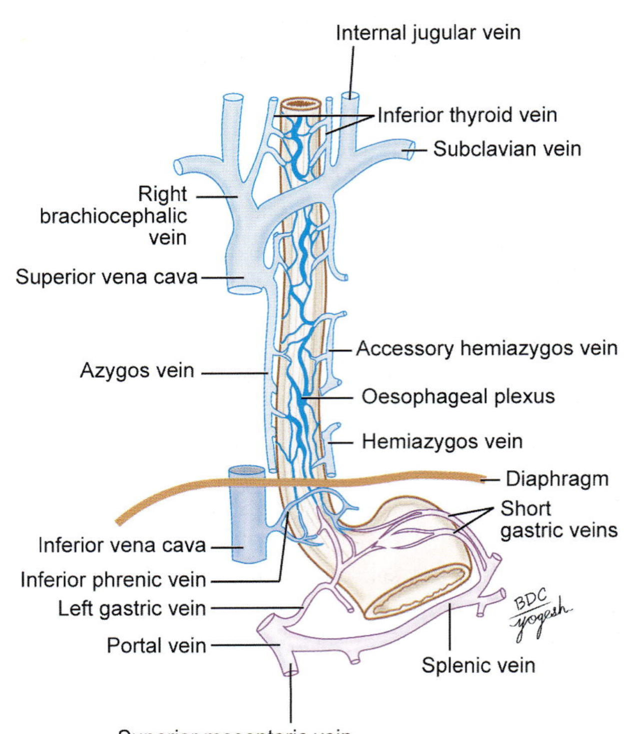

Fig. 20.11: Venous drainage of oesophagus

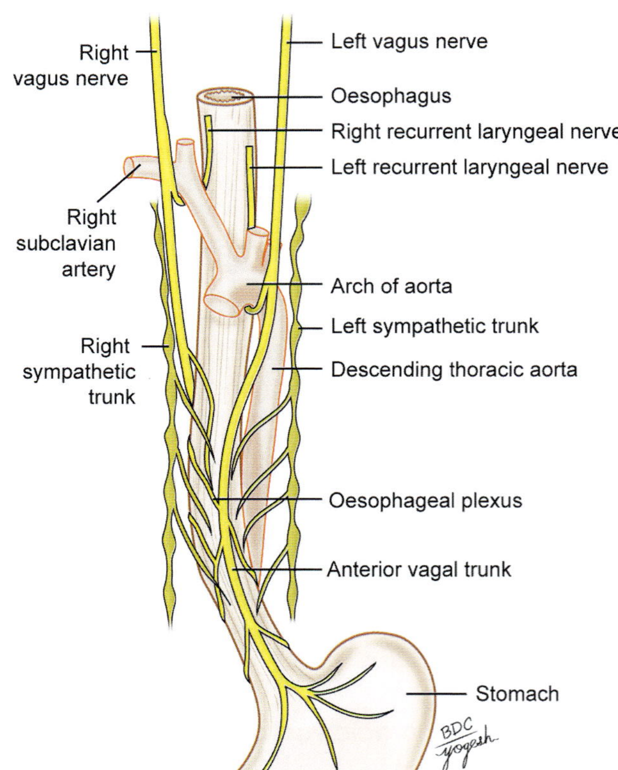

Fig. 20.12: Nerve supply of oesophagus

Venous Drainage

1. Cervical part into inferior thyroid vein (Fig. 20.11).
2. Thoracic part into azygos and hemiazygos veins.
3. Abdominal part into left gastric vein (portal vein) and into hemiazygos vein (vena cava). Thus, abdominal part of oesophagus is the site of *portosystemic anastomosis*.

Lymphatic Drainage

The cervical part drains to the deep cervical nodes, the thoracic part to the posterior mediastinal nodes, and the abdominal part to the left gastric nodes.

Nerve Supply (Fig. 20.12)

1. ***Parasympathetic nerves:*** The upper half of the oesophagus is supplied by the recurrent laryngeal nerves, and the lower half by the oesophageal plexus formed mainly by the two vagi. Parasympathetic nerves are sensory, motor and secretomotor to the oesophagus.
2. ***Sympathetic nerves:*** For upper half of oesophagus, the fibres come from middle cervical ganglion and run with inferior thyroid arteries. For lower half, the fibres come directly from upper four thoracic ganglia, to form oesophageal plexus before supplying the oesophagus. Sympathetic nerves are vasomotor.

The ***oesophageal plexus*** is formed mainly by the parasympathetic through vagi but sympathetic fibres are also present. Towards the lower end of the oesophagus, the vagal fibres form the anterior and posterior gastric nerves which enter the abdomen through the oesophageal opening of the diaphragm.

HISTOLOGY OF OESOPHAGUS

Oesophagus has the following layers (Fig. 20.13, Flowchart 20.3):

1. *Mucosa*: It consists of stratified squamous epithelium (nonkeratinized), lamina propria, and muscularis mucosa (thick, longitudinal smooth muscles).
2. *Submucosa*: It consists of dense irregular connective tissue with elastic fibers and compound tubuloalveolar glands.
3. *Muscularis externa*: In upper third of oesophagus, it has skeletal muscle fibers in middle third, both skeletal and smooth muscle fibers whereas in lower third only smooth muscle fibers.
4. *Adventitia*: Oesophagus is surrounded by connective tissue. Only at the lowest 1 inch, it is surrounded by serosa (peritoneum).

CLINICAL ANATOMY

- ***Oesophageal varices:*** In portal hypertension, the communications between the portal and systemic veins draining the lower end of the oesophagus dilate. These dilatations are called *oesophageal varices.* Rupture of these varices can cause serious haematemesis or vomiting of blood. The oesophageal varices can be visualised radiographically by barium swallow; they produce worm-like shadows (Fig. 20.14).
- Left atrial enlargement as in mitral stenosis can also be visualised by barium swallow. The enlarged atrium causes a shallow depression on the front of the oesophagus. Barium swallow also helps in the diagnosis of oesophageal strictures, carcinoma and achalasia cardia.
- ***Oesophagoscopy:*** It is the visualization of interior of oesophagus using oesophagoscope. The normal indentations on the oesophagus should be kept in mind during oesophagoscopy.
- ***Tracheo-oesophageal fistula:*** Improper separation of the trachea from the oesophagus during development gives rise to tracheo-oesophageal fistula (Fig. 20.15).
- ***Achalasia cardia:*** The lower end of the oesophagus is normally kept closed. It is opened by the stimulus of a food bolus. In case of neuromuscular incoordination, the lower end of the oesophagus fails to dilate with the arrival of food which, therefore, accumulates in the oesophagus. This condition of neuromuscular

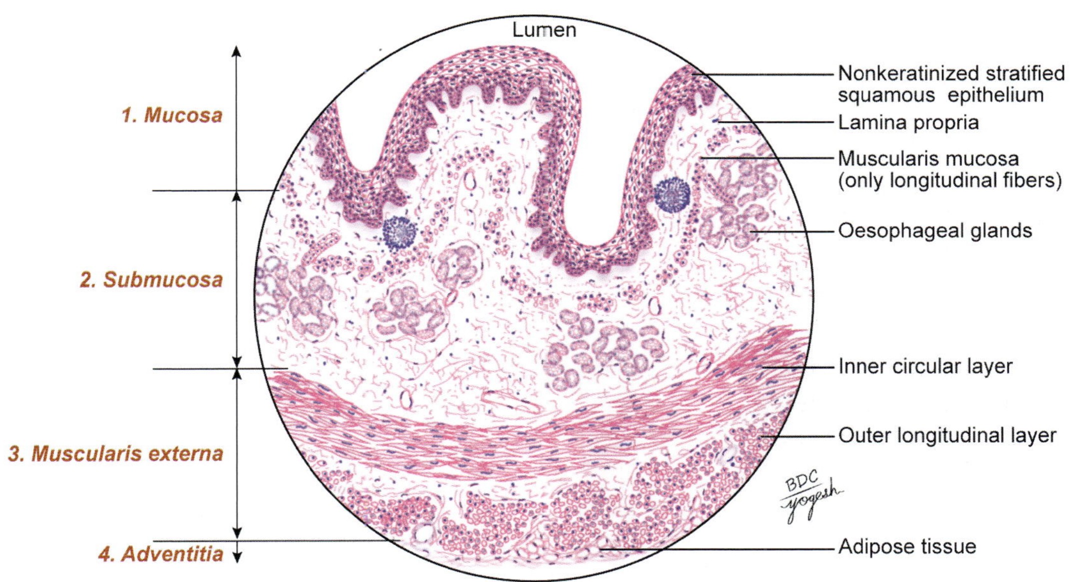

Fig. 20.13: Histology of oesophagus

Flowchart 20.3: Histology of oesophagus

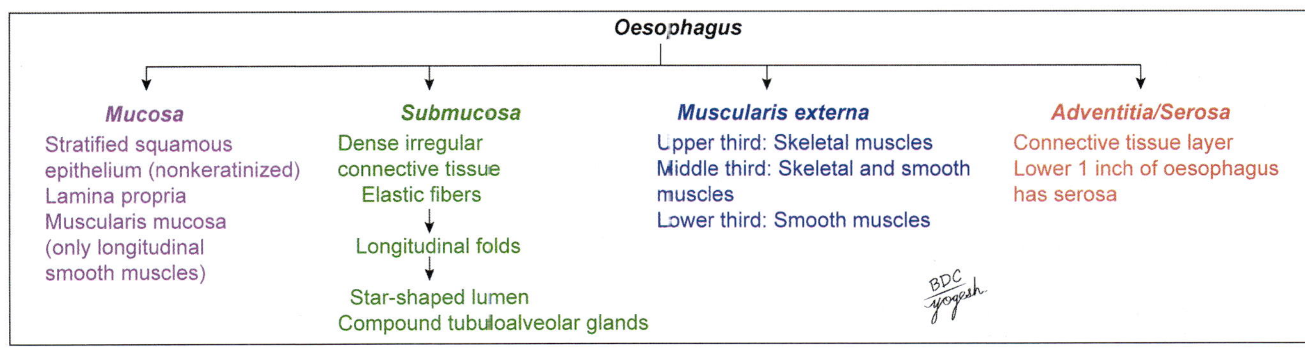

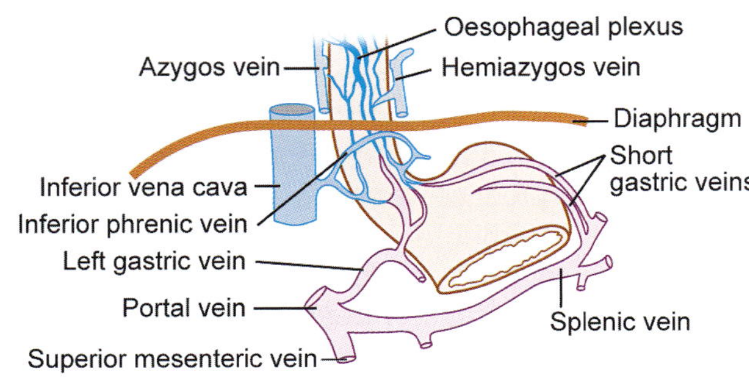

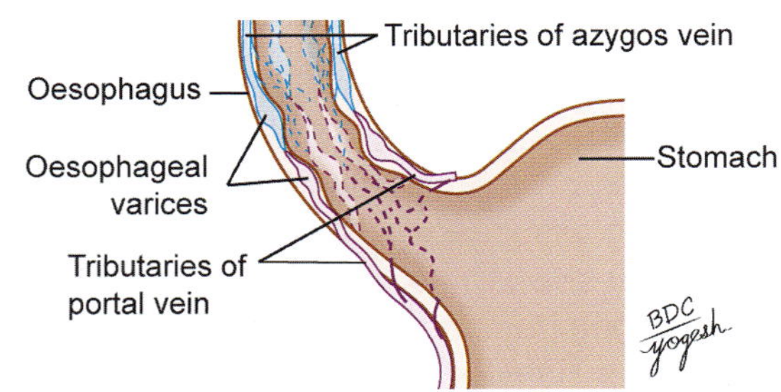

Fig. 20.14: Oesophageal varices

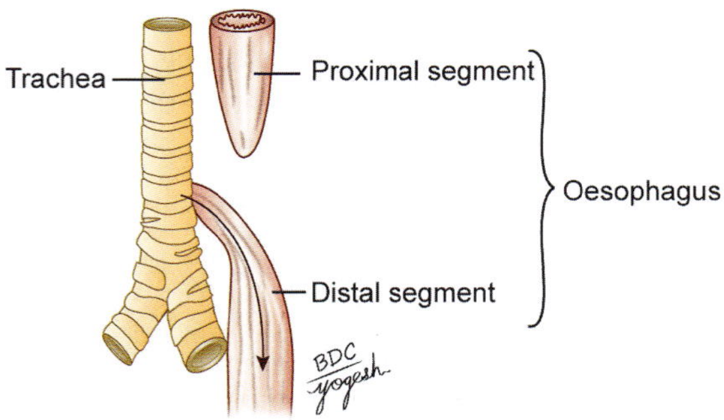

Fig. 20.15: Tracheoesophageal fistula (*Source*: Textbook of Human Embryology, 2/e, by Yogesh Sontakke)

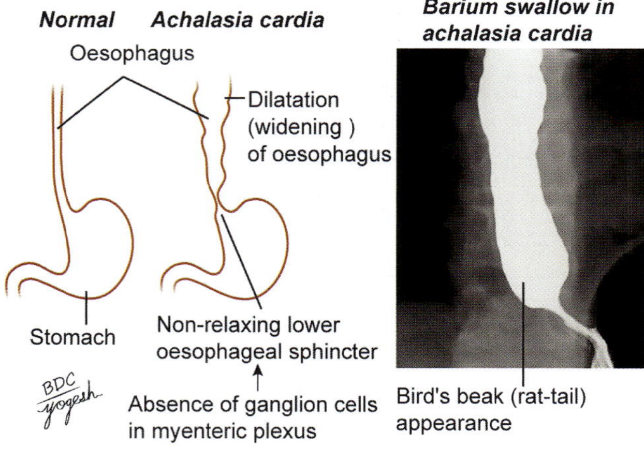

Fig. 20.16: Achalasia cardia

incoordination characterised by inability of the oesophagus to dilate is known as '*achalasia cardia*'. It may be due to congenital absence of nerve cells in wall of oesophagus (Fig. 20.16).

- Compression of the oesophagus in cases of mediastinal syndrome causes ***dysphagia*** or difficulty in swallowing.
- ***Referred pain of oesophagus (heart burn):*** Oesophageal pain is carried by sympathetic fibers (T4 and T5 segments). The pain of oesophagitis is felt in the region of chest wall supplied by T4 and T5 spinal nerves lower thoracic and epigastric region. It may be difficult to differentiate oesophageal pain from the anginal pain.
- ***Carcinoma of oesophagus:*** It occurs mostly in the lower part of oesophagus. It produces difficulty in swallowing.
- ***Barrett's oesophagus:*** In Barrett's oesophagus, lining epithelium of oesophagus changes from stratified squamous to simple columnar epithelium with goblet cells. The main cause of Barrett's oesophagus is GERD. This is precancerous condition.

Competency:

AN23.2 Describe and demonstrate the extent, relations, tributaries of thoracic duct and enumerate its applied anatomy.

THORACIC DUCT

Features

The thoracic duct is the largest lymphatic vessel in the body.

Extent: It extends from the upper part of the abdomen to the lower part of the neck, crossing the posterior and superior parts of the mediastinum.

Length: It is about 45 cm/18 inch long and 5 mm wide.

Appearance: It has a beaded appearance because of the presence of many valves in its lumen (Fig. 20.17, Flowchart 20.4).

Course

1. The thoracic duct begins as a continuation of the upper end of the cisterna chyli near the lower border of the twelfth thoracic vertebra and enters the thorax through the aortic opening of the diaphragm.
2. It then ascends through the posterior mediastinum from level of 12th thoracic vertebra to 5th thoracic vertebra, where it crosses from the right side to the left side. Then it courses through the superior mediastinum along the left edge of the oesophagus and reaches the neck.
3. In the neck, it arches laterally at the level of the transverse process of 7th cervical vertebra. Finally it descends in front of the 1st part of the left subclavian artery and ends by opening into the angle of junction between the left subclavian and left internal jugular veins (Fig. 20.17).

Relations

At the Aortic Opening of the Diaphragm

Anteriorly: Diaphragm

Posteriorly: Vertebral column

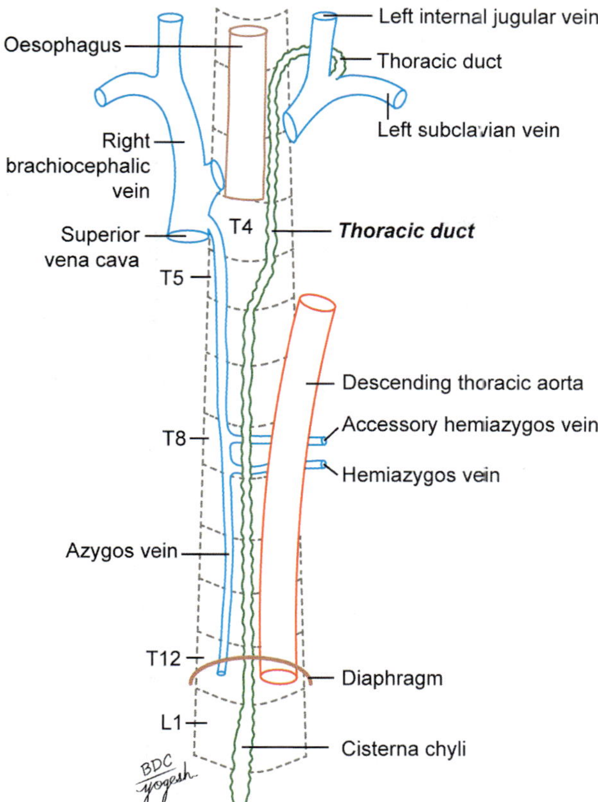

Fig. 20.17: Course of the thoracic duct

Flowchart 20.4: Thoracic duct

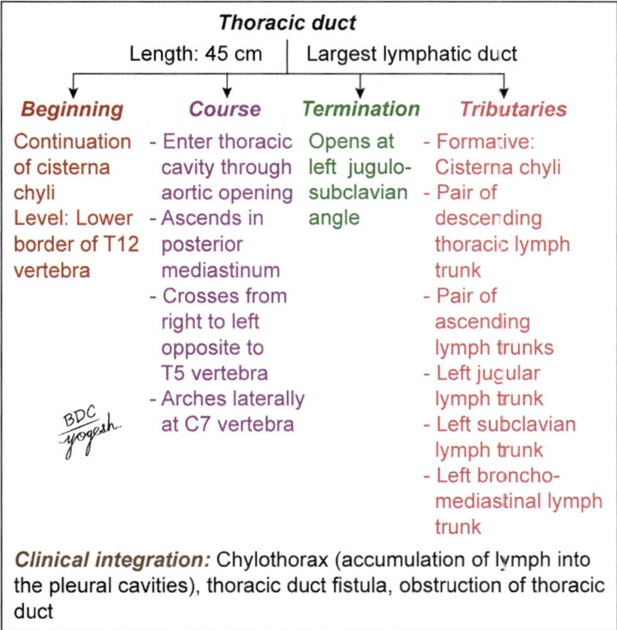

To the right: Azygos vein

To the left: Aorta.

In the Posterior Mediastinum

Anteriorly

1. Diaphragm
2. Oesophagus
3. Right pleural recess.

Posteriorly

1. Vertebral column
2. Right posterior intercostal arteries
3. Terminal parts of the hemiazygos veins.

To the right: Azygos vein

To the left: Descending thoracic aorta.

In the Superior Mediastinum

Anteriorly

1. Arch of aorta
2. The origin of the left subclavian artery.

Posteriorly: Vertebral column

To the right: Oesophagus

To the left: Pleura.

In the Neck

The thoracic duct forms an arch rising about 3–4 cm above the clavicle. The arch has the following relations.

Anteriorly

1. Left common carotid artery
2. Left vagus
3. Left internal jugular vein

Posteriorly

1. Vertebral artery and vein
2. Sympathetic trunk
3. Thyrocervical trunk and its branches
4. Left phrenic nerve
5. Medial border of the scalenus anterior
6. Prevertebral fascia covering all the structures mentioned
7. The 1st part of the left subclavian artery.

Tributaries (Fig. 20.18)

In the abdomen

- Formed by upward continuation of cisterna chyli.

In the thorax

1. A pair of descending lymph trunks – drain posterior intercostal lymph nodes of lower six intercostal lymph nodes of lower six intercostal spaces.
2. A pair of ascending lymph trunks – drain upper lumbar lymph nodes.
3. Lymph vessels from posterior mediastinal lymph nodes.

In the neck

1. Left jugular lymph trunk – drains nodes from left half of head and neck.
2. Left subclavian lymph trunk – drains lymph from the left upper limb.
3. Left bronchomediastinal lymph trunk – drains the left lung and left side of the heart.

Area of Drainage (Fig. 20.19)

- The thoracic duct drains the lymph from all the parts of body except:
  1. Right of the head and neck
  2. Right upper limb
  3. Right of chest wall
  4. Right lung and right of heart
  5. Right surface of liver.

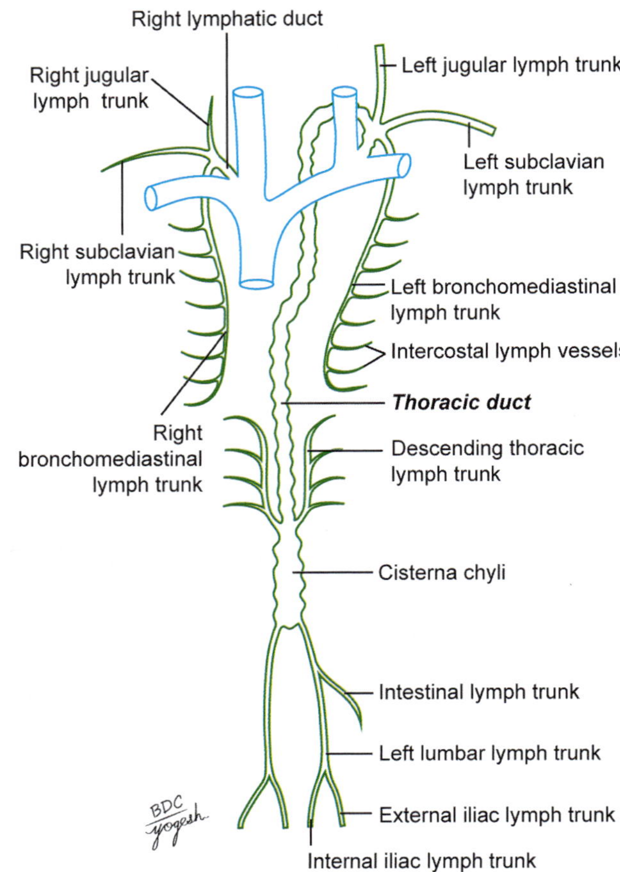

Fig. 20.18: The tributaries of the thoracic duct

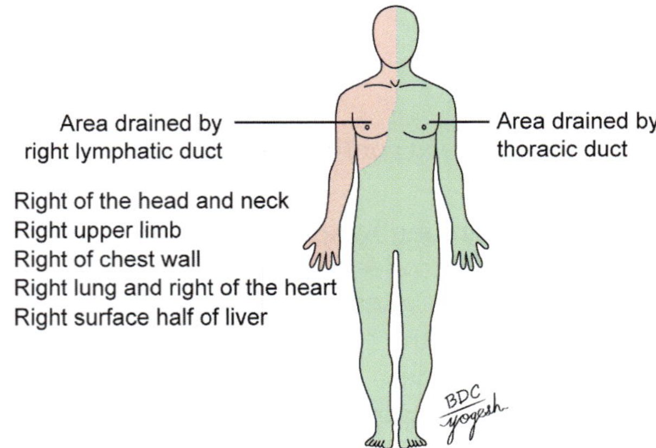

Fig. 20.19: Area of drainage of thoracic duct and right lymphatic duct

CLINICAL ANATOMY

Chylothorax: Chylothorax is the accumulation of lymph (chyle) into the pleural cavities. It may occur due to the rupture of thoracic duct (may be caused by trauma, tuberculosis, or malignancy).

***Thoracic duct fistula*:** It is the leakage of lymphatic fluid from the thoracic duct following the surgeries of the root of neck. It should be treated surgically.

***Obstruction of thoracic duct*:** Thoracic duct gets obliterated may be due to infection by microfilarial *Wuchereria bancrofti* parasite or by obstruction from external structures such as malignancies.

Facts to Remember

- Trachea contains U-shaped hyaline cartilaginous rings which are deficient posteriorly, so that the oesophagus situated behind the trachea is not compressed by trachea.
- Trachea is always patent. Carina is the most sensitive part of the trachea.
- Oesophagus is 25 cm long, like duodenum and ureter. Its maximum part about 20 cm (8 inches) lie in thoracic cavity.
- Lower part of oesophagus is a site of portocaval anastomoses and commonest site of oesophageal carcinoma.
- Achalasia cardia is a motility disorder of oesophagus due to neuromuscular incoordination.
- Thoracic duct is the largest lymphatic duct in the body. It drains lymph from both lower limbs, abdominal cavity, left side of thorax, left upper limb and left side of head and neck.
- Chylothorax is an accumulation of chyle in the pleural cavity.

BDC's Anatomy *e*-book

1. Oesophageal varices
2. Right lymphatic duct
3. Course of thoracic duct
4. Further reading
5. Viva voce questions

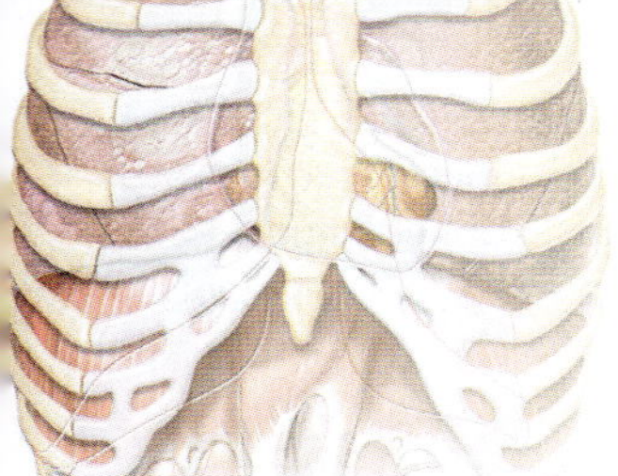

Chapter

21

Surface Marking and Radiological Anatomy of Thorax

SURFACE MARKING

Surface marking of thoracic viscera is useful for clinical examinations. This chapter includes surface markings of important thoracic viscera, such as parietal pleura, lungs, heart and cardiac valves and auscultatory areas.

The bony and soft tissue surface landmarks have been described in *see* Chapter 12.

Competency:
AN25.9 Demonstrate surface marking of lines of pleural reflection, lung borders and fissures, trachea, heart borders, apex beat and surface projection of valves of heart.

Surface Marking of Parietal Pleura

Cervical Pleura or Cupola

It is marked by a curved line extending from sternoclavicular joint (C) to the junction of medial 1/3rd and middle 1/3rd of the clavicle (A). It extends about 2.5 cm (1 inch) above the medial 1/3rd of the clavicle (B) (Figs 21.1 and 21.2).

Anterior Margin

It is also called ***costomediastinal line of pleural reflection***. It can be marked as follows:

On the right: It extends vertically downward from the right sternoclavicular joint (C) to the midpoint of the sternal angle (D). Further, it extends up to midpoint of the xiphisternal joint (E).

On the left: It extends downward from the left sternoclavicular joint to the midpoint of the sternal angle. Further, it descents vertically up to the level of the 4th costal cartilage (D1) and then it arches toward left to reach left margin of sternum. Further, it descends downward to reach the 6th costal cartilage (E1). This deviation is due to the location of the heart (bare area of the heart).

Inferior Margin

It is also called ***costodiaphragmatic line of the pleural reflection***. It can be marked as follows:

On the right: It extends laterally from the xiphisternal joint (E) and crosses the 8th rib in the midclavicular line (F), 10th rib in the midaxillary line (G), and 12th rib in

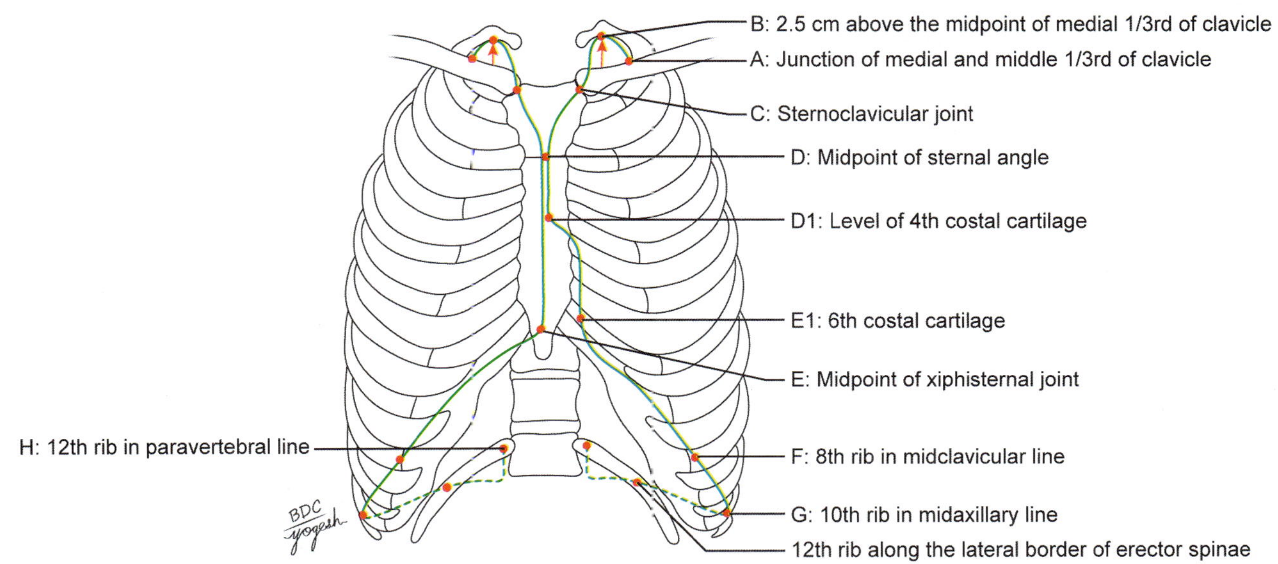

Fig. 21.1: Surface marking of the parietal pleura

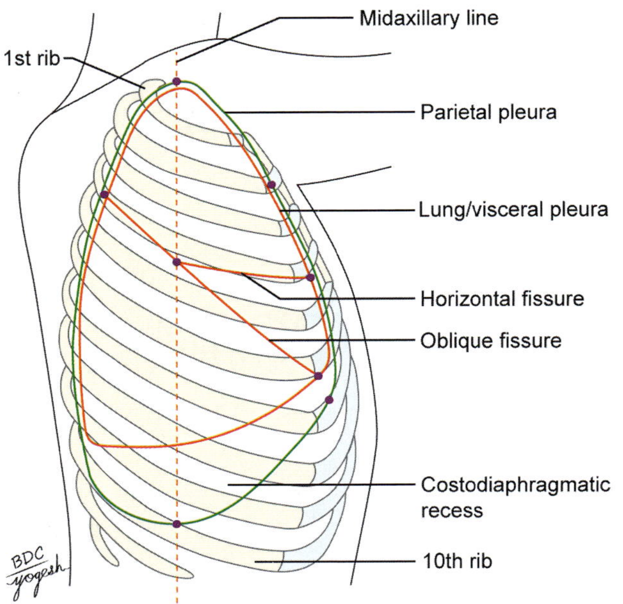

Fig. 21.2: Parietal (green) and visceral pleurae and lung (red) from the lateral aspect

paravertebral line (along the lateral border of the erector spinae muscle) (H).

On the left: It extends laterally from the left 6th costal cartilage (E1) and follows the same course as on the right (F to H).

Posterior Margins

- It is also called ***costovertebral line of reflection***. It extends as a vertical line 2 cm lateral to the spinous processes of vertebrae from C7 to T12 vertebrae (I to H). Along this line, costovertebral pleura continues with mediastinal pleura.

Note: The surface marking or the lung and visceral pleura coincides as visceral pleura is adhered to the outer surface of lungs (*see* Chapter 16 for surface marking of visceral pleura or lungs).

The parietal pleurae descend below the costal margin at three places:

a. At the right xiphicostal angle
b. At the right and left costovertebral angles
c. Below the 12th rib behind the upper poles of the kidneys.

The latter fact is of surgical importance in exposure of the kidney. The pleura may be damaged at this site (*see* Fig. 15.4).

[***Mnemonic for*** **surface markings of pleura:** '*All the even ribs, in order:* ***2, 4, 6, 8, 10, 12*** *show its route*': *Rib 2:* Both sides parietal pleura come close

Rib 4: The left pleura does a lateral shift to accommodate heart

Rib 6: Both diverge laterally

Rib 8: Midclavicular line

Rib 10: Midaxillary line

Rib12: The back]

Surface Marking of the Lungs and Visceral Pleura

Surface marking of lung is same as that of visceral pleura.

Apex (Figs 21.2 and 21.3a and b): It coincides with cervical pleura. It can be represented by convex line joining the following points:

A: Junction of middle and medial one-third of clavicle

B: Point 2.5 cm above medial end of clavicle

C: Midpoint of sternoclavicular joint.

Anterior border

On right: It runs vertically downward and marked by joining the following points:

C: Midpoint of sternoclavicular joint

D: Median plane of sternal angle

E: Median point of xiphisternal joint.

On left: It has cardiac notch. It is marked by joining

C: Midpoint of sternoclavicular joint

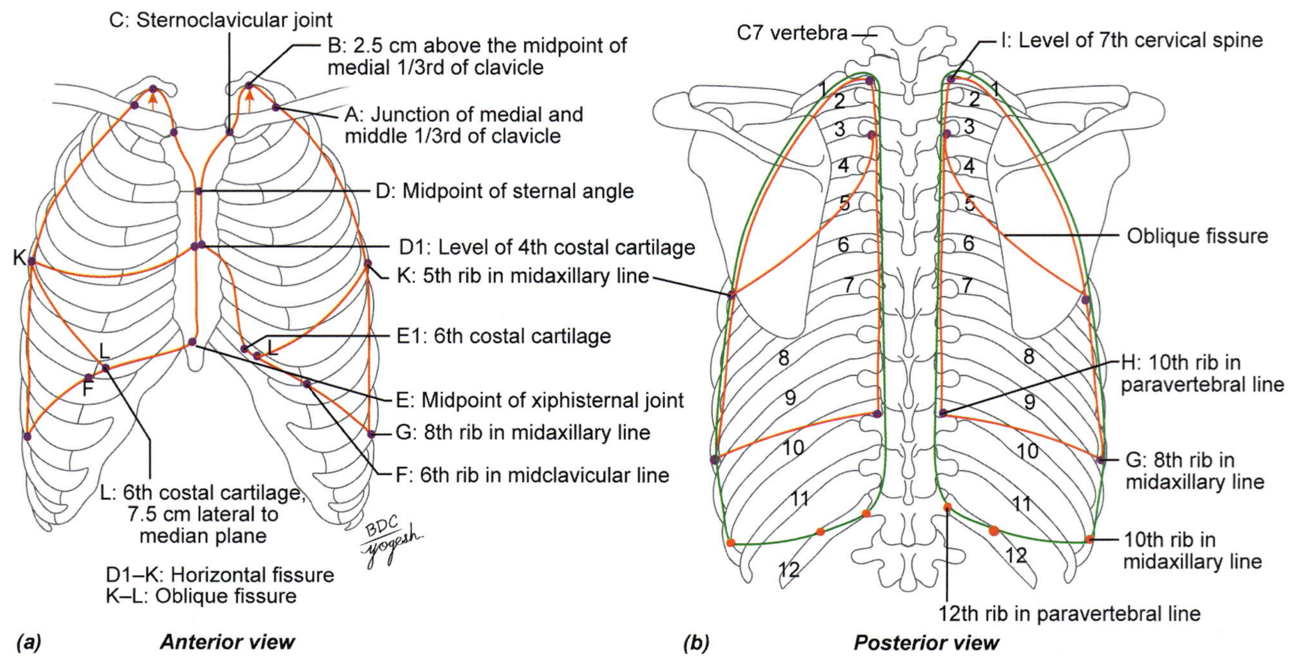

Figs 21.3a and b: Surface projection of lung or visceral pleura (red) and parietal (green): (a) Anterior view; (b) Posterior view

D: Median plane of sternal angle
D1: Median plane at the level of 4th costal cartilage and then forms convex lateral notch.
E1: At 6th costal cartilage (4 cm from median plane)

***Lower border*:** It crosses:
F: 6th rib in midclavicular line
G: 8th rib in midaxillary line
H: 10th rib in paravertebral line (2 cm lateral to 10th thoracic spine).

***Posterior border*:** It extends from
H: 10th rib in paravertebral line to
I: 7th cervical spine level in paravertebral line.

***Oblique fissure*:** It can be marked joining
J: Point 2 cm lateral to 3rd thoracic spine
K: Point on 5th rib in midaxillary line
L: 6th costal cartilage 7.5 cm lateral to median plane.

***Horizontal fissure*:** It is present only in the right lung. It can be marked by a horizontal line along the 4th costal cartilage. This line extends from anterior border (4th costal cartilage level) to the oblique fissure (at 5th rib in midaxillary line).

Area of superficial cardiac dullness: In the region of the cardiac notch, the pericardium is covered only by a double layer of pleura. The area of the cardiac notch is dull on percussion and is called the *area of superficial cardiac dullness.*

Recesses of Pleura

Between the visceral and parietal pleurae, the recesses are present.

1. ***Costodiaphragmatic recesses*** are present on both sides and are about 4–5 cm deep. The costodiaphragmatic recess is seen laterally from the lower limit of its anterior margin, so that it crosses the 8th rib in the midclavicular line (Fig. 21.2), the 10th rib in the midaxillary line, and the 12th rib at the lateral border of the sacrospinalis muscle (Fig. 21.3). Further, it passes horizontally a little below the 12th rib to the lower border of the T12 vertebra, 2 cm lateral to the upper border of the T12 spine (Fig. 21.2).
   Thus, the pleurae descend below the costal margin at three places, at the right xiphicostal angle, and at the right and left costovertebral angles below the 12th rib behind the upper poles of the kidneys. The latter fact is of surgical importance in exposure of the kidney. The pleura may be damaged at these sites (Fig. 21.2).
2. ***Costomediastinal recess*** is prominent on left side, to left of sternum between 4th and 6th costal cartilages.

Surface Marking of the Borders of the Heart

Point 1: At the lower border of the 2nd left costal cartilage about 1.3 cm from the sternal margin (Fig. 21.4).

Point 2: At the upper border of the 3rd right costal cartilage 0.8 cm from the sternal margin.

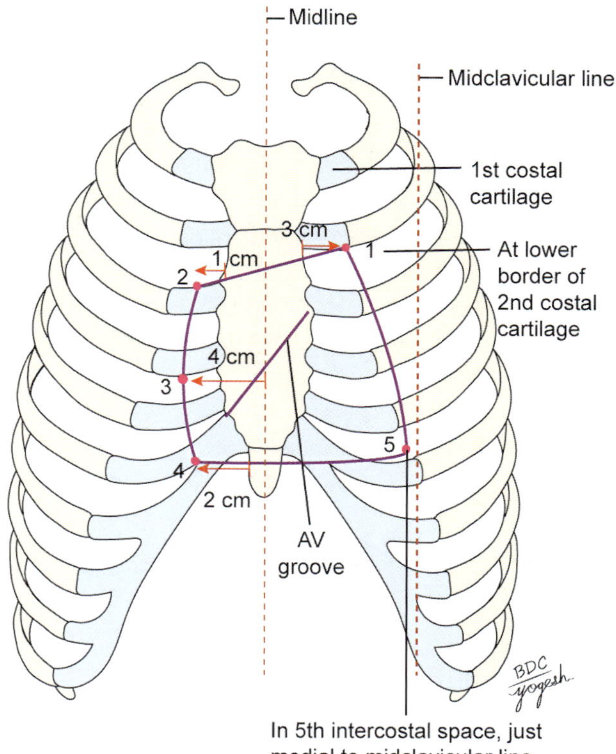

Fig. 21.4: Surface projection of the borders of the heart

Point 3: In the right 4th intercostal space 3.8 cm from median plane.

Point 4: At the lower border of the 6th right costal cartilage 2 cm from the sternal margin.

Point 5: At the apex of the heart in the left 5th intercostal space 9 cm from the midsternal line medial to left nipple.

- ***Upper border:*** Marked by joining of points 1 and 2.
- ***Right border:*** Marked by a line, slightly convex to the right, joining the points 2, 3 and 4. The maximum convexity is about 3.8 cm from the median plane in the 4th space.
- ***Inferior border:*** Marked by joining points 4 and 5.
- ***Left border:*** Marked by a line, fairly convex to the left, joining the points 1 and 5.
- **Atrioventricular groove** is marked by a line drawn from the sternal end of left 3rd costal cartilage to the sternal end of right 6th costal cartilage.
- The area of the chest wall overlying the heart is called the *precordium*.

Surface Marking of the Cardiac Valves and the Auscultatory Areas

Sound produced by closure of the valves of the heart can be heard using a stethoscope. The sound arising in relation to a particular valve are best heard not directly over the valve, but at areas situated some distance away from the valve in the direction of blood flow through it. These are called auscultatory areas. The position of the valves in relation to the surface of the body, and of the auscultatory areas is given in Table 21.1 and Fig. 21.5.

TABLE 21.1: Surface marking of the cardiac valves and the sites of the auscultatory areas (Fig. 21.6)

Valve	*Diameter of orifice*	*Surface marking*	*Auscultatory area*
Pulmonary	2.5 cm	A horizontal line, 2.5 cm long, behind the upper border of the 3rd left costal cartilage and adjoining part of the sternum	2nd left intercostal space near the sternum
Aortic	2.5 cm	A slightly oblique line, 2.5 cm long, behind the left half of the sternum at the level of the lower border of the left 3rd costal cartilage	2nd right costal cartilage near the sternum
Mitral	3 cm	An oblique line, 3 cm long, behind the left half of the sternum opposite the left 4th costal cartilage	Cardiac apex
Tricuspid	4 cm	Most oblique of all valves, being nearly vertical, 4 cm long, behind the right half of the sternum opposite the 4th and 5th spaces	Lower end of the sternum

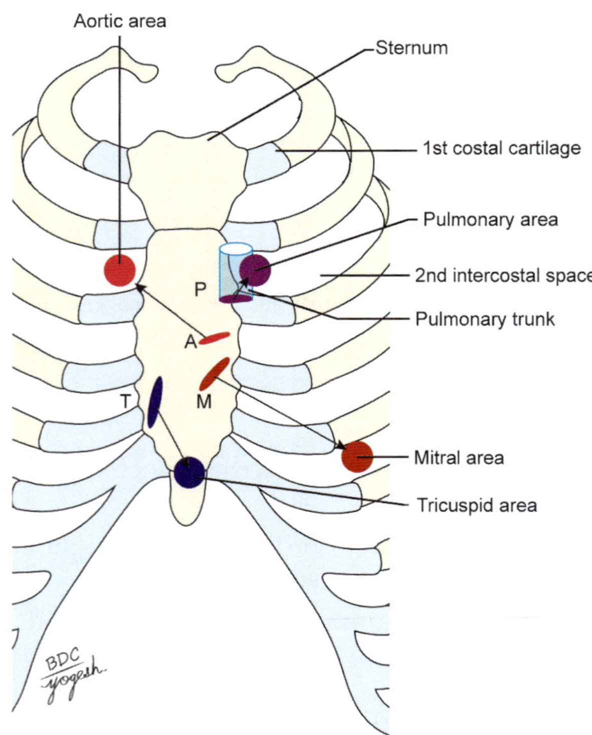

Fig. 21.5: Surface projection of the cardiac valves. The position of the auscultatory areas is also shown

Arteries

Pulmonary Trunk

1. First mark the pulmonary valve by a horizontal line 2.5 cm long, mainly along the upper border of the left 3rd costal cartilage and partly over the adjoining part of the sternum (Fig. 21.6).
2. Then mark the pulmonary trunk by two parallel lines 2.5 cm apart from the pulmonary orifice upwards to the left 2nd costal cartilage.

Ascending Aorta

1. First mark the aortic orifice by a slightly oblique line 2.5 cm long running downwards and to the right over the left half of the sternum beginning at the level of the lower border of the left 3rd costal cartilage (Fig. 21.6).
2. Then mark the ascending aorta by two parallel lines 2.5 cm apart from the aortic orifice upwards to the right half of the sternal angle (Fig. 21.6).

Arch of the Aorta

Arch of the aorta lies behind the lower half of the manubrium sterni.

Its upper convex border is marked by a line which begins at the right end of the sternal angle, arches upwards and to the left through the centre of the manubrium, and ends at the sternal end of the left 2nd costal cartilage.

Note that the beginning and the end of the arch lie at the same level. When marked on the surface as described above, the arch looks much smaller than it actually is because of foreshortening (Fig. 21.8).

Descending Thoracic Aorta

Descending thoracic aorta is marked by two parallel lines 2.5 cm apart, which begin at the sternal end of the left 2nd costal cartilage, pass downwards and medially, and end in the median plane 2.5 cm above the transpyloric plane (Fig. 21.6).

Brachiocephalic Artery

Brachiocephalic artery is marked by a broad line extending from the centre of the manubrium to the right sternoclavicular joint (Fig. 21.6).

Left Common Carotid Artery

The thoracic part of this artery is marked by a broad line extending from a point a little to the left of the centre of the manubrium to the left sternoclavicular joint.

Left Subclavian Artery

The thoracic part of the left subclavian artery is marked by a broad vertical line along the left border of the manubrium a little to the left of the left common carotid artery.

Internal Mammary (Thoracic) Artery

It is marked by joining the following points (Fig. 21.7)

- First point 1 cm above the sternal end of the clavicle, 3.5 cm from the median plane.
- Next points 2–7 marked over the upper 6 costal cartilages at a distance of 1.25 cm from the lateral sternal border.
- The last point 8 is marked in the 6th intercostal space 1.25 cm from the lateral sternal border, here, artery divides into musculophrenic, and superior epigastric arteries.

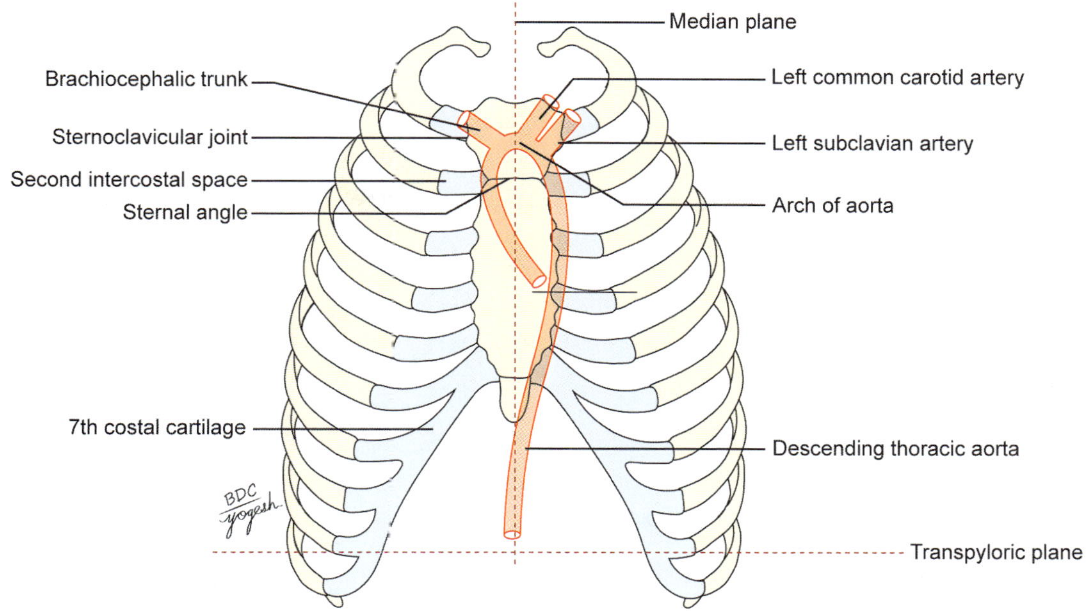

Fig. 21.6: Surface marking of major arteries of thorax

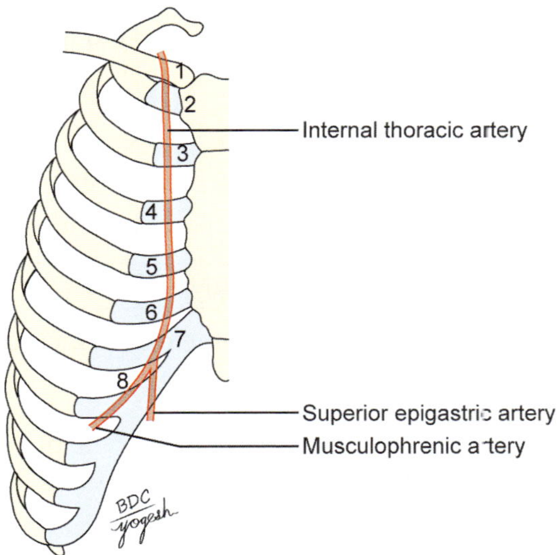

Fig. 21.7: Surface marking of internal thoracic artery (1st–8th costal cartilages)

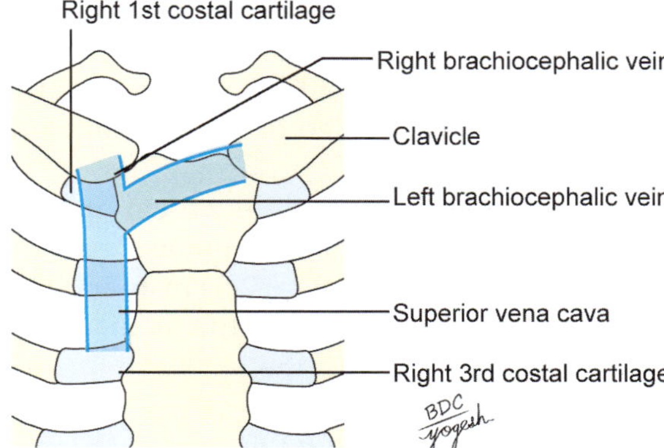

Fig. 21.8: Surface marking of veins of thorax

Veins

Superior Vena Cava

Superior vena cava is marked by two parallel lines 2 cm apart, drawn from the lower border of the right 1st costal cartilage to the upper border of the 3rd right costal cartilage, overlapping the right margin of the sternum (Fig. 21.8).

Right Brachiocephalic Vein

It is marked by two parallel lines 1.5 cm apart, drawn from the medial end of the right clavicle to the lower border of the right 1st costal cartilage close to the sternum (Fig. 21.8).

Left Brachiocephalic Vein

It is marked by two parallel lines 1.5 cm apart, drawn from the medial end of the left clavicle to the lower border of the 1st right costal cartilage. It crosses the left sternoclavicular joint and the upper half of the manubrium (Fig. 21.8).

Trachea and Principal Bronchi

Trachea (Thoracic Part)

Trachea is marked by two parallel lines 2 cm apart, drawn from the lower border of the cricoid cartilage (2 cm below the thyroid notch) to the manubriosternal angle, inclining slightly to the right (Fig. 21.9).

Right Bronchus

Right bronchus is marked by a broad line running downwards and to the right for 2.5 cm from the lower end of the trachea to the sternal end of the right 3rd costal cartilage.

Left Bronchus

Left bronchus is marked by a broad line running downwards and to the left for 5 cm from the lower end of the trachea to the left 3rd costal cartilage 4 cm from the median plane (Fig. 21.9).

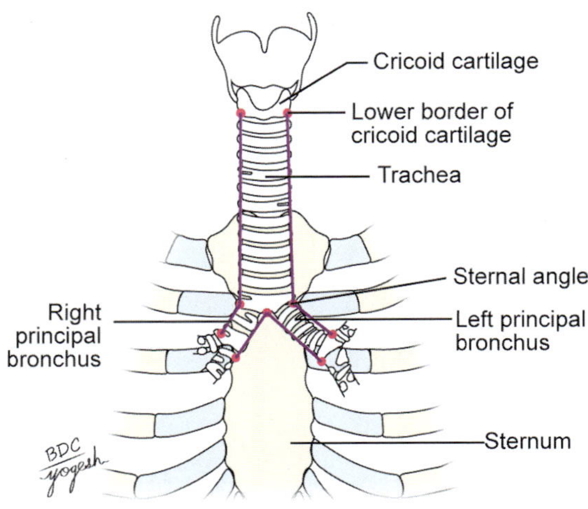

Fig. 21.9: Surface marking of trachea and principal bronchi

Oesophagus

It is marked by one on each side two parallel lines 2.5 cm apart by joining the following points:

1. Two points (one on each side) 2.5 cm apart at the lower border of the cricoid cartilage across the median plane (Fig. 21.10).
2. Two points (one on each side) 2.5 cm apart at the root of the neck a little to the left of the median plane one on each side.
3. Two points (one on each side) 2.5 cm apart at the sternal angle across the median plane.
4. Two points (one on each side) 2.5 cm apart at the left 7th costal cartilage 2.5 cm from the median plane.

Thoracic Duct

It is marked by joining the following points.

Point 1: 2 cm above the transpyloric plane slightly to the right of the median plane (Fig. 21.11).

Point 2: 2 cm to right of median plane below manubrio-sternal angle.

Point 3: Across to left side at same level.

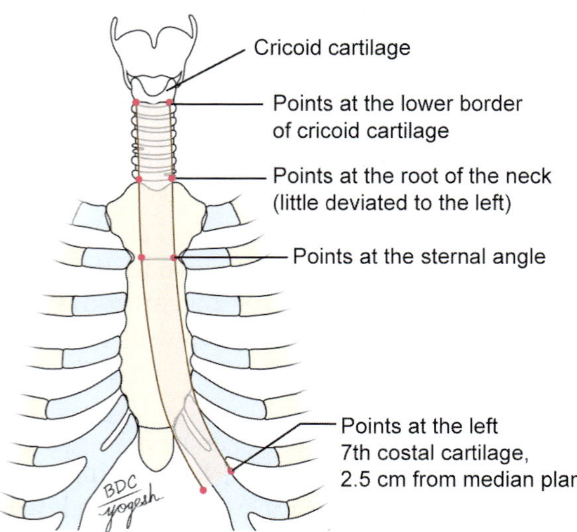

Fig. 21.10: Surface marking of oesophagus

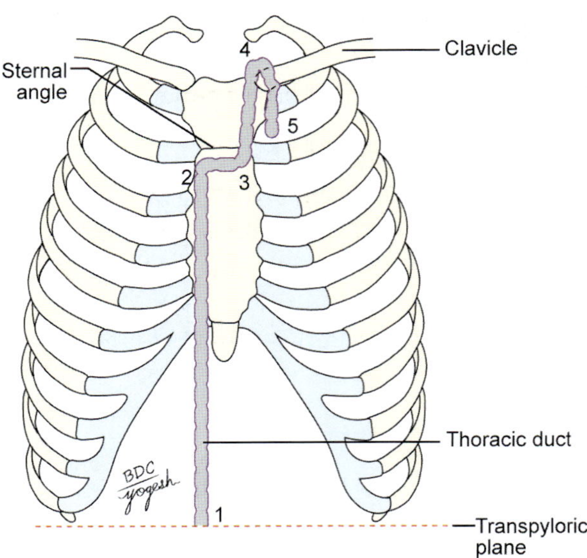

Fig. 21.11: Surface marking of thoracic duct

Point 4: 2.5 cm above the left clavicle 2 cm from the median plane.

Point 5: Just above the sternal angle 1.3 cm to the left of the median plane.

Competency:
AN25.7 Identify structures seen on a plain X-ray chest (PA view).

RADIOLOGICAL ANATOMY

Radiological examination of thoracic cage includes:

1. Plane radiographs
2. Contrast radiographs

- *Plane radiographs* include (Fig. 21.12):
  1. Posteroanterior view (PA)
  2. Anteroposterior view (AP)

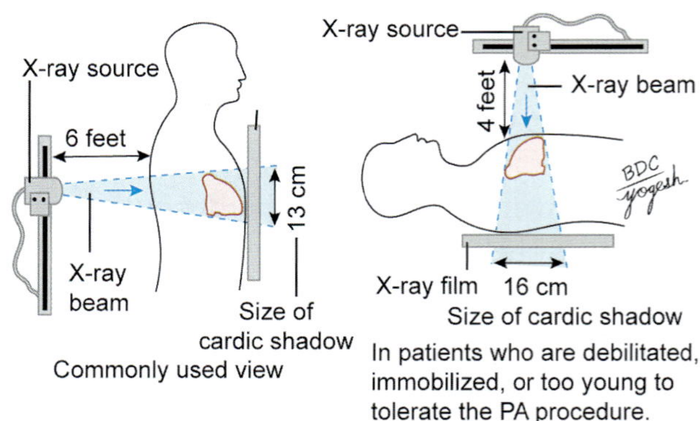

Fig. 21.12: Position of patent for chest radiograph

3. Right lateral view
4. Left lateral view

Figure 21.12 shows positions of patient for AP and PA views.

- Contrast radiographs include:
  1. Bronchography — to visualize bronchial tree
  2. Angiogram — to visualize large vessels
  3. Coronary angiography — to visualize coronary arteries
  4. Barium swallow – to visualize oesophagus.

PA VIEW OF CHEST

The most commonly taken radiographs are described as posteroanterior (PA) views. X-rays travel from posterior to the anterior side. A study of such radiographs gives information about the lungs, the diaphragm, the mediastinum, the trachea, and the skeleton of the region (Fig. 21.13). Take radiograph keeping both hands on waist to clear lung fields from scapula.

Following structures have to be examined in PA view of the thorax:

Soft Tissues

1. *Nipples* in both the sexes may be seen over the lung fields.
2. The *female breasts* will also be visualised over the lower part of the lung fields (Fig. 21.14). The extent of the overlap varies according to the size and pendulance of the breasts.

Bones

1. The bones of the *vertebrae* are partially visible. Costotransverse joints are seen on each side.
2. The posterior parts of the *ribs* are better seen because of the large amounts of calcium contained in them. The ribs get wider and thinner as they pass anteriorly. Costal cartilages are not seen unless these are calcified.
3. The medial borders of the *scapulae* may overlap the periphery of the lung fields.

Trachea

1. Trachea is seen as air-filled shadow in the midline of the neck. It lies opposite the lower cervical and upper thoracic vertebrae (Fig. 21.13).

Diaphragm

1. Diaphragm casts *dome-shaped* shadows on the two sides. The shadow on the right side is little higher than on the left side.
2. The angles where diaphragm meets the thoracic cage are the *costophrenic angles*—the right and the left. Under the left costophrenic angle is mostly the gas in the stomach, while under the right angle is the smooth shadow of the liver.

Lungs

1. The dense shadows are cast by the lung roots due to the presence of the large bronchi, pulmonary vessels, bronchial vessels and lymph nodes. The lungs readily permit the passage of the X-rays and are seen as translucent shadows during full inspiration.
2. Both blood vessels and bronchi are seen as series of shadows radiating from the *lung roots*. The smaller bronchi are not seen.
3. The lung is divided into *three zones*—upper zone is from the apex till the 2nd costal cartilage. Middle zone extends from the 2nd to the 4th costal cartilage. It includes the hilar region. Lower zone extends from the 4th costal cartilage till the bases of the lungs.

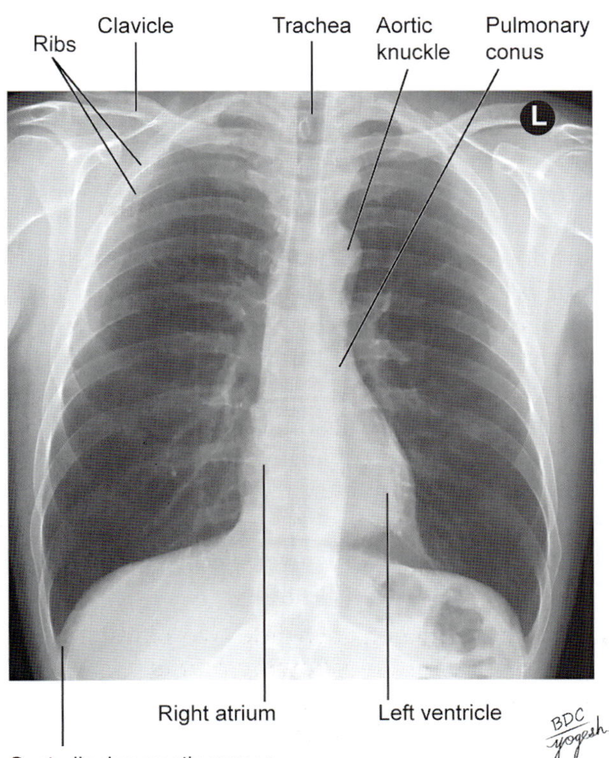

Fig. 21.13: Posteroanterior view of the male thorax

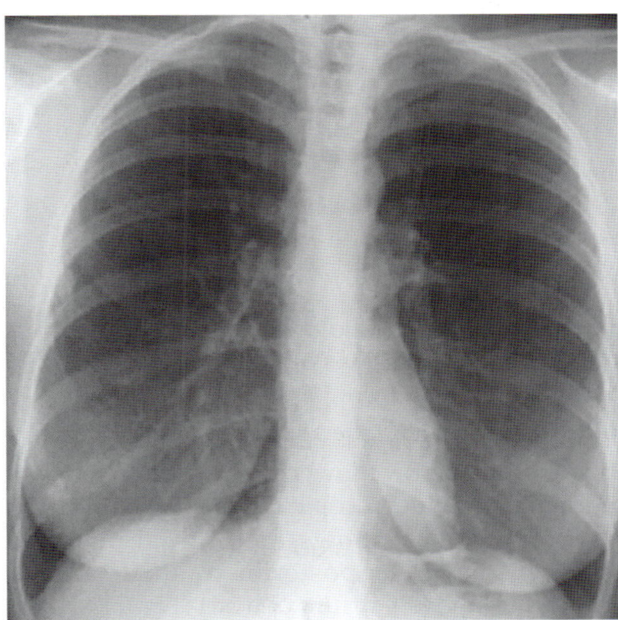

Fig. 21.14: Posteroanterior view of the female thorax

Mediastinum

1. Shadow is produced by the superimpositions of structures in the mediastinum. It is chiefly produced by the *heart* and the vessels entering or leaving the heart.
2. The ***transverse diameter of heart*** is half the transverse diameter of the thoracic cage. During inspiration, heart descends down and acquires tubular shape.
3. ***Right border*** of the mediastinal shadow is formed from above downwards by right brachiocephalic vein, superior vena cava, right atrium and inferior vena cava.
4. The ***left border*** of mediastinal shadow is formed from above downwards by aortic arch (***aortic knuckle***), left margin of pulmonary trunk, left auricle and left ventricle.
5. The ***inferior border*** of the mediastinal shadow blends with the liver and diaphragm.

Gas in Stomach

1. There may be a radiolucent or dark shadow under the left dome of diaphragm due to the gas (air) in the fundus of the stomach.

Mediastinal Shift

1. It is the deviation of the central mediastinal shadow to one of the sides. Mediastinal shift may occur on the side of the disease in case of lung fibrosis, lung collapse, and soon. It may be on the opposite side of the disease in case of pleural effusion.

Competency:
AN25.8 Identify and describe in brief a barium swallow.

Barium Swallow

Barium swallow is a radiological study of pharynx and oesophagus, up to the level of the stomach with the help of contrast.

Procedure: About 100–200 cc 50% suspension of barium sulphate is to be swallowed 2–3 times with patient standing behind fluoroscopic screen.

Barium swallow shows the normal position of ***oesophagus*** as it lies posterior to aortic arch, left bronchus and the left atrium of heart (Fig. 21.15).

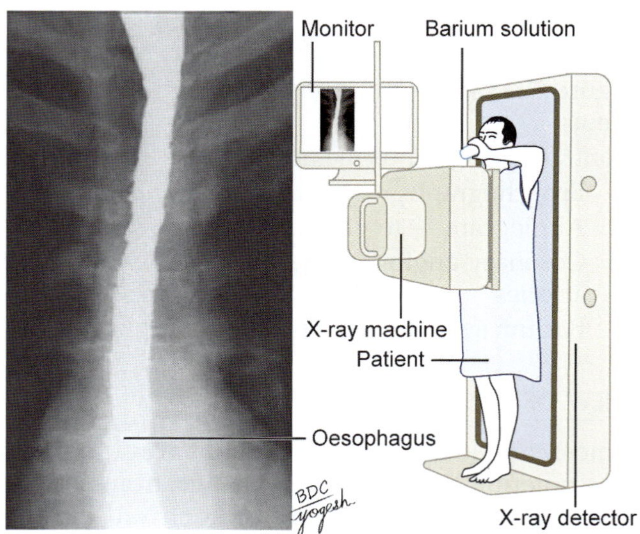

Fig. 21.15: Barium swallow

Normal barium swallow: In the right oblique view, oesophagus shows three normal impressions:
1. Aortic arch — uppermost
2. Left principal branches — middle
3. Left atrium — lower.

Conditions and specific appearance:
1. Oesophageal carcinoma — rat tail appearance of oesophagus.
2. Achalasia cardia — bird-beak sign.
3. Diffuse oesophageal spasm, nutcracker oesophagus — cork-screw appearance.

TOMOGRAPHY

Tomography is a radiological technique by which radiograms of selected layers (depths) of the body can be made. Tomography is helpful in locating deeply situated small lesions which are not seen in the usual radiograms.

BDC's Anatomy *e*-book
1. Barium swallow
2. Further reading
3. Viva voce questions

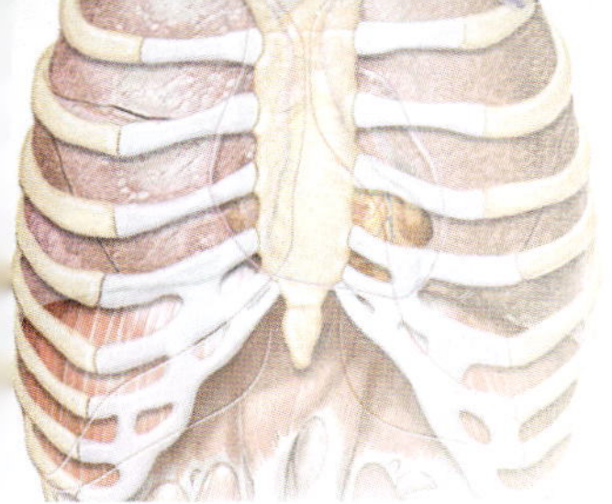

Appendix 2

Autonomic Nervous System and Arteries of Thorax

AUTONOMIC NERVOUS SYSTEM

The autonomic nervous system comprises sympathetic and parasympathetic components. ***Sympathetic component*** is active during *fright, flight or fight*. During any of these activities, the pupils dilate, skin gets pale, blood pressure rises, blood vessels of skeletal muscles, heart, and brain dilate. The person is tense and gets tired soon (Fig. A2.1). There is hardly any activity in the digestive tracts due to which the individual does not feel hungry. ***Parasympathetic component*** has the opposite effects of sympathetic component. This component is sympathetic to the digestive tract. In its activity digestion and metabolism of food occurs. Heart beats normally. Person is relaxed and can do creative work.

Autonomic nervous system is controlled by brainstem and cerebral hemispheres. These include reticular formation of brainstem, thalamic and hypothalamic nuclei, limbic lobe and prefrontal cortex including the ascending and descending tracts interconnecting these regions.

Sympathetic Nervous System

Sympathetic nervous system is the larger of the two components of autonomic nervous system. It consists of two ganglionated trunks, their branches, prevertebral ganglia, plexuses.

It supplies all the viscera of thorax, abdomen and pelvis, including the blood vessels of head and neck, brain, limbs, skin and the sweat glands as well as arrector pilorum muscle of skin of the whole body.

The ***preganglionic fibres*** are the axons of neurons situated in the lateral horns of T1–L2 segments of spinal cord. They leave spinal cord through their respective ventral roots, to pass in their nerve trunks, and beginning of ventral rami via ***white ramus communicans*** (wrc). There are 14 white rami communicantes on each side. These fibres can have following alternative routes:

1. They relay in the ganglion of the sympathetic trunks, postganglionic fibres pass via the ***grey rami communicantes*** and get distributed to the blood vessels of muscles, skin, sweat glands and to arrector pili muscles (Fig. A2.2).
2. These may pass through the corresponding ganglion and ascend to a ganglion higher before terminating in the above manner.
3. These may pass through the corresponding ganglion and descend to a ganglion lower and then terminate in the above manner.
4. These may synapse in the corresponding ganglia and pass medially to the viscera like heart, lungs, oesophagus.
5. These white rami communicantes (wrc) pass to corresponding ganglia and emerge from these as wrc (unrelayed) in the form of ***splanchnic nerves*** to supply abdominal and pelvic viscera after synapsing in the ganglia situated in the abdominal cavity. Some fibres of splanchnic nerves pass express to ***adrenal medulla***.

Sympathetic trunk on either side of the body extends from cervical region to the coccygeal region where both

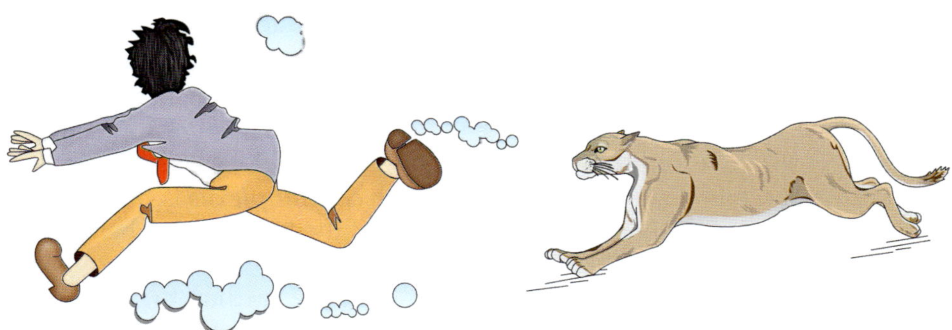

Fig. A2.1: Actions of sympathetic system

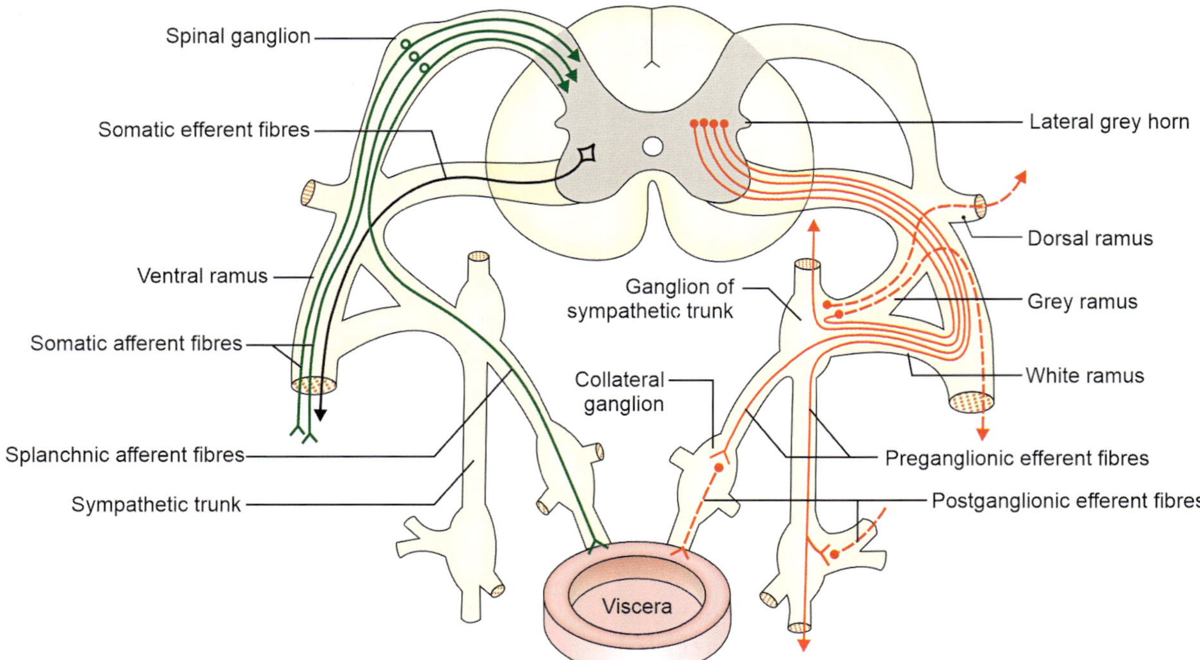

Fig. A2.2: Pathways of sympathetic and somatic nerves: Splanchnic afferent fibres and somatic afferent fibres (green); sympathetic preganglionic efferent fibres (red); sympathetic postganglionic efferent fibres (red dotted); and somatic efferent fibres (black)

trunks fuse to form a single ***ganglion impar***. Sympathetic trunk has cervical, thoracic, lumbar, sacral and coccygeal parts.

Thoracic Part of Sympathetic Trunk

There are usually ***11 ganglia*** on the sympathetic trunk of thoracic part. The 1st ganglion lies on neck of 1st rib and is usually fused with inferior cervical ganglion and forms ***stellate ganglion***. The lower ones lie on the heads of the ribs.

The sympathetic trunk continues with its abdominal part by passing behind the medial arcuate ligament. The ganglia are connected with the respective spinal nerves via the white ramus communicans (from the spinal nerve to the ganglion) and the grey ramus communicans (from the ganglion to the spinal nerve, i.e. ganglion gives grey).

Branches

1. ***Grey rami communicantes*** to all the spinal nerves, i.e. T1–T12. The postganglionic fibres pass along the spinal nerves to supply cutaneous blood vessels, sweat glands and arrector pili muscles.
2. Some white rami communicantes from T1 to T5 ganglia travel up to the cervical part of sympathetic trunk to relay in the three cervical ganglia. Fibres from the lower thoracic ganglia T10–L2 pass down as preganglionic fibres to relay in the lumbar or sacral ganglia.
3. The first five thoracic ganglia give postganglionic fibres to heart, lungs, aorta and oesophagus.
4. Lower eight ganglia give fibres which are preganglionic (unrelayed) for the supply of abdominal viscera. These are called ***splanchnic (visceral) nerves***. Ganglia 5–9 give fibres which constitute ***greater splanchnic nerve***. Some fibres reach *adrenal medulla*. Ganglia 9–10 give fibres that constitute ***lesser splanchnic nerve***. Ganglion 11 gives fibres that constitute ***lowest splanchnic nerve***.

Nerve Supply of Heart

1. *Parasympathetic nerves* reach the heart via the vagus. These are cardioinhibitory; on stimulation, they slow down the heart rate (*see* Flowchart 18.10).
2. *Sympathetic nerves* are derived from the upper 4–5 thoracic segments of the spinal cord. These are cardioacceleratory, and on stimulation, they increase the heart rate, and also dilate the coronary arteries.

Both parasympathetic and sympathetic nerves form the superficial and deep cardiac plexuses, the branches of which run along the coronary arteries to reach the myocardium.

1. ***Superficial cardiac plexus*** is situated below the arch of the aorta in front of the right pulmonary artery. It is formed by:
   a. The superior cervical cardiac branch of the left sympathetic chain.
   b. The inferior cervical cardiac branch of the left vagus nerve.

   Branches: Superficial cardiac plexus gives:
   a. Branch to the right coronary artery
   b. Communicating branch to deep cardiac plexus
   c. Communicating branch to the left anterior pulmonary plexus (*see* Fig. 18.36).
2. ***Deep cardiac plexus*** is situated in front of the bifurcation of the trachea, and behind the arch of the aorta. It is formed by:
   a. All the cardiac branches derived from all the cervical and upper thoracic ganglia of the sympathetic chain.

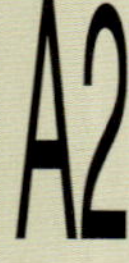

b. Cardiac branches of the vagus and recurrent laryngeal nerves, except those which form the superficial plexus.

Branches: Deep cardiac plexus comprises right and left half that gives the following branches:

a. To the right and left atria.
b. Right and left coronary artery through right and left coronary plexus.
c. Communicating branch to the right and left anterior pulmonary plexus.

Separate branches are given to the atria.

CLINICAL ANATOMY

- ***Cardiac pain*** is an ischaemic pain caused by incomplete obstruction of a coronary artery.
  Pathway: Axons of pain fibres conveyed by the sensory sympathetic cardiac nerves reach thoracic T1–T5 segments of spinal cord mostly through the dorsal root ganglia of the left side. Since these dorsal root ganglia also receive sensory impulses from the medial side of arm, forearm and upper part of front of chest, the pain gets referred to these areas.
- Viscera have low amount of sensory output, whereas skin is an area of high amount of sensory output. So pain arising from area of low sensory output area is projected as coming from high sensory output area.

Nerve Supply of Lungs

The lungs are supplied by the sympathetic and parasympathetic fibers as follows:

1. Parasympathetic nerves are derived from the vagus. These fibres are (*see* Flowchart 16.3):
   a. Motor to the bronchial muscles, and on stimulation cause bronchospasm.
   b. Secretomotor to the mucous glands of the bronchial tree.
   c. Sensory fibres are responsible for the stretch reflex of the lungs, and for the cough reflex.
2. Sympathetic nerves are derived from second to fifth sympathetic ganglia. These are inhibitory to the smooth muscle and glands of the bronchial tree. That is how sympathomimetic drugs, like adrenaline, cause bronchodilatation and relieve symptoms of bronchial asthma.

Both parasympathetic and sympathetic nerves first form anterior and posterior pulmonary plexuses situated in front of and behind the lung roots: From the plexuses, nerves are distributed to the lungs along the blood vessels and bronchi (*see* Fig. 16.4).

ARTERIES

The arteries of thorax are internal thoracic artery, ascending aorta, arch of aorta, descending thoracic aorta and coronary arteries. These have been described with their origin, course, termination and area of distribution in Tables A2.2 and A2.3.

NUMERICALS

- Anteroposterior diameter of inlet of thorax—5 cm.
- Transverse diameter of inlet of thorax—10 cm.
- Suprasternal notch—T2 vertebra.
- Sternal angle—disc between T4 and T5 vertebrae. 2nd costal cartilage articulates with the sternum.
- Xiphisternal joint—T9 vertebra.
- Subcostal angle—between sternal attachments of 7th costal cartilages.
- Vertebra prominence—7th cervical spine.
- Superior angle of scapula—level of T2 spine.

TABLE A2.1: Components of deep cardiac plexus

Right half	*Left half*
Superior, middle, inferior cervical cardiac branches of right sympathetic trunk	Only middle and inferior branches
Cardiac branches of T2–T4 ganglia of right side	Same
Superior and inferior cervical cardiac branches of right vagus	Only the superior cervical cardiac branch of left vagus
Thoracic cardiac branch of right vagus	Same
Two branches of right recurrent laryngeal nerve arising from neck region	Same, but coming from thoracic region

TABLE A2.2: Arteries of thorax

Artery	*Origin, course and termination*	*Branches*
Internal thoracic	Arises from inferior aspect of 1st part of subclavian artery. Its origin lies 2 cm above the sternal end of the clavicle. It runs downwards, forwards and medially behind the clavicle and behind the 1–6 costal cartilages and 1–5 intercostal spaces to terminate in the 6th intercostal space by dividing into superior epigastric and musculophrenic arteries	1. Pericardiophrenic artery 2. Mediastinal branches 3. Anterior intercostal arteries 4. Perforating branches: In females, perforating branches of 2nd, 3rd, and 4th intercostal spaces are larger and supply the breast 5. Superior epigastric artery 6. Musculophrenic artery
Two anterior intercostal arteries	Two arteries, each arises in 1–6 upper intercostal spaces from internal thoracic artery	Supply muscles of the 1–6 intercostal spaces and parietal pleura

(*Contd.*)

TABLE A2.2: Arteries of thorax *(Contd.)*

Artery	*Origin, course and termination*	*Branches*
Superior epigastric artery	Terminal branch of internal thoracic artery. Enters the rectus sheath and ends by anastomosing with inferior epigastric artery, a branch of external iliac artery	Supplies the content and walls of the rectus sheath
Musculophrenic artery	This is also the terminal branch of internal thoracic artery. Ends by giving 2 anterior intercostal arteries in 7–9 intercostal spaces	Two anterior intercostal arteries for 7th, 8th, and 9th intercostal spaces
Ascending aorta	Arises from the upper end of left ventricle. It continues as the arch of aorta at the sternal end of upper border of 2nd right costal cartilage. At the root of aorta, there are three dilatations of the vessel wall called the aortic sinuses. These are anterior, left posterior and right posterior	1. Right coronary artery 2. Left coronary artery
Arch of aorta (*see* Fig. 19.2)	It begins behind the upper border of 2nd right sternochondral joint. Runs upwards, backwards and to left across the left side of bifurcation of trachea. Then it passes behind the left bronchus and on the left side of body of T4 vertebra by becoming descending thoracic aorta	1. Brachiocephalic (innominate) artery 2. Left common carotid artery 3. Left subclavian artery 4. Occasional branch — thyroidea ima artery
Brachiocephalic artery	1st branch of arch of aorta. Runs upwards and soon divides into right common carotid and right subclavian arteries	Right common carotid artery Right subclavian artery
Descending thoracic aorta	Begins on the left side of the lower border of body of T4 vertebra. Descends with inclination to right and ends at the lower border of T12 vertebra by continuing as abdominal aorta	1. Nine pairs of posterior intercostal arteries for 3rd – 11th intercostal spaces) 2. Subcostal artery (one on each side) 3. Two left bronchial arteries 4. Oesophageal pericardial mediastinal branches 5. Superior phrenic arteries for diaphragm.
3–11 posterior intercostal arteries (*see* Fig. 14.9)	3–11 posterior intercostal arteries of both right and left sides arise from the descending thoracic aorta.	Muscular branches Collateral branch
Superior phrenic arteries	Two branches of descending aorta. End in the superior surface of diaphragm. These arteries anastomose with branches of musculophrenic and pericardiacophrenic arteries	Supply the thoracoabdominal diaphragm

TABLE A2.3: Comparison of right and left coronary arteries

Right coronary artery (*see* Fig. 18.28)	***Left coronary artery*** (*see* Fig. 18.28)
Origin: Anterior aortic sinus of ascending aorta	Left posterior aortic sinus of ascending aorta
Course: Between pulmonary trunk and right auricle	Between pulmonary trunk and left auricle
Descends in atrioventricular groove on the right side	Descends in atrioventricular groove on the left side
Turns at the inferior border to run in posterior part of atrioventricular groove	Turns at left border to run in posterior part of atrioventricular groove. It is called circumflex branch
Termination: Ends by anastomosing with the circumflex branch of left coronary artery	Its circumflex branch ends by anastomosing with right coronary artery
Branches: To right atrium, right ventricle (marginal artery) and posterior interventricular branch for both ventricles and posterior one-third of interventricular septa	Left atrium, left ventricle and anterior interventricular branch for both ventricles and anterior two-thirds of interventricular septa. Anterior interventricular branch ends by anastomosing with posterior interventricular branch
Supplies sinuatrial node, atrioventricular (AV) node, AV bundle, right branch of AV bundle including its Purkinje fibres	Supplies left branch of atrioventricular bundle including its Purkinje fibres

- Root of spine of scapula—level of T3 spine.
- Inferior angle of scapula—level of T7 spine.
- Length of oesophagus—25 cm
  - Cervical part—4 cm
  - Thoracic part—20 cm
  - Abdominal part—1.25 cm
  - Beginning of oesophagus—C6 vertebra
  - Termination of oesophagus—T11 vertebra
- Beginning of trachea—C6 vertebra:
  - Length of trachea—10–15 cm.
  - Length of right principal bronchus—2.5 cm.
  - Length of left principal bronchus—5 cm.

BDC's Anatomy *e*-book

1. Typical intercostal nerve
2. Atypical intercostal nerves
3. Clinical terms

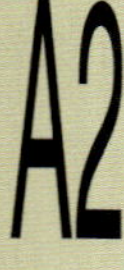

Index

C

D

E

F

G

H